AF412264

WILEY HANDBOOK OF

CURRENT AND EMERGING DRUG THERAPIES

VOLUME 7

WILEY HANDBOOK OF CURRENT AND EMERGING DRUG THERAPIES

Editorial Staff

Vice President, STM Books: **Janet Bailey**

Editorial Director: **Sean Pidgeon**

Director, Book Production and Manufacturing: **Camille P. Carter**

Production Manager: **Shirley Thomas**

Illustration Manager: **Dean Gonzalez**

Developmental Editor: **Natanya Civjan**

Production Editor: **Kristen Parrish**

Editorial Program Coordinator: **Surlan Murrell**

WILEY HANDBOOK OF

CURRENT AND EMERGING DRUG THERAPIES

VOLUME 7

The *Wiley Handbook of Current and Emerging Drug Therapies* is available online at *www.interscience.wiley.com/mrw/cedt*

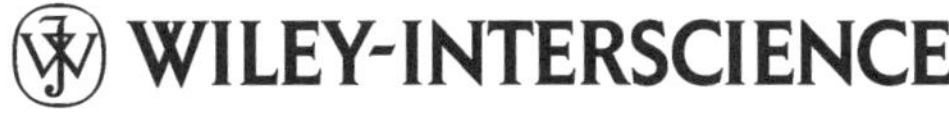

WILEY-INTERSCIENCE

A John Wiley & Sons, Inc., Publication

Contents

CARDIOLOGY

Peripheral Arterial Disease

ETIOLOGY AND PATHOPHYSIOLOGY

Introduction

Peripheral arterial disease (PAD) results primarily from atherosclerosis affecting the conduit arteries that supply the extremities and is characterized by a reduction in blood flow to the lower limbs. Manifestations of PAD include fatigue and pain or muscle ache in the legs on ambulation. Such symptoms, known as *intermittent claudication* (IC), lead to reduced mobility and impaired quality of life (QOL). As PAD progresses, patients may develop pain at rest, and, ultimately, the viability of the limb may be threatened by critical limb ischemia (CLI), in which ulceration and gangrene may occur. PAD is considered a major marker for systemic ischemic events such as stroke and myocardial infarction (MI).

Structure of the Normal Blood Vessel Wall

The healthy blood vessel wall comprises three layers of cells (Figure 1). The adventitia, the outermost layer, is made of connective tissue that contains nerves and capillaries. The adventitia is separated from the middle layer, or media, by the external elastic lamina. The media is composed of sheets of vascular smooth-muscle cells (VSMCs), collagen fibrils, and proteoglycans (components of the extracellular matrix [ECM]). The internal elastic lamina separates the media from

Wiley Handbook of Current and Emerging Drug Therapies, Volumes 5–8
Copyright © 2007 Decision Resources, Inc. Published by John Wiley & Sons, Inc.

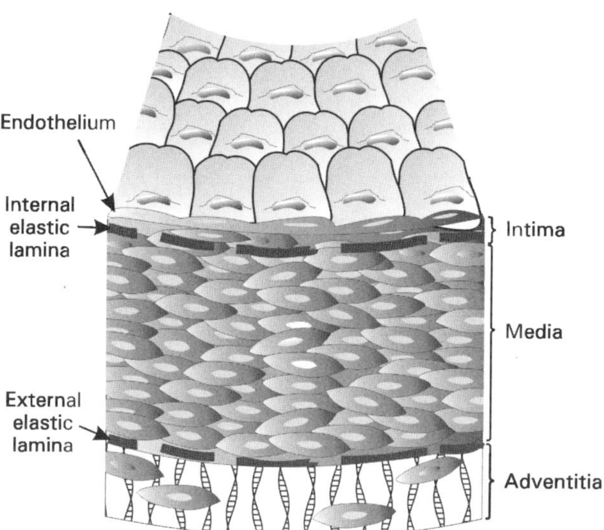

FIGURE 1. *Structure of a healthy artery wall.*

the innermost layer of the vessel wall: the intima. Composed of a single layer of endothelial cells, the intima forms a smooth, uninterrupted surface that serves as the interface between the bloodstream and vascular tissue. The endothelial cells modulate the activity of circulating blood components, and this intimal layer is the site where atherosclerotic lesions form.

Pathophysiology

Plaque Rupture: Arterial Occlusion and Its Causes. PAD is considered to be a manifestation of underlying atherosclerosis in the peripheral vascular bed. It is the development of atherosclerotic lesions and their subsequent rupture that initiates the formation of a blood clot (thrombus) and can eventually lead to arterial narrowing (stenosis) or occlusion (Figure 2). Depending on the site and size of the thrombus formed, the resulting morbidity can lead to acute events, such as MI.

A complex interaction occurs between elements involved in the pathogenesis of PAD; the exact roles of proatherogenic risk factors, mechanisms such as the oxidative modification of lipoproteins, and processes of vascular adaptation are not yet fully understood. Nevertheless, chronic inflammation is implicated at every stage of atherogenesis. Inflammatory pathways unify several of the mechanisms that are presumed to be causes of PAD, such as endothelial dysfunction, platelet activation, lipoprotein oxidation, and thrombosis.

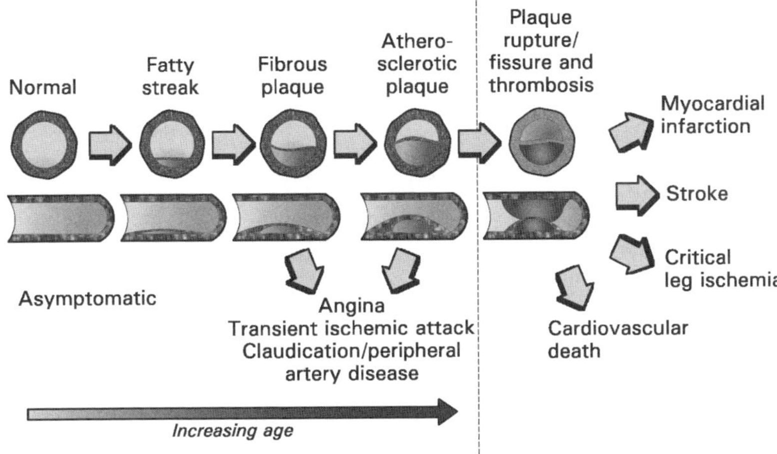

FIGURE 2. *The formation and progression of atherosclerotic lesions.*

Endothelial Dysfunction: Response-to-Injury Hypothesis. Several hypotheses propose explanations for atherosclerosis pathophysiology. The widely accepted response-to-injury hypothesis focuses on damage to endothelial cells. Normally, endothelial cells maintain vascular homeostasis through control of vasoactive and inflammatory substances, but endothelium may become damaged by mechanical stresses within the vessel that result from turbulent blood flow. These damaged endothelial cells promote a proinflammatory response that includes the upregulation of adhesion molecules (including intercellular adhesion molecule-1 [ICAM-1]) and generation of chemokines (Pradhan AD, 2002). In turn, these molecules encourage the recruitment of leukocytes. If the inflammatory response is maintained through continued stimulation, VSMCs begin to migrate and proliferate into the intimal layer. Together with the accumulation and adhesion of macrophages and lymphocytes from circulating blood, such processes mark the transformation from early- to late-stage lesion. VSMCs and macrophages produce ECM metalloproteinases (MMPs), whose deposition in the affected area forces restructuring of the lesion, so that it becomes covered by a fibrous cap, or plaque. Growth of the fibrous plaque results in vascular remodeling, arterial stenosis, and blood-flow irregularities, thereby altering the flow of blood. Once the integrity of an unstable plaque is breached, its prothrombotic contents are released and the clotting process begins.

Endothelial Dysfunction: Platelet Activation and Aggregation. An important component of atherogenesis is platelet adhesion. It occurs during the inflammatory responses that follow endothelial damage and subsequent to plaque rupture. At the site of injury, platelets can attach to collagen fibrils in vascular subendothelium, to dysfunctional endothelium, and to macrophages associated with the arterial wall. The binding process, which triggers platelet activation, is

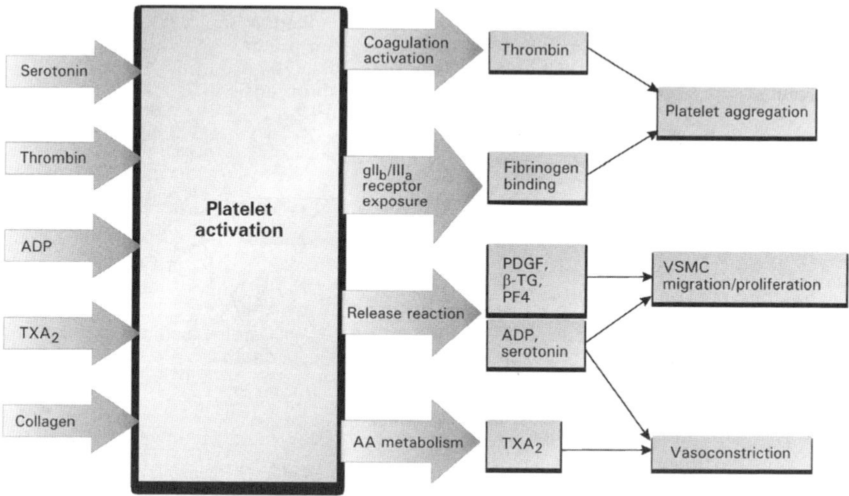

TXA$_2$ = Thromboxane A2; ADP = Adenosine diphosphate; PDGF = Platelet-derived growth factor; β-TG = β-thromboglobulin; PF4 = Platelet factor 4; AA = Arachidonic acid; VSMC = Vascular smooth muscle cell.

FIGURE 3. *Components of platelet activation.*

governed by gpIb/IX receptors and von Willebrand factor (vWF). In a similar fashion, glycoproteins gIIb/IIIa, assisted by fibrinogen, direct platelet aggregation. During and after platelet aggregation, platelets release several substances, including adenosine diphosphate (ADP), serotonin, thromboxane A$_2$ (TXA$_2$), platelet-derived growth-factor (PDGF), platelet factor 4 (PF4), and β-thromboglobulin (β-TG). These substances, through a continuous feedback loop, can initiate a cascade of further platelet activation, vasoconstriction, thrombosis, and mitogenesis and recruit additional platelets into a growing thrombus. See Figure 3.

The interconnectivity of inflammation and endothelial dysfunction is demonstrated by the fact that platelets themselves are a source of inflammatory mediators. Activated platelets express CD40 ligand (CD40L) and prompt endothelial cells to produce chemokines and express adhesion molecules (Henn V, 1998). Studies show that CD40 may be involved in atherogenesis by contributing to leukocyte adhesion and cytokine-induced inflammation (Schonbeck U, 2001).

Endothelial Dysfunction: Reduced Vasodilation and the Role of Nitric Oxide. In addition to provoking an inflammatory response, dysfunction of the endothelium diminishes the production of autocrine and paracrine modulators, such as nitric oxide (NO) and prostaglandin, which help to regulate vasodilation, vasoconstriction, thrombosis, and anticoagulation. NO, produced by endothelial NO synthase (eNOS), also partially mediates leukocyte binding to arterial walls. Moreover, decreased NO can cause SMC proliferation and migration, enhancing platelet activation. The reduced bioavailability of NO and prostaglandin, both potent vasodilators, is considered a prime factor in inducing a prothrombotic state.

In patients with established PAD, lower urinary nitrite excretion rates—a surrogate marker of systemic NO formation—relate to the severity of the disease (Boger RH, 1997). Impaired eNOS activity due to eNOS inhibitors, such as L-arginine, is one possible mechanism by which systemic NO levels are reduced. In an analysis of ten patients with CLI, an infusion of L-arginine was shown to increase femoral arterial blood flow by 43% (Bode-Boger SM, 1996).

Oxidative Modification: Oxidized LDL and Inflammation. The inflammatory potential of oxidized LDL (ox:LDL) is an alternative theory used to explain atherogenesis and was previously distinguished from the response-to-injury hypothesis. However, as the pathophysiology of atherosclerotic arterial disease becomes further elucidated, it has become clear that lipoprotein modification and endothelial dysfunction are not mutually exclusive.

Foam cells (macrophages that have taken up low-density lipoprotein [LDL]) are the hallmark of early atherosclerotic lesions. Consequently, LDL uptake is essential to early lesion generation, and this process has come under intense scrutiny by researchers. In the vessel wall, LDL becomes available for oxidation by free radicals to ox:LDL. These free radicals are produced by inflammatory cells such as monocytes and macrophages, by VSMCs, and by endothelial cells. Oxidation changes LDL charge, thereby increasing affinity between ox:LDL and the macrophage scavenger receptor to which it binds. The uptake of ox:LDL by the scavenger receptor is three to ten times more efficient than alternative pathways of native LDL uptake. This process explains why foam cells are able to form at early stages in lesion development, when LDL content may be relatively low.

Ox:LDL has numerous proatherogenic actions, some of which are shared with the pathogenesis of endothelial injury. In an action particularly relevant to plaque formation, ox:LDL activates endothelial cells and induces endothelial secretion of chemotactic factors that encourage further influx of monocytes and T lymphocytes, thereby expanding the inflammatory response. In addition, ox:LDL can enhance smooth-muscle mitogenesis and thereby promote vessel remodeling and plaque rupture.

Emerging Mechanisms Implicated in the Pathophysiology of PAD

Angiogenic Growth Factors. Development of collateral vessels is a key response to muscle ischemia instigated by PAD. Collateral vessels can reduce ischemic symptoms, such as IC, and their deterioration. The mechanism of collateral vessel development involves the release of angiogenic factors, such as vascular endothelial growth factor (VEGF). Several studies have demonstrated upregulation of VEGF and other angiogenic factors, such as fibroblast growth factor (FGF) and hepatocyte growth factor (HGF), in patients with PAD (Belgore FM, 2001; Padua RR, 1995; Roller RE, 2001). Recently, the injection of bovine eNOS DNA induced therapeutic angiogenesis, suggesting that upregulation of local VEGF expression by NO promotes angiogenesis (Namba T, 2003). However, an improved understanding of the regulation of angiogenic growth factors in neovascularization may be needed if growth-factor-based treatment strategies can obtain regulatory approval.

Endothelial Progenitor Cells (EPCs). Bone-marrow-derived EPCs have been shown to participate in endothelium repair and therefore attenuate the pathogenesis of atherosclerosis (Hill JM, 2003). One study of 15 smokers, of particular relevance to PAD, showed that smoking cessation increased the levels of EPCs (Kondo T, 2004). Other evidence that links the downregulation of EPCs with higher C-reactive protein (CRP) levels indicates that additional investigation into the role of EPCs may provide important insight into the pathophysiology of PAD.

Pathophysiology of Limb Ischemia. Severe, symptomatic PAD is characterized by reduced distal pressure and flow to the lower extremities. In patients with IC, injury to muscles from ischemia-reperfusion causes muscle fiber denervation. Common symptoms of IC include transient pain or ache that develops in the leg upon exercising. This pain usually occurs in the calf but may develop elsewhere in the limb (e.g., thigh, hip). Similar symptoms related to exertion can occur in the arm.

However, as demonstrated by the large number of asymptomatic PAD patients, the relationship between ischemic symptoms and pressure drop across the affected limbs is weak. Aside from hemodynamic influences, alterations of skeletal muscle have been shown to play an important physiological role in limb ischemia. Skeletal muscle ischemia affects muscle metabolism, leading to the accumulation of intermediates of oxidative metabolism such as acylcarnitines. Resting skeletal muscle acylcarnitine content is inversely related to functional impairment in PAD (Hiatt WR, 1996). Improvement of exercise performance has also been associated with plasma levels of acylcarnitine. Figure 4 shows the pathways involved in acylcarnitine metabolism.

Etiology

PAD, coronary artery disease (CAD), and cerebrovascular disease (CVD) often coexist as manifestations of atherosclerosis. Of 381 patients who presented at the Cleveland Clinic between 1978 and 1981 for elective peripheral vascular surgery, 90% had disease in the coronary arteries on angiography (Hertzer NR, 1984). Although the link with CVD is not as strong, one in three CVD patients also suffers from PAD (Aronow WS, 1994). Consequently, experts believe that the risk factors for CAD and CVD also predispose people to the development of PAD; however, the impact of a particular factor on disease pathogenesis in the peripheral extremities differs from its impact in the coronary vasculature. Smoking and diabetes have been shown to confer the greatest risk for early or aggressive development of PAD (Jonason T, 1987).

Risk factors are commonly defined as *nonmodifiable* or *modifiable*. Nonmodifiable risk factors include advancing age, ethnicity, and male gender. Modifiable risk factors are discussed in the following section.

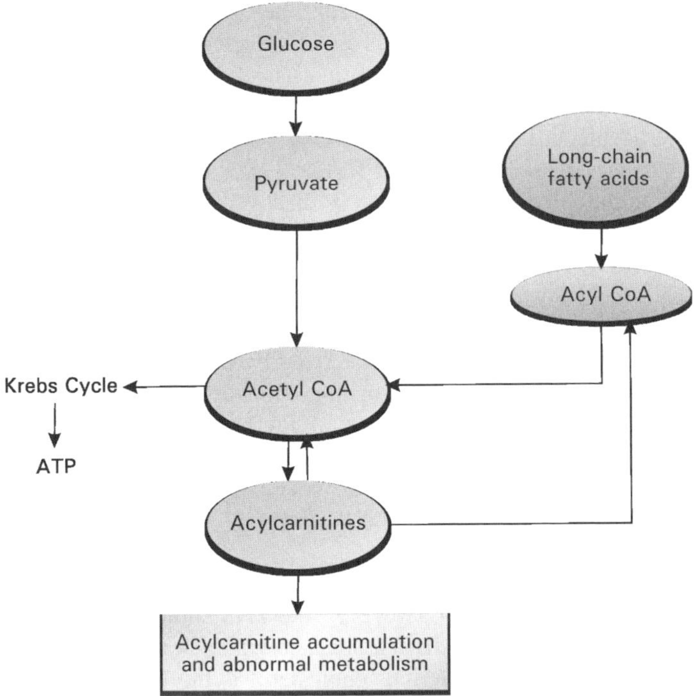

ATP = Adenosine triphosphate.

FIGURE 4. *Pathways involved in acylcarnitine metabolism.*

Modifiable Risk Factors

Smoking. The relationship between smoking and PAD has long been recognized, and its association with this disease may be stronger than the relationship between smoking and CAD. Data from the Framingham Heart Study (FHS) suggest that the risk of a cardiovascular event for smokers at all ages was almost double in PAD compared with CAD (Kannel WB, 1985), and diagnosis of PAD is made up to a decade earlier in smokers than in nonsmokers (Fowkes FGR, 1992). Continued cigarette smoking enhances the risk of progression from stable IC to severe limb ischemia and amputation and diminishes the likelihood of successful revascularization (Ingolfsson IO, 1994). Effects of smoking, such as the promotion of vasoconstriction via reduced NO (Thomas SR, 2003), can induce platelet reactivity and produce factors that decrease fibrinolysis, such as TXA_2 (Fitzgerald GA, 1988). Other pathogenic outcomes result from smoking-induced endothelial damage and increased lipid permeability of the vessel wall (Krupski WC, 1991).

Diabetes Mellitus. The exact pathophysiological process of PAD development in diabetics is unclear. Decreased renal function in diabetic patients has also been identified as an independent risk factor for atherosclerosis of the carotid arteries (Ishimura IE, 2001). Increased levels of blood glucose may lead to abnormal modifications of lipoproteins and to formation of advanced glycated end products (AGEs). AGEs cause endothelial dysfunction and damage, which are part of the atherogenic process. Changes in eNOS secretion and levels of clotting factors or other risk-associated blood factors (such as homocysteine) also cause damage. In addition, researchers recently discovered that glucose increases the expression of the macrophage scavenger receptor. This effect would increase the uptake of ox:LDL and foam-cell formation, resulting in heightened atherogenic effects. This mechanism may explain why diabetics develop more aggressive atherosclerotic disease than nondiabetics. Insulin resistance plays a key role in "metabolic syndrome," which is characterized by the concurrent presentation of conditions that include obesity, non-insulin-dependent diabetes, hyperlipidemia, hypertension, and CVD. The incidence of PAD appears to be about twice as common in diabetic patients as in nondiabetics (Reaven GM, 1988). In addition, the rate of IC in men with glycosuria has been shown to be 3.5-fold higher than the rate in nondiabetic men (Kannel WB, 1985).

Dyslipidemia. Conflicting evidence exists regarding the exact relationship between dyslipidemia and PAD. However, the FHS shows that a fasting cholesterol level greater than 270 mg/dL is associated with a doubling of incidence, and the ratio of total cholesterol to HDL cholesterol is the best predictor of occurrence of PAD (Kannel WB, 1970). Hypertriglyceridemia is also associated with PAD progression (Smith I, 1996), and lipoprotein [a] is a significant, independent risk factor for the disease (Cheng SWK, 1997).

Hypertension. The FHS shows a convincing link between hypertension and PAD: hypertension poses a 2.5-fold, age-adjusted risk for males and a 3.9-fold risk for females (Kannel WB, 1985), but other studies have shown no association between PAD and hypertension. Such different findings are attributed to the complex cause-and-effect relationship between hypertension and PAD. Some researchers suggest that hypertension may delay the onset of symptoms by elevating the central perfusion pressure in patients with PAD (Dormandy JA, 2000). The benefit for PAD patients of reducing blood pressure is underlined by a recent retrospective analysis of the Appropriate Blood-Pressure Control in Diabetes (ABCD) trial (Mehler PS, 2003). Intensive therapeutic blood pressure management significantly reduced the risk of cardiovascular events in patients with PAD and concomitant diabetes.

Inflammatory Markers as Measures of Risk

C-Reactive Protein. C-reactive protein (CRP) is involved in the body's response to inflammation or injury as part of the acute-phase response. An analysis of 14,916 healthy men participating in the Physician's Health Study (PHS) showed that CRP level was predictive of risk of MI when considered alone; combined with measurements of other lipid parameters, CRP level significantly improved risk prediction compared with lipid parameters alone (Ridker PM, 1998). CRP has also been shown to predict future risk of developing symptomatic PAD in apparently healthy men (Ridker PM, 1998).

Homocysteine. Homocysteine is an amino acid generated during protein breakdown that has been proposed as a putative marker of PAD risk. Elevated levels of homocysteine can be attributed to inherited enzyme and acquired vitamin deficiencies (Kuan Y-M, 2002) and may be a stronger risk factor for PAD than CAD. The incidence of hyperhomocysteinemia is as high as 60% in patients with vascular disease, compared with a "normal" level of 1% in the general population (Currie IC, 1996). Hyperhomocysteinemia has also been detected at high levels (28–30%) in patients with premature PAD (Boers GHJ, 1985). In a recent study of 6880 patients, elevated levels of homocysteine were related to the presence of PAD but not significantly to CAD or CVD (Darius H, 2003).

Other studies have reported conflicting results that appear to minimize the link between hyperhomocysteinemia and PAD. In 212 women with PAD, elevated levels of homocysteine were not significantly associated with an increased risk of PAD (Bloemenkamp DG, 2002).

Other Inflammatory Markers. Levels of D-dimer, another putative marker of PAD, were independently associated with the ankle-brachial index (ABI), an indicator of the presence and severity of PAD (McDermott MM, 2003[a]). In this study of 601 patients, CRP was associated with participants who had a prior history of CAD or CVD.

CURRENT THERAPIES

Patients with peripheral arterial disease (PAD) are optimally treated with a combination of therapies that relieve symptoms, address cardiovascular risk, and encourage lifestyle modification. Initial treatment goals for patients with stage II PAD aim to ameliorate the symptoms of intermittent claudication (IC). Walking distance is a required primary end point in pivotal clinical trials submitted for regulatory approval of drugs for the treatment of IC. Usually, the initial claudication distance (ICD; the distance when patients first notice pain, sometimes referred to as the pain-free walking distance) and absolute claudication distance (ACD; the distance at which patients can no longer walk because of pain, sometimes referred to as the maximal walking distance) are used. Occasionally, walking time may be measured instead of walking distance.

Often the exertional limb symptoms of IC can be successfully reduced through a combination of exercise programs and vasoactive treatments such as cilostazol (Otsuka Pharmaceutical's [Tokyo, Japan] Pletaal/Pletal) and naftidrofuryl (Merck's [Whitehouse Station, New Jersey] Praxilene/Dusodril). Patients with stage III or IV PAD, also known as critical limb ischemia (CLI), may receive parenterally administered prostaglandin analogues.

Antiplatelet agents such as aspirin (Bayer Pharmaceuticals's [West Haven, Connecticut] Bayer Aspirin, generics) and clopidogrel (Bristol-Myers Squibb

[North Billerica, Massachusetts]/Sanofi-Aventis's [Tokyo, Japan] Plavix) may also assist in symptom relief. They are also prescribed to reduce rates of subsequent cardiovascular ischemic events in all patients with PAD.

PAD is increasingly recognized as a marker for generalized atherosclerosis and is closely associated with coronary and cerebrovascular disease. Therefore, physicians seek to reduce cardiovascular risk. Interventions invariably include weight loss in obese patients, complete smoking cessation, the achievement of glycemic control in diabetics, normalization of elevated blood pressure, and reductions in cholesterol (especially low-density lipoprotein [LDL] cholesterol) to guideline levels. Table 1 lists the principal therapies currently used to treat PAD.

Several other established agents have been investigated or used to treat PAD, and most have shown limited efficacy in clinical studies. These compounds include the alpha blocker buflomedil (Abbott Laboratories's [Abbott Park, Illinois], Bufedil), which is most extensively prescribed in several European markets, particularly France.

In severe cases, PAD patients with acute limb ischemia (ALI; a sudden decrease or worsening in limb perfusion causing a threat to extremity viability [Dormandy JA, 2000]) require invasive procedures such as angioplasty, stenting, or surgery; these measures are merely outlined here.

Vasoactive Therapies

Overview. Treatment alternatives for the alleviation of PAD symptoms are limited to older vasodilators such as naftidrofuryl (Merck's Praxilene/Drofuril, generics) and pentoxifylline (Sanofi-Aventis's Trental/Elorgan, generics), often with ambiguous effects on IC; only one agent—cilostazol—has been introduced in recent years for this indication.

Mechanism of Action. Arterial walls located downstream of a stenosis or occlusion dilate in response to the ischemia induced by exercise. However, the dilation is due to endogenous factors and is not affected by older vasodilators. Instead, vasoactive agents used for PAD treatment are thought to decrease resistance in other vessels, thereby redirecting blood flow away from ischemic tissue. Vasodilators may also lower systemic blood pressure and thereby reduce perfusion pressure. Furthermore, the vasoactive treatments used to relieve the symptoms of IC decrease platelet aggregation, which may counteract occlusion.

Formulation. The majority of patients who are prescribed vasoactive treatments take them orally two or three times daily—the oral route is preferable to other routes of administration. Cilostazol, the newest drug in this class, is available only in an oral formulation. Nevertheless, the older agent pentoxifylline is available in several formulations, thus allowing flexibility in determining a treatment strategy; parenteral administration is often initiated in outpatients who are later weaned onto the oral form. An intravenous (IV) formulation of naftidrofuryl was withdrawn in 1995 owing to the incidence of adverse effects.

TABLE 1. Current Therapies Used for Treatment of Peripheral Arterial Disease

Agent	Company/Brand	Daily Dose	Availability
Vasoactive therapies			
Cilostazol	Otsuka's Pletaal/ Pletal, generics	100 mg bid	US, UK, J
Pentoxifylline	Aventis Pharma's Trental/ Elorgan, generics	400 mg tid	US, F, G, I, S, UK
5-HT$_2$ receptor antagonists			
Naftidrofuryl	Merck's Praxilene/Dusodril, generics	200 mg tid	F, G, I, S, UK
Sarpogrelate hydrochloride	Mitsubishi Pharma's Anplag	50–100 mg tid	J
Prostaglandin analogues			
Alprostadil	Pfizer/Schwarz Pharma's Prostin VR/Prostavasin, Ono's Prostandin	60 µg IV for 2 hours daily, 5 days per week for 4 weeks	US, F, G, I, S, UK, J
Beraprost	Toray's Dorner, Kaken's Procyclin	60–120 µg tid	J
Iloprost	Schering AG's Ilomedin/Ilomedine	Intermittent IV infusion, titrated from 0.5–2.0 ng/kg/min for 2–4 weeks, infusions over 6 hours daily	F, G, I, S
Cyclooxygenase-1 inhibitors			
Aspirin	Bayer's Bayer Aspirin, generics	75–300 mg qd	US, F, G, I, S, UK, J
Adenosine diphosphate receptor antagonists			
Clopidogrel	Bristol-Myers Squibb/ Sanofi-Aventis's Plavix	75 mg qd	US, F, G, I, S, UK, J
Ticlopidine	Sanofi-Aventis's Ticlid/ Tiklid/Tiklyd, Sigma-Tau's Ticlodone, Daiichi's Panaldine	250 mg bid	US, F, G, I, S, J
Statins			
Atorvastatin	Pfizer's Lipitor/Tahor/ Sortis/Torvast/ Cardyl	10–80 mg qd	US, F, G, I, S, UK, J
Simvastatin	Merck's Zocor/ Sinvacor, Boehringer Ingelheim's Denan, generics	10–80 mg qd	US, F, G, I, S, UK, J

(continued overleaf)

TABLE 1. (*continued*)

Agent	Company/Brand	Daily Dose	Availability
Angiotensin-converting enzyme inhibitors			
Ramipril	King Pharmaceuticals/Aventis's Altace/Delix/Tritace	1.25–5 mg	US, F, G, I, S, UK
Quinapril	Pfizer's Accupro/ Acuitel/Accuprin/Acuprel, Sanofi-Aventis's Korec, generics	2.5–20 mg	F, G, I, S, UK, J

US = United States; F = France; G = Germany; I = Italy; S = Spain; UK = United Kingdom; J = Japan.
IV = Intravenous; bid = Twice daily; qd = Once daily; tid = Thrice daily.

Cilostazol. Cilostazol (Otsuka's Pletaal/Pletal) is the only new agent for PAD to reach the market in recent years; it was approved in 1988 in Japan and other Asian countries for arterial occlusive disorders and in 1999 in the United States for the treatment of IC symptoms. The first European introduction of cilostazol occurred in June 2002 in the United Kingdom for relief of stage II PAD. Otsuka is seeking authorization in other European Union countries under the mutual recognition procedure, in which the United Kingdom will act as the reference member state. During the procedure, some of the concerned member states requested additional clinical data; Otsuka had had plans to submit these data by mid 2005, but at the time of composing this reference, no new information from Otsuka has been announced.

However, Otsuka lost its U.S. market exclusivity for cilostazol in 2004 and will face generic competition in that country because five abbreviated new drug applications (ANDAs) for cilostazol were approved by the FDA in November 2004. To combat this competition, Otsuka has entered into an agreement with Prasco Laboratories (Cincinnati, Ohio) that authorizes Prasco to produce a branded generic version of cilostazol.

Cilostazol, a quinolinone derivative, is a type IIIA phosphodiesterase (PDE) inhibitor that increases cyclic adenosine monophosphate (cAMP) concentrations. Like other vasoactive agents, cilostazol decreases platelet aggregation and contraction of vascular smooth-muscle cells (VSMCs) (Liu Y, 2001). However, as previously discussed, these two effects alone are not sufficient to alleviate IC, so the role of cilostazol in symptom relief in not clear. The agent has also been shown to induce a positive effect on serum lipids, reducing triglyceride levels and increasing high-density lipoprotein (HDL) cholesterol levels (Liu Y, 2001).

Researchers examined 516 men and women aged 40 or older who had moderately severe IC and were randomized to receive cilostazol 100 mg or 50 mg or placebo orally twice per day. At week 24, the improvement in ICD was 59% in the 100 mg cilostazol group, 48% in the 50 mg group, and 20% in the placebo group. Patients in the 100 mg group doubled their ACD at 24 weeks to 259 meters (Beebe HG, 1999). A meta-analysis of eight trials involving 2,702

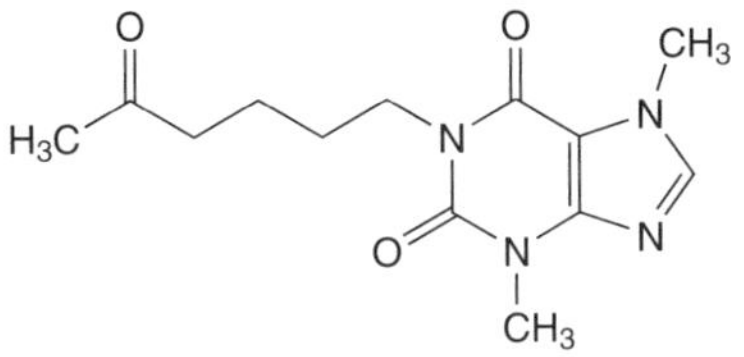

FIGURE 5. Structure of pentoxifylline.

patients showed that cilostazol consistently improves ACD and ICD. The level of improvement over periods between 12 and 24 weeks ranged from 50% to 67%. Furthermore, cilostazol decreased triglycerides by 15.8% and increased HDL cholesterol by 12.8% (Thompson PD, 2002).

A recent study sponsored by Otsuka examined the effects on bleeding time of cilostazol alone or in combination with aspirin and/or clopidogrel. Patients underwent a series of two-week regimens prescribed as follows: washout; 325 mg aspirin daily; aspirin plus 100 mg cilostazol twice daily; washout; cilostazol; cilostazol plus 75 mg clopidogrel daily; washout; clopidogrel; clopidogrel plus aspirin; clopidogrel, aspirin, and cilostazol. At the end of each treatment phase, bleeding time was measured. When cilostazol is added to aspirin, to clopidogrel, or to both antiplatelet agents, there is no additional increase in bleeding time. Because its antiplatelet effects are weak, cilostazol appears to be safe to use in combination with aspirin or clopidogrel (Wilhite DB, 2003).

The most common adverse effects associated with cilostazol are headache, which occurred in 34% of patients, and diarrhea, which occurred in 12% (Beebe HG, 1999). This agent is also contraindicated in patients with congestive heart failure owing to the detrimental effects on survival shown by earlier PDE inhibitors.

Pentoxifylline. Pentoxifylline (Sanofi-Aventis's Trental/Elorgan, generics) (Figure 5) is marketed worldwide as a treatment for peripheral and cerebral vascular disorders, Raynaud's syndrome (a peripheral venous disease in which blood vessels spasm in the fingers, toes, ears, or nose, usually brought on by exposure to cold), and stroke. It was the first drug to receive FDA approval specifically for the treatment of IC and has been available in Europe since 1972 and in the United States since 1984.

Pentoxifylline is a trisubstituted xanthine derivative. Its metabolites improve erythrocyte deformability, reduce blood viscosity, and decrease platelet reactivity and plasma hypercoagulability (Dawson DL, 2001).

Data supporting the use of pentoxifylline for IC are weak. Although meta-analyses demonstrated that the agent was more effective than placebo in improving ICD, such effects have often been relatively small. An analysis of six double-blind trials found that the agent was associated with an increased ICD of 21 meters and an ACD of 44 meters (Girolami B, 1999). However, many studies of pentoxifylline predate current design and reporting recommendations.

Pentoxifylline and cilostazol are the only two agents currently approved by the FDA for symptom alleviation of IC in the United States. The first head-to-head trial of these two agents was published in 2000. ACD and ICD were assessed in 698 patients who were receiving either cilostazol (100 mg orally twice per day), pentoxifylline (400 mg orally three times per day), or placebo. After 24 weeks, the increase in ACD was 107, 64, and 65 meters in the cilostazol, pentoxifylline, and placebo groups, respectively. Thus, while cilostazol provided clear benefits in relieving the symptoms of IC, pentoxifylline was shown to be no better than placebo (Dawson DL, 2000).

5-HT$_2$ Receptor Antagonists

Overview. The concept of treating PAD by antagonizing 5-HT$_2$ serotonin receptors is well established; naftidrofuryl has been available in Europe for more than three decades. After a decade of use in Japan, sarpogrelate (Mitsubishi Pharma's [Osaka, Japan] Anplag) is being developed for the European market.

Mechanism of Action. There are at least 15 types and subtypes of serotonin receptors, but the 5-HT$_2$ subtypes predominate in the cardiovascular system. When platelets are activated, they release serotonin that acts as a potent local vasoconstrictor and also enhances platelet aggregation. By selectively occupying platelet serotonin receptors, 5-HT$_2$ antagonists inhibit aggregation of platelets and relax VSMCs.

Naftidrofuryl. Naftidrofuryl oxalate is a serotonin (5-HT$_2$) receptor antagonist with vasodilator and antiplatelet effects. The agent has been marketed widely in Europe since the late 1960s but is not available in the United States or Japan.

A placebo-controlled study in 221 patients with IC shows that 200 mg naftidrofuryl treatment thrice daily is both statistically and clinically relevant. After six months, treated patients demonstrated a 92% improvement in ICD versus 17% for placebo and an 83% improvement in ACD versus 14% for placebo. The incidence of adverse events was similar in both groups (Kieffer E, 2001). Furthermore, pooled results from three studies in 754 patients demonstrated that 200 mg naftidrofuryl thrice daily significantly improved patients' quality of life (QOL) (Spengel F, 2002). However, other studies have shown varying degrees of benefit. A meta-analysis of four double-blind trials demonstrated that naftidrofuryl increased pain-free walking by 59 meters and ACD by 71 meters, leading the authors to conclude that, like pentoxifylline, naftidrofuryl had conferred only modest treatment benefit (Girolami B, 1999).

Sarpogrelate Hydrochloride. In 1993, Tokyo's Tanabe received the initial authorization to market sarpogrelate hydrochloride in Japan for treatment of chronic arterial occlusive disease. The company merged with the Mitsubishi Chemical Corporation in 1999 to form Mitsubishi Pharma, which is now the marketing authorization holder for this agent. In January 2004, Phase II clinical trials were under way in the United Kingdom for the treatment of IC.

Sarpogrelate has higher affinity for the $5\text{-}HT_{2A}$-receptor subtype than other $5\text{-}HT_2$ antagonists, such as ketanserin, which may explain why sarpogrelate's antiplatelet aggregation effects are 50-fold stronger than those of ketanserin (Mizuno, 2000).

To support its Japanese approval, sarpogrelate was compared with ticlopidine in a double-blind study of 161 patients with chronic PAD manifested by ischemic ulcers. For six weeks, the patients received 100 mg sarpogrelate thrice daily, 100 mg ticlopidine five times daily, or placebo. Patients were assessed and given a global improvement rating based on ulcer size, granulation, pain, and psychroesthesia. Improved scores were seen in 64% of sarpogrelate patients and 52% of ticlopidine patients, but this difference was not statistically significant. There was a significant difference in the safety of the two agents: administration of the trial drug was evaluated as safe in 93% of sarpogrelate patients and 77% of ticlopidine patients. Adverse events experienced by patients receiving sarpogrelate included abdominal pain, nausea, and GI hemorrhage (Furukawa K, 1991).

Prostaglandin Analogues

Overview. Prostaglandins have long been recognized as potent vasodilators and inhibitors of platelet aggregation. On the basis of their physiological effects, prostaglandin E_1 (PGE_1) and prostacyclin I_2 (PGI_2) have been used for more than 20 years to treat advanced CLI. The goal is to relieve rest pain, heal ischemic ulcers, and reduce the rate of amputation. Few studies of the effects of prostaglandins on IC have been made, and it is unclear whether patients with stage II PAD benefit from PGE_1 or PGI_2 therapy. Although PGI_2 is very potent, it is an unstable molecule; this instability has led to the development of more stable analogues such as beraprost (Toray Industries's [Tokyo, Japan] Dorner) and iloprost (Schering AG's [Berlin, Germany] Ilomedin). In Japan, physicians also use limaprost (Ono Pharmaceutical's [Osaka, Japan] Opalmon, Dainippon Pharmaceutical's [Osaka Japan] Prorenal), an oral PGE_1 derivative approved since 1988 for treatment of various ischemic symptoms such as ulcer, pain, and coldness of the hands and feet associated with thromboangiitis obliterans.

Mechanism of Action. Prostaglandins are biologically active fatty acid derivatives of arachidonic acid. They are extremely potent, endogenous, regulatory substances that are synthesized and released for immediate, local action on specific G-protein-coupled receptors found in most tissues of the body. PGE_1 and PGI_2 are vasodilators that are synthesized in vascular endothelium, which forms the inner lining of cells in all blood vessels. PGI_2 is the most potent vasodilator prostaglandin known: approximately 30 times more potent than PGE_1. Both PGE_1 and PGI_2 are also antiplatelet agents. By binding to the EP_1 and IP receptors respectively, PGE_1 and PGI_2 activate adenylyl cyclase, which in turn increases platelet concentrations of cAMP that inhibit platelet aggregation at elevated intracellular concentrations (Harker LA, 1986; Samuelsson B, 1975).

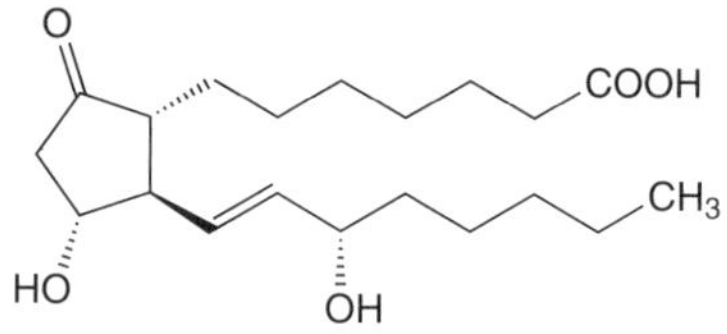

FIGURE 6. Structure of alprostadil.

Formulation. PGE_1 is rapidly inactivated in the lungs, and PGI_2 is degraded by the gastrointestinal tract before it can be absorbed; therefore, prostaglandins and their analogues must be given parenterally. Originally, intra-arterial administration into the obstructed artery was employed, but this is no longer considered an appropriate delivery system for PAD treatment; instead, large doses are administered intravenously. An oral formulation of PGI_2 is also available in some markets and is used extensively in Japan for the symptomatic alleviation of IC. This agent is not marketed in Western Europe or the United States.

Alprostadil. PGE_1 as alprostadil a-cyclodextrin (Pfizer/Schwarz Pharma's [Milwaukee, Wisconsin] Prostin VR/Prostavasin, Ono's Prostandin) (Figure 6) is indicated for use in treatment of ulceration of the extremities, necrosis, and rest pain. The agent has been marketed worldwide for cardiovascular indications, skin ulcers, and erectile dysfunction, and it is administered intravenously.

In a multicenter, randomized trial studying the effect of PGE_1 on CLI, 1,560 patients received either daily IV infusions of 60 mg PGE_1 ($n = 771$) or placebo ($n = 789$) during hospitalization. At hospital discharge, there was a modest reduction in composite outcome (death and peripheral and cerebro/cardiovascular illness) events in the PGE_1 group compared with the control group (63.9% versus 73.6%), but this difference was not significant at six months. Clinical benefit with alprostadil was therefore apparent in the short term but declined over time (ICAI Study Group, 1999). Other trials have shown PGE_1 to be ineffective in ulcer healing (Schuler JJ, 1984).

Data on efficacy in patients in earlier stages of PAD are limited, but alprostadil has demonstrated some benefit. In a 44-patient, randomized study, 40 μg PGE_1 administered over two hours twice daily, combined with intensive exercise, produced a significantly more effective (604%) and sustained improvement in ICD in comparison with exercise alone (119%) or exercise combined with twice-daily, 200 mg, IV-administered pentoxifylline (105%) (Scheffler P, 1994). In a comparative study with iloprost (see the "Iloprost" section) in diabetics, patients treated with PGE_1 had a considerably poorer outcome than patients treated with iloprost, but side effects such as headache, flushing, and gastrointestinal symptoms were more common with iloprost (73.9%) than with PGE_1 (31.0%) (Altstaedt HO, 1993).

Beraprost. Beraprost (Toray's Dorner, Kaken Pharmaceuticals [Tokyo, Japan] Procyclin) (Figure 7), an oral prostacyclin PGI_2 derivative, was launched in

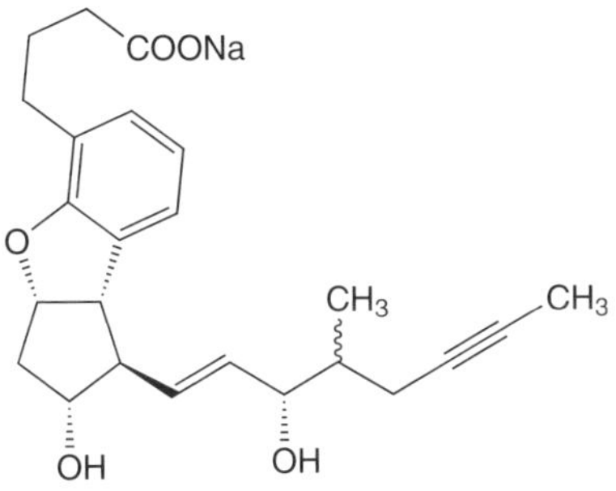

FIGURE 7. *Structure of beraprost.*

Japan in 1992 for the treatment of PAD and pulmonary arterial hypertension. Beraprost is comarketed in Japan by Toray, Kaken, and Tamanouchi Pharmaceutical (Tokyo, Japan) and is licensed by United Therapeutics Corporation (Silver Spring, Maryland) for distribution in the United States. Aventis Pharmaceuticals, Inc. (Bridgewater, New Jersey) is the licensee for Europe, but the company suspended research on the agent following rejection in France of a regulatory dossier that had been submitted in 1998.

European Phase III clinical trials of beraprost showed that the agent has beneficial effects both on CVD events and in symptomatic treatment of IC. In the Beraprost Claudication Investigation (BERCI) 2 study, 424 patients were randomly assigned to placebo or beraprost (Besse B, 1999; Lièvre M, 2000). The double-blind trial showed that 40 mg of beraprost three times daily improved ICD by 81.5% (compared with 52.0% in the placebo group) and ACD by 60.1% (compared with 35.0% in the placebo group). Patients on beraprost experienced fewer vascular events than patients on placebo (4.8% versus 8.9%) and reported greater improvements in QOL. However, a similar U.S. study failed to duplicate the European findings, and United Therapeutics discontinued development for IC. An explanation for the difference offered by one of the study directors was variation imposed by beraprost's limited half-life of 45 minutes.

During the BERCI 2 study, adverse events were experienced by 16.7% of patients treated with beraprost and 7% of patients receiving placebo. The most common adverse events in the beraprost group were headache (6.2%) and vasodilation (5.3%) (Lièvre M, 2000).

Sales of beraprost in Japan are supported by a continuing trial program. For example, a recently published study involving 40 diabetic patients with arteriosclerosis obliterans (ASO) who were administered six 20 mg tablets daily for six months. At both three and six months, ABI had significantly increased, and symptoms such as lack of feeling in the lower extremities were significantly reduced. One in four patients increased ambulatory distance approximately three-fold (Toyota T, 2002).

Development of the immediate-release form of beraprost for PAD is not proceeding in the United States and Europe, although United Therapeutics is

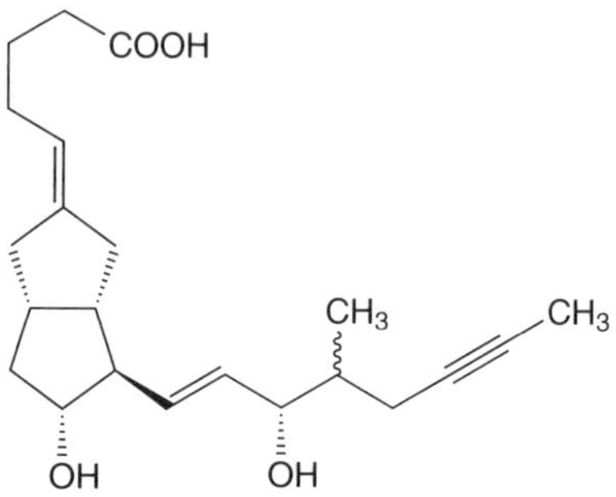

FIGURE 8. *Structure of iloprost.*

developing a sustained-release formulation. Investigations of this formulation are at the preclinical stage.

Iloprost. Iloprost (Schering AG's Ilomedin/Ilomedine) (Figure 8), a stable analogue of epoprostenol (prostacyclin; PGI_2), is marketed in Europe, excluding the United Kingdom, for IV treatment of CLI when patients are at risk of amputation, or require surgical intervention, and for patients with severe Raynaud's syndrome.

Schering reported the results of an open study of iloprost in 853 patients who were in Fontaine stages III and IV; these patients were treated with iloprost infusions for six hours daily for up to 42 days. Response rates were 66.0% in stage III patients and 41.8% in stage IV patients; at six-month follow-up, 71.4% and 66.2%, respectively, of the initial responders remained free from rest pain and showed complete or partial healing of trophic lesions (Staben P, 1996).

This agent is reserved for severe, inoperable cases and patients in severe pain. A sustained-release oral preparation was developed for outpatient therapy, but its administration showed no clear benefit following one-year treatment of patients with advanced, severe leg ischemia (Oral Iloprost in Severe Leg Ischaemia Study Group, 2000).

Practical problems associated with IV administration and variable efficacy hinder the more widespread use of current parenteral prostacyclins. This situation is likely to persist, limiting use principally to hospitalized patients with advanced PAD symptoms such as CLI. Also, associated with iloprost treatment are numerous adverse events that can be attributed to its vasodilatory action. In Schering's open study of iloprost, 83.2% and 86.0% of Fontaine stages III and IV patients, respectively, experienced adverse events that included headache, nausea, flush, and gastrointestinal symptoms, but these events mostly occurred during the titration phase (Staben P, 1996).

Cyclooxygenase-1 Inhibitors

Overview. PAD is associated with platelet hyperaggregability; enhanced platelet activation may contribute substantially to the morbidity and mortality related to adverse outcomes such as myocardial infarction (MI), stroke, and vascular death. Cyclooxygenase-1 (COX-1) inhibitors—notably aspirin (Bayer's Aspirin, generics)—have been shown to reduce the incidence of such outcomes in patients with vascular disease.

Mechanism of Action. Platelet agonists such as collagen, adenosine diphosphate, and thrombin lead to the synthesis of thromboxane (TX) A_2. TXA_2 amplifies the activation signal from the agonists and induces irreversible platelet aggregation. Aspirin permanently inhibits the enzyme COX-1, which is responsible for the formation of prostaglandin H_2 (PGH_2) from arachidonic acid. PGH_2 is the precursor of TXA_2 (Patrono C, 2004).

Formulation. Antiplatelet agents are used in both oral and parenteral forms to treat PAD. Oral agents are used principally in a secondary and, to some extent, symptomatic role in patients with Fontaine stage II and later stages of disease. Parenteral agents are used in more severe cases of CLI.

Aspirin. Aspirin (Bayer's Bayer Aspirin, generics) (Figure 9) is the most widely used antiplatelet agent in PAD. Although it confers little symptomatic benefit either in pain relief or improved walking distance (Ciocon JO, 1997), aspirin may modify the progression of lower extremity arterial insufficiency and reduce the incidence of associated cardiovascular events.

In a study of 240 patients treated for two years with placebo, aspirin (330 mg), or dipyridamole (75 mg) plus aspirin (330 mg), disease progression was most marked in the placebo-treated group, reduced in the aspirin-treated group, and seen least in the dipyridamole and aspirin group (Hess H, 1985). However, other investigators have concluded that evidence for this combination versus aspirin alone is not convincing (Hirsh J, 1995).

One of the major applications for aspirin use in patients with PAD is the prevention of death and disability from stroke and MI. In a meta-analysis conducted by the Antiplatelet Trialists' Collaboration, data from a subgroup analysis of 16,000 "high-risk" patients (including those with PAD) demonstrated that 6% of patients suffered a vascular event while on antiplatelet therapy versus 8% of patients on control—a one-year benefit of 20 vascular events avoided per 1000 patients treated. The most widely tested regimen was "medium-dose" (75–325 mg per day) aspirin (Antiplatelet Trialists' Collaboration, 1994).

Some patients cannot tolerate aspirin, either because of an allergic reaction or because of gastrointestinal side effects.

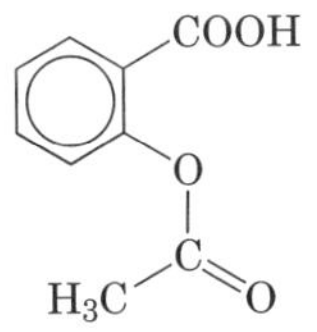

FIGURE 9. *Structure of aspirin.*

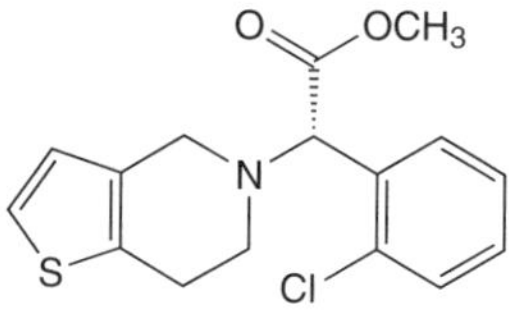

FIGURE 10. *Structure of clopidogrel.*

Adenosine Diphosphate Receptor Antagonists

Overview. Agents that inhibit platelet aggregation via a mechanism different from that of aspirin may avoid some of its side effects and thereby gain a portion of the aspirin market. Clopidogrel and ticlopidine (Sanofi-Aventis's Ticlid, Daiichi Pharmaceutical's [Tokyo, Japan] generics) are the major alternative antiplatelet agents in current use.

Mechanism of Action. Clopidogrel and ticlopidine are structurally related thienopyridines that, unlike aspirin, have no direct effects on arachidonic acid metabolism. The agents of this class bind to P2 purinoreceptors and antagonize stimulation of adenylyl cyclase by adenosine diphosphate (ADP). This selective interaction irreversibly inhibits ADP-induced platelet activation and aggregation (Patrono C, 2004).

Clopidogrel. Clopidogrel (Bristol-Myers Squibb/Sanofi-Aventis's Plavix) (Figure 10) has been marketed in the United States and Europe since gaining regulatory approval in 1997 and 1998; in both territories, clopidogrel is indicated for the reduction of atherosclerotic events in patients suffering from acute coronary syndrome, MI, stroke, or established PAD. In Japan, Daiichi Pharmaceutical has completed Phase III trials with clopidogrel. The company had planned to file an NDA in Japan in 2000, but this procedure was delayed until the end of 2003.

In January 2005, clopidogrel was approved in Japan and is now expected to be launched in the second quarter of 2006.

The key study providing clinical evidence to support the use of clopidogrel for secondary prevention in PAD is the Clopidogrel Versus Aspirin in Patients at Risk of Ischemic Events (CAPRIE) trial. This study involved 19,185 people who had a recent MI (within the previous 35 days), a recent stroke (within the previous one to six months), or PAD. Patients received either clopidogrel (75 mg per day) or aspirin (325 mg per day). Researchers found that the subsequent annual rate of adverse events was 5.32% in the clopidogrel-treated group, compared with 5.83% in the aspirin-treated group. This difference represented an 8.7% risk reduction in the clopidogrel-treated group over and above the 25% reduction currently accepted with aspirin. The study also showed that the risk of neutropenia with clopidogrel was 0.10% versus 0.17% for aspirin (CAPRIE Steering Committee, 1996).

These results demonstrated that long-term administration of clopidogrel was effective in preventing ischemic events in patients with atherosclerotic vascular disease, including PAD. Subgroup analysis revealed that much of the benefit associated with clopidogrel was observed in the group that presented with symptomatic disease. The relative risk reduction of vascular events (classified as "qualifying disorders") in favor of clopidogrel was 3.7% for AMI, 7.3% for ischemic stroke, and 23.8% for PAD (CAPRIE Steering Committee, 1996). Furthermore, treatment with clopidogrel resulted in a significant decrease in the need for rehospitalization for ischemic events or bleeding compared with aspirin (1502 versus 1673 cases) (Bhatt DL, 2000).

The CAPRIE study demonstrated that clopidogrel-treated patients experience less frequent GI upset, abnormal liver function, and GI hemorrhage than patients who receive aspirin, but more frequent diarrhea, pruritis, and rash. Neutropenia and thrombocytopenia occurred rarely and at similar rates in both groups (CAPRIE Steering Committee, 1996). Tolerability of clopidogrel is superior to that of ticlopidine (Bertrand ME, 2000).

The Clopidogrel in Unstable Angina to Prevent Recurrent Events (CURE) study examined the benefit of dual antiplatelet therapy and demonstrated that long-term treatment with clopidogrel in addition to aspirin was superior to aspirin alone in the prevention of major vascular ischemic events in patients with unstable angina or non-Q-wave MI (Hacke W, 2002). As in the case of other secondary therapy regimens used in PAD patients, physicians may well extrapolate CHD results to PAD, especially in patients considered to be high-risk.

Sanofi-Aventis and Bristol-Myers Squibb are supporting two new clinical trials of clopidogrel in PAD patients. For 42 months, the Clopidogrel for High Atherothrombotic Risk and Ischemic Stabilization, Management, and Avoidance (CHARISMA) trial will evaluate the safety and efficacy of clopidogrel plus aspirin versus 75–162 mg aspirin alone in 15,603 patients with coronary or cerebrovascular disease, PAD, or major cardiovascular risk factors (Bhatt DL, 2004). CHARISMA is expected to be completed during 2006. The second trial will examine the role of clopidogrel in patients who have had surgical intervention to treat PAD: over a 24-month period, the Clopidogrel and Aspirin in Bypass Surgery for Peripheral Arterial Disease (CASPAR) trial will investigate the rate of patency and survival in 1460 PAD patients treated with clopidogrel plus aspirin versus 75–100 mg aspirin alone after bypass grafting. The investigators plan to end CASPAR in 2008.

Ticlopidine. Available in all of the major pharmaceutical markets except the United Kingdom, ticlopidine (Sanofi-Aventis's Ticlid/Tiklid/Tyclid, Sigma-Tau Pharmaceuticals's [Gaithersburg, Maryland] Ticlodone) (Figure 11) is used in the treatment of IC, in secondary prevention of stroke, and in combination with aspirin to prevent restenosis after stenting. Ticlopidine was never authorized in the United Kingdom but was used on a named-patient basis for prophylaxis following intracoronary stenting. However, after the 2002 approval of clopidogrel throughout Europe via the centralized procedure, the use of ticlopidine was discontinued in the United Kingdom in February 2003.

Early studies demonstrated ticlopidine's beneficial effects in providing progressive and sustained improvement in ICD, ACD, and ABI (Arcan JC, 1988;

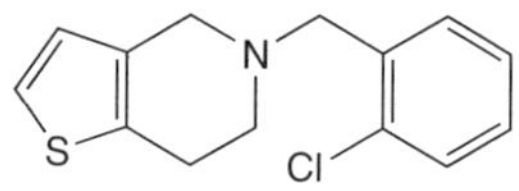

FIGURE 11. Structure of ticlopidine.

Balsano F, 1989). A meta-analysis of PAD studies demonstrated that a significant reduction (from 9% to 3%) in fatal and nonfatal cardiovascular events was observed in patients treated with ticlopidine compared with those treated with placebo (Boissel JP, 1989). Over a seven-year period, ticlopidine (250 mg twice daily) also reduced the need for vascular reconstructive surgery in PAD cases by some 50% (Bergqvist D, 1995). An earlier analysis of this same study concluded that the agent reduced high morbidity and mortality rates in both cardiovascular and cerebrovascular disease (Janzon L, 1990).

Like patients taking clopidogrel, patients taking ticlopidine experience diarrhea and rash more often than patients taking aspirin. However, ticlopidine use is constrained by a higher incidence of serious adverse events than are seen following clopidogrel treatment: neutropenia occurs in 2.3% of ticlopidine patients; thrombotic thrombocytopenic purpura affects 1 in 2000–4000 patients (Bennett CL, 1998; Hankey GJ, 2000).

Statins

Overview. Because PAD patients may suffer multiple concomitant disorders, secondary prevention of cardiovascular events motivated the use of statins first in patients considered to be at high risk, such as patients with Fontaine stage III or IV disease. Following several studies of the effect of this drug class on IC, statins are given increasingly to patients with stage II PAD.

Seven statins are marketed worldwide: atorvastatin (Pfizer's [New York, New York] Lipitor), fluvastatin (Novartis's [Basel, Switzerland] Lescol), lovastatin (Merck's Mevacor), pitavastatin (Sankyo [Tokyo, Japan]/Kowa's [Tokyo, Japan] Livalo), pravastatin (Bristol-Myers Squibb's Pravachol), rosuvastatin (AstraZeneca's [Wilmington, Delaware] Crestor), and simvastatin (Merck's Zocor). This section focuses on atorvastatin and simvastatin, which have been specifically investigated in IC patients. Nevertheless, there is evidence that any statin improves leg function in patients with symptomatic PAD regardless of the dose administered or patient cholesterol levels (McDermott MM, 2003[b]), and physicians may favor other members of the statin class.

Mechanism of Action. Statins are structurally similar to the cholesterol precursor HMG-CoA; they act as competitive inhibitors of HMG-CoA reductase, the rate-limiting enzyme in cholesterol biosynthesis. Statins act to inhibit the conversion of hydroxymethyglutaryl to mevalonic acid. In response to reduced hepatic cholesterol biosynthesis, activation of the transcription factor sterol regulatory element binding protein (SREBP) upregulates LDL receptor gene expression, which leads to enhanced clearing of serum lipids by the liver (Liao JK, 2003).

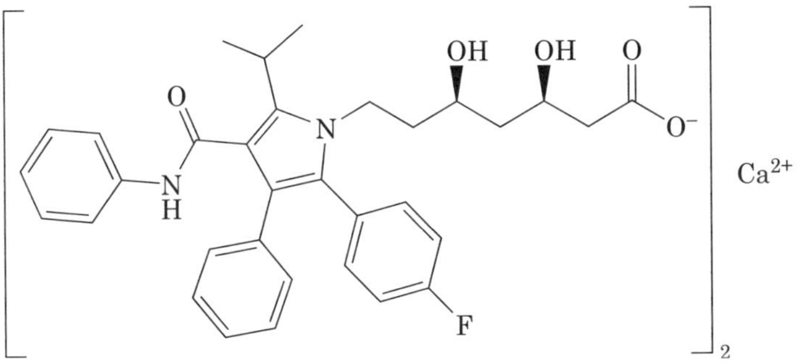

FIGURE 12. Structure of atorvastatin.

Statins are commonly believed to confer additional beneficial effects on cardiovascular health, independently of their cholesterol-lowering activities. Termed pleiotropic effects, these actions stem from the statins' ability to modify endothelial function, possibly by promoting the production of nitric oxide and inhibiting the production of inflammatory molecules in the endothelium (Wassmann S, 2004). This class effect of the statins may reduce inflammation, stabilize atherosclerotic plaques, inhibit platelet aggregation, and improve blood flow, all of which act to prevent coronary events.

Atorvastatin. Pfizer has marketed atorvastatin (Pfizer's Lipitor/Tahor/Sortis/Torvast/Cardyl) (Figure 12) in the United States, Europe, and Japan since 1997.

Like other agents in the statin class, atorvastatin acts to competitively inhibit HMG-CoA reductase, the rate-limiting enzyme in cholesterol biosynthesis. A therapeutic response is seen within two weeks of treatment; the maximum response is usually achieved at four weeks of therapy, and this response is maintained throughout chronic administration. Pleiotropic actions of atorvastatin have been observed in several recent studies, including improvements in endothelial function in both diabetic and nondiabetic patients and in atherosclerotic plaque color and morphology (Wassmann S, 2004; Dalla NE, 2003; Takano M, 2003).

Like simvastatin, atorvastatin has been shown to improve walking distance in patients with IC. In the Treatment of PAD with Moderate or Intensive Lipid Lowering study (TREADMILL), sponsored by Pfizer, 354 patients were treated for 12 months with atorvastatin, either 10 or 80 mg per day, or with placebo. Patients receiving 80 mg atorvastatin showed an improvement in pain-free walking time of 61%, compared with 33% for placebo. There was no significant difference between the pain-free walking time of patients treated with 10 mg atorvastatin and that of placebo-treated patients (Mohler ER, 2003).

Although the statins are generally well tolerated and cause few side effects, the safety profile of these agents has come under increased scrutiny in recent years following the withdrawal of cerivastatin (Bayer's Lipobay) in August 2001. Bayer withdrew cerivastatin after higher doses were linked to cases of life-threatening rhabdomyolysis (the destruction of skeletal muscle) that led to 31 deaths in the

United States; 12 of the patients who died were receiving concomitant therapy with the fibrate gemfibrozil (Pfizer's Lopid). These deaths led to a review of the safety of statins and the issue of new guidelines on their use (Pasternak RC, 2002). Because the symptoms of rhabdomyolysis may include leg pain, it is possible that this rare adverse event could be confused with symptomatic IC in PAD patients.

Simvastatin. Simvastatin (Merck's Zocor/Sinvacor, Boehringer Ingelheim's Denan, generics) (Figure 13) was launched in Europe in 1988 and in the United States and Japan in 1992. One of its indications is the reduction of cardiovascular mortality and morbidity in patients with manifest atherosclerotic cardiovascular disease. Therefore, its use in treatment of PAD is authorized.

Simvastatin competitively inhibits HMG-CoA reductase, the rate-limiting enzyme in cholesterol biosynthesis. Pleiotropic effects, such as improvements in endothelial function, have been demonstrated in studies of simvastatin (Pereira EC, 2003; Rezaie-Majid A, 2003).

According to the Scandinavian Simvastatin Survival Study (4 S), a 1.0% decrease in LDL is associated with a 1.7% reduction in risk of a CHD event (Pedersen TR, 2001). Further analysis of this study found that simvastatin (Merck's Zocor) reduces the risk of new or worsening IC by 38%. Such effects suggest a general antiatherosclerotic effect not limited solely to the coronary bed (Pedersen TR, 1998).

The Medical Research Council/British Heart Foundation (MRC/BHF) Heart Protection Study (HPS) of 20,536 U.K. adults at high risk of a major vascular event, including 2,701 with PAD, reported a 25% reduction in the incidence of ischemic stroke in patients treated with 40 mg/day simvastatin (Heart Protection Study Collaborative Group, 2002). This study led directly to a new indication for simvastatin: prevention of mortality and morbidity in patients at risk of cardiovascular events, including patients with PAD. This revision was approved in both Europe and the United States in 2003.

In an Italian study of 86 patients with stage II PAD and total cholesterol levels greater than 200 mg/dL, 43 were given 40 mg simvastatin per day; the other 43 received placebo. ACD and ICD were assessed at the start of the study and after

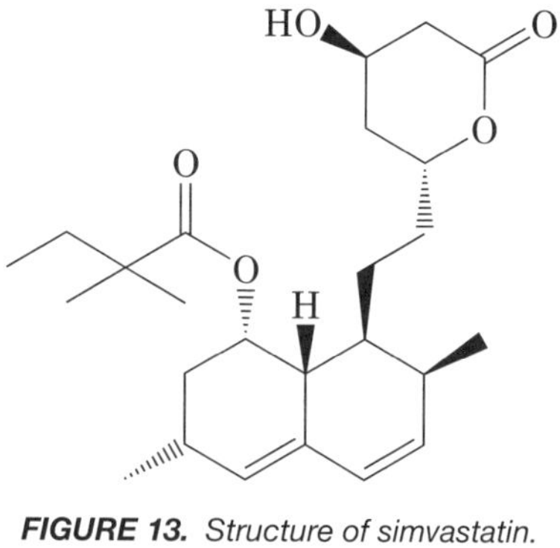

FIGURE 13. *Structure of simvastatin.*

three and six months of treatment. Initially, patients from both treatment groups were able to walk 72–74 meters without pain and 93–96 meters in total. After six months, patients who were receiving simvastatin had significantly increased their ICD and ACD to 190 meters and 230 meters, respectively. In contrast, the corresponding distances in the placebo group were only 100 meters and 104 meters (Mondillo S, 2003).

W. S. Aronow and colleagues used treadmill exercise time to gauge the benefits of simvastatin in stage II PAD patients. Sixty-nine patients aged 60 or older who were receiving cilostazol for treatment of IC and had LDL cholesterol levels of 125 mg/dL or higher were given 40 mg simvastatin per day or placebo. After six and twelve months, treadmill exercise time increased significantly by 24% and 42%, respectively, in patients receiving simvastatin. No significant change in exercise time occurred in the placebo group over the course of the study (Aronow WS, 2003).

Angiotensin-Converting Enzyme Inhibitors

Overview. As a result of the Heart Outcomes Prevention Evaluation (HOPE) study, angiotensin-converting enzyme (ACE) inhibitors (ACEIs) are increasingly used in prevention of cardiovascular events, irrespective of their antihypertensive effects. ACEIs are involved in preventing cell proliferation, reducing platelet aggregation, and enhancing fibrinolysis (Lonn EM, 1998).

Mechanism of Action. ACEIs lower blood pressure by inhibiting the vasoconstrictive action of the renin-angiotensin-aldosterone system (RAAS). Pharmacologically, ACEIs prevent the angiotensin-converting enzyme (ACE) from converting angiotensin I (AI) into angiotensin II (AII), a potent vasoconstrictive agent. Blocking the production of AII—and subsequently, aldosterone—increases cardiac output and reduces sodium and water retention. AII has several additional unwanted actions in the vasculature that are combated by ACEI therapy. AII causes contraction of the VSMCs lining the vascular wall, an action that ultimately leads to hypertrophy (an increase in cell size) and hyperplasia (an increase in cell number). This action manifests as a thickening of the arterial wall and a narrowing of the lumen—developments that generate an increase in the peripheral resistance of the vasculature. AII also increases production of reactive oxygen species, which in turn increase vasoconstriction and damage the endothelial wall (Sowers JR, 2002). Treatment with ACEIs also reduces the breakdown of the vasodilator bradykinin, an action that, in turn, upregulates endothelial nitric oxide synthase (ecNOS) activity, which means that the endothelium produces nitric oxide (NO) that promotes vasodilation. However, bradykinin accumulation results in cough, a side effect of ACE inhibition evident in 10–20% of patients.

Ramipril. Ramipril (King Pharmaceuticals [Bristol, Tennessee] Aventis's Altace/Delix/Tritace) (Figure 14) was launched in France in 1989 and was approved in the United States in 1991 for hypertension. In 2000, the FDA

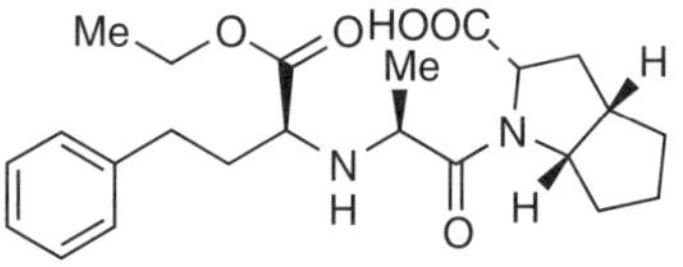

FIGURE 14. Structure of ramipril.

expanded its labeling as a result of the HOPE study. Ramipril is now indicated in patients aged 55 years or older who are at high risk of developing a major cardiovascular event because of a history of coronary artery disease (CAD), stroke, peripheral vascular disease (PVD; comprises venous and arterial disease), or diabetes that is accompanied by at least one other cardiovascular risk factor: hypertension, elevated total serum cholesterol, low HDL, or cigarette smoking. Ramipril helps reduce the risk of MI, stroke, or death from cardiovascular causes. It can be used in addition to other required treatments (such as antihypertensive, antiplatelet, or lipid-lowering therapy) and is available in all markets under study except Japan.

The HOPE study involved 9,541 high-risk patients with clinical symptoms associated with atherosclerosis (Dagenais GR, 2001). Over a five-year follow-up period, patients taking ramipril experienced a 20.3% reduction in the combined primary end point of MI, stroke, or cardiovascular death. Furthermore, their risk of death from cardiovascular events declined by approximately 25%. The therapeutic implications of the HOPE study resulted in FDA and European approval of ramipril for use in high-risk atherosclerotic patients, including reduction of risk of MI, stroke, cardiovascular death, or need for revascularization procedures in PAD patients aged 55 years or older. When PAD patients involved in the HOPE trial were studied in more detail, the investigators found that ramipril reduced the risk of cardiovascular events in all groups of patients with symptomatic and asymptomatic PAD. The percentage incidences of the primary end point of cardiovascular death, MI, or stroke in symptomatic PAD patients receiving ramipril or placebo were 20.1% and 25.8%, respectively. A similar event reduction was noted in asymptomatic patients: 13.6% of patients treated with ramipril reached the primary end point, compared with 17.0% of placebo-treated patients (Östergren J, 2004).

Quinapril. Quinapril (Pfizer's Accupro/Acuitel/Accuprin/Acuprel, Sanofi-Aventis's Korec, generics) (Figure 15) was approved in the United States in 1991 for hypertension and is also available in Japan and throughout Europe.

The Quinapril Ischemic Event Trial (QUIET) was designed to test the hypothesis that quinapril given at 20 mg per day would reduce ischemic events caused by atherosclerosis; research has suggested that AII plays an important role in the development of coronary atherosclerosis and ischemic events. A total of 1,750 patients were randomized to quinapril or placebo and followed for an average of 27 months. The incidence of ischemic events was similar in both groups: 38%. Quinapril did not significantly affect the overall progression of coronary

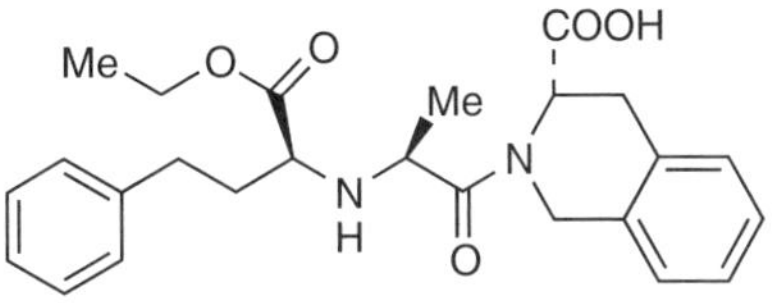

FIGURE 15. *Structure of quinapril.*

atherosclerosis. However, the study authors indicated that QUIET had several limitations, the most significant being the sample size and the resultant lack of statistical power to detect a reduction in ischemic events (Pitt B, 2001).

Nonpharmacological Approaches

Exercise Programs. Specific exercise training for PAD patients can be carried out at home, but physical training programs should be structured and preferably supervised.

An example would be an intensive exercise program conducted under standardized conditions, such as two (morning and afternoon) sessions of supervised aerobic activity for 30 minutes, followed by two cycles of treadmill exercise, each amounting to 66% of the ACD. Studies demonstrate that better results are obtained when patients exercise until moderate claudication pain is reached (Cachovan M, 1994).

A meta-analysis of 21 studies found that, following exercise rehabilitation programs, the mean ICD increased by 179% to 351 meters, while the mean ACD increased by 122% to 723 meters. Optimal improvements were obtained when patients exercised for at least three supervised sessions of more than 30 minutes duration every week for six months or more (Gardner AW, 1995). Another systematic review and meta-analysis of 15 trials involving 250 patients with IC suggests that exercise improves maximal walking time by 150% (Leng GC, 2000).

Exercise training has the advantage of being safe, noninvasive, and cost-effective. However, supervised programs are available at comparatively few centers, so treatment of IC will likely continue to rely heavily on pharmacotherapy.

Nutritional Supplements. Attention might also be paid to the role of nutrition and nutritional supplements, especially in obese patients. Some clinicians recommend supplements that are considered comparatively safe and inexpensive, such as L-arginine and carnitine, in addition to exercise and pharmacotherapeutic interventions.

One peripheral, vasculature-related condition that is significant in PAD is an impairment of the vasodilator mechanism, due in part to abnormalities of the NO synthase pathway. The effects of nutritional supplements that act on this pathway (and thus are beneficial in PAD) are attributed to antioxidant properties and improvement in vascular relaxation due to preservation of endothelium-derived NO (Cooke JP, 2000). Studies are under way to confirm the benefit of such therapies, but the data that support exercise, cilostazol, and revascularization are stronger.

Revascularization and Surgical Procedures. In addition to the use of parenteral prostaglandins (see "Prostaglandin Analogues"), treatment options for more-severe cases of PAD—patients presenting with CLI—include revascularization and surgical procedures. Indications include progressive and limiting IC that detracts significantly from QOL, rest pain, dermal ulceration, and gangrene.

Percutaneous transluminal angioplasty (PTA) offers a minimally invasive method of improving blood flow to the limb. In this procedure, a catheter is inserted into the artery and a balloon at the catheter tip is dilated to expand the occluded area; a stent is then positioned to maintain vessel patency. However, patency rates vary, depending on the number, site, and extent of occlusions, and the long-term outlook for such intervention remains inferior to that of open surgical techniques. The more distal the occlusion, the lower the patency rates; three-year rates are less than 60% following infrainguinal angioplasty and stenting (Ouriel K, 2001). Proponents argue that the decline in patency is offset by the less invasive nature of the interventions and resultant reduced morbidity, compared with open surgery, and that the procedure can be repeated. Intra-arterial thrombolysis is performed prior to intervention; agents such as urokinase and alteplase are infused directly into the occluding thrombus. Heparins—in particular, low-molecular weight heparin (LMWH)—may also be used to improve disease staging prior to the revascularization procedure.

Reconstructive surgery is rarely indicated in patients with IC alone because the risk of major amputation is low, but it is the treatment of choice for patients with chronic CLI. Two main approaches are applied in PAD: endarterectomy and bypass grafting. Endarterectomy (resection of thickened intima of major arteries) is performed when stenosis is localized—for example, short localized lesions in the deep femoral arteries. With longer occlusions, patency rates are unsatisfactory and bypass grafting is more appropriate. In these cases, the common procedures are aortofemoral and infrainguinal bypass surgery.

Systemic anticoagulation with heparin is invariably used in patients undergoing lower extremity arterial reconstructive procedures; aspirin is given to patients undergoing bypass to improve graft patency. Warfarin may also be used in patients believed to be at high risk for graft thrombosis.

EMERGING THERAPIES

One of the most striking aspects of drug development for the treatment of peripheral arterial disease (PAD) is the relative paucity of new approaches, especially when compared with other areas of cardiovascular medicine.

Of the limited number of new approaches being developed, most are of one of two types: skeletal muscle metabolic modulators and angiogenesis-promoting growth factors. Skeletal muscle metabolic modulators represent the most advanced area of development. Although offering the prospect of improved localized metabolism in the leg, the compounds in development display only modest benefit.

Growth factors that promote angiogenesis offer the prospect of stimulating collateral blood vessel development in the diseased limb and are likely to make a greater impact on PAD therapy. However, much work remains to be done in the development of these agents.

This review of emerging therapies focuses on medicinal products for the treatment of chronic PAD and products that address the underlying causes of the disease. Some important therapies are in development for treatment of acute limb ischemia (ALI), notably alfimeprase (Nuvelo/Amgen), but because ALI affects only approximately 100,000 patients each year in the United States, a discussion of such agents is beyond the scope of this section. Table 2 lists emerging therapies for the treatment of PAD.

Skeletal Muscle Metabolic Modulators

Overview. Metabolic modulation may potentially circumvent the problem of tissue hypoxia by modifying tissue metabolism and promoting glucose over fatty-acid oxidation.

Mechanism of Action. Intermittent claudication (IC) is associated with altered muscle metabolism and accumulation of acylcarnitines in skeletal muscles. Acylcarnitines are intermediates of oxidative metabolism of fatty acids and are formed from acylCoA in a reversible reaction. In PAD patients, there is a positive correlation between accumulation of acylcarnitines and walking impairment (Hiatt WR, 2001[b]). Skeletal muscle metabolic modulators restore the equilibrium of the reversible reaction and thus relieve the buildup of acylcarnitines.

Propionyl-L-Carnitine. Sigma-Tau is developing oral and intravenous (IV) forms of the endogenous organic amine propionyl-L-carnitine (PLC). Registered in Italy as Dromos, PLC is indicated for peripheral vascular and muscle disorders; elsewhere in Europe, the agent is in Phase III studies. In the United States, PLC has completed Phase III trials for IC, and, at the time of composing this reference, a new drug application (NDA) dossier is still in preparation.

IC is associated with altered muscle metabolism and accumulation of acylcarnitines in skeletal muscles (Hiatt WR, 2001[b]). PLC affects the metabolic actions of carnitine in skeletal muscles by normalizing oxidative metabolism under conditions of hypoxic stress.

The European Multicenter Study on PLC in IC conducted a 12-month evaluation of 485 patients randomized into drug-treated and placebo groups. Results suggest that PLC provides significant improvement of absolute claudication distance (ACD; the distance at which patients can no longer walk because of pain, sometimes referred to as the maximal walking distance) in "moderately severe" claudication (defined as walking distance of less than 250 meters before the

TABLE 2. Emerging Therapies in Development for Peripheral Arterial Disease

Compound	Development Phase	Marketing Company
Skeletal muscle metabolic modulators		
Propionyl-L-carnitine		
United States	PR	Sigma-Tau Ind. Farm. Riunite
Europe	R	Sigma-Tau Ind. Farm. Riunite
Japan	—	—
Ranolazine		
United States	PR	CV Therapeutics
Europe	PR	CV Therapeutics
Japan	—	—
Growth factors		
Ad$_{GV}$VEGF$_{121.10}$		
United States	S	GenVec
Europe	—	—
Japan	—	—
VEGF$_{165}$		
United States	—	—
Europe	II	Valentis
Japan	—	—
HGF (DS-992)		
United States	II	AnGes MG/Daiichi
Europe	—	—
Japan	III	AnGes MG/Daiichi
rFGF-2		
United States	II	Chiron
Europe	—	—
Japan	—	—
NV1FGF		
United States	II	Sanofi-Aventis/Gencell
Europe	II	Sanofi-Aventis/Gencell
Japan	—	—
Phosphodiesterase inhibitors		
NM-702		
United States	II	Nissan Chemical/Taisho
Europe	—	—
Japan	I	Nissan Chemical/Taisho
TXA$_2$ antagonists		
Z-335		
United States	—	—
Europe	—	—
Japan	I	Zeria Pharmaceutical
Prostaglandin analogues		
Ecraprost (Circulase)		
United States	III	Mitsubishi Pharma
Europe	—	—
Japan	II	Mitsubishi Pharma

TABLE 2. (*continued*)

Compound	Development Phase	Marketing Company
Liprostin		
United States	II	Endovasc
Europe	II	Endovasc
Japan	—	—
Immune-modulation therapies		
Celacade (Vasocare)		
United States	III	Vasogen
Europe	III	Vasogen
Japan	—	—

PR = Preregistered; R = Registered; S = Suspended.

patient experiences pain): 44% improvement compared with placebo (Brevetti G, 1999). However, for patients experiencing pain at a walking distance of more than 250 meters (the majority of IC patients), no significant difference was observed between PLC and placebo.

The researchers found similar rates of discontinuation of therapy owing to side effects in the PLC and placebo groups; however, the PLC group reported overall fewer discontinuations due to vascular events (38 events compared with 98 in the placebo group). The PLC and placebo groups did not differ with respect to the need for amputation and revascularization, but a smaller proportion of PLC-treated patients developed rest pain compared with placebo patients (2.1% compared with 4.1%).

In a recent trial, 155 patients with an ankle-brachial index (ABI) of less than 0.9 were randomized into placebo and PLC groups (Hiatt WR, 2001[a]). They were evaluated over a period of six months for effects on exercise performance. Patients receiving PLC demonstrated a 26% improvement in ACD and reported better quality of life (QOL) than patients receiving placebo.

PLC's greatest benefit is its safety profile; it provokes very few side effects. However, its ability to prevent cardiovascular disease (CVD) risk factors has not been studied, and it does not appear to significantly modify the disease.

Ranolazine. CV Therapeutics is developing ranolazine, a partial fatty-acid oxidation (pFOX) inhibitor licensed from Roche Bioscience (Basel, Switzerland). CV Therapeutics, Inc., (Palo Alto, California) has partnered with Innovex to commercialize ranolazine in the United States under the brand name Ranexa; an NDA dossier was submitted in December 2002. The primary target for development is the treatment of chronic stable angina; the agent is also under active development for congestive heart failure. In late 2003, the FDA asked CV Therapeutics to provide additional safety data; the FDA was concerned about delayed cardiac repolarization because prolongation of the QT interval had been observed in all patient populations studied. The FDA also had reservations about potential testicular toxicity because fertility was impaired in rats treated with ranolazine.

In August 2004, CV Therapeutics announced the initiation of two new studies drawn up in consultation with the FDA; if successful, these studies would support approval of ranolazine for treatment of chronic stable angina (ERICA study) and acute coronary syndromes (MERLIN study).

At the time of composing this reference, the ERICA data have become available and results from MERLIN may be available in the fourth quarter of 2006 or the first quarter of 2007, according to CV Therapeutics.

In the ERICA study, a hundred and sixty-five patients with chronic angina who had more than three angina attacks weekly, despite at least two weeks treatment with 10 mg amlodipine daily (the maximum labeled dose), were randomized to receive placebo or 1,000 mg ranolazine twice daily for six weeks. Patients continued amlodipine at a daily dose of 10 mg; long-acting nitrates were allowed as background therapy at the start of the study and were used by nearly half the patients. The primary end point of ERICA was angina frequency. Data presented at the 2005 AHA meeting showed that ranolazine significantly reduced weekly angina frequency, compared with placebo ($p = 0.028$). Patients who experienced 4.5 or more angina attacks each week benefited most from ranolazine. In these severely afflicted patients, the frequency of angina attacks and need for sublingual nitroglycerin use were significantly reduced over the six-week treatment period. Ranolazine was well tolerated, and there were no cases of syncope during the study.

In Europe, CV Therapeutics submitted a dossier to the EMEA, under the centralized procedure, in March 2004.

Ranolazine is thought to act by shifting energy metabolism from free fatty acid to glucose oxidation during stress, enabling tissues to produce more energy per unit of oxygen consumed. Preclinical data have confirmed that ranolazine reduces myocardial ischemic injury in various animal models (Schofield RS, 2002).

In 2001, CV Therapeutics reported data from a Phase III study in 823 patients with stable angina. In this trial, ranolazine significantly increased symptom-limited exercise duration at 12 weeks by an average of 116 seconds—an increase of 26% compared with placebo. Minor side effects occurred in 33% of treated patents (versus 26% with placebo); the side effects most commonly reported were constipation, nausea, dizziness, and asthenia. The incidence of serious adverse events was 7% in ranolazine-treated patients.

The primary focus of CV Therapeutics' development activity with ranolazine is chronic stable angina. Two studies in patients with intermittent claudication were included in the NDA submitted to the FDA, but they involved only 48 patients and were not used to support efficacy claims.

Growth Factors

Overview. Prospective gene therapy products for PAD are intended to promote angiogenesis, a natural biological process that results in the growth of additional (collateral) blood vessels, thus restoring adequate blood flow to oxygen-deprived tissues. Most such gene-based development targets growth factors. Growth factors provide angiogenesis therapy for PAD, promoting growth and proliferation of blood vessels from existing vascular structures, thereby increasing tissue perfusion (Lederman RJ, 2002). Research on angiogenesis in this area has focused on several targets, three of which are described here: vascular endothelial growth factors (VEGFs), hepatocyte growth factor (HGF), and fibroblast growth factors (FGFs).

Stimulation of angiogenesis by gene transfer offers the prospect of an effective symptomatic treatment for PAD patients, but fundamental issues remain regarding the development of growth factors. These issues will need to be addressed in Phase II studies that identify the optimal route of administration, dosage, duration of effect, and frequency of application.

Differences in safety and efficacy between the various growth factors may well emerge—for example, differences between acidic and basic molecules. Another consideration that may influence development is that patients may require subsequent courses of treatment. This requirement may limit the use of growth factors that employ viral vectors because such growth factors may precipitate an immunologic response in patients whose antibodies have been raised after the first infusion.

Growth factors could provide effective symptom relief because they allow blood to be transported directly to the afflicted leg through new arteries. This approach could also reduce the need for invasive procedures, resulting in fewer hospitalizations. However, growth factors are unlikely to achieve widespread application owing to potentially life-threatening side effects that are more significant than side effects caused by the combination of cilostazol (Otsuka's Pletaal/Pletal) and clopidogrel (Bristol-Myers Squibb/Sanofi-Aventis's Plavix). Patients receiving growth factors would have to be monitored for cancer and other angiogenesis-based diseases owing to a potentially higher systemic risk of tumor and plaque growth. Therefore, use of growth factors is likely to be reserved for patients with severer symptoms, particularly those who are not candidates for standard revascularization procedures. Furthermore, growth factors do not address the primary end point of disease modification by reducing the risk of cardiovascular events (e.g., stroke, MI) or preventing the progression of atherosclerosis.

Currently, no gene therapies are available in the major pharmaceutical markets. Transfer of genetic material into humans for in vivo expression is in its infancy and will be subject to some of the most stringent licensing requirements of any class of therapeutic agent. In addition, public concerns about genetic modification have great influence in the regulatory arena. Only one such agent is currently in Phase III clinical studies: AnGes MG's *HGF* gene therapy DS-992.

Mechanism of Action. Angiogenesis (the formation of new blood vessels) is a multistep process involving the proliferation, migration, adhesion, and tube-forming activity of endothelial cells, which form the inner lining of cells in all blood vessels. In healthy tissue, this process is controlled by angiogenic (angiogenesis-promoting) factors such as VEGFs, HGF, and FGFs. Gene therapy approaches to PAD treatment involve local expression of growth factors that stimulate new blood vessel formation in and around the occluded arteries. This collateral vessel development allows bypass of the obstruction, reperfusion of damaged tissue, and improved blood flow in the hypoperfused tissue.

VEGF receptors are found on endothelial cells, monocytes, and hematopoietic stem cells. Activation of the receptors by VEGFs stimulates proliferation, migration, and tube formation, thus leading to the development of new collateral channels. HGF also has effects on endothelial cells and hematopoietic stem cells, despite its misleading name. FGF therapy has aroused much interest because this group of growth factors stimulates migration and proliferation of various vascular cell types, such as smooth-muscle cells and fibroblasts, in addition to endothelial cells (Losordo DW, 2004).

Ad$_{GV}$VEG$_{121.10}$. GenVec, Inc. (Gaithersburg, Maryland) is developing $Ad_{GV}VEGF_{121.10}$ (BioBypass), an adenovirally delivered VEGF gene licensed from Scios. The agent was being developed for the treatment of coronary artery disease (CAD) and PAD. A lot of interest surrounded BioBypass, and it was touted as one of the most promising gene therapies in development.

GenVec enjoyed a successful Phase I, open-label, dose-escalating study involving 33 patients with severe debilitating PAD, who were given 20 local intramuscular injections of $Ad_{GV}VEGF_{121.10}$. Early indications of efficacy were observed, with a 77% improvement in ACD seen in the treatment group at 12 months (Rajagopalan S, 2001). However, the results of the Phase II Regional Angiogenesis with Vascular Endothelial Growth Factor (RAVE) study, involving 107 patients with moderate to severe PAD, were much less favorable. The double-blind, placebo-controlled trial assessed peak walking time (PWT); the primary end point was PWT at 12 weeks after 20 local, intramuscular injections of $Ad_{GV}VEGF_{121.10}$. After 12 weeks, there was no difference in PWT between patients treated with placebo, low-dose $Ad_{GV}VEGF_{121.10}$. (4×10^9 PU), or high-dose $Ad_{GV}VEGF_{121}.10$ (4×10^{10} PU) (Rajagopalan S, 2003). A result of these disappointing data was GenVec's announcement that it would no longer develop BioBypass for PAD, although it would continue to pursue the CAD indication. This was a particularly high-profile failure for a gene therapy regimen from which great things had been expected.

VEGF$_{165}$. Valentis, Inc. (Burlingame, California) has developed a gene therapy (VLTS-934) consisting of a plasmid-encoding $VEGF_{165}$ formulated with a proprietary cationic lipid delivery system (DOTMA). In parallel, Valentis is developing a combination of endothelial locus-1 (*Del-1*) with a 5% solution of $VEGF_{165}$ in a gene-based therapy called VLTS-589, or Deltavasc. The *Del-1* gene facilitates angiogenesis by binding to the a5b3 integrin receptor, inhibiting endothelial cell death and promoting vascular growth.

A single administration of the *Del-1* gene in muscle had effects on development of new blood vessels in animal models that were similar to the effects of a comparator $VEGF_{165}$ gene. According to Valentis, acute toxicities were observed with the $VEGF_{165}$ gene in dose-response studies but were not observed with the *Del-1* gene at similar doses, suggesting that the latter agent may be safer than $VEGF_{165}$.

Preliminary data from a Phase II clinical trial of Deltavasc versus VLTS-934 alone were reported at the American Heart Association (AHA) Scientific Sessions in November 2004. One hundred patients with bilateral PAD, with ABIs <0.80 in each leg and suffering from IC, were randomized to receive either 84 mg of Deltavasc or a 5% solution of VLTS-934 alone. The treatments were administered as a course of 21 intramuscular injections in each leg in a distributed pattern of concentric rings, three above the knee and two below the knee. After 90 days, the VLTS-934 and Deltavasc patients had a significant increase in exercise tolerance from baselines of 34% and 32%, respectively. The ABI increased in both treatment groups: by 0.059 (VLTS-934) and 0.048 (Deltavasc). Both Deltavasc and VLTS-934 were well tolerated (Rajagopalan S, 2004). The 180-day safety and efficacy data were expected to be announced in early 2005; but at the time of composing this reference, no new data seem to be available.

In March 2005, a Phase IIb trial in PAD began, and Valentis anticipates that the results will be available in July 2006. These results will be followed by the initiation of pivotal Phase III trials. On the basis of the 90-day results, it appears that the *Del-1* component of Deltavasc does not synergize with $VEGF_{165}$.

HGF. AnGes MG, Inc. (Osaka, Japan, formerly MedGene Bioscience) is developing DS-992, an *HGF* gene therapy, for the treatment of PAD and ischemic heart disease in Japan, Europe, and the United States. Daiichi Pharmaceutical has the marketing and distribution rights for the PAD indication in each of those territories. Trials with PAD patients have reached Phase II and Phase III in the United States and Japan, respectively. Patients with severe symptomatic stages II-IV PAD are the target population.

The first part of the open-label Phase I/IIa study of DS-992 involved six patients with chronic PAD who were treated with two 2 mg doses of naked *HGF* plasmid DNA. The doses were separated by four weeks. Treatment with DS-992 reduced leg pain in five of the patients who had improved blood circulation in their lower extremities as measured by transcutaneous arterial partial pressure of oxygen changes before and after stimulation with oxygen. The mean ABI increased from 0.426 at baseline to 0.626 after four weeks and to 0.596 after eight weeks. Angiogenesis was confirmed in five patients who were examined with angiography imaging, and three of the four patients with ulceration showed a 25% or more alleviation of symptoms and reduction of ulcer size (Morishita R, 2004). Data from the second part of the study were presented at the Therapeutic Angiogenesis and Wound Healing-IBC International Conference in November 2004. Seventeen patients with critical limb ischemia (CLI) were treated with 2 mg and 4 mg doses of DS-992. Six months after treatment, the mean ABI increase ranged from 0.4 to 0.6. Some patients experienced a reduction in rest pain and ulcer size. A multicenter Phase III trial to evaluate the efficacy of DS-992 in patients with PAD stage III or IV was begun in Japan in 2004.

An ongoing Phase II dose-finding study for DS-992, involving 100 patients who have been administered two doses (0.4 mg and 4 mg), will compare two versus three repeat administrations. The study was expected to be completed in the third quarter of 2005 (Morishita R, 2004), but at the time of composing this reference, no new data are yet available.

FGF-2. The most advanced growth factor therapy is recombinant fibroblast growth factor-2 (rFGF-2), also known as basic fibroblast growth factor (bFGF 2), which is marketed in Japan as Fiblast (trafermin), a topical spray for treatment of dermal ulcers, by Kaken Pharmaceuticals under license from Scios Inc. (Fremont, California). Rights to trafermin were granted to Chiron Corporation (Emeryville, California) in 1999. Chiron subsequently developed recombinant FGF-2 for the treatment of PAD in the United States but discontinued this program in March 2003. In Japan, an intramuscular formulation of rFGF-2 is being developed for stage IV PAD.

FGF-2 is a powerful mitogen that stimulates migration and proliferation of various vascular cell types, such as smooth-muscle cells and fibroblasts (unlike VEGF, which is specific for endothelial cells), thus favoring the development of thicker-walled structures. FGF-2 stimulates endothelial-cell production of matrix metalloproteinases required for vessel remodeling. FGF-2 is a nitric oxide-dependent vasodilator that is upregulated by hypoxia and has additional properties that protect against ischemia-reperfusion injury. And FGF-2's high-affinity binding to heparin sulfates on the surfaces of endothelial cells prolongs its tissue half-life and pharmacodynamic profile at the FGF-2 receptor.

Chiron supported the randomized, double-blind, placebo-controlled Therapeutic Angiogenesis with Recombinant Fibroblast Growth Factor-2 for Intermittent Claudication (TRAFFIC) study. This Phase II trial involved 190 patients with moderate to severe claudication (ABI less than 0.8). rFGF-2 was administered intra-arterially on days 1 and 30 of the trial in either a single dose or a double dose of 30 µg/kg body weight. With single-dose rFGF-2 infusion, peak walking time (PWT) at 90 days exceeded the PWT of placebo by 195%. Serious adverse events were similar in all groups; side effects included hypotension and protein-uria. The investigators concluded that the study findings provided evidence of clinically therapeutic angiogenesis (Lederman RJ, 2002).

NV1FGF. Sanofi-Aventis and Aventis Gencell (Hayward, California) are developing an acidic, nonviral type 1 *FGF* (*NV1FGF*), targeted at patients with unreconstructable, end-stage PAD (Fontaine stages III/IV). Gencell has initiated a collection of trials for *NV1FGF1*, called the Therapeutic Angiogenesis Leg Ischemia Study for Management of Arteriopathy and Nonhealing Ulcers (TALISMAN) program, which comprises five Phases I and II trials.

In a Phase I dose-escalating study in 51 patients, preliminary results showed a significant reduction in pain and aggregate ulcer size, compared with pretreatment baseline values. A significant increase in ABI was also observed. Of 29 patients with nonhealing ulcers at entry, 20 (69%) demonstrated complete or partial ulcer healing at six months. At three months following *NV1FGF* treatment, 33% of

36 patients who were evaluated arteriographically had evidence of new blood vessel development. Although 66 serious adverse events were reported, only four patients had adverse effects, such as injection site or other pain and peripheral edema, that were attributed to treatment (Comerota AJ, 2002).

In May 2004, Gencell gave an update on TALISMAN at the SMi Angiogenesis meeting in London, stating that the PM201 Phase II trial in stages III and IV PAD and the PM211 Phase II trial in stage II PAD had begun enrollment in Europe and the United States, with results due in early 2006.

In October 2005, clinical data were presented at the 13th European Society of Gene Therapy congress in Prague, Czech Republic. In February 2006, Sanofi-Aventis announced that Phase IIb data would be available in March 2006 and that Phase III trials would begin later in 2006.

Phosphodiesterase Inhibitors

Overview. The success of cilostazol has validated phosphodiesterase (PDE) as a therapeutic target for treatment of IC. Many PDE inhibitors are in development for a wide range of cardiovascular diseases, but only Nissan Chemical Industries (Tokyo, Japan)/Taisho Pharmaceutical's (Tokyo, Japan) NM-702 is being pursued specifically for PAD indications.

Mechanism of Action. Like cilostazol, NM-702 inhibits PDE III, which degrades cyclic adenosine monophosphate (cAMP). By increasing the cAMP concentration, NM-702 decreases platelet aggregation and contraction of vascular smooth-muscle cells (VSMCs). In addition, NM-702 has inhibitory effects on PDE V and thromboxane synthetase. PDE V degrades cyclic guanosine monophosphate (cGMP); elevation of cGMP is recognized as a cause of relaxation of smooth muscle cells and inhibition of platelets. Thromboxane (TX) A_2 induces platelet aggregation; therefore, inhibition of thromboxane synthetase, the enzyme that synthesizes TXA_2 from prostaglandin H_2 (PGH_2), also contributes to the antiplatelet effects of NM-702.

NM-702. NM-702 was originally developed by the Welfide Corporation (Osaka, Japan, formerly Yoshitomi), which later merged with Mitsubishi-Tokyo Pharmaceuticals to form Mitsubishi Pharma Corporation. In September 2002, Mitsubishi Pharma terminated the development of NM-702, but Nissan Chemical Industries and Taisho Pharmaceutical announced that they were to codevelop NM-702 for Japanese and U.S. markets. Nissan Chemical is seeking to outlicense development and commercialization rights to NM-702 in Europe.

At the American Heart Association (AHA) meeting in November 2003, W.R. Hiatt and colleagues presented data from a Phase IIb clinical trial of NM-702 in IC patients aged 50 years or older. The multicenter, double-blind U.S. study evaluated 206 patients who were treated with placebo or with 1 mg, 2 mg, or 4 mg NM-702 twice daily for 12 weeks. The percentage change in PWT was 29.0% for the placebo group and 23.0%, 17.8%, and 58.7%, respectively, for the

1 mg, 2 mg, and 4 mg NM-702 groups. NM-702 also improved patient-assessed QOL. No severe adverse events were observed in the trial (Hiatt WR, 2003).

Following this successful trial, another Phase IIb trial of NM-702 began in November 2003 in the United States. The study was designed to evaluate PWT after 24 weeks of treatment with NM-702 at doses of 4 mg and 8 mg.

The 2005 annual report of Nissan Chemical states that in the United States, Phase III trials are due to start in 2006, with a view to a market launch 2008–2009 while Japanese Phase III studies will start in 2006/2007, with a launch target of 2010–2011.

TXA$_2$ Antagonists

Overview. As with all antiplatelet agents, assessing the risk of gastrointestinal side effects, including bleeding, with aspirin (Bayer's Bayer Aspirin, generics) and aspirin-like compounds is crucial in determining their future success.

Mechanism of Action. TXA$_2$ is involved in platelet aggregation. By inhibiting this pathway, TXA$_2$ antagonists block activation of platelets. However, TXA$_2$ is farther down the activation cascade than cyclooxygenase-1 (COX-1), which is the target of aspirin. Therefore, TXA$_2$ antagonists have a more specific effect on platelets and may cause fewer adverse events, such as prolonged bleeding (Tanaka T, 1998).

Z-335. Zeria Pharmaceutical (Tokyo, Japan) is developing Z-335, an oral thromboxane A$_2$ antagonist, as a prospective once-daily antiplatelet agent for the treatment and prevention of PAD. The agent prevents arterial thrombosis through its antiplatelet action by blocking thromboxane A$_2$ receptor activation. Z-335 is under investigation in a randomized, double-blind Phase II trial in Japan in patients with IC.

Preclinical data revealed that, unlike cilostazol's effects, Z-335's effects persisted for 16 hours and that the agent inhibited platelet aggregation in induced arterial thrombosis (Tanaka T, 2000). In a Phase I study, investigators concluded, based on a once-daily regimen, that Z-335 was safe and provided long-lasting blockade of thromboxane A2 receptors (Matsuno H, 2002).

Prostaglandin Analogues

Overview. Use of prostaglandin analogues in Western countries has been limited by the need for parenteral administration—in particular, the requirement for infusions of up to six hours. This requirement has restricted application to hospitalized patients with severe disease. Parenteral administration reflects the short half-life of the prostacyclin analogues marketed to date; this aspect of the agent is cited as a reason for the failure of oral beraprost in a key U.S. clinical trial (see "Current Therapies").

Although sales of the novel parenteral forms may grow at the expense of existing infusible prostacyclins and may expand Western markets to an extent by facilitating use in outpatient departments, these products are likely to be used only in patients with the most severe disease (i.e., patients in Fontaine stages III and IV). These agents may make more of an impact in Japan, which is a receptive market for prostaglandin analogues in PAD.

Mechanism of Action. As discussed in the "Current Therapies" section, the prostaglandins PGE_1 and PGI_2 are extremely potent, endogenous vasodilators and antiplatelet agents that are synthesized and act in vascular endothelium (Harker LA, 1986; Samuelsson B, 1975).

Formulation. Developments in this therapy class have concentrated on extending the half-life of analogues to produce more-convenient oral and parenteral formulations. Furthermore, in the case of oral formulations, researchers hope to produce more consistently effective treatments for PAD. Most efforts have been directed at encapsulating prostaglandins in lipid microspheres or liposome, thereby facilitating sustained release.

Ecraprost. Mitsubishi Pharma is developing ecraprost (Circulase), a parenteral prostaglandin E_1 pro-drug incorporated into liposomes. Phase II and III trials in PAD are under way in Japan and the United States, respectively, with the latter being undertaken by Alpha Therapeutic Corporation (Los Angeles, California), a Mitsubishi subsidiary.

In a Phase II multicenter study conducted in the United Kingdom, 80 patients with symptomatic IC and an ACD of less than 300 meters received bolus injections of ecraprost in various regimens. At eight weeks post treatment, 50% of patients in the treatment group achieved a clinically significant 30% increase over baseline in initial claudication distance (ICD; the distance when patients first notice pain, sometimes referred to as the pain-free walking distance [PFWD]), compared with 33% for placebo. Median dose-related increases in PFWDs were 20.9 meters in one treatment group, compared with 0 meters for placebo. Improvements in QOL were also reported with ecraprost (Belch JJF, 1997).

Liprostin. Endovasc, Inc. (Montgomery, Texas) is developing Liprostin, a liposome-encapsulated form of PGE_1, as a prospective treatment for PAD. The agent is delivered directly into the vessel wall via the same catheters that are used during angioplasty or stent procedures.

Endovasc issued a press release in August 2004 with details of a Phase II clinical trial that evaluated the effects of Liprostin in patients with stages II/III PAD. The patients were classified as Fontaine's stage II or III, and most were older than age 40. Each patient was treated six times with Liprostin. Seventy-three patients completed the trial and showed significant improvements in both ACD and ICD during the 12-week trial. ACD increased by more than 100%, and the average ICD increased by almost 200%. In addition, patient-assessed QOL improved as indicated by increases in overall walking distance and walking speed. Patients showed a significant improvement in partial pressure of oxygen in their extremities when transcutaneous oxygen pressure was monitored. These data suggest that Liprostin may also be used to treat ischemic ulcers in patients with severe PAD. All the improvements observed in patients during the trial were sustained during the one-month, post-treatment evaluation period, thus indicating that the encapsulated delivery prolongs the period of time in which Liprostin is active.

Phase II clinical trials are ongoing in several European countries, including Italy, but no data have been published at this time. Endovasc is currently preparing for Phase III clinical trials.

In April 2005, Endovasc met with the FDA to further define the clinical development strategy for Liprostin and submitted Phase II data to the agency. According to Endovasc's Web site, discussion on Phase III trials are under way with contract research organizations.

Immune-Modulation Therapies

Overview. As discussed in the "Etiology and Pathophysiology" section, PAD is a symptomatic manifestation of atherosclerosis. The implication of inflammatory pathways in the development and progression of atherosclerosis is well established. This fact raised the possibility of treating PAD by targeting the immune cells responsible for the inflammatory response. Vasogen is developing an immune-modulation therapy called Celacade (also known as Vasocare) as a potential treatment for PAD and atherosclerosis.

Mechanism of Action. Celacade therapy is designed to combat the deleterious effects of uncontrolled inflammation. In inflammatory disorders, such as in the blood vessel wall in atherosclerosis, activated immune system cells accumulate and release cytokines and other inflammatory mediators that kill healthy cells and damage surrounding tissue. The Celacade process involves the intramuscular readministration of whole blood subjected to heat, ozonation, and ultraviolet irradiation that oxidatively stresses cells, inducing senescence. Senescent cells are known to undergo apoptosis, the process that triggers the immune system to beneficially modulate cytokines and other mediators of inflammation.

Celacade. Vasogen (Toronto, Ontario, Canada) intends to gain marketing authorization for Celacade in North America and Western Europe and has carried out clinical trials in both these territories. Vasogen has already been granted approval under medical device regulations in the European Union, but before it can be launched, a combination product such as Celacade will also require examination under the legislation governing medicinal products.

In a Phase II, placebo-controlled study in 81 patients conducted at two centers in the United Kingdom, 67% of patients receiving treatment achieved a greater than 50% improvement in ICD at 24 weeks, compared with 42% in the placebo group. The treatment group increased its ICD from a median 65 meters at baseline to 140 meters at nine weeks post treatment, compared with a 40-meter improvement seen in the placebo group. The results were supported by QOL measurements (McGrath C, 2002).

Building on these promising results, 500 patients aged 40 or older with stage II PAD had enrolled in a double-blind, randomized, placebo-controlled Phase III study. The trial had become known as the Study of Immune Modulation Therapy in Peripheral Arterial Disease and Intermittent Claudication Outcomes (SIMPADICO). Inclusion criteria for the trial included an ABI $\leq$ 0.85 and an ACD of $\geq$ 50 meters. The primary end point of the trial was the change in ACD over six months. The combined incidence of cardiovascular events and QOL were also to be evaluated.

SIMPADICO was terminated in August 2005 because the independent monitoring committee concluded that there was insufficient evidence of efficacy.

REFERENCES

Abbott RD, et al. Ankle brachial blood pressure in men 70 years of age and the risk of coronary heart disease. *American Journal of Cardiology*. 2000;**86**:280–284.

Altstaedt HO, et al. Treatment of patients with peripheral arterial occlusive disease Fontaine stage IV with intravenous iloprost and PGE1: a randomized open controlled study. *Prostaglandins, Leukotrienes, and Essential Fatty Acids*. 1993;**49**(2):573–578.

Antiplatelet Trialists' Collaboration. Collaborative overview of randomized trials of antiplatelet therapy—I: Prevention of death, myocardial infarction, and stroke by prolonged antiplatelet therapy in various categories of patients. *British Medical Journal*. 1994;**308**(6921):81–106.

Antithrombotic Trialists' Collaboration. Collaborative meta-analysis of randomised trials of antiplatelet therapy for prevention of death, myocardial infarction, and stroke in high risk patients. *British Medical Journal*. 2002;**324**(7329):71–86.

Arcan JC, et al. Multicenter double-blind study of ticlopidine in the treatment of intermittent claudication and the prevention of its complications. *Angiology*. 1988;**39**(9):802–811.

Aronow WS, Ahn C. Prevalence of coexistence of coronary artery disease, peripheral arterial disease, and atherothrombotic brain infarction in men and women > or = 62 years of age. *American Journal of Cardiology*. 1994;**74**(1):64–65.

Aronow WS, et al. Effect of simvastatin versus placebo on treadmill exercise time until the onset of intermittent claudication in older patients with peripheral arterial disease at six months and at one year after treatment. *American Journal of Cardiology*. 2003;**92**(6):711–712.

Baiton D, et al. Peripheral vascular disease: consequences for survival and association with risk factors in the Speedwell Prospective Heart Disease Study. *British Heart Journal*. 1994;**72**:128–137.

Balkau B, et al. Epidemiology of peripheral arterial disease. *Journal of Cardiovascular Pharmacology*. 1994;**23**(suppl 3):S8–S16.

Balsano F, et al. Ticlopidine in the treatment of intermittent claudication: a 21-month double-blind trial. *Journal of Laboratory and Clinical Medicine*. 1989;**114**(1):84–91.

Becker GJ, et al. The importance of increasing public and physician awareness of peripheral arterial disease. *Journal of Vascular and Interventional Radiology*. 2002;**13**:7–11.

Beebe HG, et al. A new pharmacological treatment for intermittent claudication: results of a randomized, multicenter trial. *Archives of Internal Medicine*. 1999;**159**(17): 2041–2050.

Beebe H. Intermittent claudication: effective medical management of a common circulatory problem. *American Journal of Cardiology*. 2001;**87**:14D–18D.

Belch JJF, et al. Randomized, double-blind, placebo-controlled study evaluating the efficacy and safety of AS-013, a prostaglandin E1 pro-drug in patients with intermittent claudication. *Circulation*. 1997;**95**:2298–2302.

Belch JJF, et al. Critical issues in peripheral arterial disease detection and management: a call to action. *Archives of Internal Medicine*. 2003;**163**(8):884–892.

Belgore FM, et al. Measurement of free and complexed soluble vascular endothelial growth factor receptor, Flt-1, in fluid samples: development and application of two new immunoassays. *Clinical Science*. 2001;**100**(5):567–575.

Bennett CL, et al. Thrombotic thrombocytopenic purpura associated with ticlopidine. A review of 60 cases. *Annals of Internal Medicine*. 1998;**128**(7):541–544.

Bennett C, et al. Thrombotic thrombocytopenic purpura associated with clopidogrel. *New England Journal of Medicine*. 2000;**342**:1773–1777.

Bergqvist D, et al. Reduction of requirement for leg vascular surgery during long-term treatment of claudicant patients with ticlopidine: results from the Swedish Ticlopidine Multicentre Study (STIMS). *European Journal of Vascular and Endovascular Surgery*. 1995;**10**(1):69–76.

Bertrand ME, et al. Double-blind study of the safety of clopidogrel with and without a loading dose in combination with aspirin compared with ticlopidine in combination with aspirin after coronary stenting: the clopidogrel aspirin stent international cooperative study (CLASSICS). *Circulation*. 2000;**102**(6):624–629.

Besse B, et al. Beraprost sodium, an effective treatment for peripheral arterial disease: results of BERCI 2, a randomized, placebo-controlled, double-blind study. *Journal of the American College of Cardiology*. 1999;**33**(suppl A):277A.

Bhatt DL, et al. Reduction in the need for hospitalization for recurrent ischemic events and bleeding with clopidogrel instead of aspirin. CAPRIE investigators. *American Heart Journal*. 2000;**140**(1):67–73.

Bhatt DL, et al. Clopidogrel added to aspirin versus aspirin alone in secondary prevention and high-risk primary prevention: rationale and design of the Clopidogrel for High Atherothrombotic Risk and Ischemic Stabilization, Management, and Avoidance (CHARISMA) trial. *American Heart Journal*. 2004;**148**(2):263–268.

Bloemenkamp DG, et al. Novel risk factors for peripheral arterial disease in young women. *American Journal of Medicine*. 2002;**113**(6):462–467.

Boccalon H, et al. Assessment of the prevalence of atherosclerotic lower limb arteriopathy in France as a systolic index in a vascular risk population. *Journal des Maladies Vasculaires*. 2000;**25**:38–46.

Bode-Boger SM, et al. L-arginine induces nitric oxide-dependent vasodilation in patients with critical limb ischemia. A randomized, controlled study. *Circulation*. 1996;**93**(1): 85–90.

Boers GHJ, et al. Heterozygotes for homocysteinuria in premature peripheral and cerebral occlusive arterial disease. *New England Journal of Medicine*. 1985;**313**:709–715.

Boger RH, et al. Biochemical evidence for impaired nitric oxide synthesis in patients with peripheral arterial occlusive disease. *Circulation*. 1997;**95**(8):2068–2074.

Boissel JP, et al. Is it possible to reduce the risk of cardiovascular events in subjects suffering from intermittent claudication of the lower limbs? *Thrombosis and Haemostasis*. 1989;**62**(2):681–685.

Bongard V, et al. Prévalence et prise en charge des patients avec antécédents athérothrombotiques dans le cadre des consultations de médicine générale en France: Resultats de l'enquete ECLAT 1. *Archives des Maladies du Coeur et des Vaisseaux*. 2003;**96**:833–840.

Breek JC, et al. Quality of life in patients with intermittent claudication using the World Health Organisation (WHO) questionnaire. *European Journal of Vascular and Endovascular Surgery*. 2001;**21**(2):118–122.

Brevetti G, et al. European multicenter study on propionyl-L-carnitine in intermittent claudication. *Journal of the American College of Cardiology*. 1999;**34**:1618–1624.

Brevetti G, et al. Prevalence, risk factors and cardiovascular comorbidity in symptomatic peripheral arterial disease in Italy. *Atherosclerosis*. 2004;**175**:131–138.

Burns P, et al. What constitutes best medical therapy for peripheral arterial disease? *European Journal of Vascular and Endovascular Surgery*. 2002;**24**(1):6–12.

Cachovan M, et al. The effectiveness of standardized exercise training in intermittent claudication. *Wiener Klinische Wochenschrift*. 1994;**106**(16):517–520.

CAPRIE Steering Committee. A randomised, blinded trial of clopidogrel versus aspirin in patients at risk of ischemic events (CAPRIE). *Lancet*. 1996;**348**:1329–1339.

Chacón-Quevedo A, et al. Comparative evaluation of pentoxifylline, buflomedil, and nifedipine in the treatment of intermittent claudication of the lower limbs. *Angiology Journal of Vascular Disease*. 1994;**45**:647–653.

Cheanvechai V, et al. Incidence of peripheral vascular disease in women: Is it different from that in men? *Journal of Thoracic and Cardiovascular Surgery*. 2004;**127**: 314–317.

Cheng SWK, et al. Lipoprotein (a) and its relationship to risk factors and severity of atherosclerotic peripheral vascular disease. *European Journal of Vascular and Endovascular Surgery*. 1997;**14**:17–23.

Cimminiello C. PAD: epidemiology and pathophysiology. *Thrombosis Research*. 2002; **106**:V295–V301.

Ciocon JO, et al. A comparison between aspirin and pentoxifylline in relieving claudication due to peripheral vascular disease in the elderly. *Angiology*. 1997;**48**(3):237–240.

Clagett GP, et al. Antithrombotic therapy in peripheral arterial occlusive disease: the Seventh ACCP Conference on Antithrombotic and Thrombolytic Therapy. *Chest*. 2004;**126**(suppl 3):609S–626S.

Collins TC, et al. The prevalence of peripheral arterial disease in a racially diverse population. *Archives of Internal Medicine*. 2003;**163**:1469–1474.

Comerota AJ, et al. Naked plasmid DNA encoding fibroblast growth factor type 1 for the treatment of end-stage unreconstructible lower extremity ischemia: preliminary results of a Phase I trial. *Journal of Vascular Surgery*. 2002;**35**(5):930–936.

Coni N, et al. Prevalence of lower extremity arterial disease among elderly people in the community. *British Journal of General Practice*. 1992;**42**:149–152.

Cooke JP. Does ADMA cause endothelial dysfunction? *Arteriosclerosis, Thrombosis, and Vascular Biology*. 2000;**20**(9):2032–2037.

Creager MA. Medical management of peripheral arterial disease. *Cardiology in Review*. 2001;**9**:238–245.

Creager MA, et al. American Heart Association. Atherosclerotic vascular disease conference: Writing Group V: medical decision making and therapy. *Circulation*. 2004; **109**(21):2634–2642.

Criqui MH, et al. The prevalence of peripheral arterial disease in a defined population. *Circulation*. 1985;**71**:510–515. [a]

Criqui MH, et al. The sensitivity, specificity and predictive value of traditional clinical evaluation of peripheral arterial disease: results from noninvasive testing in a defined population. *Circulation*. 1985;**71**:516–522. [b]

Criqui MH, et al. Peripheral arterial disease in large vessels is epidemiologically distinct from small vessel disease. *American Journal of Epidemiology*. 1989;**129**:1110–1119.

Criqui MH, et al. Mortality over a period of 10 years in patients with peripheral arterial disease. *New England Journal of Medicine*. 1992;**326**:381–386.

Currie IC, et al. Homocysteine: an independent risk factor for the failure of vascular intervention. *British Journal of Surgery*. 1996;**83**:1238–1241.

Cui R, et al. Ankle-arm blood pressure index and cardiovascular risk factors in elderly Japanese men. *Hypertension Research*. 2003;**28**:377–382.

Dagenais GR, et al. Effects of ramipril on coronary events in high-risk persons: results of the Heart Outcomes Prevention Evaluation Study. *Circulation*. 2001;**104**:522–526.

Dalla NE, et al. Atorvastatin improves metabolic control and endothelial function in type 2 diabetic patients: a placebo-controlled study. *Journal of Endocrinology Investigation*. 2003: **26**:73–78.

Darius H, et al. Are elevated homocysteine plasma levels related to peripheral arterial disease? Results from a cross-sectional study of 6880 primary care patients. *European Journal of Clinical Investigation*. 2003;**33**(9):751–757.

Dawson DL, et al. Cilostazol has beneficial effects in treatment of intermittent claudication. Results from a multicenter, randomized, prospective, double-blind trial. *Circulation*. 1998;**98**:678–686.

Dawson DL, et al. A comparison of cilostazol and pentoxifylline for treating intermittent claudication. *American Journal of Medicine*. 2000;**109**(7):523–530.

Dawson DL. Comparative effects of cilostazol and other therapies for intermittent claudication. *American Journal of Cardiology*. 2001;**87**(12A):19D–27D.

Dey S, Mukherjee D. Clinical perspectives on the role of anti-platelet and statin therapy in patients with vascular diseases. *Current Vascular Pharmacology*. 2003;**1**(3):329–333.

Diehm C, et al. High prevalence of peripheral arterial disease and co-morbidity in 6880 primary care patients: cross-sectional study. *Atherosclerosis*. 2004;**172**:95–105.

Dixon A, Mossialos E, eds. *European Observatory on Health Care Systems. Health Care Systems in Eight Countries: trends and challenges*. London, UK. London School of Economics & Political Science. 2002.

Donnelly R. Assessment and management of intermittent claudication: importance of secondary prevention. *International Journal of Clinical Practice Supplement*. April 2001:2–9.

Dormandy J. The natural history of claudication: risk to life and limb. *Seminars in Vascular Surgery*. 1999;**12**:123–137.

Dormandy JA, et al. Management of peripheral arterial disease (PAD). TASC Working Group. Trans-Atlantic Inter-Society Consensus (TASC). *Journal of Vascular Surgery*. 2000;**31**(1 Pt 2):S1–S296.

FitzGerald GA, et al. Cigarette smoking and hemostatic function. *American Heart Journal*. 1988;**115**(1):267–271.

Fowkes FGR, et al. Edinburgh Artery Study: prevalence of asymptomatic and symptomatic peripheral arterial disease in the general population. *International Journal of Epidemiology*. 1991;**20**:384–392.

Fowkes FGR, et al. Smoking, lipids, glucose intolerance and blood pressure as risk factors for peripheral atherosclerosis compared with ischemic heart disease in the Edinburgh Artery Study. *American Journal of Epidemiology*. 1992;**135**:331–340.

Fowkes FGR. Epidemiology of peripheral vascular disease. *Atherosclerosis*. 1997;**131**(suppl):s29–s31.

Fowkes FGR. Epidemiological research on peripheral vascular disease. *Journal of Clinical Epidemiology*. 2001;**54**:863–868.

Fowler B, et al. Prevalence of peripheral arterial disease: persistence of excess risk in former smokers. *Australian and New Zealand Journal of Public Health*. 2002;**26**:219–224.

Fox KM, et al. Efficacy of perindopril in reduction of cardiovascular events among patients with stable coronary artery disease: randomised, double-blind, placebo-controlled, multicentre trial (the EUROPA study). *Lancet*. 2003;**362**(9386):782–788.

Furukawa K, et al. Therapeutic effects of sarpogrelate hydrochloride (MCI-9042) on chronic arterial occlusive diseases—a double-blind comparison with ticlopidine hydrochloride. *Rinsho Iyaku*. 1991;**7**(8):1747–1770.

Gallotta G, et al. Prevalence of peripheral arterial disease in an elderly rural population of southern Italy. *Gerontology*. 1997;**43**:289–295.

Gardner AW, Poehlman ET. Exercise rehabilitation programs for the treatment of claudication pain. A meta-analysis. *Journal of the American Medical Association*. 1995;**274**:975–980.

Gent M, et al. A randomized, blinded trial of clopidogrel versus aspirin in patients at risk of ischemic events (CAPRIE). *Lancet*. 1996;**348**:1329–1339.

Gey DC, et al. Management of peripheral arterial disease. *American Family Physician*. 2004;**69**(3):525–532.

Girolami B, et al. Treatment of intermittent claudication with physical training, smoking cessation, pentoxifylline, or nafronyl: a meta-analysis. *Archives of Internal Medicine*. 1999;**159**(4):337–345.

Gotoh F, et al. Cilostazol stroke prevention study: a placebo-controlled double-blind trial for secondary prevention of cerebral infarction. *Journal of Stroke and Cerebrovascular Disease*. 2000;**9**:147–157.

Gregg EW, et al. Prevalence of lower-extremity disease in the U.S. adult population $\geq$ 40 years of age with and without diabetes. *Diabetes Care*. 2004;**27**:1591–1597.

Hacke W. From CURE to MATCH: ADP receptor antagonists as the treatment of choice for high-risk atherothrombotic patients. *Cerebrovascular Diseases*. 2002;**13**(suppl 1): 22–26.

Hankey GJ, et al. Thienopyridine derivatives (ticlopidine, clopidogrel) versus aspirin for preventing stroke and other serious vascular events in high vascular risk patients. *Cochrane Database of Systematic Reviews*. 2000;(2):CD001246.

Harker LA, Fuster V. Pharmacology of platelet inhibitors. *Journal of the American College of Cardiology*. 1986;**8**(6 suppl B):21B–32B.

HCUPnet, Healthcare Cost and Utilization Project. Agency for Healthcare Research and Quality, Rockville, MD. http://www.ahrq.gov/HCUPnet/ Accessed October 2004.

Heart Protection Study Collaborative Group. MRC/BHF Heart Protection Study of cholesterol lowering with simvastatin in 20,536 high risk individuals: a randomized placebo-controlled trial. *Lancet*. 2002;**360**:7–22.

Heidrich H, et al. Frequency of asymptomatic peripheral arterial disease in patients entering the department of general and internal medicine of a general care hospital. *Vasa*. 2004;**33**:63–67.

Henn V, et al. CD40 ligand on activated platelets triggers an inflammatory reaction of endothelial cells. *Nature*. 1998;**391**(6667):591–594.

Hennekens CH, et al. Additive benefits of pravastatin and aspirin to decrease risks of cardiovascular disease: randomized and observational comparisons of secondary prevention trials and their meta-analyses. *Archives of Internal Medicine*. 2004; **164**(1):40–44.

Hertzer NR, et al. Coronary artery disease in peripheral vascular patients; a classification of 1,000 coronary angiograms and results of surgical management. *Annals of Surgery*. 1984;**199**:223–233.

Hess H, et al. Drug-induced inhibition of platelet function delays progression of peripheral occlusive arterial disease. A prospective double-blind arteriographically controlled trial. *Lancet*. 1985(8426):415–419.

Hiatt WR, et al. Effect of exercise training on skeletal muscle histology and metabolism in peripheral arterial disease. *Journal of Applied Physiology*. 1996;**81**(2):780–788.

Hiatt WR, et al. Propionyl-L-carnitine improves exercise performance and functional status in patients with claudication. *American Journal of Medicine*. 2001;**110**(8):616–622. [a]

Hiatt WR. New treatment options in intermittent claudication: the U.S. experience. *International Journal of Clinical Practice Supplement*. 2001;**119**:20–27. [b]

Hiatt WR. Medical treatment of peripheral arterial disease and claudication. *New England Journal of Medicine*. 2001;**344**:1608–1621. [c]

Hiatt WR, et al. Benefit of NM-702, a phosphodiesterase inhibitor, in the treatment of claudication. Scientific Sessions of the American Heart Association; November 12, 2003. Abstract 2876.

Higgins JP, Higgins JA. Epidemiology of peripheral arterial disease in women. *Journal of Epidemiology*. 2003;**13**:1–14.

Hill JM, et al. Circulating endothelial progenitor cells, vascular function, and cardiovascular risk. *New England Journal of Medicine*. 2003;**348**(7):593–600.

Hirsh J, et al. Aspirin and other platelet-active drugs. The relationship among dose, effectiveness, and side effects. *Chest*. 1995;**108**(4 suppl):247S–257S.

Hirsch AT, et al. Peripheral arterial disease detection, awareness and treatment in primary care. *Journal of the American Medical Association*. 2001;**286**:1317–1324. [a]

Hirsch AT, et al. PAD awareness, risk, and treatment: new resources for survival—the USA PARTNERS program. *Vascular Medicine*. 2001;**6**(3 suppl):9–12. [b]

Hirsch AT, et al. Mandate for creation of a national peripheral arterial disease public awareness program: an opportunity to improve cardiovascular health. *Journal of Vascular Surgery*. 2004;**39**(2):474–481.

Hood SC. Management of intermittent claudication with pentoxifylline: meta-analysis of randomized controlled trials. *Canadian Medical Association Journal*. 1996;**155**: 1053–1059.

Hooi JD, et al. The prognosis of non-critical limb ischaemia: a systematic review of population-based evidence. *British Journal of General Practice*. 1999;**49**:49–55.

Hooi JD, et al. Asymptomatic peripheral arterial occlusive disease and erection problems. *British Journal of General Practice*. 2001;**51**:404. [a]

Hooi JD, et al. Incidence of and risk factors for asymptomatic peripheral arterial occlusive disease: a longitudinal study. *American Journal of Epidemiology*. 2001;**153**:666–672. [b]

Hooi JD, et al. Asymptomatic peripheral arterial occlusive disease predicted cardiovascular morbidity and mortality in a 7-year follow-up study. *Journal of Clinical Epidemiology*. 2004;**57**:294–300.

ICAI Study Group. Prostanoids for chronic critical leg ischemia. A randomized, controlled, open-label trial with prostaglandin E1. *Annals of Internal Medicine*. 1999;**130**(5): 412–421.

Ingolfsson IO, et al. A marked decline in the prevalence and incidence of intermittent claudication in Icelandic men 1968–1986: a strong relationship to smoking and serum cholesterol—the Reykjavik Study. *Journal of Clinical Epidemiology*. 1994;**47**(11): 1237–1243.

Ishimura IE, et al. Renal insufficiency accelerates atherosclerosis in patients with type 2 diabetes mellitus. *American Journal of Kidney Disease*. 2001;**38**:S186–S190.

Janzon L, et al. Prevention of myocardial infarction and stroke in patients with intermittent claudication; effects of ticlopidine. Results from STIMS, the Swedish Ticlopidine Multicentre Study. *Journal of Internal Medicine*. 1990;**227**(5):301–308.

Johnsen MC. Evaluation of Legs For Life National Screening and Awareness Program for Peripheral Vascular Disease: results of a follow-up survey of screening participants. *Journal of Vascular and Interventional Radiology*. 2002;**13**(1):25–35.

Jonason T, Bergstrom R. Cessation of smoking in patients with intermittent claudication. Effects on the risk of peripheral vascular complications, myocardial infarction and mortality. *Acta Medica Scandinavica*. 1987;**221**(3):253–260. Abstract.

June EB, et al. Peripheral arterial disease in diabetic and nondiabetic patients. A comparison of severity and outcome. *Diabetes Care*. 2001;**24**:1433–1437.

Kannel WB, et al. Intermittent claudication: incidence in the Framingham study. *Circulation*. 1970;**41**:875–883.

Kannel WB, McGee DL. Update on some epidemiologic features of intermittent claudication: the Framingham Study. *Journal of the American Geriatric Society*. 1985; **33**(1):13–18.

Kawarada O, et al. Carotid stenosis and peripheral artery disease in Japanese patients with coronary artery disease undergoing coronary artery bypass grafting. *Circulation Journal*. 2003;**67**:1003–1006.

Kieffer E, et al. A new study demonstrates the efficacy of naftidrofuryl in the treatment of intermittent claudication. Findings of the Naftidrofuryl Clinical Ischemia Study (NCIS). *International Angiology*. 2001;**20**(1):58–65.

Kitamura A, et al. Prevalence and correlates of carotid atherosclerosis among elderly Japanese men. *Atherosclerosis*. 2004;**172**:353–359.

Klevsgård R, et al. Quality of life associated with varying degrees of chronic lower limb ischaemia: comparison with a healthy sample. *European Journal of Vascular and Endovascular Surgery*. 1999;**17**:319–325.

Klevsgård R, et al. The effects of successful intervention on quality of life in patients with varying degrees of lower-limb ischaemia. *European Journal of Vascular and Endovascular Surgery*. 2000;**19**:238–245.

Kondo T, et al. Smoking cessation rapidly increases circulating progenitor cells in peripheral blood in chronic smokers. *Arteriosclerosis, Thrombosis, and Vascular Biology*. 2004;**24**(8):1442–1447.

Krupski WC. The peripheral vascular consequences of smoking. *Annals of Vascular Surgery*. 1991;**5**(3):291–304.

Kuan Y-M, et al. Homocysteine: an etiological contributor to peripheral vascular arterial disease. *Australian and New Zealand Journal of Surgery*. 2002;**72**(9):668.

Lacroix P, et al. Validation d'une traduction française du questionnaire d'Édimburg au sein d'une population de consultants en médicine générale. *Archives des Maladies du Coeur et des Vaisseaux*. 2002;**95**:596–600.

Lederman RJ, et al. Therapeutic angiogenesis with recombinant fibroblast growth factor-2 for intermittent claudication (the TRAFFIC study): a randomized trial. *Lancet*. 2002;**359**(9323):2053–2058.

Leng GC, et al. The Edinburgh Claudication Questionnaire: an improved version of the WHO/Rose Questionnaire for use in epidemiological surveys. *Journal of Clinical Epidemiology*. 1992;**45**:1101–1109.

Leng GC, et al. Accuracy and reproducibility of duplex ultrasonography in grading femoropopliteal stenosis. *Journal of Vascular Surgery*. 1993;**17**:510–517.

Leng GC, et al. Use of ankle brachial pressure index to predict cardiovascular events and death: a cohort study. *British Medical Journal*. 1996;**313**(7070):1440–1443.

Leng GC, et al. Exercise for intermittent claudication. *Cochrane Database of Systematic Reviews*. 2000;(2):CD000990.

Levy PJ. Premature lower extremity atherosclerosis: clinical aspects. *American Journal of Medical Sciences*. 2002;**323**:11–16.

Liao D, et al. Lower heart rate variability is associated with the development of coronary heart disease in individuals with diabetes: the Atherosclerosis Risk in Communities (ARIC) study. *Diabetes*. 2002;**51**(12):3524–3531.

Liao JK. Role of statin pleiotropism in acute coronary syndromes and stroke. *International Journal of Clinical Practice*. 2003;**134**:51–57.

Liévre M, et al. Oral beraprost sodium, a prostaglandin I(2) analogue, for intermittent claudication: a double-blind, randomized, multicenter controlled trial. Beraprost et Claudication Intermittente (BERCI) Research Group. *Circulation*. 2000;**102**(4):426–431.

Liu Y, et al. Cilostazol (Pletal): a dual inhibitor of cyclic nucleotide phosphodiesterase type 3 and adenosine uptake. *Cardiovascular Drug Review*. 2001;**19**(4):369–386.

Lonn EM, Yusuf S. Emerging approaches in the prevention of atherosclerotic cardiovascular diseases. *International Journal of Clinical Practice (Supplement)*. 1998;**94**:7–19.

Losordo DW, Dimmeler S. Therapeutic angiogenesis and vasculogenesis for ischemic disease: part I: angiogenic cytokines. *Circulation*. 2004;**109**(21):2487–2491.

Mallikaarjun S, et al. Interaction potential and tolerability of the coadministration of cilostazol and aspirin. *Clinical Pharmacokinesis*. 1999;**37**(suppl 2):87–93.

Marchand G. Épidémiologie et facteurs de risqué de l'artériopathie oblitérante des membres inférieurs. *Annales de Cardiologie et d'Angeiologie (Paris)*. 2001;**50**:119–127.

Matsuno H, et al. Pharmacokinetic and pharmacodynamic properties of a new thromboxane receptor antagonist (Z-335) after single and multiple oral administrations to healthy volunteers. *Journal of Clinical Pharmacology*. 2002;**42**(7):782–790.

McDermott MM, et al. Exertional leg symptoms other than intermittent claudication are common in peripheral arterial disease. *Archives of Internal Medicine*. 1999;**159**:387–392. [a]

McDermott MM. Ankle brachial index as a predictor of outcomes in peripheral arterial disease. *Journal of Laboratory Clinical Medicine*. 1999;**133**:33–40. [b]

McDermott MM, et al. Leg symptoms in peripheral arterial disease: associated clinical characteristics and functional impairment. *Journal of the American Medical Association*. 2001;**286**(13):1599–1606.

McDermott MM, et al. The ankle brachial index is associated with leg function and physical activity: The Walking and Leg Circulation study. *Annals of Internal Medicine*. 2002;**136**:873–883.

McDermott MM, et al. Relation of levels of hemostatic factors and inflammatory markers to the ankle brachial index. *American Journal of Cardiology*. 2003;**92**(2):194–199. [a]

McDermott MM, et al. Statin use and leg functioning in patients with and without lower-extremity peripheral arterial disease. *Circulation*. 2003;**107**(5):757–761. [b]

McGrath C, et al. A randomised, double-blind, placebo-controlled study to determine the efficacy of immune modulation therapy in the treatment of patients suffering from peripheral arterial occlusive disease with intermittent claudication. *European Journal of Vascular and Endovascular Surgery*. 2002;**23**:381–387.

Meijer WT, et al. Peripheral arterial disease in the elderly: the Rotterdam Study. *Arteriosclerosis, Thrombosis, and Vascular Biology*. 1998;**18**:185–192.

Mehler PS, et al. Intensive blood pressure control reduces the risk of cardiovascular events in patients with peripheral arterial disease and type 2 diabetes. *Circulation*. 2003;**107**(5):753–756.

Menotti A, et al. Coronary heart disease incidence in northern and southern European populations: a reanalysis of the seven countries study for a European coronary risk chart. *Heart*. 2000;**84**:238–244.

Mizuno A, et al. Synthesis and serotonin 2 (5-HT2) receptor antagonist activity of 5-aminoalkyl-substituted pyrrolo[3,2-*c*]azepines and related compounds. *Chemical and Pharmaceutical Bulletin*. 2000;**48**(5) 623–635.

Mohler ER. Peripheral arterial disease. Identification and implications. *Archives of Internal Medicine*. 2003;**163**:2306–2314. [a]

Mohler ER, et al. Cholesterol reduction with atorvastatin improves walking distance in patients with peripheral arterial disease. *Circulation*. 2003;**108**(12):1481–1486. [b]

Mondillo S, et al. Effects of simvastatin on walking performance and symptoms of intermittent claudication in hypercholesterolemic patients with peripheral vascular disease. *American Journal of Medicine*. 2003;**114**(5):359–364.

Morishita R, et al. Safety evaluation of clinical gene therapy using hepatocyte growth factor to treat peripheral arterial disease. *Hypertension*. 2004;**44**(2):203–209.

Müller I, et al. Effects of statins on platelet inhibition by a high loading dose of clopidogrel. *Circulation*. 2003;**108**(18):2195–2197.

Murabito JM, et al. Prevalence and clinical correlates of peripheral arterial disease in the Framingham Offspring Study. *American Heart Journal*. 2002;**143**:961–965.

Murabito JM, et al. The ankle-brachial index in the elderly and risk of stroke, coronary disease and death. The Framingham Study. *Archives of Internal Medicine*. 2003;**163**: 1939–1942.

Namba T, et al. Angiogenesis induced by endothelial nitric oxide synthase gene through vascular endothelial growth factor expression in a rat hindlimb ischemia model. *Circulation*. 2003;**108**(18):2250–2257.

Nair N, et al. Proteomic profiling of PAD—towards a new diagnostic modality. Society for Vascular Medicine and Biology 15th Annual Scientific Sessions; June 4–5, 2004; Anaheim, CA.

Ness J, et al. Risk factors for symptomatic peripheral arterial disease in older persons in an academic hospital based geriatrics practice. *Journal of the American Geriatrics Society*. 2000;**48**:312–314.

Newman AB, et al. Ankle-arm index as a marker of atherosclerosis in the Cardiovascular Health Study. *Circulation*. 1993;**88**:837–845.

Newman AB, et al. Ankle-arm index as a predictor of cardiovascular disease and mortality in the Cardiovascular Health Study. *Arteriosclerosis, Thrombosis, and Vascular Biology*. 1999;**19**:538–545.

Newman AB. Peripheral arterial disease: insights from population studies of older adults. *Journal of the American Geriatrics Society*. 2000;**48**:1157–1162.

Novo S, et al. Prevalence of risk factors in patients with peripheral arterial disease. A clinical and epidemiological evaluation. *International Angiology*. 1992;**11**(3):218–229.

O'Hare AM. High prevalence of peripheral arterial disease in persons with renal insufficiency. Results from the National Health and Nutrition Examination Survey 1999–2000. *Circulation*. 2004;**109**; 320–323.

Ogren M, et al. Low ankle-brachial pressure index in 68-year-old men: prevalence, risk factors and prognosis. *European Journal of Vascular and Endovascular Surgery*. 1993: **7**:500–506.

Oral Iloprost in Severe Leg Ischaemia Study Group. Two randomised and placebo-controlled studies of an oral prostacyclin analogue (Iloprost) in severe leg ischaemia. *European Journal of Vascular and Endovascular Surgery*. 2000;**20**(4):358–362.

Östergren J, et al. Impact of ramipril in patients with evidence of clinical or subclinical peripheral arterial disease. *European Heart Journal*. 2004;**25**(1):17–24.

Ouriel K. Peripheral arterial disease. *Lancet*. 2001;**358**:1257–1264.

Padua RR, et al. Basic fibroblast growth factor is cardioprotective in ischemia-reperfusion injury. *Molecular and Cellular Biochemistry*. 1995;**143**(2):129–135.

Pasternak RC. ACC/AHA/NHLBI clinical advisory on the use and safety of statins. *Journal of American College of Cardiology*. 2002;**40**(3):567–572.

Patrono C, et al. Platelet-active drugs: the relationships among dose, effectiveness, and side effects. *Chest*. 2001;**119**(suppl 1):39S–63S.

Patrono C, et al. Expert consensus document on the use of antiplatelet agents. The task force on the use of antiplatelet agents in patients with atherosclerotic cardiovascular disease of the European Society of Cardiology. *European Heart Journal*. 2004;**25**(2):166–181.

Pedersen TR, et al. Effect of simvastatin on ischemic signs and symptoms in the Scandinavian Simvastatin Survival Study (4S). *American Journal of Cardiology*. 1998;**81**(3): 333–335.

Pedersen TR. Pro and con: low-density lipoprotein cholesterol lowering is and will be the key to the future of lipid management. *American Journal of Cardiology*. 2001; **87**(5 suppl 1):8–12.

Pentecost MJ, et al. Guidelines for peripheral percutaneous transluminal angioplasty of the abdominal aorta and lower extremity vessels. *Circulation*. 1994;**89**(1):511–531.

Pereira EC, et al. Effects of simvastatin and L-arginine on vasodilation, nitric oxide metabolites and endogenous NOS inhibitors in hypercholestrolemic subjects. *Free Radical Research*. 2003;**37**:529–536.

Physicians' Desk Reference. 56th Edition, 2002. Thomson Healthcare.

Pitt B, et al. The QUinapril Ischemic Event Trial (QUIET): evaluation of chronic ACE inhibitor therapy in patients with ischemic heart disease and preserved left ventricular function. *American Journal of Cardiology*. 2001;**87**(9):1058–1063.

Population Division of the Department of Economic and Social Affairs of the United Nations Secretariat. *World Population Prospects: The 2002 Revision*, Vol. II, *The Sex and Age Distribution of Populations* (United Nations publication, Sales No. E.03.XIII.7), 2003.

Pradhan AD, et al. Soluble intercellular adhesion molecule-1, soluble vascular adhesion molecule-1, and the development of symptomatic peripheral arterial disease in men. *Circulation*. 2002;**106**(7):820–825.

Pratt C. Analysis of the cilostazol safety database. *American Journal of Cardiology*. 2001;**87**:28D–33D.

Rajagopalan S, et al. A Phase I study of intramuscular administration of CI-1023 (ADGVVEGF121.10) in patients with peripheral vascular disease. *Circulation*. 2001;**104**:A262.

Rajagopalan S, et al. Regional angiogenesis with vascular endothelial growth factor in peripheral arterial disease: a phase II randomized, double-blind, controlled study of adenoviral delivery of vascular endothelial growth factor 121 in patients with disabling intermittent claudication. *Circulation*. 2003;**108**(16):1933–1938.

Rajagopalan S, et al. A Phase II multicenter, randomized, double-blind, placebo-controlled trial of plasmid Del-1 (Developmentally regulated Endothelial Locus 1) in subjects with intermittent claudication secondary to peripheral arterial disease: DELTA1-PAD. Scientific Sessions of the American Heart Association; November 8, 2004. Abstract 2439.

Rashid M, et al. AT-1015, a newly synthesized 5-HT2 receptor antagonist, dissociates slowly from the 5-HT2 receptor sites in rabbit cerebral cortex membrane. *Journal of Pharmacy and Pharmacology*. 2002;**54**(8):1123–1128.

Reaven GM. Banting lecture: role of insulin resistance in human disease. *Diabetes*. 1988;**37**:1595–1607.

Reunanen A, et al. Prevalence of intermittent claudication and its effect on mortality. *Acta Medica Scandinavica*. 1982;**211**:249–256.

Rezaie-Majid A, et al. Simvastatin reduces the expression of adhesion molecules in circulating monocytes from hypercholestrolemic patients. *Arteriosclerosis, Thrombosis and Vascular Biology*. 2003;**23**:397–403.

Ridker PM, et al. Plasma concentration of C-reactive protein and risk of developing peripheral vascular disease. *Circulation*. 1998;**97**(5):425–8.

Roller RE, et al. Oxidative stress and increase of vascular endothelial growth factor in plasma of patients with peripheral arterial occlusive disease. *Thrombosis and Haemostasis*. 2001;**85**(2):368.

Samuelsson B, et al. Prostaglandins. *Annual Review of Biochemistry*. 1975;**44**:669–695.

Savader SJ, et al. The Legs For Life Screening for Peripheral Vascular Disease: results of a prospective study designed to improve patient compliance with physician recommendations. *Journal of Vascular and Interventional Radiology*. 2001;**12**(10):1149–1155.

Scheffler P, et al. Intensive vascular training in stage IIb of peripheral arterial occlusive disease. The additive effects of intravenous prostaglandin E1 or intravenous pentoxifylline during training. *Circulation*. 1994;**90**(2):818–822.

Schmieder F, et al. Intermittent claudication: magnitude of the problem, patient evaluation, and therapeutic strategies. *American Journal of Cardiology*. 2001;**87**:3D–13D.

Schofield RS, et al. The use of ranolazine in cardiovascular disease. *Expert Opinion on Investigational Drugs*. 2002;**11**(1):117–123.

Schonbeck U, Libby P. CD40 signalling and plaque instability. *Circulation Research*. 2001;**89**(12):1092–1103.

Schuler JJ, et al. Efficacy of prostaglandin E1 in the treatment of lower-extremity ischemic ulcers secondary to peripheral vascular occlusive disease. Results of a prospective randomized, double-blind, multicenter clinical trial. *Journal of Vascular Surgery*. 1984;**1**(1):160–170.

Scott-Okafor HR, et al. Lower extremity strength deficits in peripheral arterial occlusive disease patients with intermittent claudication. *Angiology*. 2001;**52**:7–14.

Second European Consensus Document on Chronic Leg Ischemia. *European Journal of Vascular Surgery*. 1992;**6**(suppl A):1–32.

Selvin E, Erlinger T. Prevalence of and risk factors for peripheral arterial disease in the United States. Results from the National Health and Nutrition Examination Survey, 1999–2000. *Circulation*. 2004;**110**:738–743.

Sharrett AR, et al. Smoking and diabetes differ in their associations with subclinical atherosclerosis and coronary heart disease - the ARIC study. *Atherosclerosis*. 2004;**172**:143–149.

Smith GD. Intermittent claudication, heart disease risk factors, and mortality. The Whitehall Study. *Circulation*. 1990;**82**:1925–1931.

Smith I, et al. The influence of smoking cessation and hypertriglyceridaemia on the progression of peripheral arterial disease and the onset of critical ischaemia. *European Journal of Vascular and Endovascular Surgery*. 1996;**11**(4):402–408.

Sowers JR. Hypertension, angiotensin II and oxidative stress. *New England Journal of Medicine*. 2002;**346**(25):1999–2001.

Spengel F, et al. Findings of the naftidrofuryl in quality of life (NIQOL) European study program. *International Angiology*. 2002;**21**(1):20–27.

Staben P, Albring M. Treatment of patients with peripheral arterial occlusive disease Fontaine stage III and IV with intravenous iloprost: an open study in 900 patients. *Prostaglandins, Leukotrienes, and Essential Fatty Acids*. 1996;**54**(5):327–333.

Stoffers HE, et al. The prevalence of asymptomatic and unrecognized peripheral arterial occlusive disease. *International Journal of Epidemiology*. 1996;**25**:282–290.

Takano M, et al. Changes in coronary plaque color and morphology by lipid-lowering therapy with atorvastatin:serial evaluation by coronary angioscopy. *Journal of the American College of Cardiology*. 2003;**42**:687–689.

Tanaka T, et al. A new thromboxane receptor antagonist, Z-335, ameliorates experimental thrombosis without prolonging the rat tail bleeding time. *Thrombosis Research*. 1998;**91**(5):229–235.

Tanaka T, et al. Z-335, a new thromboxane A(2) receptor antagonist, prevents arterial thrombosis induced by ferric chloride in rats. *European Journal of Pharmacology*. 2000;**401**(3):413–418.

The Global Lower Extremity Amputation Study Group. Epidemiology of lower extremity amputation in centres in Europe, North America and East Asia. *British Journal of Surgery*. 2000;**87**:328–337.

Thomas SR, et al. Oxidative stress and endothelial nitric oxide bioactivity. *Antioxidants & Redox Signaling*. 2003;**5**(2):181–194.

Thompson PD, et al. Meta-analysis of results from eight randomized, placebo-controlled trials on the effect of cilostazol on patients with intermittent claudication. *American Journal of Cardiology*. 2002;**90**(12):1314–1319.

Toyota T, et al. Effects of beraprost sodium (Dorner) in patients with diabetes mellitus complicated by chronic arterial obstruction. *Angiology*. 2002;**53**(1):7–13.

Tunstall-Pedoe H, et al. Contribution of trends in survival and coronary event rates to changes in coronary heart disease mortality: 10-year results from 37 WHO MONICA Project populations. *Lancet*. 1999;**353**:1547–1557.

Ueshima H, et al. Differences in cardiovascular disease risk factors between Japanese in Japan and Japanese-Americans in Hawaii: the INTERLIPID study. *Journal of Human Hypertension*. 2003;**17**:631–639.

Verhaeghe R. Epidemiology and prognosis of peripheral obliterative arteriopathy. *Drugs*. 1998;**56**(suppl 3):1–10.

Vogt MT, et al. Prevalence and correlates of lower-extremity arterial disease in elderly women. *American Journal of Epidemiology*. 1993;**137**:559–68. [a]

Vogt MT, et al. Decreased ankle/arm blood pressure index and mortality in elderly women. *Journal of the American Medical Association*. 1993;**270**:465–469. [b]

Wassmann S, et al. Effect of atorvastatin 80 mg on endothelial cell function (forearm blood flow) in patients with pretreatment serum low-density lipoprotein cholesterol levels <130 mg/dL. *American Journal of Cardiology*. 2004: **93**; 84–88.

Watanabe H, et al. Westernization of lifestyle markedly increases carotid intima-media wall thickness (IMT) in Japanese people. *Atherosclerosis*. 2003;**166**:67–72.

Weitz JI, et al. American Heart Association Scientific Statement: diagnosis and treatment of chronic arterial insufficiency of the lower extremities: a critical review. *Circulation*. 1996;**94**:3026–3049.

Wienbergen H, et al. Comparison of clinical benefits of clopidogrel therapy in patients with acute coronary syndromes taking atorvastatin versus other statin therapies. *American Journal of Cardiology*. 2003;**92**(3):285–288.

Weiner SD, et al. Peripheral arterial disease. Medical management in primary care practice. *Geriatrics*. 2001;**56**:20–22, 25–26, 29–30.

Wilhite DB, et al. Managing PAD with multiple platelet inhibitors: the effect of combination therapy on bleeding time. *Journal of Vascular Surgery*. 2003;**38**(4):710–713.

Yusuf S, et al. Effects of clopidogrel in addition to aspirin in patients with acute coronary syndromes without ST-segment elevation. *The New England Journal of Medicine*. 2001;**345**:494–502.

Zheng ZJ, et al. Associations of ankle-brachial index with clinical coronary heart disease, stroke and preclinical carotid and popliteal atherosclerosis: the Atherosclerosis Risk in Communities (ARIC) Study. *Atherosclerosis*. 1997;**131**:115–125.

Post-Myocardial Infarction

ETIOLOGY AND PATHOPHYSIOLOGY

Introduction

Post-myocardial infarction (PMI) is defined as the state that exists after a patient has survived at least 48 hours after damage to the myocardium resulting from an acute myocardial infarction (AMI). PMI is recognized as a significant contributor to morbidity and mortality for patients who have survived a prior acute event. Analysis indicates that within six years of a recognized myocardial infarction (MI), 18% of men and 35% of women will have a subsequent MI; 7% of men and 6% of women will experience sudden death (American Heart Association, 2002). An initial attack invariably damages the heart, leaving it susceptible to future infarction, heart failure, and dysfunction. Hence, pharmacotherapy and cardiac rehabilitation are essential to reduce the patient's risk of a recurrent MI and improve the efficiency of the damaged heart.

Pathophysiology

To fully understand the PMI disease state, it is essential to understand the under-lying disease process leading to AMI. Coronary artery disease (CAD)—athero-sclerosis of the coronary arteries—underlies most AMIs. The development of atherosclerotic lesions and their subsequent rupture initiates the formation of a

Wiley Handbook of Current and Emerging Drug Therapies, Volumes 5–8
Copyright © 2007 Decision Resources, Inc. Published by John Wiley & Sons, Inc.

thrombus that can eventually occlude the vessel. If the vessel is a coronary artery (one of the major vessels feeding the heart), the heart is endangered. The blockage causes ischemia, in which a lack of oxygen caused by decreased blood flow can lead to tissue death and thus AMI.

Atherosclerotic Lesions. Atherosclerosis results from the formation of atherosclerotic lesions, which advance through three main stages:

- Initiation of the atherosclerotic lesion.
- Lesion growth and progressive occlusion of the vessel lumen.
- Rupture of the atherosclerotic lesion and the formation of an occlusive thrombus, which leads to ischemia and MI.

Atherosclerotic lesions are made up of three main components: lipids, cells such as macrophages and lymphocytes, and extracellular matrix (ECM) components. Figure 1 depicts the sequence of atherosclerotic plaque formation.

Initiation of the Atherosclerotic Lesion. The early atherosclerotic lesion, often referred to as a primary lesion or "fatty streak," can develop as early as the first decade of life. This lesion does not necessarily develop into an atherosclerotic plaque—in fact, it can regress as well as grow. Primary lesions appear as accumulations of lipid-engorged macrophages (sometimes called "foam cells" because of their appearance under the microscope) just below the surface of the artery wall.

Alterations in the properties of the endothelium (the layer of endothelial cells that line the vessel wall) are fundamental to the initiation of the lesion. Both physical stresses such as turbulent blood flow and chemical stresses such as circulating

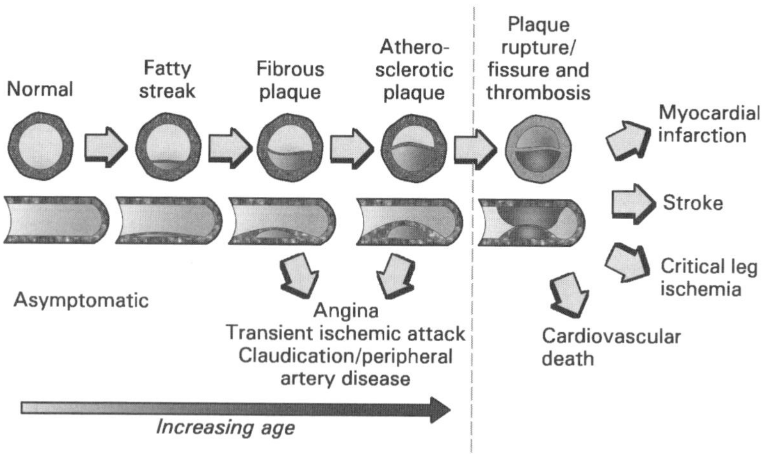

FIGURE 1. *Formation of atherosclerotic plaque.*

modified low-density lipoprotein (LDL) (see "The Role of Lipoproteins"), toxins from cigarette smoke, and bacterial or viral pathogens can cause these alterations (Ross R, 1999; Folsom AR, 2001). In response, endothelial cells promote a pro-inflammatory response, including the upregulation of adhesion molecules that encourage the attachment of circulating inflammatory cells such as lymphocytes and monocytes. Concurrently, the endothelial layer becomes more permeable to large molecules such as LDL that can penetrate the artery wall.

Lesion Growth and Progressive Occlusion of the Vessel Lumen. After the monocytes and lymphocytes have attached to the endothelium, they migrate into the artery wall. The monocytes differentiate into macrophages, proliferate, and take up modified LDL. This action stimulates the macrophages to secrete factors that encourage the migration into the lesion of a third type of cell, the vascular smooth-muscle cell (VSMC). These cells have mainly contractile properties, but they also produce and secrete components of the ECM such as collagen and fibronectin.

The atherosclerotic lesion continues to grow in size because of the influx of cells and the increase in ECM and lipid. The lesion projects into the lumen of the vessel, increasing both occlusion of the vessel and turbulent blood flow within it. As the plaque ages, it can undergo angiogenesis (new blood vessel growth). In some cases, hemorrhages into the lesion lead to the formation of small clots (thrombi) that become incorporated into the lesion, contributing to its overall growth.

The lipid pool within the lesion also grows as the lipid-containing macrophages die and release their intracellular lipid stores into the core of the lesion. Ultimately, the center of the plaque becomes necrotic and calcified. Atherosclerotic plaques with a central lipid pool and an overlying fibrous layer of ECM are referred to as fibrous lesions, which have very different clinical outcomes depending on whether they are stable or unstable.

Rupture of the Atherosclerotic Lesion and Formation of an Occlusive Thrombus. Some plaques are more prone to rupture than others, depending on the size of the lipid core and the integrity of the fibrous cap that overlies it. Foremost among several factors involved in the shift from a stable to an unstable atherosclerotic plaque is the integrity of this overlying fibrous cap.

Macrophages within the plaque produce enzymes called matrix metalloproteinases (MMPs), which can degrade the ECM laid down by the VSMCs. The macrophages predominate at the shoulder regions of the plaque, and, consequently, these areas are richest in these degradatory MMPs. The shoulder regions also bear most of the physical stress caused by blood flow within the artery; this stress is often exacerbated where atherosclerotic lesions that project into the vessel lumen result in more turbulent blood flow. As the ECM in these shoulder regions is degraded, the fibrous cap is subject to increased physical pressure and becomes prone to rupture.

Within the plaque are several procoagulant factors that can stimulate the formation of blood clots. When a plaque ruptures, a small tear appears in the fibrous cap, exposing a procoagulant surface that initiates the clotting process. If the exposed area is initially limited, the clot that forms in response will likely also be limited and may not lead to an acute event. If the plaque ruptures more extensively, a much larger area is exposed and the thrombus that forms on top may completely block the vessel. If this happens in a coronary artery, the outcome is an MI.

The Role of Lipoproteins. The key role of lipoproteins in CAD is illustrated by the findings of myriad studies, all of which indicate that modifying serum lipoprotein levels decreases the risk of adverse cardiac events such as AMI.

Approximately 70% of blood lipoprotein exists as LDL. The amount of LDL that accumulates in the lesion correlates positively with levels of circulating LDL. Once inside the artery wall, LDL undergoes oxidation to form oxidized LDL (ox:LDL). Ox:LDL has pro-inflammatory activity, stimulating endothelial cells to recruit other inflammatory cells into the lesion, thereby contributing to the lesion's overall growth and progression. Macrophages take up ox:LDL via the "scavenger receptor" on the cell surface and encourage VSMC migration into the lesion.

High-density lipoprotein (HDL) plays a different yet equally important role in modifying the atherosclerotic process. This lipoprotein is often termed "good cholesterol": the lower the LDL:HDL ratio, the lower the risk of heart disease. HDL retards LDL oxidation and can remove cholesterol from atherosclerotic plaques through the reverse cholesterol transport process (Asztalos BF, 2003; Brewer HB, 2003). In this process, plasma HDL takes up cholesterol from tissues, such as fibroblasts and macrophages. Cholesterol is subsequently esterified to form cholesteryl ester by lecithin-cholesterol acyltransferase (LCAT), resulting in the production of mature, spherical HDL. Cholesterol is also taken up from triglyceride-rich lipoproteins in a process mediated by cholesteryl ester transfer protein (CETP).

Cholesterol is returned to the liver by several routes. First, cholesteryl esters may be transferred from HDL to LDL or intermediate-density lipoprotein (IDL) by CETP. These lipoproteins undergo metabolism and subsequent uptake by the liver. Another route involves HDL particles or free cholesterol being taken up directly by the liver.

The Role of Platelets. Platelets are the first component of the blood to adhere when a thrombogenic (clot-promoting) surface is exposed. Platelets progress through a three-step process of adherence, activation, and aggregation. Adherence to the vessel wall occurs in the wake of endothelial cell damage or plaque rupture and is dependent on von Willebrand Factor (vWF), which is released from the endothelial cells upon activation. vWF facilitates the adherence of the platelets to the vessel wall at sites of high shear stress where blood flows through the damaged passageway. The released vWF attaches to the subendothelial collagen and then binds to a receptor on the platelet membrane, thus anchoring the platelet to the subendothelium (Ruggeri ZM, 2003).

Once attached, the platelets become activated and release adenosine diphosphate (ADP), which recruits other platelets to the same site and causes them to stick together, forming a platelet-platelet aggregate. ADP is also released by erythrocytes (red blood cells) and endothelial cells, contributing to ongoing activation and aggregation of platelets, as shown in Figure 2. Further platelet activation involves changes in the platelet plasma membrane that result in the release of additional platelet agonists and an increase in the aggregation and coagulation factors necessary to generate the platelet- and fibrin-rich thrombus, also known as the primary hemostatic plug.

Like ADP, thromboxane A_2 (TXA_2) is released from activated platelets; its function, too, is to activate other platelets, thereby prompting those platelets to adhere to the existing aggregation of platelets. Figure 3 shows how the arachidonic acid cascade produces TXA_2 within a platelet. The process begins in activated platelets when membrane-bound phospholipids are broken down by the enzyme phospholipase A_2 to form free arachidonic acid. The enzyme cyclooxygenase (COX) further metabolizes the arachidonic acid to form the intermediate prostaglandin G_2 (PGG_2). Another enzyme, thromboxane synthetase, converts PGG_2 into the vasoactive TXA_2—the substance that, upon release, promotes platelet aggregation and hence thrombus formation. The normal physiological role of this process is to stem bleeding in the event of injury, but within the vasculature, the thrombus can occlude the vessel, giving rise to ischemia and, ultimately, infarction.

Perhaps the most critical component of thrombogenesis is the glycoprotein IIb/IIIa (gpIIb/IIIa) receptor. In platelet aggregation, fibrinogen attaches to

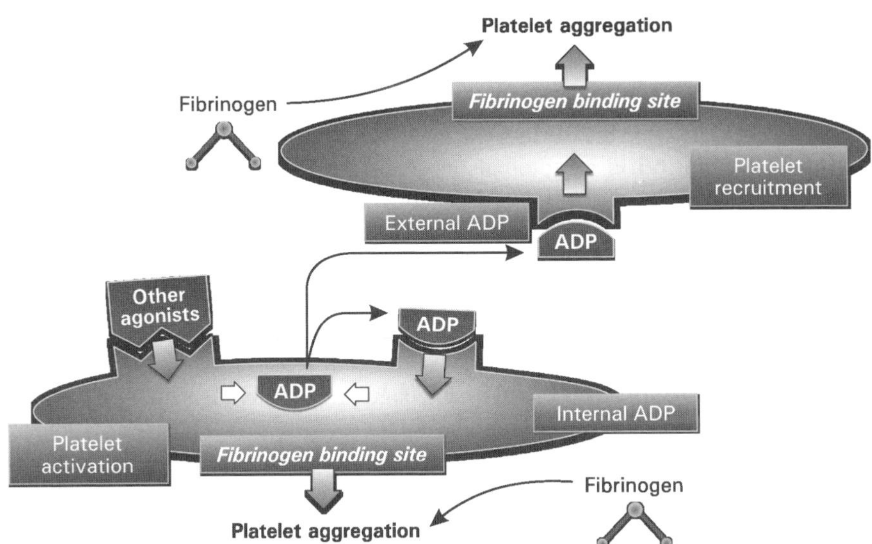

FIGURE 2. *Platelet activation and aggregation mechanisms.*

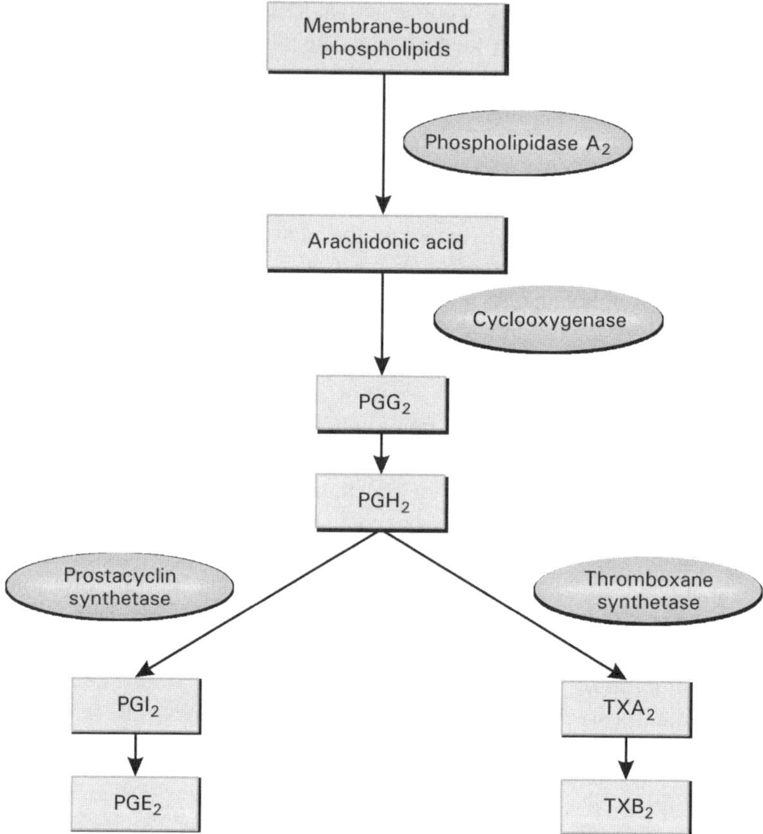

FIGURE 3. *Formation of thromboxane and prostaglandins from arachidonic acid.*

gpIIb/IIIa receptors on the surface of each neighboring platelet. Upon platelet activation, the gpIIb/IIIa receptor also becomes activated, and more gpIIb/IIIa receptors are mobilized from internal stores to the surface. These receptors then bind additional vWF as well as fibrinogen, which leads to more platelet binding—and so the process of platelet aggregation within the vessel escalates. This platelet activation process presents novel opportunities for therapeutic intervention (see "Emerging Therapies").

The Role of Coagulation. The human coagulation system is usually described as a cascade of reactions in which the factor activated in one step catalyzes activation of the factor in the following step and ultimately results in the formation of an insoluble clot to stem the loss of blood in response to injury. The coagulation cascade is shown in Figure 4.

The same cascade is responsible for clot formation in an atherosclerotic setting. Some patients show enhanced coagulation activity after AMI, and thrombi can

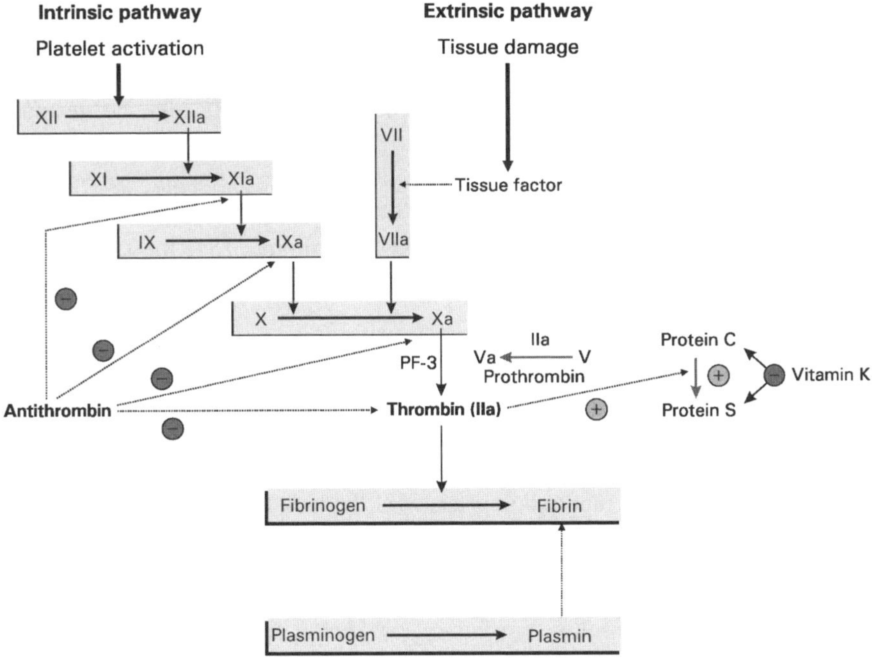

FIGURE 4. *Major reactions of the coagulation cascade.*

persist at the site of the lesion, with coagulation activity increased for months after the initial event. The coagulation cascade is divided into two pathways: (1) the intrinsic, in which all relevant components are found within the blood, and (2) the extrinsic, in which some components are found outside the blood within the vessel wall and damaged tissues. Both pathways ultimately converge at the point where prothrombin is converted to thrombin. Thrombin, in turn, converts soluble fibrinogen into insoluble fibrin strands, which are incorporated into the clot structure. Methods of inhibiting thrombin have been investigated, mainly with the aim of preventing the formation of new clots after AMI and thereby reducing the risk of subsequent infarction.

Etiology

The total recovery time following an AMI is approximately six months, depending on the severity of the infarction. In the days and months following an AMI, the heart undergoes several changes as the healing process begins and the heart adapts to the damage that has occurred. The myocardium around the ischemic area thins as the infarcted tissue dies off; because of this thinning, patients can be more prone to heart rupture. Within three months of the AMI, the ischemic area is replaced by scar tissue beneath which the endocardium has thickened. That area of the heart consequently loses some or all of its ability to function, to the detriment of its overall performance. Determinants of whether a patient is likely to suffer another AMI include the following:

- The extent and severity of the ischemic area perfusing the residual myocardium, as already described.
- Left ventricular (LV) function. As discussed in the following sections, this factor may be the most critical of the three.
- The susceptibility of a patient to serious arrhythmias. (See the later section "Arrhythmias and Sudden Cardiac Death.")

The balance of these factors primarily predicts the extent of symptoms and short- and long-term survival following an MI.

Left Ventricular Remodeling and Dysfunction. Perhaps the most critical risk to the heart, during and after an infarction, arises from the loss of myocytes (muscle cells). In an attempt to compensate for the loss, the left ventricle changes in size and shape, a process known as ventricular remodeling (VR), which can ultimately lead to LV dysfunction. Up to 40% of all MIs are associated with LV dysfunction (Kober L, 1998).

Immediately following myocyte injury, the infarct area expands as the inter-myocyte scaffolding structure that holds the cells together degrades. The result is ventricular dilation, wall thinning, and increased wall stresses. Concurrently, these changes stimulate intracellular signaling of the renin-angiotensin-aldosterone system (RAAS) and the sympathetic nervous system. Alterations in ventricular architecture follow, as the ECM forms a collagen scar. Ventricular remodeling can continue for several months until the distending forces are offset by the holding strength of the collagen scar.

Researchers believe that VR is an adaptive response to the initial AMI in which the heart attempts to pump the same amount of blood with each beat even though the damage from the AMI has reduced its contractility. Current therapies such as revascularization techniques are decreasing the amount of VR in PMI patients, but VR still poses a serious problem for some PMI sufferers.

Prognostic Significance of Left Ventricular Ejection Fraction. As LV volume enlarges due to VR there is a concomitant fall in the left ventricular ejection fraction (LVEF) (the ratio of the volume of blood remaining in the left ventricle at the end of ventricular contraction to the total volume of the ventricle when filled). Hence, LVEF is a marker of the remodeling process and has been shown to be a strong predictor of clinical outcomes (White HD, 1987).

Mortality varies dramatically depending on the LVEF. The normal LVEF range is 56–78%. Where LVEF exceeds 50%, the mortality rate is 3%; in those patients whose LVEF is reduced to less than 30% (as is the case for approximately 25% of PMI patients), the mortality rate exceeds 40%. An LVEF of less than 30% is particularly likely to result from serious AMIs, such as ST-segment-elevation myocardial infarction (STEMI). Experts recommend that patients with an LVEF value of less than 15% should not be considered for trials because they tend to die from the failure of the heart to pump blood sufficiently.

Influential Factors in Ventricular Remodeling

Infarct Size. In patients with VR, the extent of remodeling is related to infarct size (the area of necrosis caused by the ischemic damage). The Survival and Ventricular Enlargement (SAVE) trial showed that infarct size at two weeks is a strong predictor of subsequent remodeling (Connors KF, 1995; Pfeffer MA, 1992; St. John Sutton M, 1997). In an estimated 25–33% of AMI survivors, VR develops into congestive heart failure (CHF), but only recently have some of the processes involved been elucidated. VR can also result in poor relaxation of the ventricle during diastole (the relaxation portion of the heartbeat), an effect that can lead to postinfarction heart failure.

Renin-Angiotensin-Aldosterone System. Angiotensin-converting enzyme (ACE) is a ubiquitous enzyme found in particularly high concentrations in the blood vessels. ACE is responsible for the formation of the potent vasoconstrictor angiotensin II (AII), which is associated with remodeling of the heart after AMI. For this reason, ACE inhibitors are effective at reducing VR in PMI patients. Another important function of ACE is in the breakdown of the potent vasodilator bradykinin (Figure 5), which researchers suggest is cardioprotective. Thus, inhibiting ACE has a twofold effect: It reduces ACE-associated cardiac remodeling and increases the levels of the endogenous vasodilator bradykinin, thereby creating a cardioprotective effect.

The ACE gene is polymorphic, which means it commonly exists in more than one form. Two forms, or alleles, of the ACE gene are known to exist. An insertion of 287 nucleotide base pairs is present in one but absent in the other. Where the insertion is present, the allele is termed I; without the insertion, it is termed D. Each person has two ACE alleles, so three combinations, or genotypes, are possible: ACE-II, ACE-DD, or ACE-ID. Those with the ACE-DD genotype have twice the amount of ACE than those with ACE-II. In a survey of 610 individuals, the ACE-DD genotype were 34% more likely to have had an MI than were those with ACE-ID or ACE-II. The ACE-DD genotype is also more common in patients undergoing heart transplantation for ischemic heart failure (Ghidh-Jain M, 1998).

However, a much larger population study of 4629 MI patients and 5934 healthy controls did not confirm a strong association between the ACE-DD genotype and an increased risk of MI, and did not find genotype predictive of survival. However, the researchers could not rule out a small (10–15%) increase in the risk of MI with the ACE-DD genotype (Keavney B, 2000).

AII acts on two major receptor subtypes: AT1 and AT2. Most of the potent cardiovascular effects of AII are mediated through the AT1 receptor, which has also been isolated in the kidney, brain, and adrenal glands.

One proposed mechanism for VR is that stretching of the cell membrane in response to a change in the degree of stretch of the cardiac muscle cells before

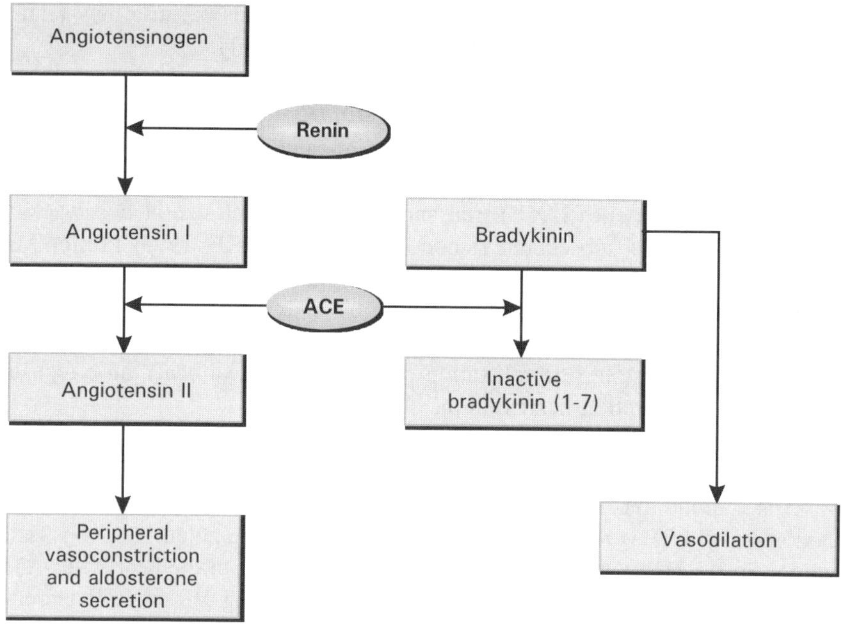

FIGURE 5. *Mechanism of action of angiotensin-converting enzyme.*

contraction seen in the PMI heart causes the release of AII from the myocytes. This AII then binds to AII receptors, most notably the AT1 receptor subgroup. Researchers surmise that this process ultimately results in activation of transcription factors and stimulation of further protein synthesis, which contributes to cardiac hypertrophy. Excess proliferation (hyperplasia) of VSMCs is also stimulated by AII and could well contribute to occlusion of the blood vessels, leading to further ischemia. This mechanism of action would explain why ACE inhibitors are effective in reducing VR in PMI patients, given that ACE is required for the formation of AII from its precursor angiotensin I (AI).

Sympathetic Nervous System. After an acute myocardial event, the sympathetic nervous system (SNS) is stimulated as a compensatory measure in response to reduced cardiac output (CO). SNS stimulation activates the RAAS system and promotes further VR and life-threatening arrhythmias. (See the "Arrhythmias and Sudden Cardiac Death" section for more on arrhythmias.) The SNS has other deleterious effects on cardiac rehabilitation by inducing arterial and venous vasoconstriction, increasing cardiac load, and causing the release of renin, which upregulates RAAS activity (Cody RJ, 1997). Although the mechanisms of action of beta-blockade agents in PMI patients are incompletely understood, they may play a role in interfering with the pathophysiology of SNS activation. (See the "Current Therapies" section.)

Arrhythmias and Sudden Cardiac Death. Sudden cardiac death (SCD) is death resulting from abrupt loss of heart function (cardiac arrest). It accounts for approximately a quarter of a million deaths each year in the United States alone. The most common cause of cardiac arrest leading to SCD is arrhythmia, the rapid or chaotic beating of the diseased heart. There are different kinds of arrhythmias, including tachycardia (rapid beating of the heart), bradycardia (slow beating of the heart), and fibrillation (uncoordinated contraction) of the ventricles or atria of the heart.

Arrhythmia-associated SCD commonly occurs within 24 hours after the onset of symptoms and is the leading cause of death during the early stages of the PMI period. Postmortem studies have shown that up to 75% of people suffering SCD had a previous, healed MI, making SCD a significant potential outcome in the PMI population (Myerburg RJ, 1997).

The prognostic significance of each type of arrhythmia is dependent on time of onset after the initial MI. More than 50% of SCDs in the PMI population are due to ventricular tachycardia and ventricular fibrillation (VF). Ventricular tachycardias are observed in 40% of patients with AMI, and most take place within the first 24–48 hours after the AMI. Some cases may require aggressive therapy or an implantable defibrillator. An antiarrhythmic drug is sometimes given in the short term. Long-term therapy is indicated only if the tachycardia occurs for more than 48 hours from AMI.

Ventricular fibrillation can develop 48–72 hours following AMI symptom onset. The Gruppo Italiano per lo Studio della Sopravvivenza nell' Infarto (GISSI) trial showed VF to be associated with a high in-hospital mortality rate (10.8%, versus 5.9% for AMI patients without VF) (Franzosi MG, 1998; Volpi A, 1998; Volpi A, 2001). Until recently, prophylactic lidocaine was sometimes prescribed to ward off VF, even though the agent has never been proved to reduce mortality and, in fact, may do more harm than good.

A more serious arrhythmia that can occur after AMI is atrioventricular (AV) block. The AV node is a small structure that slows conduction in the heart from the atria (the heart's upper chambers) to the ventricles (the lower chambers) and is responsible for the time lag between atrial and ventricular beats. However, because it is a small structure, even a minimal degree of ischemia can have a significant pathological effect and cause heart block, which may lead to syncope and cardiac arrest. The mortality rate of patients with complete AV block associated with an anterior MI can reach 75%; for those with AV block and inferior infarction, the mortality rate is 25–40%. Electrical pacing (via the implantation of a pacemaker) may benefit some of these patients, but for those with large infarcts, the prognosis is usually poor.

The etiologies of the arrhythmias vary. Several factors have been associated with the initiation of arrhythmias: regional ischemia, electrolyte imbalances, hypotension, and the use of drugs such as digitalis. Supraventricular arrhythmias can be caused by atrial ischemia and by the effects of excess stretch and distension of the atrial myocardium, which occur as a result of the increased atrial pressure.

Accelerated idioventricular rhythm (or slow ventricular tachycardia) is associated with sinus bradycardia and occurs in 25% of patients who experience an AMI (in particular, those who experience an inferoposterior infarction).

Traditional Risk Factors. In addition to the risks for PMI that arise from an initial AMI as discussed in the previous sections, the classic risk factors for cardiovascular disease (CVD), such as diabetes, hypertension, high LDL levels, tobacco smoking, and obesity, apply to patients at risk for a recurrent event. Each of these risk factors can be a target of efforts to improve outcomes for PMI patients. Diabetes and hypertension, in particular, are targets for pharmacotherapy.

The East-West study in Finland studied outcomes for diabetic and nondiabetic PMI patients (Haffner SM, 1998). The seven-year incidence of recurrent MI was 45% for diabetics versus 18.8% for patients who had suffered a prior MI but did not have diabetes. Insulin resistance also plays a pathological role in disease progression by upregulating both the RAAS and SNS pathways, and thus encouraging VR.

Studies have also demonstrated a compelling correlation between PMI and hypertension. In a follow-up study of 1,093 AMI patients, postdischarge mortality rates for patients with antecedent hypertension were 9.5% versus 5.5% for nonhypertensive (normotensive) patients (Richards AM, 2002). Hypertension also increased the risk of subsequent heart failure, with 12.4% of hypertensive patients readmitted to the hospital with the condition, versus 5.5% of normotensive patients. Recent analysis of 456 patients from the Survival and Ventricular Enlargement (SAVE) trial revealed that hypertension is associated with a doubling of the risk of LV dilation and consequently is a significant risk factor for heart failure (Kenchaiah S, 2004).

CURRENT THERAPIES

Treatment approaches after a myocardial infarction (MI) focus on three main objectives. The first goal is to reopen the occluded vessel as quickly as possible, using thrombolytic agents or mechanical revascularization. The second is to limit the immediate complications of MI, such as recurrent MI and arrhythmias. The third objective, and the most relevant in terms of long-term treatment post-MI, is the secondary prevention of post-myocardial infarction (PMI) cardiovascular events through lifestyle alteration and pharmacotherapy.

Major drug classes used for the long-term management of PMI patients include antiplatelet agents, beta blockers, angiotensin-converting enzyme (ACE) inhibitors, angiotensin II receptor antagonists (AIIRAs), and statins (HMG-CoA reductase inhibitors). Clinical trial data convincingly demonstrate the benefits of these agents in the treatment of PMI, including improved patient outcomes and survival. However, despite well-established American Heart Association (AHA), American College of Cardiology (ACC), and European Society of Cardiology

(ESC) guidelines recommending use of these agents, data indicate that almost all drug classes are underprescribed or incorrectly dosed in the PMI population. These data come from the European Action on Secondary and Primary Prevention through Intervention to Reduce Events (EUROASPIRE) study, the Multinational Monitoring of Trends and Determinants in Cardiovascular Disease (MONICA) study, the Cooperative Cardiovascular Project (CCP), and the United States National Registry.

This section describes a range of current secondary prevention strategies, including pharmacotherapy with commonly used agents and lifestyle modification. Table 1 summarizes the therapies currently used for PMI. Few therapies are specifically indicated to treat PMI; instead, most therapies are licensed to treat components of the PMI state (e.g., hypertension, dyslipidemia) and are used off-label in PMI.

Although not covered extensively here, some PMI patients are given oral anticoagulants, such as the vitamin K antagonist warfarin (generics). Because data have shown no benefit to prescribing warfarin with aspirin over aspirin alone (Fiore LD, 2002; Herlitz J, 2004), oral anticoagulants are usually reserved for patients with a low left ventricular ejection fraction (LVEF), with an intolerance to aspirin, or with complications such as atrial fibrillation (AF). In addition, some patients are discharged receiving sublingual or transdermal nitrates to relieve angina-like symptoms.

Antiplatelet Agents

Overview. All antiplatelet agents reduce the risk of thrombosis by preventing platelet aggregation. Antiplatelet agents commonly used for the treatment of PMI include the cyclooxygenase (COX) inhibitor aspirin (Bayer Pharmaceutical's [West Haven, Connecticut] Bayer Aspirin, generics) and the thienopyridine adenosine diphosphate (ADP) receptor antagonists clopidogrel (Sanofi-Aventis [Tokyo, Japan]/Bristol-Myers Squibb's [North Billerica, Massachusetts] Plavix, Bristol-Myers Squibb's Iscover) and ticlopidine (Roche's [Basel, Switzerland] Ticlid, Sanofi-Aventis's Ticlid). Aspirin is prescribed prophylactically to limit reocclusion of damaged arteries—or new blockages—by thrombogenesis.

Mechanism of Action. Aspirin exerts its antithrombotic effects through inhibition of cyclooxygenase-1 (COX-1). COX-1 catalyzes the synthesis of prostaglandins, including thromboxane A_2, an intermediate in the ADP receptor-mediated coagulation pathway that promotes platelet aggregation.

Ticlopidine and clopidogrel both inhibit ADP-induced fibrinogen binding to platelets during platelet aggregation. Platelet activation releases ADP which, when bound to adenylate cyclase-coupled P2 purinoreceptors on the platelet surface, triggers a signaling cascade that generates further platelet activation and aggregation (Figure 2). Antagonism of ADP binding to its receptor by thienopyridines such as clopidogrel and ticlopidine inhibits platelet activation and aggregation during thrombus formation.

TABLE 1. Current Therapies Used for Post-Myocardial Infarction

Agent	Company/Brand	Dose	Availability
Antiplatelet agents			
Aspirin	Bayer's Aspirin, generics	75–300 mg qd	US, F, G, I, S, UK, J
Clopidogrel	Sanofi-Aventis/Bristol-Myers Squibb's Plavix, Bristol-Myers Squibb's Iscover	75 mg qd	US, F, G, I, S, UK,
Ticlopidine	Roche's Ticlid, Sanofi-Aventis's Ticlid/Tiklyd/Tiklid	250 mg bid	US, F, G, I, S, UK, J
Beta blockers			
Atenolol	AstraZeneca's Tenormin/Tenormine, Schwarz Pharma's Seles Beta, Merck's Isopress, generics	50–100 mg qd	US, F, G, I, S, UK, J
Metoprolol succinate	AstraZeneca's Toprol XL/Beloken/ Selozok	50–100 mg qd	US, F, G, I, S, UK, J
Metoprolol tartrate	Novartis's Lopressor, AstraZeneca's Seloken/ Betaloc, generics	100–450 mg	US, F, G, I, S, UK, J
Carvedilol	Roche's Kredex/Dilatrend/Coropres/ Eucardic, Roche/GlaxoSmithKline's Coreg, Altana's Querto	50–100 mg qd	US, F, G, I, S, UK, J
Angiotensin-converting enzyme inhibitors			
Ramipril	Sanofi-Aventis's Altace/Triatec/Acovil/ Tritace/Delix, AstraZeneca's Vesdil/ Unipril	5–20 mg qd or bid	US, F, G, I, S, UK
Enalapril	Boehringer Ingelheim's Pres, Merck's Vasotec/Xanef/ Enapren/Innovace, Sigma-Tau's Naprilene, Schwarz Pharma's Neotensin, generics	5–20 mg qd or bid	US, F, G, I, S, UK, J
Lisinopril	AstraZeneca's Zestril/Acerbon, Bristol-Myers Squibb's Carace/Coric, Merck's Prinivil, generics	5–10 mg qd or bid	US, F, G, I, S, UK, J
Captopril	Bristol-Myers Squibb's Lopirin/ Capoten, Sanofi-Aventis's Alopresin, generics	25–50 mg bid or tid	US, F, G, I, S, UK, J

TABLE 1. (*continued*)

Agent	Company/Brand	Dose	Availability
Fosinopril sodium	Merck's Fozitec, Schwarz Pharma's Dynacil, Bristol-Myers Squibb's Monopril/Fosinorm/ Tensogard/Fosinil/ Staril	20 mg qd or bid	US, F, G, I, S, UK,
Angiotensin II receptor antagonists			
Losartan	Merck's Cozaar/Lozaar, Sigma-Tau's Losaprex	25–100 mg qd or bid	US, F, G, I, S, UK, J
Valsartan	Novartis's Diovan/Tareg, Sanofi-Aventis's Nisis, Schwarz Pharma's Provas	80–320 mg qd or bid	US, F, G, I, S, UK, J
Statins			
Simvastatin	Merck's Zocor/Sinvacor, Boehringer Ingelheim's Denan, Banyu's Lipovas	10–40 mg qd	US, F, G, I, S, UK, J
Pravastatin	Bristol-Myers Squibb's Pravachol/ Elisor/Pravasin/Selectin/ Lipostat, Sanofi-Aventis's Vasten, Sankyo's Sanaprav/Mevalotin	10–40 mg qd	US, F, G, I, S, UK, J
Atorvastatin	Pfizer's Lipitor/ Tahor/Sortis/ Torvast/Cardyl	10–80 mg qd	US, F, G, I, S, UK, J
Rosuvastatin	AstraZeneca's Crestor	5–40 mg qd	US, F, I, UK
Pitavastatin	Nissan/Kowa Kogyo/ Novartis/ Sankyo's Livalo	1–4 mg qd	J
Lovastatin	Merck's Mevacor/Mevinacor, Merck/Schwarz Pharma's Liposcler	20–80 mg qd	US, G, S, J
Fluvastatin	Novartis's Lescol/Locol/Lochol, Solvay's Digaril	20–40 mg qd	US, F, G, I, S, UK, J
Cholesterol absorption inhibitors			
Ezetimibe	Merck and Schering-Plough's Zetia/Ezeterol	10 mg qd	US, F, G, S, UK

Bid = Twice daily; qd = Once daily; tid = Three times daily.
US = United States; F = France; G = Germany; I = Italy; S = Spain; UK = United Kingdom; J = Japan.

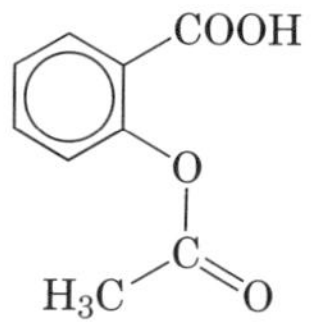

FIGURE 6. Structure of aspirin.

Aspirin. Acetylsalicylic acid (Bayer's Aspirin, generics) (Figure 6) has been widely available for more than 100 years. As already mentioned, aspirin exerts its antithrombotic effects through inhibition of COX-1. Current ACC/AHA guidelines for the management of patients with acute myocardial infarction (AMI) continue to recognize the administration of aspirin (160–325 mg/day) for an indefinite period as the most important therapy for patients following AMI (Ryan TJ, 2002).

One trial with positive evidence for the use of aspirin in PMI was the Persantine-Aspirin Reinfarction Study (PARIS). This study compared the efficacy and safety of a combination of dipyridamole (Boehringer Ingelheim's [Ingelheim, Germany] Persantine, another antiplatelet agent) and aspirin or aspirin alone with placebo in 2026 PMI patients for three years (PARIS investigators, 1980). There was a trend toward improved survival rates both for the combination and single drug compared with placebo. Coronary events were significantly lower in the combination group compared with placebo during the first 24 months of treatment; significant reductions in the aspirin group occurred only at 8 and 24 months. Similar results were obtained in the 3128-patient follow-up PARIS II study (Klimt CR, 1986). However, the Aspirin Myocardial Infarction Study (AMIS), which randomized 4,524 PMI patients to 1.0 g aspirin daily or placebo, found a statistically nonsignificant increase in mortality in the drug-treated group (10.8% versus 9.7%). There was a nonsignificant trend of a lower incidence of nonfatal MI in the aspirin group (6.3%) compared with placebo (8.1%) (AMIS Research Group, 1980).

More recently, the Coumadin Aspirin Reinfarction Study (CARS) demonstrated that 3,393 PMI patients randomized to receive aspirin (160 mg/day) had a lower incidence of ischemic stroke than 2028 patients receiving an aspirin/warfarin (80 mg/1 mg) combination, although this reduction did not reach statistical significance (0.6% versus 1.1%; $p = 0.0534$) (O'Connor CM, 2001). The Combined Hemotherapy and Mortality Prevention (CHAMP) study enrolled 5059 patients within 14 days of an MI to a similar treatment regimen used in the CARS study (Fiore LD, 2002). No significant differences in the rates of stroke, mortality, or recurrent MI were seen between the high-dose aspirin and the low-dose aspirin/warfarin groups. Similarly, there was no benefit observed by adding warfarin to aspirin therapy in the 3300-patient Low-Dose Warfarin and Aspirin (LoWASA) trial (Herlitz J, 2004).

The Antiplatelet Trialists' Collaboration reviewed 174 trials involving approximately 100,000 patients. This study identified a 25% reduction in vascular events—including nonfatal MI, nonfatal stroke, or vascular death—following prolonged treatment with aspirin (Antiplatelet Trialists' Collaboration, 1994).

Although the antiplatelet activity of aspirin is mediated through COX-1, COX-1 also catalyzes the synthesis of the prostaglandin PGE_2, which normally protects the gastric mucosa. Inhibition of PGE_2 synthesis can generate gastric side effects, including ulceration of the mucosa and gastric bleeding; long-term aspirin therapy damages the gastrointestinal (GI) tract, particularly the stomach. Some PMI patients are intolerant of aspirin, either because of allergic reaction or GI side effects. Nonetheless, aspirin continues to be recommended in all aspirin-tolerant patients.

Clopidogrel. Clopidogrel (Sanofi-Aventis/Bristol-Myers Squibb's Plavix, Bristol-Myers Squibb's Iscover) (Figure 7) was first launched in the United States and Europe in 1998. This agent is a more potent antiplatelet agent than aspirin, inhibiting ADP-induced fibrinogen binding during platelet aggregation; it also lacks the GI side effects of aspirin.

Clopidogrel antagonizes stimulation of adenylyl cyclase by adenosine diphosphate (ADP) on the surface of platelets. This selective interaction irreversibly inhibits ADP-induced platelet activation and aggregation.

The Clopidogrel Versus Aspirin in Patients at Risk of Ischemic Events (CAPRIE) trial—a key study supporting the use of clopidogrel for prevention of subsequent cardiovascular events in secondary prevention populations (including PMI)—demonstrated the superiority of clopidogrel (75 mg/day) over aspirin treatment (325 mg/day). In 19,185 patients with peripheral arterial disease (PAD), a recent MI (within the previous 35 days), or a recent stroke (within the previous one to six months), clopidogrel treatment conferred an 8.7% reduction in risk of cardiovascular events over that seen for aspirin. Clopidogrel was effective in preventing ischemic events in patients with atherosclerotic vascular disease including PMI. Subgroup analysis revealed that much of the benefit associated with clopidogrel was observed in the group presenting with symptomatic disease. The relative risk reduction of vascular events was 3.7% for AMI, 7.3% for ischemic stroke, and 23.8% for PAD, in favor of clopidogrel. The risk of neutropenia with clopidogrel was 0.10%, compared with 0.17% for aspirin (CAPRIE Steering Committee, 1996). Furthermore, treatment with clopidogrel resulted in a significant decrease in the need for rehospitalization for ischemic events or bleeding compared with aspirin (1502 versus 1673 cases) (Bhatt DL, 2000).

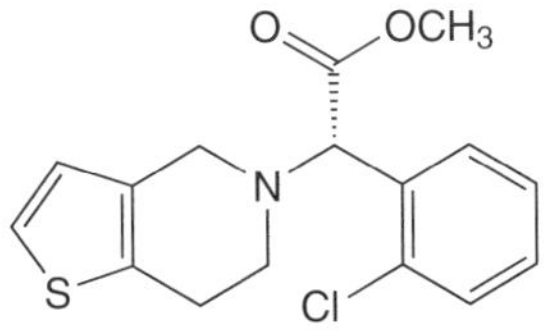

FIGURE 7. *Structure of clopidogrel.*

Analysis of data from the multinational Clopidogrel in Unstable Angina to Prevent Recurrent Events (CURE) trial—in which 12,562 patients hospitalized within 24 hours of onset of non-ST-elevation acute coronary syndromes (ACS) were randomized to either clopidogrel (75 mg/day) plus aspirin (75–325 mg/day) or placebo plus aspirin (75–325 mg/day) and followed for up to one year postevent—identified an incremental 19.1% reduction in risk of cardiovascular death, MI, and stroke following aspirin and clopidogrel treatment versus aspirin alone. Trial investigators concluded that, despite a 33% increase in bleeding episodes in the active group, the benefits of clopidogrel and aspirin combination treatment outweigh the risks; combination treatment could prevent between 50,000 and 100,000 new MIs, strokes, and deaths every year (CURE Trial Investigators, 2001).

The Clopidogrel for Reduction of Events During Observation (CREDO) study evaluated the benefit of clopidogrel pretreatment and long-term clopidogrel and aspirin treatment following percutaneous coronary intervention (PCI); 2116 patients scheduled to undergo PCI were randomized to receive either placebo ($n = 1063$) or a 300 mg loading dose of clopidogrel ($n = 1053$) 3–24 hours before PCI. During the 28 days following PCI, all patients received clopidogrel (75 mg/day) and aspirin (325 mg/day), and for the remaining 11 months of the study, patients received either placebo or clopidogrel (75 mg/day) in addition to aspirin (81–325 mg/day) and other standard therapies. The primary 28-day end point was a composite of death, heart attack, or urgent target revascularization (UTVR), and the principal one-year end point was a composite of death, heart attack, or stroke. Treatment with clopidogrel 3–24 hours before PCI generated a (nonsignificant) 18.5% relative reduction in risk of death, heart attack, or UTVR relative to placebo; when patients were treated at least 6 hours prior to PCI, the relative risk reduction increased to 38.6%. Long-term clopidogrel therapy was associated with a significant 26.9% relative reduction in the composite one-year end point; risk of major bleeding increased, although not significantly, relative to placebo (Steinhubl SR, 2002).

Clopidogrel is indicated for the prophylaxis of thrombosis-related cardiovascular events. It has several advantages over ticlopidine (discussed next), including a superior pharmacokinetic profile and longer half-life, allowing once-daily dosing of clopidogrel versus twice-daily dosing for ticlopidine. Additionally, clopidogrel has increased potency and a lower risk of neutropenia, a potentially life-threatening decrease in white blood cell count, relative to ticlopidine. Neutropenia is thought to severely affect up to 1% of patients taking ticlopidine (Flores-Runk P, 1993).

Ticlopidine. Ticlopidine (Roche's Ticlid, Sanofi-Aventis's Ticlid) (Figure 8) has been available in the United States and Europe since the early 1990s. It has a similar mechanism of action to clopidogrel, in that it inhibits platelet aggregation by inhibiting ADP-induced fibrinogen binding.

Unlike trial data on clopidogrel, data on ticlopidine indicate that it is not superior to aspirin. The report from the second cycle of the Antiplatelet Trialists'

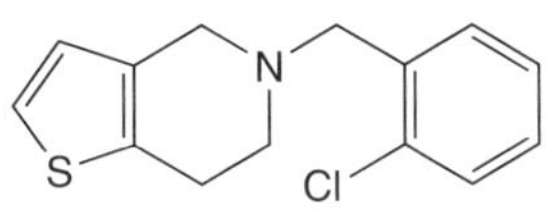

FIGURE 8. *Structure of ticlopidine.*

Collaboration showed no significant difference between ticlopidine and aspirin combination therapy and aspirin monotherapy in three separate trials. This finding was confirmed in a group of 4696 survivors of AMI, in which treatment with 500 mg/day of ticlopidine compared with 160 mg/day of aspirin resulted in no difference in rate of mortality, recurrent MI, stroke, or angina (Scrutino D, 2001).

In the PMI setting, ticlopidine is most commonly used as a short-term treatment after coronary stent emplacement. Treatment with aspirin and ticlopidine resulted in a lower rate of stent thrombosis than with aspirin alone or a combination of aspirin and warfarin in the 1653-patient Stent Anticoagulation Restenosis Study (STARS), although there were more hemorrhagic complications than with aspirin alone (Leon MB, 1998). A recent study in 883 patients with ST-segment-elevation myocardial infarction (STEMI) undergoing primary stenting showed no difference in long-term clinical outcome between clopidogrel and ticlopidine as adjunctive antiplatelet therapy (De Luca G, 2004). In a recent meta-analysis, however, aspirin with ticlopidine was found to be significantly less efficient at preventing the primary end point of death or nonfatal MI than aspirin and clopidogrel in 11,688 patients undergoing coronary stenting (Casella G, 2003).

The safety profile of ticlopidine severely restricts its use; the drug is associated with a higher adverse event rate than aspirin. One of the most serious adverse events associated with ticlopidine is the development of neutropenia. Pooled data from the Canadian American Ticlopidine Study (CATS) and the Ticlopidine Aspirin Stroke Study (TASS) suggest neutropenia occurs in approximately 1.3% of patients, compared with 0.1% in aspirin-treated patients (Gent M, 1989; Bellavance A, 1993). For this reason, hematological monitoring at two-week intervals of all patients taking ticlopidine is recommended.

Beta Blockers

Overview. The value of blockading beta adrenergic stimuli during PMI treatment is well recognized; current AHA guidelines recommend beta blockers as first-line anti-ischemic therapy in PMI patients, and a large number of trials support the benefits of beta blockers in improving morbidity and mortality in PMI. The CCP in the United States examined the medical records of more than 200,000 Medicare patients who had experienced AMI. It reported a 40% improvement in survival rates in the 69,338 patients whose AMI was treated with beta blockers, with apparently little difference in the effect on overall mortality according to which specific agents were used (Gottlieb SS, 2001). Prescribing beta blockers provides major benefits to PMI patients, and these drugs appear to be particularly useful in patients who have suffered AMI and are experiencing left ventricular dysfunction (LVD) or ventricular arrhythmias.

Beta blockers are contraindicated in patients who have asthma, chronic obstructive pulmonary disease (COPD), peripheral vascular disease (PVD), diabetes, or heart failure.

Mechanism of Action. Beta blockers act by inhibiting sympathetic innervation of the heart via the β-adrenoreceptor. The receptors comprise three subgroups—β_1, β_2, and β_3—of which the β_1 receptor is the most significant in terms of regulating cardiac inotropy (force or energy of contraction) and chronotropy (time or rate of contraction). Although beta blockers are also vasoconstrictive, the net effect is to reduce blood pressure (BP) by reducing heart rate and cardiac output. Different beta blockers have varying supplementary effects. Some agents—such as atenolol (AstraZeneca [Wilmington, Delaware] Tenormin, Schwarz Pharma's [Milwaukee, Wisconsin] Seles Beta, Merck's [Whitehouse Station, New Jersey] Isopress, generics), metoprolol (AstraZeneca's Toprol XL, Novartis's [Basel, Switzerland] Lopressor, generics), and bisoprolol fumarate (Merck KGaA's Cardicor, Wyeth's [Madison, New Jersey] Zebeta, generics)—are more cardioselective than others and exert a greater action on β_1 receptors.

Common side effects of all beta blockers include fatigue, insomnia, and impotence.

Atenolol. Atenolol (AstraZeneca's Tenormin, Schwarz Pharma's Seles Beta, Merck's Isopress, generics) (Figure 9) was first approved by the FDA in 1981 and is now available in generic form in all seven of the major pharmaceutical markets (United States, France, Germany, Italy, Spain, United Kingdom, and Japan).

Atenolol is a selective β_1 adrenoreceptor blocker with a rapid onset of action.

In the Global Utilization of Streptokinase and t-PA for Occluded Coronary Arteries-I (GUSTO-I) trial, PMI patients receiving atenolol along with thrombolytic therapy ($n = 30,771$) had significantly lower 30-day mortality rates than PMI patients not receiving atenolol ($n = 10,073$) (Pfisterer M, 1998).

A recent analysis in the United States compared the effects of different beta blockers on mortality in 201,752 survivors of AMI (Gottileb SS, 2001). Overall, beta blockade was associated with a 40% improvement in survival. At two years, mortality rates with metoprolol and atenolol (both selective beta blockers) were virtually identical (13.5% and 13.4%, respectively), but these rates were slightly higher with propranolol (Wyeth/AstaZeneca's Inderal, generics) (15.9%).

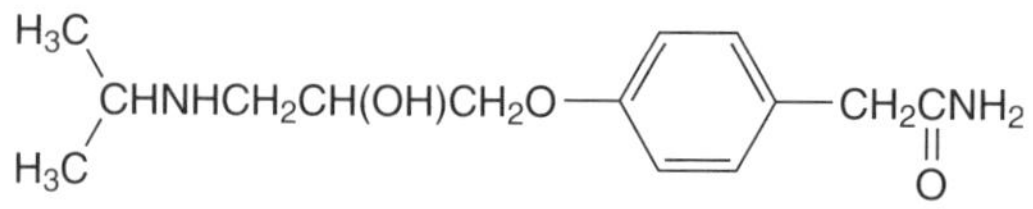

FIGURE 9. *Structure of atenolol.*

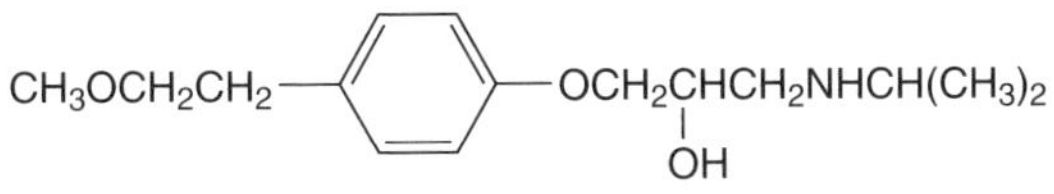

$$CH_3OCH_2CH_2 - \underset{}{\bigcirc} - OCH_2\underset{\underset{OH}{|}}{C}HCH_2NHCH(CH_3)_2$$

FIGURE 10. *Structure of metoprolol.*

Metoprolol Succinate and Metoprolol Tartrate. Metoprolol (Figure 10) was first launched in the United States in 1978 and is now available in generic form in all of the major pharmaceutical markets. Metoprolol is a selective β_1 adrenoreceptor blocker available as an extended-release (ER) succinate salt (AstraZeneca's Toprol XL/Beloken/Selozok) or the immediate-release (IR) tartrate salt (Novartis's Lopressor, AstraZeneca's Seloken/Betaloc, generics). The advantage of metoprolol succinate is its once-daily regimen; metoprolol tartrate requires twice-daily dosing in some instances.

Metoprolol is a selective β_1 adrenoreceptor blocker.

The benefit of using metoprolol in a PMI population was first demonstrated in a small study of 201 survivors of AMI. Patients randomized to metoprolol (100 mg twice daily) had a significantly lower incidence of nonfatal reinfarction at 36 months than did the placebo arm (11.7% versus 21.1%, $p > 0.05$) (Olsson G, 1985). In Japan, the first trials to investigate the effects of beta blockers in PMI patients mainly used metoprolol and showed a 36% reduction in mortality and a 56% reduction in cardiac events (Ishikawa K, 2000). A Scandinavian study to investigate the effects of beta blockers on long-term mortality in 2161 PMI patients showed that among patients prescribed metoprolol at doses of 200 mg, 100 mg, and 50 mg, the five-year mortality rates were 24%, 33%, and 43%, respectively, suggesting that higher doses of metoprolol may be more protective (Herlitz J, 2001).

Carvedilol. The most recently launched beta blocker is carvedilol (Roche's Kredex, Roche/GlaxoSmithKline's [Brentford, Middlesex, United Kingdom] Coreg, ALTANA, Inc.'s [Melville, New York] Querto) (Figure 11), a nonselective alpha and beta adrenoreceptor blocker. Carvedilol is under license to Eisai (for hypertension) and to Daiichi (for cardiac failure) in Japan. Carvedilol is indicated for the treatment of hypertension and heart failure, but is also used in PMI patients.

The Carvedilol Post Infarction Survival Control in Left Ventricular Dysfunction (CAPRICORN) trial investigated the addition of carvedilol to the widely

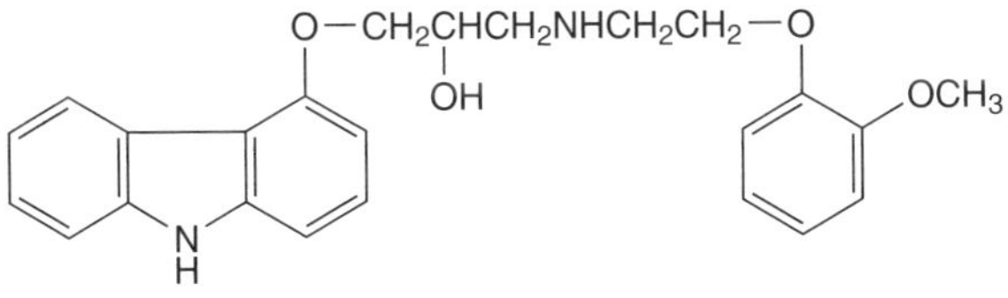

FIGURE 11. *Structure of carvedilol.*

used combination of ACE inhibitors, aspirin, and statins in PMI patients with LVD. A total of 1959 patients presenting with LVD of less than 40% (mean 33%) following MI were randomized to receive either carvedilol ($n = 975$) or placebo ($n = 984$) in addition to standard ACE inhibitor, aspirin, and statin treatment regimens. Over a mean follow-up period of 15 months, carvedilol treatment was associated with an absolute risk reduction of 3.4% for all-cause mortality (from 15.3% with placebo to 11.9% with carvedilol), equating to a relative risk reduction of 23%. Additionally, the incidence of recurrent MI was reduced from 5.8% with placebo to 2.3%, a relative risk reduction of 41% (Dargie HJ, 2001; Otterstad JE, 2002).

Angiotensin-Converting Enzyme Inhibitors

Overview. Results from trials involving more than 100,000 PMI patients have demonstrated the efficacy of angiotensin-converting enzyme (ACE) inhibitors in reducing mortality. ACE inhibitors appear to have significant benefits when given immediately after MI. Researchers believe that ACE inhibitors inhibit the left ventricular remodeling that can occur post MI, although the precise mechanism by which this effect is achieved is not fully understood, (Reynolds G, 1996).

Current ACC/AHA guidelines recommend that ACE inhibitors be started within the first 24 hours of an MI and be continued for four to six weeks afterward.

ACE inhibitors are particularly beneficial in PMI patients who have suffered an MI of the anterior heart wall, those with an LVEF less than 40%, or those with signs of heart failure.

A common side effect of ACE inhibitor use is a dry, nonproductive cough, which can occur in 5–20% of patients. ACE inhibitors are contraindicated in pregnancy. (The FDA has rated this class of drugs as Pregnancy Category C [risk cannot be ruled out] in the first trimester] and Category D [published documentation of risk exists] for the second and third trimesters.) ACE inhibitors are also contraindicated for patients with serious renal stenosis or widespread vascular lesions in the kidney due to potentially decreased renal perfusion. A further concern is angioedema (swelling and accumulation of fluid in the deep layer of the skin and the connective tissue that underlies mucous membranes); although angioedema occurs in 0.1% of all patients taking ACE inhibitors, it is three times more common in black patients.

Some literature suggests that an adverse interaction between aspirin and ACE inhibitors may exist. Detrimental ACE inhibitor/aspirin interactions have been reported in 1 out of 5 trials in hypertension, 1 out of 4 trials in coronary heart disease, and 9 out of 13 trials in congestive heart failure (CHF) (Meune C, 2000). However, the authors of this meta-analysis cite the need for prospective trials to definitively establish this connection.

Mechanism of Action. ACE inhibitors lower blood pressure by inhibiting the vasoconstrictive action of the renin-angiotensin-aldosterone system (RAAS).

Additionally, ACE inhibitors are known to have some action in preventing cell proliferation, reducing platelet aggregation, and enhancing fibrinolysis (Lonn EM, 1998) as well as in promoting collateral vessel development and improving prognosis in coronary artery bypass graft (CABG) patients (O'Keefe JH, 2001). Pharmacologically, ACE inhibitors act to prevent the conversion of angiotensin I into angiotensin II (AII)—a potent vasoconstrictive agent—by ACE. AII is also known to stimulate contraction of the vascular smooth-muscle cells (VSMCs) lining the vascular wall, an action ultimately leading to hypertrophy (an increase in cell size) and hyperplasia (an increase in cell number). This action manifests as a thickening of the arterial wall and a narrowing of the lumen that generates an increase in the peripheral resistance of the vasculature. AII also increases production of excess reactive oxygen species, which in turn increase vasoconstriction and damage the endothelial wall (Sowers JR, 2002).

Independently of their action on the RAAS, ACE inhibitors reduce breakdown of the vasodilator bradykinin, high levels of which are responsible for the cough frequently associated with ACE inhibitor prescription. However, high levels of bradykinin may also have positive effects on cardiovascular health; bradykinin, acting through ACE-bradykinin type 2 [B(2)] receptors, is thought to potentiate the insulin responsiveness of both adipocytes and muscle fibers. Transduction of the bradykinin signal via this receptor reduces tyrosine kinase-mediated inactivation of the insulin receptor (McCarty MF, 2003) and upregulates B(2) receptor expression (Tom B, 2003). These actions limit the development of diabetes by limiting insulin resistance in the adipocytes, which in turn has a beneficial effect on blood lipid profile; data from the Heart Outcomes Prevention Evaluation (HOPE) study indicate that ACE inhibitors may reduce the risk of patients developing type 2 diabetes (Dagenais GR, 2001), a common cardiovascular risk factor in secondary prevention populations such as PMI.

Ramipril. Ramipril (Sanofi-Aventis's Altace, AstraZeneca's Vesdil) (Figure 12) was first launched in France in 1989 and was approved in the United States in 1991. Ramipril is available in the United States and Europe, but not in Japan, where it is under review in CHF following MI. Following oral administration, ramipril is converted to the active form, ramiprilat, by hepatic cleavage of an ester group. Ramilprilat's mechanism of action is as described in the previous "Mechanism of Action" section.

Ramipril was evaluated in the Acute Infarction Ramipril Efficacy (AIRE) study, which involved 2006 PMI patients with evidence of heart failure. Patients

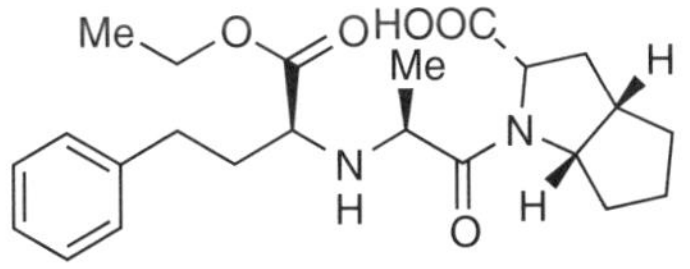

FIGURE 12. *Structure of ramipril.*

were randomized and given twice-daily 5 mg doses of oral ramipril or placebo. After an average follow-up time of 15 months, total mortality was reduced by 27% in the ramipril group. AIRE also demonstrated significant reduction in progression to serious or resistant heart failure, recurrent AMI, or stroke (AIRE Study Investigators, 1993). A follow-up of the AIRE study (AIREX) indicated a reduction in relative risk of 36% in the ramipril-treated group three years after the end of the AIRE study period (Hall AS, 1997).

The use of ramipril in PMI patients is supported by positive data demonstrating its efficacy in PMI patients, particularly those at high risk of further cardiovascular events. The HOPE study involved 9541 high-risk subjects with clinical symptoms associated with atherosclerosis. Over a five-year follow-up period, patients taking ramipril experienced a 20.3% reduction in the combined primary end point of MI, stroke, or cardiovascular death. Furthermore, their risk of death from cardiovascular events declined by approximately 25%. In 2000, the FDA expanded ramipril's labeling as a result of the HOPE study. Other ACE inhibitors are under investigation to determine whether ramipril's antiatherosclerotic effects are class-related.

Enalapril. Enalapril (Boehringer Ingelheim's Pres, Merck's Vasotec, Sigma Tau's [Rome, Italy] Naprilene, Schwarz Pharma's Neotensin, generics) (Figure 13) was approved in the United States in December 1985 and has since become available in Europe and Japan. This compound has a moderate-range half-life (11 hours) and requires less frequent dosing than other ACE inhibitors such as captopril, a trait that may improve compliance. Enalapril's mechanism of action is as described in the "Mechanism of Action" section for ACE inhibitors.

Large-scale clinical trials of enalapril, such as the Studies of Left-Ventricular Dysfunction (SOLVD) (SOLVD Investigators, 1991) and the Cooperative North Scandinavian Enalapril Survival Study (CONSENSUS) (CONSENSUS Trial Study Group, 1987), have focused on CHF. However, the ACE Inhibitor Comparative Trial in Cardiac Infarction and LV Function (PRACTICAL) trial—a randomized, placebo-controlled trial in 225 patients suffering recent MI—demonstrated that enalapril reduces mortality at 90 days and at 12 months post-MI (Foy SG, 1994). These results followed the disappointing CONSENSUS II trial, in which 6090 patients with AMI and hypertension (blood pressure greater than 100/60 mm Hg) were randomized to treatment with either enalapril or placebo within 24 hours of the onset of symptoms. Mortality rates in the two groups at 6 months were not significantly different (10.2% versus 11.0%,

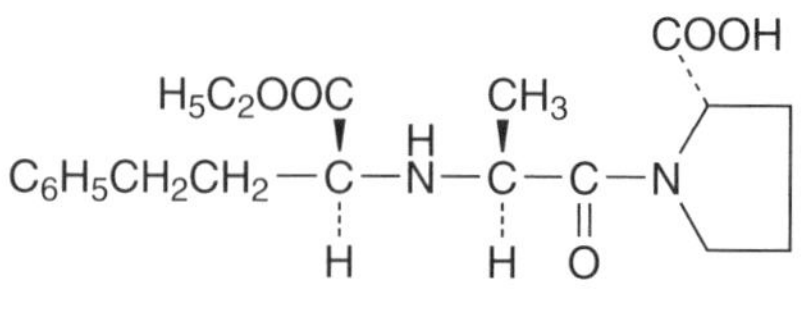

FIGURE 13. *Structure of enalapril.*

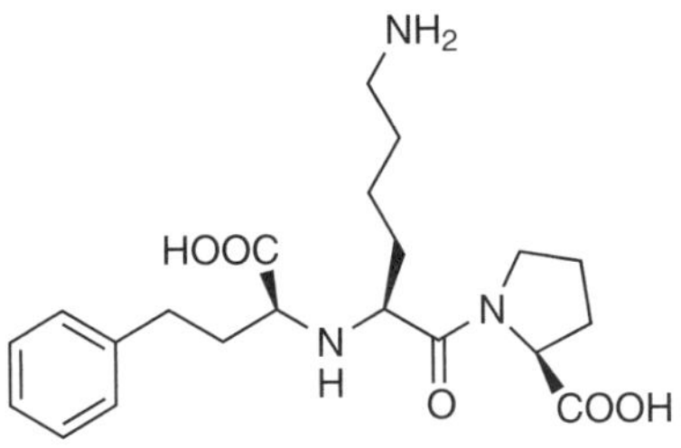

FIGURE 14. Structure of lisinopril.

respectively). However, death due to progressive heart failure was less frequent in the enalapril group compared with placebo (3.4% versus 4.3%, $p = 0.06$) (Swedberg K, 1992[b]).

Lisinopril. Lisinopril (AstraZeneca's Zestril, Bristol-Myers Squibb's Carace, Merck's Prinivil, generics) (Figure 14), along with ramipril and enalapril, is among the ACE inhibitors most frequently prescribed to PMI patients. The FDA approved lisinopril in December 1987 for use as an antihypertensive agent; the agent is now available in all of the major pharmaceutical markets. Lisinopril's mechanism of action is as described in the "Mechanism of Action" section for ACE inhibitors.

The 19,394-patient Gruppo Italiano per lo Studio della Sopravvivenza nell'Infarto Miocardico (GISSI)-3 trial investigated the relative effectiveness of six weeks of oral lisinopril, a nitrate (glycerol trinitrate, generics), both, or neither in PMI patients. Patients also received standard treatment with aspirin and/or beta blockers. Lisinopril, alone or with a nitrate, significantly reduced mortality, heart failure, and LVD. Mortality among patients treated only with lisinopril was 6.3%, versus 7.1% for those receiving placebo. The group receiving only nitrates demonstrated no beneficial effects on end points at 42 days post-MI (GISSI-3 Study Group, 1994). In addition, subsequent analysis of GISSI-3 data determined that lisinopril does not interact detrimentally with aspirin. The authors concluded that lisinopril is safe and effective when given early after the onset of MI, regardless of a coprescription of aspirin (Latini R, 2000).

Subgroup analysis of GISSI-3 did, however, identify detrimental effects of excessive blood pressure reduction in PMI. Although lisinopril significantly reduced the risk of lethal events in the 10,661 normotensive patients, an increased rate of lethal events was identified in 7362 hypertensive patients (Avanzini F, 2002). The authors identified a subgroup of 1165 hypertensive patients with a low baseline systolic blood pressure, increased mortality rates following cardiogenic shock on the first day of lisinopril treatment, and a persistent death trend after six weeks. Physicians may be reassured by the more recent Survival of Myocardial Infarction Long-term Evaluation-2 (SMILE-2) study, which randomized 1,024 thrombolyzed patients with AMI to either zofenopril (Bristol-Myers

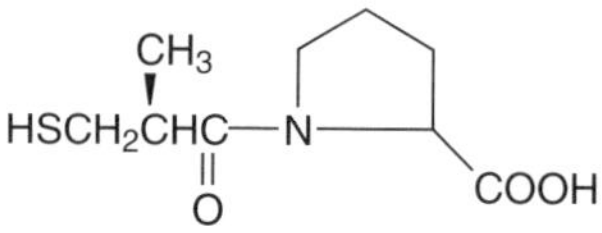

$$HSCH_2CHC\text{—}N \qquad \overset{CH_3}{\underset{O}{|}} \qquad COOH$$

FIGURE 15. *Structure of captopril.*

Squibb/Menarini's [Florence, Italy] Zofenil) or lisinopril, starting within 12 hours of completion of thrombolytic therapy and continuing for 42 days. The overall incidence of severe hypotension was low in both study groups (10.9% with zofenopril and 11.7% with lisinopril, $p = 0.38$) (Borghi C, 2003). Nonetheless, caution is recommended when using lisinopril during the first six weeks of PMI treatment in patients with a history of hypertension but low systolic blood pressure.

Captopril. Captopril (Bristol-Myers Squibb's Lopirin, Sanofi-Aventis' Alopresin, generics) (Figure 15) is available in all of the major pharmaceutical markets for the treatment of PMI. This ACE inhibitor has a relatively short half-life (approximately two to three hours) and so requires dosing two or three times daily. Its mechanism of action is as described in the "Mechanism of Action" section for ACE inhibitors.

Captopril's use in the PMI population is supported by results of the large International Study of Infarct Survival (ISIS-4) trial, in which captopril, compared with placebo, reduced mortality by 7% after the first five weeks—an effect that was maintained over the first year (ISIS-4 Collaborative Group, 1995). Additionally, the 2,231-patient Survival and Ventricular Enlargement (SAVE) trial showed that long-term captopril treatment resulted in a 19% reduction in mortality rate, a 25% reduction in the risk of recurrent MI, and a 32% reduction in risk of death following recurrent MI (Pfeffer MA, 1992).

Evidence supporting the use of captopril in PMI patients was provided by the Optimal Trial in Myocardial Infarction with the Angiotensin II Antagonist Losartan (OPTIMAAL). This study randomized 5,477 patients with confirmed MI and heart failure (HF) to losartan (titrated to 50 mg once daily) or captopril (titrated to 50 mg three times daily). After a mean follow-up of 2.7 years, mortality in the captopril group was lower than in the losartan group (16% versus 18%, $p = 0.07$) (Dickstein K, 2002). Losartan was significantly better tolerated than captopril, suggesting that, when adjusted for compliance, the effect on mortality in favor of captopril may be even greater. The authors concluded that although the difference in total mortality in favor of captopril is not significant, captopril should remain the preferred treatment in PMI.

Fosinopril Sodium. Fosinopril (Merck's Fozitec, Schwarz Pharma's Dynacil, Bristol-Myers Squibb's Monopril) (Figure 16) has been available in Europe and the United States (but not Japan) since the early 1990s. The long half-life of this drug (approximately 12 hours) allows for once-daily dosing, giving it an

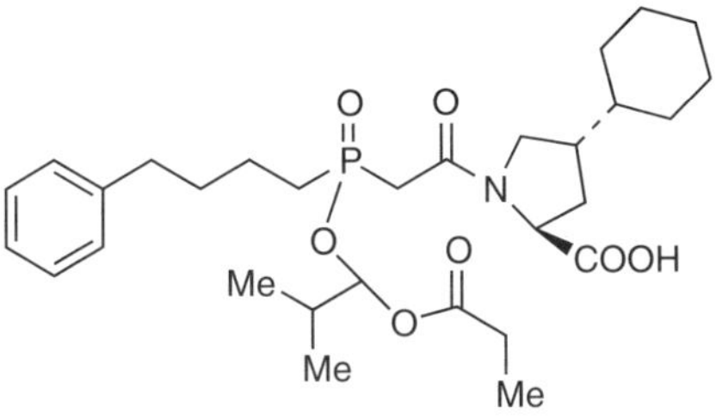

FIGURE 16. *Structure of fosinopril.*

advantage over some older agents in this class. Fosinopril's mechanism of action is as described in the "Mechanism of Action" section for ACE inhibitors.

The efficacy of fosinopril in the PMI population was assessed in the Fosinopril in Acute Myocardial Infarction Study (FAMIS). FAMIS researchers investigated 285 patients with anterior AMI receiving active treatment with fosinopril or placebo. Treatment was continued for three months, and treated patients showed a reduction in the two-year combined prevalence of death or moderate to severe CHF, despite having a worse clinical profile at baseline (Borghi C, 1998).

Angiotensin II Receptor Antagonists

Overview. Six AIIRAs are marketed for hypertension, but losartan (Merck's Cozaar, Sigma-Tau's Losaprex) and valsartan (Novartis's Diovan, Sanofi-Aventis's Nisis, Schwarz Pharma's Provas) are the most commonly used in PMI patients. Only limited data on the relative efficacy of these agents in PMI are currently available. However, clinical trials have demonstrated that AIIRAs possess efficacy equivalent to—but not superior to—that of ACE inhibitors in several other indications. For example, the Evaluation of Losartan in the Elderly II (ELITE II) trial failed to detect a difference between losartan and the ACE inhibitor captopril for their effects on all-cause mortality in elderly patients with CHF (Pitt B, 2000).

Mechanism of Action. AIIRAs, like ACE inhibitors, act on the RAAS; however, AIIRAs selectively antagonize the angiotensin II receptor subtype 1 (AT1) instead of blocking AII generation. The principal benefit of AIIRAs over ACE inhibitors is their benign side-effect profile: AIIRAs are not associated with cough. Although AIIRAs are well tolerated in all age-groups, showing side effects similar to placebo, angioedema and orthostatic hypotension have been observed in some patients (Mazzolai L, 1999).

Losartan. Launched in 1995, losartan (Merck's Cozaar, Sigma Tau's Losaprex) (Figure 17) was the first AIIRA to market for hypertension. In vivo, losartan is metabolized to produce an active carboxylic acid metabolite. Its mechanism of action is common to all AIIRAs, as described previously.

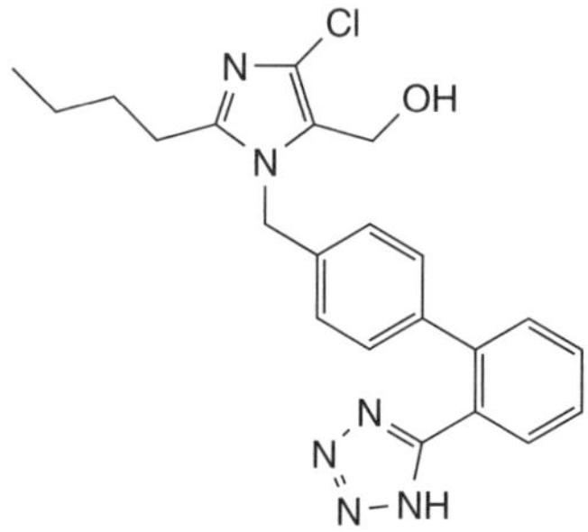

FIGURE 17. Structure of losartan.

The OPTIMAAL trial addressed the relative efficacy of Losartan and the ACE inhibitor captopril in PMI. A total of 5477 patients aged 50 or older (mean 67) with confirmed MI and heart failure (HF) during anterior infarction or reinfarction were randomly assigned and titrated to a target dose of losartan (50 mg once daily) or captopril (50 mg three times daily). After a mean follow-up of 2.7 years, mortality in the captopril group was lower than in the losartan group (16% versus 18%, $p = 0.07$) (Dickstein K, 2002). Losartan was significantly better tolerated than captopril, suggesting that, when adjusted for compliance, the effect on mortality in favor of captopril may be even greater. The authors concluded that, although the difference in total mortality in favor of captopril is not significant, captopril should remain the preferred treatment in PMI, with losartan use being restricted to patients who cannot tolerate ACE inhibitors.

Valsartan. Valsartan (Novartis's Diovan, Sanofi-Aventis's Nisis, Schwarz Pharma's Provas) (Figure 18) was launched for hypertension in the United States and various European countries (including France, Germany, and the United Kingdom) in 1996–1997 and Japan in 2000. In October 2004, valsartan was licensed in the United Kingdom for use in patients who had suffered an MI. In August 2005, Novartis was finally granted approval of valsartan in PMI from the FDA, which back in October 2002 had already approved this agent for use

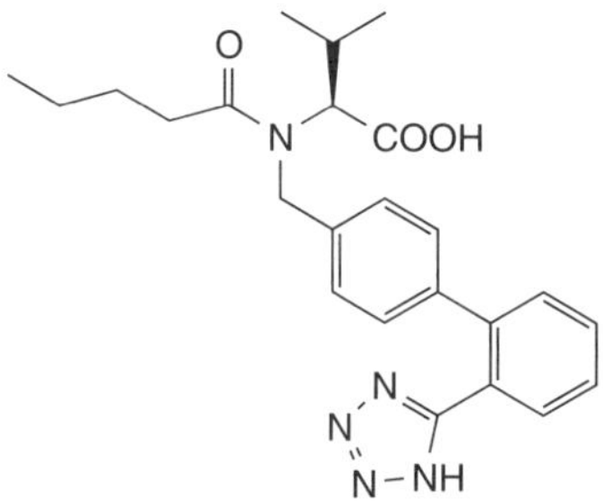

FIGURE 18. Structure of valsartan.

in CHF as a treatment for patients who cannot tolerate ACE inhibitors. Unlike losartan, valsartan does not require metabolism to an active form. Its mechanism of action is common to all AIIRAs, as described previously.

Approval for CHF was granted based on data from the Valsartan Heart Failure Trial (Val-HeFT), which assessed all-cause mortality in patients with HF. In Val-HeFT, 5010 HF patients taking angiotensin-converting enzyme inhibitors (ACEIs) and/or beta blockers were randomized into valsartan and placebo groups. Two-year follow-up results indicate that valsartan had no effect on total mortality compared with placebo, but the combined end point of all-cause morbidity and mortality dropped by 13.3%. ACE inhibitor-intolerant patients benefited most from valsartan; in patients already receiving beta blockers, the overall treatment effect was significantly less (Burnier M, 2001; Coats AJ, 2001).

The efficacy of valsartan in a PMI population was recently demonstrated in the Valsartan in Acute Myocardial Infarction Trial (VALIANT), an active control study in 14,500 patients with MI, associated HF, or left ventricular dysfunction. VALIANT randomized patients 0.5 to 10 days after AMI to one of three treatment arms; standard treatment (aspirin or other antiplatelet agents, beta blockers, statins, and diuretics) plus valsartan, standard treatment plus captopril, or standard treatment plus valsartan and captopril. No significant differences in mortality between treatment groups were observed at two years; however, patients receiving the captopril and valsartan combination suffered more adverse events (Pfeffer MA, 2003). The authors concluded that valsartan is as effective as captopril in patients who are at high risk for cardiovascular events after MI and that there was no advantage in combining the two medications.

Statins

PMI patients typically present with coronary artery disease (CAD), which is often the cause of their original MI. Because cholesterol plays an important role in the formation, progression, and rupture of atherosclerotic plaques, lowering plasma cholesterol (particularly low-density lipoprotein [LDL]) could help reduce atherosclerosis and the risk of subsequent MI. Statins (HMG-CoA reductase inhibitors) are the core component of lipid-lowering therapy. Physicians now almost universally recognize the importance of lowering LDL cholesterol in preventing future cardiac events in the PMI population and the pivotal role of statins in achieving this aim. ACC/AHA guidelines recommend that statins be prescribed to MI patients at discharge. Clear evidence exists for the benefit of statin therapy in PMI and other ACS (Wright RS, 2002).

Mechanism of Action. Statins are structurally similar to the cholesterol precursor HMG-CoA and act as competitive inhibitors of HMG-CoA reductase, the rate-limiting enzyme in cholesterol biosynthesis; statins inhibit the conversion of hydroxymethyglutaryl to mevalonic acid. In response to reduced hepatic cholesterol biosynthesis, activation of the transcription factor sterol regulatory element binding protein (SREBP) upregulates LDL receptor gene expression, which leads to enhanced clearing of serum lipids (Liao JK, 2003). Statins are thought to confer additional beneficial effects on cardiovascular health independently of their cholesterol-lowering activities. Termed *pleiotropic effects*, these actions stem from statins' ability to modify endothelial function, possibly by promoting the production of nitric oxide and inhibiting the production of inflammatory molecules in the endothelium (Wassmann S, 2001). This class effect of statins may reduce inflammation, stabilize atherosclerotic plaques, inhibit platelet aggregation, and improve blood flow, all of which act to prevent subsequent coronary events. Although poorly understood at present, these effects are under study and should support the use of statins in many cardiovascular secondary prevention populations, irrespective of starting lipid levels.

Simvastatin. Simvastatin (Merck's Zocor, Boehringer Ingelheim's Denan, Banyu Pharmaceutical's [Tokyo, Japan] Lipovas) (Figure 19) was first launched in Europe in 1989 and in the United States and Japan in 1991. Simvastatin competitively inhibits HMG-CoA reductase, the rate-limiting enzyme in cholesterol biosynthesis. Pleiotropic effects, such as improvement in endothelial function, have also been demonstrated in studies of simvastatin (Pereira EC, 2003; Rezaie-Majid A, 2003).

The efficacy of simvastatin in PMI was confirmed in the landmark Scandinavian Simvastatin Survival Study (4S), a double-blind, placebo-controlled study in 4444 patients with either previous MI or angina pectoris and evidence of dyslipidemia. Patients were randomized to receive either simvastatin (20–40 mg/day) or placebo for a period of five years. At the end of the trial, simvastatin treatment conferred a 25% reduction in total serum cholesterol (TSC) relative to placebo. LDL fell by 35%, and the risk of major coronary events dropped 34%. The investigators also noted a 10% fall in triglycerides (TGs) and an 8% rise in high-density lipoprotein (HDL) (Scandinavian Simvastatin Survival Study Group, 1994). Subsequent subgroup analysis of the 3525 PMI patients who participated in 4 S identified that simvastatin treatment conferred a relative (versus placebo) risk reduction of 38%, 39%, and 42%, respectively, in patients defined as being at low, medium, and high risk for a cardiovascular event (Wilhelmsen L, 2001).

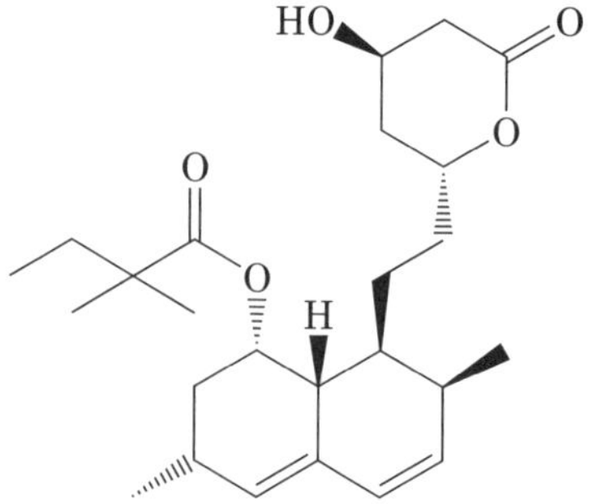

FIGURE 19. *Structure of simvastatin.*

Despite the plethora of trial data demonstrating the benefit of simvastatin therapy in secondary prevention, the recent A to Z trial, which compared early intensive intervention with simvastatin to a delayed conservative strategy in patients with ACS, has provided disappointing results. A total of 22,497 patients with ACS were treated with either 40 mg/day of simvastatin for 1 month followed by 80 mg/day for up to 24 months (aggressive strategy), or placebo for 4 months followed by 20 mg/day simvastatin (conservative strategy). The aggressive strategy failed to show a significant decrease in events compared with the conservative strategy in the first phase of the trial; of the patients receiving the conservative strategy, 16.7% experienced the primary end points of cardiovascular death, nonfatal MI readmission for ACS, or stroke, compared with 14.4% in the aggressive treatment arm ($p = 0.14$). From 4 months through the end of the study the primary end points were significantly reduced in the aggressive treatment arm ($p = 0.02$). However, myopathy was more common in the aggressive arm (De Lemos, JA, 2004). The lack of early benefit of early aggressive simvastatin therapy, together with an increase in the rate of side-effects is in contrast to studies of aggressive atorvastatin therapy such as PROVE-IT and MIRACL (see atorvastatin, covered later in this section), a fact that may well be exploited by Pfizer when marketing atorvastatin in the PMI population.

Pravastatin. Pravastatin (Bristol-Myers Squibb's Pravachol, Sanofi-Aventis's Vasten, Sankyo Pharma's [Parsippany, New Jersey] Mevalotin) (Figure 20) was first launched by in Japan in 1989, and subsequently launched in the United States in 1991.

Pravastatin competitively inhibits HMG-CoA reductase, and pleiotropic effects have been demonstrated in pravastatin treatment (Mulder HJ, 2003). Unlike other statins, pravastatin is not extensively metabolized by P450 isoenzymes and therefore does not compete with agents such as cyclosporin, thereby enhancing its value in renal transplant patients. Also, pravastatin does not appear to be as toxic to muscles as some other statins because it is less readily absorbed. Therefore, for patients who have myositis (inflammation of muscle tissue) but do not

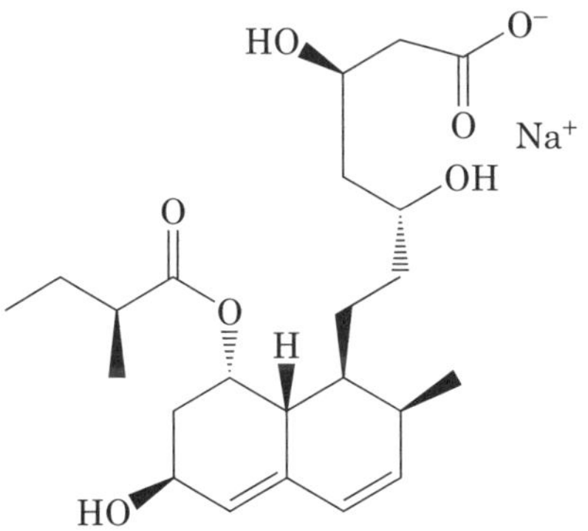

FIGURE 20. Structure of pravastatin.

have a high creatine phosphokinase (CPK) level (indicative of muscle damage), pravastatin may be the drug of choice.

The five-year placebo-controlled Cholesterol and Recurrent Events (CARE) trial evaluated pravastatin's efficacy in a secondary prevention setting. CARE's 4,159 CAD patients, who had mean LDL cholesterol levels of 139 mg/dL and had survived an AMI, were randomized to 40 mg/day of pravastatin or placebo. At the end of the trial, the pravastatin-treated group showed a 28% reduction in LDL and a 20% reduction in total cholesterol level. Compared with the placebo group, the treatment group experienced a 24% reduction in fatal CAD and nonfatal AMI (Pfeffer MA, 1995).

The Long-Term Intervention with Pravastatin in Ischemic Disease (LIPID) study involved 9014 patients with a history of unstable angina or AMI and normal to high cholesterol. In the 5754 patients with diagnosed MI, pravastatin (40 mg/day) reduced the risk of mortality by 21% (Tonkin AM, 2000).

Although not as efficacious in lowering LDL as some newer statins, pravastatin is supported by a strong evidence base in both primary and secondary care. A recent meta-analysis of secondary prevention trials with pravastatin examined the additive beneficial effects of pravastatin and aspirin therapy (Hennekens CH, 2004). The relative risk reductions for fatal or nonfatal MI were 31% for pravastatin plus aspirin versus aspirin alone and 26% for pravastatin plus aspirin versus pravastatin alone. In August 2003, Bristol-Myers Squibb launched its combination blister pack (two pills packed together) pravastatin/aspirin (Pravigard PAC) in the United States for secondary prevention only, at the same price as branded pravastatin.

Atorvastatin. Atorvastatin (Pfizer's [New York, New York] Lipitor) (Figure 21) reached the U.S. and European markets in February 1997 and was launched in Japan in 2000. In August 2004, the FDA extended atorvastatin's label to include "the prevention of cardiovascular disease by reducing heart attack risk in people with normal to mildly elevated cholesterol levels who have other cardiovascular risk factors." This agent's mechanism of action is as described in the "Mechanism of Action" section for statins.

A growing body of evidence supports the use of atorvastatin in high-risk populations. The Myocardial Ischemia Reduction with Aggressive Cholesterol Lowering (MIRACL) trial set out to investigate whether aggressive cholesterol lowering in the period just after AMI would reduce the occurrence of the early events that are responsible for most mortality in the PMI population (Schwartz GG, 2001). The MIRACL trial showed a 40% reduction in LDL levels and a 16% reduction in the risk of recurrent ischemic events, primarily by reducing the risk of recurrent symptomatic ischemia that required hospitalization. The 80 mg/day dose of atorvastatin showed greater absolute lowering of LDL levels than was previously achieved in the 4 S (36%), CARE (28%), or LIPID (25%) studies, but it should be noted that the timing of therapy and follow-up in these trials differ.

In March 2004, data were presented from the Pravastatin or Atorvastatin Evaluation and Infection Therapy trial (PROVE IT [TIMI-22]) at the American

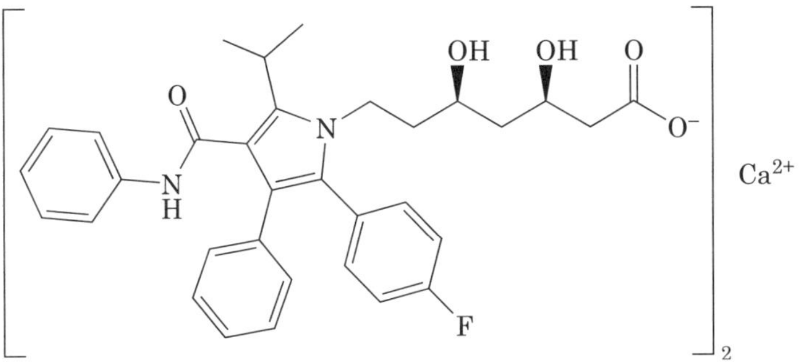

FIGURE 21. *Structure of atorvastatin calcium.*

College of Cardiology Annual Scientific Session in New Orleans (Cannon CP, 2004). This trial compared treatment with pravastatin 40 mg/day (standard therapy) or atorvastatin 80 mg/day (aggressive therapy) in 4,162 patients with a confirmed MI up to ten days previously, with a follow-up of up to 2.5 years. For the combined incidence rates of all-cause mortality, nonfatal MI, and urgent revascularization, the group receiving aggressive atorvastatin treatment showed a highly significant reduction compared with the standard therapy group (16.7% versus 12.9%, risk reduction = 25%, $p = 0.0004$). More patients in the aggressive therapy arm experienced myalgia, although none of the myalgia cases were severe. Also, a significantly higher number of patients receiving aggressive therapy had alanine aminotransferase levels three times the upper limit of normal than the standard therapy group (3.3% versus 1.1%, $p < 0.001$). This trial clearly demonstrated that PMI patients can benefit from early intervention with high-dose atorvastatin. Using a similar treatment regimen, the Reversing Atherosclerosis with Aggressive Lipid Lowering (REVERSAL) study in 654 patients with CAD demonstrated that high-dose atorvastatin (80 mg) therapy led to a statistically nonsignificant improvement in atheroma volume as measured by intravascular ultrasound (IVUS), whereas with moderate dose pravastatin (40 mg), the atheroma volume continued to increase (Nissen S, 2003).

Recent data from the Aggressive Lipid-Lowering Initiation Ablates New Cardiac Events (ALLIANCE) trial has demonstrated an improvement in outcomes associated with aggressive atorvastatin therapy in high-risk patients. This study enrolled 2,442 patients with a history of coronary heart disease (CHD). The aim of the study was to establish whether intensive lipid-lowering with atorvastatin would reduce cardiovascular events to a greater extent than usual care (i.e., lipid-lowering treatment that includes lifestyle modifications such as diet and exercise, and drug treatment if necessary). Patients began the study on 10 mg of atorvastatin; the dose was titrated upward until an LDL cholesterol level of less than 80 mg/dL was reached. (The maximum dose of atorvastatin used was 80 mg). The investigators reported that patients taking atorvastatin experienced 47% fewer nonfatal heart attacks compared with patients receiving usual care. Patients in the atorvastatin arm also experienced a 17% reduction in overall negative cardio-vascular outcomes, including cardiac death, MIs, and strokes (Koren MJ, 2004).

Several trials of high-dose atorvastatin are ongoing, including the Incremental Decrease in Endpoints Through Aggressive Lipid Lowering (IDEAL) trial, which was initiated in April 1999 to investigate aggressive long-term therapy with atorvastatin in comparison with a conventional lipid-lowering regimen with simvastatin. The trial design required that more than 7,600 patients under the age of 78 and with current or prior MI were recruited, randomized to either atorvastatin (80 mg/day) or simvastatin (20–40 mg/day), and followed for 5.5 years.

Results were expected back in 2004 but were finally presented in November 2005. These data showed that the incidence of major coronary events did not differ significantly between the simvastatin and atorvastatin arms of the study.

Rosuvastatin. Rosuvastatin (Crestor) (Figure 22) was developed by AstraZeneca under license from Shionogi Pharmaceuticals (Osaka, Japan). This agent was launched for the treatment of hyperlipidemia in its first market, Canada, in February 2003. By the end of 2003, rosuvastatin was launched for hyperlipidemia in the United States and several European countries, including France and the United Kingdom. In October 2004, rosuvastatin received a positive recommendation from Japan's Ministry of Health, Labor, and Welfare's Advisory Food and Drugs Sanitation Council and the drug was indeed finally launched in Japan in 2005.

Germany, Spain, and Norway, however, have withdrawn from the European mutual recognition (MR) process. Launches in these countries are currently on hold as further safety data are awaited. Furthermore, due to the new reference pricing scheme for statins in Germany, AstraZeneca has expressed serious doubt as to whether rosuvastatin will ever be launched in this country. Rosuvastatin is currently in Phase III trials for atherosclerosis in the United States and Western Europe. Although AstraZeneca expects rosuvastatin to be approved for this indication in 2006, the drug is used off-label in PMI patients because of its potency and the continuing drive to achieve lipid targets in secondary prevention populations.

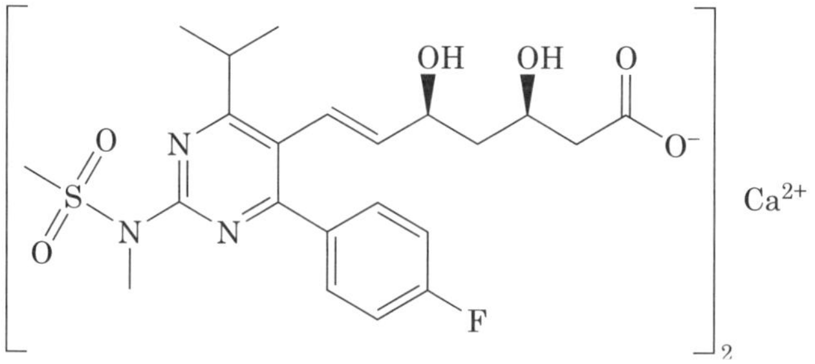

FIGURE 22. *Structure of rosuvastatin calcium.*

Rosuvastatin shares a common mechanism of action with other statins and has a low affinity for lipids (similar to that of pravastatin). As a result, rosuvastatin selectively accumulates in hepatocytes, the cell type within which statins exert their effect. In contrast to many other statins, rosuvastatin does not appear to undergo significant hepatic metabolism via the cytochrome P450 system, and has a relatively long half-life (20 hours), meaning it is effective over a longer period of time than other statins.

Rosuvastatin's main advantage over other statins is its potency. In a multi-center clinical trial, more than 500 patients with primary hypercholesterolemia were randomized to receive 5 mg or 10 mg rosuvastatin or 20 mg pravastatin or simvastatin for 12 weeks. The 5 mg and 10 mg doses of rosuvastatin reduced LDL cholesterol by 42% and 49%, respectively, compared with 28% for pravastatin and 37% for simvastatin ($p < 0.001$ and $p < 0.01$, respectively). Serum apolipoprotein B levels were also lower in the rosuvastatin-treated groups (Paoletti R, 2001). Another study treated 477 patients with rosuvastatin (5 mg or 10 mg), pravastatin (20 mg), or simvastatin (20 mg). After 12 weeks, if treatment goals were not achieved, the statin dose was titrated upward. At 12 weeks, statistically significant decreases in LDL levels were observed in the 5 mg and 10 mg rosuvastatin-treated patients compared with patients who had received 20 mg pravastatin and simvastatin (39%, 47%, 27%, and 35%, respectively; $p < 0.05$). After dose titration, 88% of the rosuvastatin 5 mg and 10 mg groups achieved their LDL cholesterol goals, compared with 60% for pravastatin and 72.5% for simvastatin. Additionally, a greater increase in HDL levels and a greater reduction in triglyceride (TG) levels were observed in patients treated with rosuvastatin (Brown WV, 2002).

The Measuring Effective Reductions in Cholesterol Using Rosuvastatin Therapy (MERCURY I) trial examined the effect of switching from other statins to rosuvastatin. This open-label study randomized 3161 high-risk patients to rosuvastatin (10 or 20 mg), atorvastatin (10 or 20 mg), simvastatin, or pravastatin treatment. After 8 weeks, one-fourth of the patients were switched to treatment with 10 mg rosuvastatin, with another one-fourth switched to 20 mg rosuvastatin for a further 8 weeks. At 16 weeks, patients switching from 10 mg atorvastatin to 10 mg rosuvastatin showed greater decreases in LDL compared with patients remaining on 10 mg atorvastatin (46% versus 38%; $p < 0.001$); more patients treated with rosuvastatin reached Third Report of the National Cholesterol Education Program (NCEP) Adult Treatment Panel (ATP III) treatment goals (46% versus 38%; $p < 0.001$). Greater increases in HDL cholesterol were also observed. However, no significant difference was observed when patients were switched from a 20 mg dose of atorvastatin (Schuster H, 2003).

The STELLAR (Statin Therapies for Elevated Lipid Levels Compared Across Doses to Rosuvastatin) study compared 10, 20, 40, and 80 mg rosuvastatin to equivalent doses of atorvastatin, simvastatin, and pravastatin in 2431 hypercholesterolemic patients. Results showed that, dose for dose, rosuvastatin lowered LDL and raised HDL to a significantly greater degree than any of the other statins (Jones PH, 2003).

AstraZeneca is also trying to differentiate rosuvastatin from atorvastatin on its comparative efficacy in raising HDL. This effect is particularly relevant to atherosclerosis and metabolic syndrome. In a subgroup analysis of the STELLAR trial of patients with diagnosed metabolic syndrome, significantly greater increases in HDL were seen in patients treated with rosuvastatin 20 mg/day than with atorvastatin 80 mg/day ($p < 0.002$). The Comparative Study with Rosuvastatin in Subjects with Metabolic Syndrome (COMETS) trial has also demonstrated the efficacy of rosuvastatin in metabolic syndrome patients. This trial compared the effects of rosuvastatin and atorvastatin (10 mg/day) with placebo over six weeks, followed by 20 mg/day of either statin for a further six weeks, in 397 metabolic syndrome patients. At six weeks, rosuvastatin led to a significantly greater reduction in LDL than atorvastatin (42% versus 36%, $p < 0.001$); this significant reduction was maintained at week 12 (Stalenhoef AFH, 2004). Levels of HDL cholesterol were also raised significantly more after rosuvastatin therapy (9.3%) than after atorvastatin treatment (4.8%).

Recent trials have demonstrated the efficacy of rosuvastatin over atorvastatin in patients with type 2 diabetes and dyslipidemia. In the 263-patient CORALL (Compare the Effect of Rosuvastatin with Atorvastatin on Apo B/Apo A-1 Ratio in Patients with Type 2 Diabetes Mellitus and Dyslipidaemia) trial, rosuvastatin 10 mg, 20 mg, and 40 mg reduced cholesterol significantly greater at 18 weeks than did atorvastatin 20 mg, 40 mg, and 80 mg (all $p < 0.05$), with 90% of patients receiving the highest dose of rosuvastatin achieving European LDL-cholesterol goals (<2.5 mmol/L), compared with 78% of those on the highest dose of atorvastatin (Wolffenbuttel BHR, 2004). Two other studies, ANDROMEDA (A Randomised, Double Blind, Double Dummy, Multicenter Phase IIIb Parallel Group Study to Compare the Efficacy and Safety of Rosuvastatin [10 mg and 20 mg] and Atorvastatin [10 mg and 20 mg] in Subjects with Type II Diabetes Mellitus) and URANUS (Use of Rosuvastatin Versus Atorvastatin in Type 2 Diabetes Mellitus Subjects) demonstrated greater reductions in C-reactive protein (CRP), TG, and non-HDL cholesterol with rosuvastatin compared with equal doses of atorvastatin (Berne C, 2004; Betteridge DJ, 2004).

Three ongoing studies in the GALAXY program are investigating the effects of rosuvastatin on atherosclerosis reflected by thickening of the arterial walls. The Measuring Effects on Intima Media Thickness: An Evaluation of Rosuvastatin (METEOR) study will evaluate rosuvastatin on the progression of carotid atherosclerosis by measuring intima media thickness (IMT) in low-risk hypercholesterolemic subjects with subclinical evidence of atherosclerosis. A Study to Evaluate the Effect of Rosuvastatin on Intravascular Ultrasound-Derived Coronary Atheroma Burden (ASTEROID) is using intravascular ultrasound (IVUS) and quantitative coronary angiography (QCA) to assess the effects of rosuvastatin on the regression of coronary atherosclerosis in patients with coronary artery disease (CAD) who require coronary angiography. The Outcome of Rosuvastatin Treatment on Carotid Artery Atheroma: A Magnetic Resonance Imaging Observation (ORION) trial is a small study ($n = 39$) examining the effect of high- and low-dose rosuvastatin on carotid atheroma volume in patients with moderate hypercholesterolemia and asymptomatic carotid stenosis.

Recruitment for METEOR and ASTEROID studies is now complete. Data from ORION were announced in April 2005 and showed that low and high doses of rosuvastatin significantly reduced the proportion of lipid-rich necrotic core the most diseased area of atherosclerotic plaques.

Despite assurances of the safety of rosuvastatin (rosuvastatin has been to reported to have an adverse-event profile similar to that of other statins and does not produce significant increases in creatinine kinase levels [Olsson AG, 2002]), ongoing concerns have tempered its early uptake. Myopathy was reported in Phase III trials in some patients receiving the 80 mg dose (Shepherd J, 2001); subsequently, AstraZeneca voluntarily withdrew this dose of rosuvastatin. Following approval, AstraZeneca was forced to issue a letter to European health professionals in June 2004 advising that all patients should be started on the 10 mg dose, and titrated to 20 mg only after four weeks. The letter also stated the 40 mg dose should only be used under specialist supervision. This letter, which also prompted the FDA to issue a reminder, followed postmarketing surveillance, which highlighted an increased risk of myopathy in certain populations (including the elderly and patients with hypothyroidism or renal insufficiency), especially at the 40 mg dose (FDA, 2004).

Other safety concerns have been raised over rosuvastatin after the report of a significant interaction between the drug and warfarin. One case report noted a patient's international normalized ratio (INR) went from a stable 2.0 to 8.0 and resulted in bruising and hematurea (Barry M, 2004). AstraZeneca has conducted a series of studies investigating potential interactions between vitamin K antagonists (the class of agents to which warfarin belongs) and rosuvastatin, and the company has emphasized that patients receiving warfarin and rosuvastatin (or any other statin) in combination should be carefully monitored. Furthermore, a significant interaction between rosuvastatin and gemfibrozil (Pfizer's Lopid/Lipur, generics) has been noted, precluding coadministration of these drugs.

Pitavastatin. Nissan Chemical Industries (Tokyo, Japan), Kowa Kyogo (Tokyo, Japan), and Novartis have codeveloped and launched pitavastatin (also known as Livalo, itavastatin/nisvastatin, and NK-104) (Figure 23). Pitavastatin was launched in Japan in September 2003 for hypercholesterolemia. Phase II trials for the treatment of hypercholesterolemia are ongoing in Europe and the United States. Although not in clinical development specifically for atherosclerosis at present, pitavastatin is likely to be used off-label for this indication in PMI patients. Sankyo shares Japanese and U.S. comarketing rights for pitavastatin with Kowa Kogyo; European marketing rights are split between Kowa Kogyo and Novartis. Kowa Kogyo has also signed a licensing agreement with Recordati to market pitavastatin in Italy.

Pitavastatin is a competitive inhibitor of HMG-CoA reductase, the rate-limiting enzyme in the cholesterol biosynthesis pathway. Although the enzymes P450-29 C and P450-28 C are involved in pitavastatin's metabolism, the agent has a low

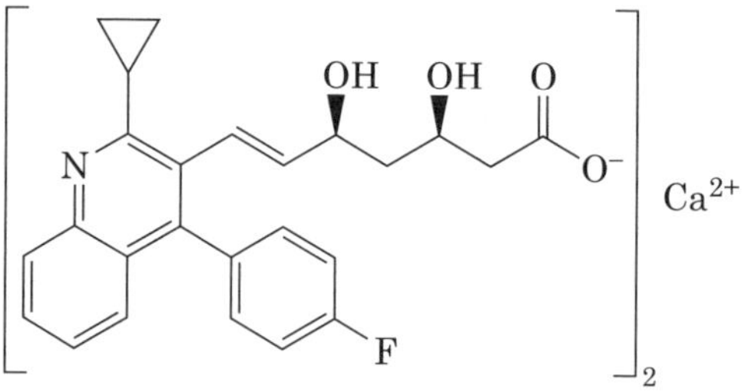

FIGURE 23. *Structure of pitavastatin calcium.*

affinity for them, thus reducing the potential for drug interactions (Kajinami K, 2003). Pitavastatin can be safely administered with fibrates, including gemfibrozil, because these drugs do not affect the agent's metabolism.

Reflecting widespread concerns about safety of the emerging statins, the Japanese Pharmaceutical and Medical Device Evaluation Centre (PMDEC) requested extended safety data for pitavastatin. Nissan submitted supplemental data in January 2002. Long-term safety data for pitavastatin are scarce. However, only one adverse reaction was noted following 122 weeks of treatment in 25 heterozygous familial hypercholesterolemia patients (Noji Y, 2002). Also, patients achieved significant reductions in LDL and total serum cholesterol (TSC) (49% and 37%, respectively) at week 12.

One 12-week, randomized, multicenter, double-blind, controlled study in 240 patients with primary hypercholesterolemia receiving pitavastatin (2 mg/day) or pravastatin (Sankyo's Mevalotin; 10 mg/day) showed LDL reductions that were significantly greater in the pitavastatin treatment arm than with pravastatin (37.6% and 18.4% decreases from baseline levels, respectively). Equivalent increases in HDL were noted in the two treatment arms, although TG reductions were significantly greater in the pitavastatin group (Saito Y, 2002). The agents exhibited similar safety profiles, although longer treatment regimens in larger populations are required to compete with the safety data acquired by pravastatin.

Lovastatin. Lovastatin (Merck's Mevacor, Schwarz Pharma's Lioscler) (Figure 24), launched in 1987, was the first statin to be approved in the United States. Sankyo and Merck developed this drug, with Merck obtaining several marketing licenses, but Sankyo's patent rights precluded launch in most Western European countries and Japan. Lovastatin is currently marketed only in the United States, Japan, Germany, and Spain. Like other statins, lovastatin is a competitive inhibitor of HMG-CoA reductase.

Lovastatin has not been fully investigated in the PMI population; however, in a primary prevention study, the 6,605-patient Air Force/Texas Coronary Atherosclerosis Prevention Study (AF/TexCAPS), lovastatin reduced the incidence of first coronary event by 37% compared with placebo (Downs JR, 1998).

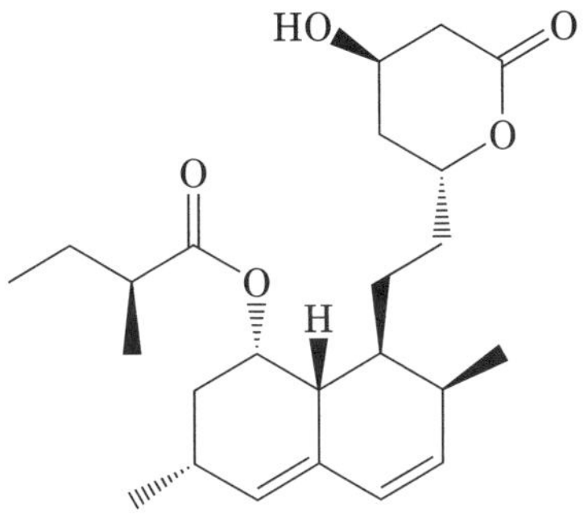

FIGURE 24. Structure of lovastatin.

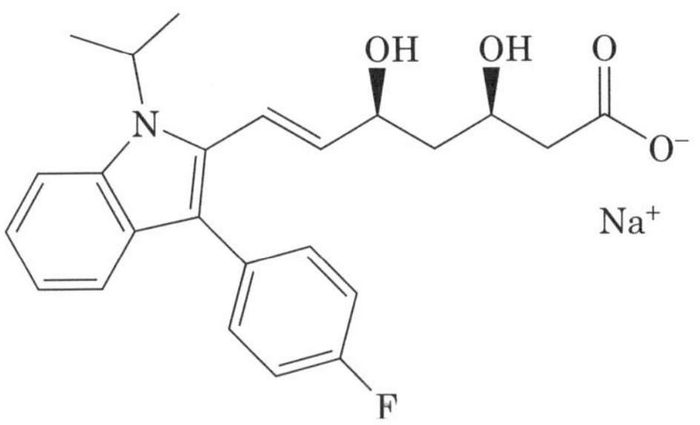

FIGURE 25. Structure of fluvastatin.

Fluvastatin. Fluvastatin (Novartis's Lescol, Solvay's [Brussels, Belgium] Digaril) (Figure 25) was launched in 1994 and is available in all of the major pharmaceutical markets. Its mechanism of action is as described in the "Mechanism of Action" section for statins.

The Fluvastatin on Risk Diminishing After Acute Myocardial Infarction (FLORIDA) study examined the effectiveness of early administration of fluvastatin (80 mg/day) following MI. This placebo-controlled trial followed 540 patients for one year post-MI; primary end points were residual myocardial ischemia at one year or clinical events (including cardiovascular death or recurrent MI). Investigators found that fluvastatin did not confer a statistically significant benefit in either end point, although following post-hoc the analysis authors concluded that the trials may have been statistically underpowered to detect the end points (Liem AH, 2002). In contrast, the Fluvastatin Angioplasty Restenosis (FLARE) trial identified a benefit of early fluvastatin treatment (relative to placebo following coronary balloon angioplasty). Patients with primary coronary artery lesion, who were scheduled to undergo elective coronary angioplasty and presented with LDL in excess of 160 mg/dL were randomized to either fluvastatin (80 mg/day, $n = 526$) or placebo ($n = 528$) two weeks prior to treatment and were followed for 40 weeks. Although fluvastatin did not reduce the rate of restenosis, it did significantly reduce the incidence of a combined end point of death and MI from 4% in the placebo group to 1.4% in the active group.

Cholesterol Absorption Inhibitors

Overview. The uptake of dietary cholesterol from the intestine presents a potential target for cholesterol-lowering agents. The use of a cholesterol absorption inhibitor in combination with a statin may result in additive or synergistic cholesterol-lowering effects because statins inhibit the endogenous hepatic production of cholesterol.

Mechanism of Action. Dietary and biliary cholesterol is absorbed in the form of bile acid micelles into enterocytes in the small intestine. Recent evidence suggests that this process is not passive; rather, it is mediated via specific cholesterol transporters. Cholesterol absorption inhibitors interfere with this process at the enterocyte brush border in the intestine.

Ezetimibe. Ezetimibe (Zetia/Ezeterol) (Figure 26) is the first selective cholesterol absorption inhibitor to reach the market. Developed as a joint venture between Merck and Schering-Plough (Kenilworth, New Jersey), it was launched in the United States and Germany in October 2002 for hypercholesterolemia. In March 2003, ezetimibe completed the European Union's MR process and was launched in the United Kingdom for hypercholesterolemia. Subsequent launches in France and Spain have followed.

Recent evidence suggests that the inhibition of cholesterol by ezetimibe is mediated through the Niemann-Pick C1 Like-1 (NCP1L1) protein, found in the brush border membrane of enterocytes. NCP1L1 knockout mice absorb less cholesterol from the gut, and cholesterol absorption is unaffected when the diet is supplemented with bile acids. Ezetimibe had no effect on serum cholesterol levels in these animals, which suggests that this protein is crucial to the drug's mechanism of action (Altmann SW, 2004).

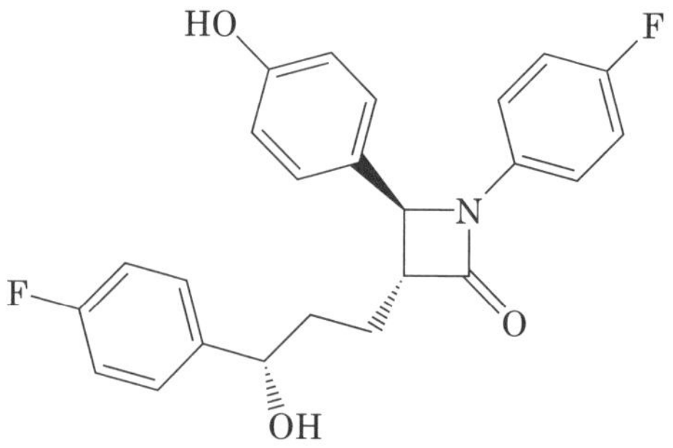

FIGURE 26. *Structure of ezetimibe.*

In a Phase III study, the effects of 10 mg/day ezetimibe versus placebo were investigated in 827 primary hypercholesterolemic patients (LDL 130–250 mg/dL, TG less than or equal to 350 mg/dL [Knopp RH, 2001]). Treatment with the drug significantly reduced LDL by 17.7% (versus a 0.8% reduction with placebo) and increased HDL by 1.0% (versus a decrease of 1.3% with placebo).

The efficacy of ezetimibe in lowering cholesterol levels has been assessed in combination with statin therapy (Gagne C, 2002[a]). Patients at high cardiovascular risk receiving statins but not achieving ATP II goals had either placebo ($n = 390$) or 10 mg/day ezetimibe ($n = 379$) added to their existing regimens. Approximately one-third of patients were receiving therapy with atorvastatin, one-third were receiving simvastatin, and one-third were receiving other statins at a range of doses. Highly significant reductions in LDL and TGs (25% versus 4%, and 14% versus 3%), coupled with significant increases in HDL (2.7% versus 1.0%), were observed in the group receiving ezetimibe when compared with placebo controls. These changes were achieved within the first two weeks of the study and persisted until the 15-week end point. Of the patients receiving ezetimibe, 71.5% reached treatment goals at the study's end point compared with 18.9% of patients receiving placebo ($p < 0.001$). The addition of ezetimibe to statin therapy was well tolerated, with no cases of myopathy reported in the ezetimibe-treated group, proving that the addition of ezetimibe to statin therapy is safe and efficacious.

In a further study (Davidson MH, 2002), 668 patients with primary hypercholesterolemia were treated with simvastatin at 10, 20, 40, or 80 mg/day; simvastatin at these doses plus 10 mg ezetimibe, ezetimibe alone, or placebo. When the doses were pooled, the simvastatin/ezetimibe treatment produced a reduction in LDL of 50% versus 36% in the group receiving simvastatin only ($p < 0.01$). TG levels fell by 24% versus 17% for simvastatin only ($p < 0.01$), and HDL_3 (a subfraction of HDL) was increased by 7.5% versus 3.8% ($p = 0.16$).

In separate studies, ezetimibe has also been evaluated in combination with a range of doses of lovastatin, pravastatin, and atorvastatin. When 192 patients receiving lovastatin and ezetimibe were compared with 220 patients receiving lovastatin only, highly significant reductions in LDL (39% versus 25%), TG (22% versus 11%) and increases in HDL3 (7% versus 3%) were observed (Kerzner B, 2003). Similarly, 255 patients with primary hypercholesterolemia receiving an ezetimibe/atorvastatin combination produced statistically significant reductions in LDL and TG (12.1% and 8.0%, respectively) and increases in HDL (3.0%) compared with atorvastatin monotherapy ($n = 248$; Ballantyne CM, 2003). A pravastatin/ezetimibe combination showed significantly different changes in LDL and TG (reductions of 13.5% and 10.0%, respectively) compared with pravastatin/placebo, while the increase in HDL was 1.4%.

More recently, ezetimibe has been shown to produce incremental decreases in LDL of approximately 16% when used in combination with 10 mg rosuvastatin compared with rosuvastatin monotherapy (Kosoglou T, 2004). Coadministration of the drugs was well tolerated.

Ezetimibe has a side-effect profile similar to that of placebo. Gastrointestinal disorders were reported in approximately 1% of patients (Gagne C, 2002). A slight increase in serum transaminases has been reported in patients receiving concurrent ezetimibe and statin therapy. Myopathy and rhabdomyolysis have not been associated with ezetimibe treatment. However, following routine postmarketing monitoring of adverse events, Merck and Schering-Plough announced that they were to include a warning that ezetimibe can cause allergic reactions, including angioedema and rash, on the label for the drug. The safety and effectiveness of ezetimibe in combination with fibrates have not yet been established.

Nonpharmacological Approaches

A patient who survives AMI is typically informed of lifestyle changes that can help prevent subsequent MI and other secondary cardiac events. AHA guidelines recommend several changes, including the complete cessation of smoking, regular physical activity, weight management, and improvements in diet.

Smoking increases serum levels of detrimental very-low-density lipoprotein (VLDL) cholesterol, lowers HDL, increases platelet aggregation, and raises fibrinogen levels, promoting thrombus formation. Evidence from the AHA, which estimates that 25–30% of patients with CHD still smoke after diagnosis, and from the EUROASPIRE II study, which shows that smoking habits prevail in 21% of patients with established CHD, highlights the difficulty of smoking cessation.

Compliance with exercise programs is generally poor. Following AMI, many patients are left unemployed or take early retirement; this transition can diminish their opportunity and inclination to engage in physical activity. Also, many PMI patients fear that exercise will provoke complications. Cardiac rehabilitation clinics can help educate PMI patients about exercise regimens that improve outcomes; however, rehabilitation schemes are not widely available in all countries. Estimates from the CCP suggest that 62–89% of patients do not receive cardiac rehabilitation; these proportions translate to 8–12 million patients in the United States.

Dietary modifications that reduce lipid intake—in particular, saturated dietary fats—complement pharmacological treatments for managing blood lipids. Results from the Lyon Diet Heart Study indicate a 50–70% reduction in recurrent heart disease in patients following a defined "Mediterranean-style" diet (Kris-Etherton P, 2001; Robertson RM, 2001). Investigators concluded that significant dietary modification generates benefits comparable to those seen with pharmaceutical intervention. However, as with other lifestyle recommendations, compliance with dietary treatment protocols remains poor.

EMERGING THERAPIES

The aim of pharmacotherapy in post-myocardial infarction (PMI) is to reduce the likelihood of the patient having a further acute coronary event. Many pharmacotherapies are available that effectively stabilize the patient, improve heart function after myocardial infarction (MI), and halt the progression of atherosclerosis, thereby reducing risk of future coronary events. Furthermore, second- or even third-line options are often available if initial therapies are ineffective. As a result, PMI is not an area of great unmet pharmacological need. Multiple agents within each drug class and upcoming patent expiries are also limiting development of "me-too" therapies within established drug classes.

There remains, however, a lack of agents that are capable of reversing atherogenesis, which is the major factor in recurrent coronary events. Drugs currently in development target multiple mechanisms responsible for atherosclerotic plaque formation, progression, and rupture. One advance that is generating special interest is the development of novel treatments for non-low-density lipoprotein (LDL) abnormalities—low levels of high-density lipoprotein (HDL) in particular.

PMI is a disease state that is often not defined consistently, which creates problems in designing clinical trials. Hence there are relatively few agents specifically in development for PMI. Instead, most emerging agents discussed in this section target specific components of PMI, such as atherosclerosis, dyslipidemia, or restenosis; once launched, these agents are likely to be used off-label in PMI. Although these emerging agents are unlikely to replace established drug classes, they may be used as adjuncts to existing therapies. The challenge will be to find the most effective and complementary combination of drugs. Table 2 lists emerging agents for the treatment of PMI and details their development phases for the cardiovascular disease (CVD) indications where there is activity.

Statin Combinations

Overview. Many combination therapies—single pills containing two or more individual drugs—are in development for cardiovascular indications. Of these, fixed-dose combinations containing a statin are the most likely to have an impact on the PMI market in the near term.

There are several rationales for developing combination pills. By combining agents with the same target (e.g., lowering LDL cholesterol), a synergistic effect may be achieved, maximizing the therapeutic effect while minimizing adverse events associated with each individual agent. Combination therapies are also being developed to aid convenience in multidrug regimens, and are also seen as a way of protecting individual agents' brand franchises.

Mechanism of Action. Single-pill combination therapies incorporate the mechanisms of action of each individual agent into a single-pill formulation, as discussed in the following sections.

Simvastatin/Ezetimibe. Merck and Schering-Plough have codeveloped a once-daily, fixed-combination tablet of the statin simvastatin (Zocor) and the cholesterol-absorption inhibitor ezetimibe (Zetia). In April 2004, the pill was launched as Inegy in Germany (which acted as the mutual recognition state for the European Union) for hypercholesterolemia. This launch was followed in

TABLE 2. Emerging Therapies in Development for Post-Myocardial Infarction

Compound	Development Phase	Marketing Company
Statin combinations		
Simvastatin/ezetimibe[a]		
United States	III	Merck/Schering-Plough
Europe	III	Merck/Schering Plough
Japan	—	—
Atorvastatin/torcetrapib		
United States	III	Pfizer
Europe	—	—
Japan	—	—
Simvastatin/niacin		
United States	III	Kos Pharmaceuticals
Europe	—	—
Japan	—	—
Cholesterol ester transfer protein inhibitors		
JTT-705		
United States	—	—
Europe	II	Japan Tobacco
Japan	I	Japan Tobacco
CETi-1		
United States	II	Avant Immunotherapeutics
Europe	—	—
Japan	—	—
Acyl CoA cholesterol acetyltransferase inhibitors		
Pactimibe		
United States	D	Sankyo/Kyoto
Europe	D	Sankyo/Kyoto
Japan	D	Sankyo/Kyoto
Eflucimibe (F-12511)		
United States	—	—
Europe	II	Pierre Fabre/Eli Lilly
Japan	—	—
Antiplatelet agents		
Prasugrel (CS-747)		
United States	II	Sankyo/Eli Lilly
Europe	II	Sankyo/Eli Lilly
Japan	I	Sankyo/Eli Lilly
NCX-4016		
United States	—	—
Europe	II	NicOx
Japan	—	—
S-18886		
United States	—	—
Europe	II	Servier
Japan	—	—
Z-335		
United States	—	—
Europe	—	—
Japan	II	Zeria Pharmaceutical

TABLE 2. (*continued*)

Compound	Development Phase	Marketing Company
Anticoagulants		
Ximelagatran (Exanta)		
United States	W	AstraZeneca
Europe	W	AstraZeneca
Japan	—	—
Reverse lipid transport pathway		
activators		
ETC-216		
United States	II	Pfizer
Europe	—	—
Japan	—	—
ETC-588		
United States	II	Pfizer
Europe	—	—
Japan	—	—
Antioxidants/vascular protectants		
AGI-1067		
United States	III	AtheroGenics
Europe	I	AtheroGenics
Japan	—	—
BO-653		
United States	II	Roche/Chugai
Europe	—	—
Japan	I	Roche/Chugai
Growth factor receptors		
BioBypass		
United States	II	GenVec
Europe	—	—
Japan	—	—
Stem-cell therapy		
MyoCell		
United States	I	Bioheart
Europe	II	Bioheart
Japan	—	—
Myoblast cell therapy		
United States	I	GenVec
Europe	—	—
Japan	—	—

[a]Currently marketed for hypercholesterolemia/dyslipidemia.
D = Discontinued; PC = Preclinical (including discovery); M = Marketed; PR = Preregistered; R = Registered; W = Withdrawn.

July by another in the United States (as Vytorin), also for hypercholesterolemia; and in June 2005, Simvastatin/Ezetimibe was launched in the United Kingdom. The fixed-dose combination is available in several dosing strengths: (simvastatin/ezetimibe) 10/10 mg, 20/10 mg, 40/10 mg, and 80/10 mg.

Operating through two different mechanisms—hydroxymethyl glutaryl (HMG)-CoA reductase inhibition (simvastatin) and inhibition of cholesterol absorption (ezetimibe)—the combination therapy promises a synergistic, cholesterol-lowering effect, improved control of triglyceride (TG) levels, and the prospect of improved patient compliance.

A trial in 100 patients (42 of whom had coronary heart disease [CHD]) with baseline LDL $\geq$130 mg/dL and TG $\geq$350 mg/dL demonstrated how coadministration of ezetimibe with ongoing simvastatin therapy can provide significantly greater LDL reduction than doubling the simvastatin dose alone: Patients prescribed simvastatin (40 mg) achieved an 11.1% change in LDL levels while a 24.5% decrease was reported for the cohort prescribed simvastatin/ezetimibe (20 mg/10 mg). Importantly, coadministration of ezetimibe and simvastatin is reported to be well tolerated, with a safety profile similar to that of simvastatin alone (Davidson MH, 2002).

A recent study compared the efficacy of the simvastatin/ezetimibe combination with that of atorvastatin in 781 patients with hypercholesterolemia. The trial lasted 24 weeks, and was divided into four six-week treatment phases, with a dose titration step at each phase. Patients were randomized to receive atorvastatin starting at 10 mg/day, titrated up to 80 mg/day, or simvastatin/ezetimibe 10 mg/10 mg, titrated up to 80 mg/10 mg. A third treatment arm started at simvastatin/ezetimibe 20 mg/10 mg, titrated to 40 mg/10 mg for two periods, then 80 mg/10 mg. Results demonstrate that at the end of the first six-week period, reductions in LDL and the mean increase in HDL were significantly greater ($p < 0.01$) for the 10/10 mg simvastatin/ezetimibe group and the 20/10 mg simvastatin/ezetimibe group than for the 10 mg atorvastatin group. At the maximum dose, the combination proved superior to atorvastatin with respect to reduction in LDL ($-59.4%$ versus $-52.5%$ change from baseline) and increase in HDL ($+12.3%$ versus $+6.5%$ change from baseline) (Ballantyne CM, 2004).

The recent issuing of more-stringent cholesterol goals by the National Cholesterol Education Program, third report of the Adult Treatment Panel (NCEP ATP III) is likely to raise confidence in simvastatin/ezetimibe, especially in the light of another recent study that investigated whether simvastatin/ezetimibe would be more effective than simvastatin monotherapy in allowing high-risk patients to achieve the NCEP ATP III LDL cholesterol goal of less than 100 mg/dL. Seven hundred and ten patients with hypercholesterolemia and CHD or CHD risk equivalents were randomized to 23 weeks' treatment with simvastatin 20 mg, simvastatin/ezetimibe 10 mg/10 mg, simvastatin/ezetimibe 20 mg/10 mg, or simvastatin/ezetimibe 40 mg/10 mg. Patients not at goal had their simvastatin doses doubled at weeks 6, 12, and/or 18, up to a maximum of 80 mg. Ezetimibe plus any dose of simvastatin produced greater reductions in LDL cholesterol and allowed more patients to achieve goal after 5 weeks ($p < 0.001$) and at the end of the study ($p < 0.001$) than simvastatin 20 mg alone. Fewer patients receiving the simvastatin/ezetimibe combination required dose titration to reach goal (Feldman T, 2004).

Additionally, Merck and Schering-Plough have announced that they are initiating a large-scale study of simvastatin/ezetimibe in a secondary prevention population; the IMPROVE IT (Improved Reduction of Outcomes: VYTORIN

Efficacy International) trial will evaluate the efficacy of simvastatin/ezetimibe (40 mg/10 mg) compared with simvastatin alone (40 mg) in reducing death and major coronary events in 10,000 patients with acute coronary syndromes (ACS) over two years. This population includes patients with unstable angina (UA), non-ST-segment-elevation acute myocardial infarction (NSTEMI), and ST-segment-elevation acute myocardial infarction (STEMI) and should provide firm evidence for prescribing simvastatin/ezetimibe in the PMI population.

Atorvastatin/Torcetrapib. Pfizer is developing a combination of the cholesterol ester transfer protein (CETP) inhibitor torcetrapib (CP-529414) and its blockbuster statin atorvastatin (Lipitor) for treatment of atherosclerosis and dyslipidemia. Torcetrapib was formerly in Phase II development as a monotherapy, but in late 2003 the atorvastatin/torcetrapib combination progressed into Phase III clinical trials in the United States, and it now seems likely the monotherapy will not be released in favor of the combination.

Pfizer has been concentrating on the atorvastatin/torcetrapib combination for the past couple of years but recently (in February 2006), the company announced that it may market torcetrapib as a single agent after all.

The dual mechanism of action—HMG-CoA reductase inhibition and CETP inhibition—will simultaneously decrease LDL and increase HDL.

Company-reported data indicate that the combination—if used across the entire statin dose range—can raise HDL by more than 50% while lowering LDL as much as 80%. In trials in which atherosclerotic patients were given 90 mg/day of torcetrapib in combination with 20 mg/day atorvastatin, the addition of torcetrapib generated an incremental 15% reduction in LDL over the reduction achieved with the statin monotherapy; the HDL-raising efficacy of torcetrapib was not adversely affected in combination with atorvastatin.

A recent single-blind, placebo-controlled clinical study investigated the actions of torcetrapib both as a monotherapy and in combination with atorvastatin (20 mg) (Brousseau ME, 2004). Nineteen patients were enrolled; nine received atorvastatin and ten did not. All subjects received placebo for the first four weeks of the study, followed by 120 mg of torcetrapib daily for an additional four weeks. Six patients in the nonatorvastatin arm received 120 mg of torcetrapib twice daily for an additional four weeks. Results showed a 61% increase in plasma HDL in the atorvastatin group following treatment with 120 mg of torcetrapib daily; a 46% increase was seen in patients not on statin therapy. Treatment with 120 mg of torcetrapib twice daily during the additional study period increased HDL by 106%. A further reduction in LDL levels of 17% was observed in the atorvastatin/torcetrapib treatment arm ($p = 0.02$). CHD is generally associated with low levels of large HDL particles and higher levels of small, dense LDL particles; in this study, the number of large HDL particles increased significantly with torcetrapib treatment. Torcetrapib was well tolerated at the doses used in this trial.

The effects of torcetrapib monotherapy have been highlighted in several clinical studies. A recently published Phase I study investigated the HDL-raising properties of torcetrapib in healthy young adults (Clark RW, 2004). Five groups of eight patients were randomized to receive 10, 30, 60, or 120 mg daily for 14 days, or 120 mg twice daily for 14 days. CETP inhibition with the agent dose-dependently increased HDL by 16–91%. In the group treated with 120 mg torcetrapib twice daily, apolipoprotein (Apo) A-I and E were elevated 27% and 66%, respectively, and ApoB was reduced 26%. Researchers noted that the effects of CETP inhibition observed in this study are similar to those observed in CETP-deficient subjects.

Pfizer is currently involved in several imaging trials in the United States that are examining changes in plaque morphology associated with torcetrapib treatment. However, whether these imaging studies will be accepted by the medical community as a surrogate to end point data is uncertain.

Simvastatin/Niacin. Kos Pharmaceuticals (Miami, Florida) is developing a combination of its extended-release niacin product, Niaspan, with simvastatin (Merck's Zocor) (Kos Pharmaceuticals, 2004). This product is likely to replace the existing product Advicor (a combination of niacin and lovastatin currently available for the treatment of hypercholesterolemia in the United States). Kos hopes to file a new drug application (NDA) for the simvastatin/niacin combination in 2006.

Simvastatin shares a common mechanism of action with all statins, as described in the "Statins" section of the "Current Therapies" section. Niacin (nicotinic acid) lowers both cholesterol and TG concentrations by inhibiting their synthesis, but the precise mechanism of action is unknown. One drawback of niacin therapy is the relatively high incidence of side effects (e.g., flushing).

The simvastatin/niacin combination (KS1-019) is in two pivotal studies. The Safety and Efficacy of a Combination of Niacin ER and Simvastatin in Patients with Dyslipidemia: A Dose-Ranging Study (SEACOAST) is a Phase III, 20-week, randomized, double-blind, multicenter, dose-escalation study that aims to randomize 525 dyslipidemic patients not achieving NCEP ATP III goals with simvastatin (20 mg, 40 mg) to combination treatment with various doses of simvastatin (up to 80 mg) and niacin (up to 2,000 mg) or simvastatin alone. The Evaluation of the Safety and Efficacy of a Combination of Niacin ER and Simvastatin in Patients with Dyslipidemia (OCEANS) study is a multicenter, Phase III, open-label, parallel group study that aims to randomize up to 1000 dyslipidemic patients currently receiving 40 mg/day of simvastatin into one of two titration schedules of up to 2000 mg/day of niacin for up to 40 weeks.

Clinical information on the simvastatin/niacin combination is currently unavailable, but information exists on the lovastatin/niacin combination. In the Advicor Versus Other Cholesterol-Modulation Agents Trial Evaluation (ADVOCATE), the effectiveness of the lovastatin/niacin combination was compared with simvastatin and atorvastatin (Bays HE, 2003). In this study, 315 dyslipidemic patients were treated over 16 weeks with escalating doses of extended-release niacin (Kos's Niaspan) combined with lovastatin (up to a maximum dose of 1000 mg/40 mg), simvastatin (10 mg–40 mg), or atorvastatin (10–40 mg).

By week 8, the niacin/lovastatin combination reduced LDL to the same degree as 10 mg atorvastatin (38%) and to a greater degree than 10 mg simvastatin (28%). Furthermore, HDL was raised by a significantly greater degree (20% versus 3% and 7%, respectively), and TG was lowered by a significantly greater amount (28% versus 15% and 10%, respectively).

Cholesteryl Ester Transfer Protein Inhibitors

Overview. Cholesteryl ester transfer protein (CETP) is a plasma protein that mediates the exchange of cholesteryl ester in high-density lipoprotein (HDL) for triglyceride (TG) in very-low-density lipoprotein (VLDL). This process decreases the level of antiatherogenic HDL and increases proatherogenic VLDL and LDL, so CETP is potentially atherogenic. The importance of HDL as a marker of CHD risk is increasing. However, some caution has been voiced, as raising HDL through CETP inhibition has not yet proved to be beneficial. Currently, only a few CETP inhibitors are in development; two agents are in early Phase II trials—discussed later—and two other CETP inhibitors, Pharmacia's SC-795 and SC-744, are in preclinical investigation.

Mechanism of Action. CETP transfers cholesterol from HDLs to VLDLs and LDLs. CETP inhibitors interfere with this cholesterol transfer and therefore have a positive effect on lipid ratios—increasing HDL and decreasing LDL levels.

JTT-705. Japan Tobacco's (Tokyo, Japan) JTT-705 is in Phase I and II trials in Japan and Europe, respectively, for hyperlipidemia. In October 2004, Japan Tobacco licensed exclusive development and commercialization rights outside Japan and South Korea to Roche.

JTT-705's mechanism of action is as described for the CETP inhibitor drug class in general; it inhibits the transfer of cholesteryl esters from HDL to proatherogenic lipid subfractions. Bioavailability studies suggest that the agent is a more effective inhibitor of CETP postprandially.

Clinical data from a Phase II study in 198 subjects with mild dyslipidemia show that treatment with JTT-705 (900 mg/day) for four weeks decreases CETP activity by 37%, raises HDL levels by 34%, and reduces LDL by 7% without affecting TG (de Grooth GJ, 2002). Other reports of clinical trial data confirm the HDL- and LDL-modifying ability of JTT-705 and also its ability to reduce TG (Schaefer E, 2003). Minor gastrointestinal side effects have been reported following treatment with JTT-705 in clinical trials. Although no clinical data on the benefits in atherosclerotic patients are available, one study in the Japanese White Rabbit model for atherosclerosis indicates that, despite strong increases in HDL, JTT-705 does not have a strong antiatherogenic effect (as measured by changes in the atheromatous area in aortic lesions) (Huang Z, 2002). The authors of that study postulate that in patients with severe hypercholesterolemia, reductions in TG or LDL may prove more important for the control of atherosclerosis.

CETi-1. CETi-1 is an anti-CETP vaccine in Phase II development in the United States by Avant Immunotherapeutics (Needham, Massachusetts) for the treatment of atherosclerosis and hyperlipidemia.

CETi-1 is a recombinant peptide containing sequences from human CETP and tetanus toxin, designed to illicit a strong response to CETP. The company hopes that the vaccine can be administered as a single immunization with once- or twice-yearly booster doses to sustain adequate antibody levels against the CETP enzyme. This would give the vaccine advantages over existing lipid-lowering drugs, especially with respect to compliance. The vaccine may also offer a favorable gastrointestinal side-effect profile compared with other antihyperlipidemics.

Avant reports that, in preclinical studies in rabbits, CETi-1 reduced atherosclerotic lesions in blood vessels by 40%. Phase I, double-blind, placebo-controlled trials in 48 subjects showed a dose response to the vaccine with no significant adverse events. Antibody response was observed as early as one week following repeat vaccination and was sustained for up to ten weeks in some subjects treated with the highest dose.

At the time of composing this reference, CETi-1 has completed Phase II trials, but its development has been set back because of formulation issues. Currently, further development has been delayed following company reports in October 2004 that the company is continuing to evaluate several new adjuvants and delivery technologies for its original formulation of its clinical candidate vaccine. The company had planned to have a CETP vaccine back in clinical trials toward the end of 2005 but this did not happen.

In a Phase II, placebo-controlled, dose-escalating clinical trial, 203 subjects with low HDL were administered four injections of CETi-1 at 0, 4, and 8 weeks, with a final booster at six months (Avant Immunotherapeutics, 2003). Three doses of CETi-1 were tested, and subgroups received concurrent statin therapy. Follow-up was for one year. Anti-CETP antibodies were detected in approximately 90% of patients. A statistically significant increase in HDL of 8.4% was observed in patients not receiving statins. However, significant changes in HDL-C were not observed in patients receiving statins. No treatment-related adverse events were reported. In light of these results, Avant was planning to reformulate the vaccine with different adjuvants to increase the immune response before proceeding with further clinical trials.

Acyl CoA Cholesterol Acetyltransferase Inhibitors

Overview. Acyl CoA cholesterol acetyltransferase (ACAT) inhibitors were once thought to hold great promise as antidyslipidemic agents. However, the number under development has diminished considerably over the past few years. The latest to be discontinued is Pfizer's avasimibe, which was the ACAT inhibitor farthest advanced in trials, and this failure has shaken confidence in the whole class. Pfizer may have elected to concentrate on development of other antiatherogenic compounds (such as the HDL mimetics discussed in the "Reverse Lipid Transport Pathway Activators" section) after the FDA requested more trials assessing the effect of avasimibe on atherosclerotic plaque deposition. This class has also suffered from fears over drug-induced adrenal toxicity and a failure of clinical trials to meet expectations raised by studies in animal models.

Mechanism of Action. The enzyme ACAT is involved in cholesterol absorption from the small intestine and in cholesterol metabolism in macrophages and the liver. ACAT inhibitors may reduce the development of atherosclerotic lesions by interfering with these mechanisms. In animal models, ACAT inhibitors inhibit foam cell formation not only by enhancing free cholesterol efflux but also by inhibiting the uptake of modified LDL. Thus, the accumulation of lipids and macrophage infiltration into the arterial wall is reduced. ACAT inhibitors may also reduce matrix metalloproteinase expression and the secretion of ApoB and ApoB-containing lipoproteins into plasma from the liver.

Pactimibe. In November 2005, pactimibe was shown to hamper the beneficial effects of statins in the prevention of atherosclerosis progression, and clinical development was discontinued.

Originally, Sankyo, in partnership with Kyoto University (Kyoto, Japan), was developing pactimibe (CS-505) for the treatment of atherosclerosis and hyperlipidemia. The compound had been in Phase II/III trials for both indications in the United States and Europe, and preparations were under way for Phase I trials in Japan. However, research seemed to be directed primarily toward development for atherosclerosis.

Pactimibe's mechanism of action was as described for the ACAT-inhibitor class in general. ACAT inhibitors demonstrate cholesterol-lowering and antiatherosclerotic activities by blocking intestinal absorption of dietary cholesterol, inhibiting hepatic secretion of VLDL, and preventing the formation of foam cells (a step in the atherogenic process) in the arterial wall. Sankyo had reported (back in 2003) that pactimibe reduced the progression of atherosclerosis in animal models by preventing cholesterol accumulation in macrophages.

However, as noted above, the drug has been discontinued.

Eflucimibe. Eli Lilly and Company (Indianapolis, Indiana) licensed eflucimibe (F-12511) from Pierre Fabre (Castres, France). The drug is currently in Phase II clinical trials in Europe for atherosclerosis and hypercholesterolemia.

Eflucimibe's mechanism of action is as described for the ACAT inhibitor class in general. ACAT inhibitors demonstrate cholesterol-lowering and antiatherosclerotic activities by blocking intestinal absorption of dietary cholesterol, inhibiting hepatic secretion of VLDL, and preventing the formation of foam cells (a step in the atherogenic process) in the arterial wall.

Treatment with eflucimibe (8 mg/kg/day) in rabbit models reduced both TSC and the incidence of atherosclerotic lesions by 50%, and significantly reduced the surface area of preatherosclerotic lesions (Rival Y, 2002). Other animal model data for eflucimibe show dose-dependent reductions in TSC and decreases in dietary cholesterol absorption of 18% (Milliat F, 2001).

Antiplatelet Agents

Overview. Aspirin continues to dominate the antiplatelet market by virtue of its low cost. However, because 10% and 15% of PMI patients are intolerant of aspirin because of either allergic reaction or gastrointestinal (GI) side effects, respectively, clopidogrel is sometimes prescribed in its place. The popularity of clopidogrel in PMI is growing, largely owing to excellent efficacy data (see the "Current Therapies" section). New agents will need to do well in head-to-head comparisons with both clopidogrel (Sanofi-Aventis/Bristol Myers Squibb's Plavix, Bristol-Myers Squibb's Iscover) and aspirin to successfully compete in this market.

Mechanism of Action. All antiplatelet agents reduce the risk of thrombosis by preventing the aggregation of platelets. Aspirin inhibits platelet cyclooxygenase-1 (COX-1), which prevents the synthesis of thromboxane A_2 (TXA_2), an intermediate in the adenosine diphosphate (ADP) receptor-mediated coagulation pathway. The currently marketed clopidogrel and ticlopidine (Roche's Ticlid, Sanofi-Aventis's Ticlid/Tiklyd/Tiklid) inhibit ADP activity by preventing its binding to the platelet receptor.

Prasugrel. Sankyo and Eli Lilly are developing prasugrel (CS-747), a P_{2T} ADP receptor antagonist, as a potential oral treatment for the secondary prevention of thrombotic cardiovascular complications in patients with ischemic strokes or acute coronary syndromes. Prasugrel is currently in Phase I trials in Japan and Phase II trials in the United States and Europe. In October 2004, Eli Lilly announced that a Phase III trial to compare the antithrombotic effects of CS-747 with clopidogrel in patients undergoing a percutaneous coronary intervention (PCI) was to be initiated before the end of 2004, but no further information has been released.

In August 2004, data from a Phase II trial comparing CS-747 and clopidogrel in patients undergoing PCI were presented at the European Society of Cardiology in Munich, Germany. The 904-patient Joint Utilization of Medications to Block Platelets Optimally (JUMBO) TIMI-26 trial compared CS-747 with clopidogrel in patients undergoing stent implantation. There were no significant differences in bleeding rates between CS-747 and clopidogrel, but a non-significantly lower number of acute coronary events occurred in patients receiving CS-747 compared with patients taking clopidogrel (7.2% versus 9.4%). CS-747 was most effective at a dose of 15 mg.

Like clopidogrel and ticlopidine, CS-747 is a thienopyridine pro-drug that generates an active metabolite (R-99224) in vivo. Following oral administration in rats, CS-747 produces more-potent antiplatelet and antithrombotic activity than clopidogrel or ticlopidine, but it also prolongs bleeding times to a greater extent (Sugidachi A, 2001).

More recently, in August 2004, data from a Phase II trial comparing CS-747 and clopidogrel in patients undergoing PCI were presented at the European Society of Cardiology in Munich, Germany. The 904-patient Joint Utilization of Medications to Block Platelets Optimally (JUMBO) TIMI-26 trial compared CS-747 with clopidogrel in patients undergoing stent implantation. There were no significant differences in bleeding rates between CS-747 and clopidogrel, but a nonsignificantly lower number of acute coronary events occurred in patients receiving CS-747 compared with clopidogrel (7.2% versus 9.4%). CS-747 was most effective at a dose of 15 mg; however, because of increased bleeding risk, Sankyo has elected to use the 10 mg dose in Phase III trials

NCX-4016. NicOx (Sophia-Antipolis, France) is developing NCX-4016, a nitric oxide (NO)-donating derivative of aspirin. The compound is currently in Phase II trials for peripheral vascular disease in France and Phase I trials in the United Kingdom for thrombosis.

NCX-4016 consists of an acetyl salicylic acid (aspirin) linked to an NO-donating moiety. The molecule exerts its therapeutic effect through inhibition of the COX-1 pathway, while the NO counteracts some of the detrimental GI side effects of aspirin, such as reduced gastric mucosal blood flow, increased tumor necrosis factor (TNF)-alpha plasma levels, and leukocyte-endothelial cell adherence.

NCX-4016 has been shown to have an improved side-effect profile compared with aspirin (Napoli C, 2001). It also may have other beneficial anti-inflammatory properties not possessed by aspirin. In a recently published study, 48 healthy subjects were treated with either NCX-4016 (800 mg twice daily [bid]), NCX-4016 plus 325 mg of aspirin, aspirin alone, or placebo for 21 days (Fiorucci S, 2004). NCX-4016 inhibited platelet aggregation to a similar extent as aspirin alone, and significantly inhibited tissue factor (TF) expression, interleukin-6, and MCP-1 in ex vivo stimulated monocytes. NCX-4016 was not associated with gastric damage and significantly reduced gastric injury when co-administered with aspirin. In an endoscopic study of 40 healthy volunteers, treatment for seven days with 400 mg or 800 mg NCX-4016 twice daily was associated with virtually no gastric or duodenal toxicity (Fiorucci S, 2003). NCX-4016 is less gastrotoxic than aspirin because it is associated with improved mucosal blood flow, which in turn leads to almost complete abolition of the ulceration and GI side effects that so frequently compromise patients on aspirin therapy. Results in rats have shown that NCX-4016 is significantly better than aspirin at reducing infarct size in the PMI heart and improves healing of the affected area (Wainwright CL, 2002; Rossoni G, 2001).

S-18886. Servier (Neuilly Sur Seine, France) is developing a TXA_2 receptor antagonist, S-18886, which is currently in Phase II clinical development in France for the treatment of CAD. Aspirin is an indirect TXA_2 inhibitor. Unlike aspirin, S-18886 preserves the production of prostacyclin—a powerful vasodilator and antiplatelet agent—in addition to blocking the effect of COX-2-mediated TXA_2 production.

According to preclinical data, S-18886 dose-dependently decreases clot weight after oral administration in rats (at doses of 0.03–1.00 mg/kg) and inhibits platelet and fibrinogen deposition in pigs significantly more than does heparin or heparin plus aspirin. Other preclinical studies found that the antithrombotic effect of S-18886 is comparable to that of clopidogrel (Osende JI, 2004).

Clinical trial data on the antithrombotic effects of S-18886 are limited. However, data from patients with CAD treated with aspirin and S-18886 show improved endothelium-dependent vasodilation compared with patients treated with aspirin alone (Belhassen L, 2003). Ancillary benefits of S-18886 include atherosclerotic lesion reduction. Preclinical studies in ApoE-deficient mice illustrate that S-18886 prevents atherosclerotic lesion development to a greater degree than does aspirin (Cayette AJ, 2000). If late-phase clinical studies confirm the ancillary benefits of S-18886 in addition to platelet inhibition, this agent could compete effectively with clopidogrel in the treatment of aspirin-intolerant patients.

Z-335. Zeria Pharmaceutical (Tokyo, Japan) is developing a TXA_2 receptor antagonist, Z-335, which is currently in Phase II clinical development in Japan for the treatment of atherosclerosis. Like other TXA_2 antagonists, Z-335 prevents coagulation by inhibiting TXA_2, an intermediate in the ADP receptor-mediated coagulation pathway

Phase I data (based on 40 mg doses administered once daily in healthy male volunteers) show Z-335 is well tolerated and provides long-lasting blockade of TXA_2 receptors (Matsuno H, 2002).

Anticoagulants

Overview. Anticoagulants are not a common PMI medication. The reluctance to prescribe them may be due to the drawbacks of currently available oral agents (e.g., warfarin has a narrow therapeutic window, a poor side-effect profile, and many food and drug interactions) and their failure so far to demonstrate superiority over antiplatelet agents in preventing thromboembolic events after MI.

Other anticoagulants that are in development for MI but are not covered here because of a lack of data or early stage of development are Sanofi-Aventis's factor Xa inhibitor otamixaban and Nuevlo's long-acting tissue factor inhibitor rNAPc2.

Mechanism of Action. All anticoagulants interfere with the clotting cascade, inhibiting the conversion of fibrinogen to insoluble fibrin—a major component of a thrombus. Warfarin and heparin, the most commonly used anticoagulants, have indirect action on the clotting cascade, interacting with factors responsible for clotting factor formation and regulation. Thrombin is responsible for catalyzing the production of fibrin from fibrinogen and, as such, is a critical mediator of thrombosis. Direct thrombin inhibitors, which inactivate both free thrombin and thrombin bound to fibrinogen, have the potential to be more potent and controllable than indirect inhibitors.

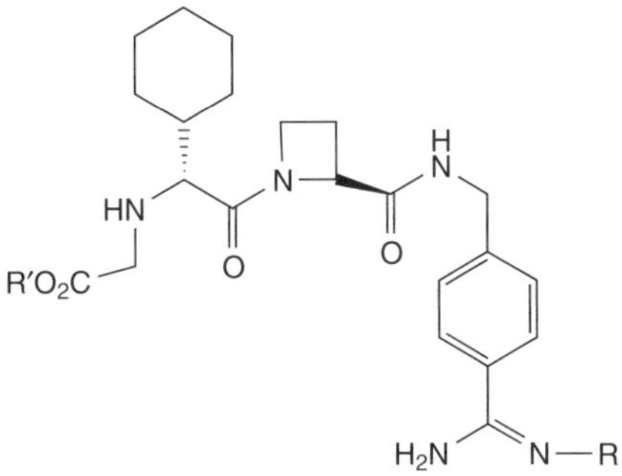

FIGURE 27. *Structure of ximelagatran* ($R = OH$, $R_1 = CH_2CH_3$).

Ximelagatran. In February 2006, AstraZeneca announced that it was withdrawing ximelagatran from all markets.

AstraZeneca's ximelagatran (Exanta) (Figure 27) was an orally active direct thrombin inhibitor in development for several cardiovascular indications, including the prevention of thrombotic complications in MI, for which it was in Phase II trials in the United States and Europe. It was in Phase III trials for atrial fibrillation (AF) in Europe and preregistered for this indication in the United States. Ximelagatran was launched in Germany for the prevention of deep vein thrombosis (DVT) after orthopedic surgery; however, in September 2004, the FDA cardiovascular and renal advisory panel did not approve recommendation of ximelagatran for the prevention or treatment of DVT or the prevention of stroke in atrial fibrillation. The advisory panel cited concerns over liver toxicity with long-term treatment and an increase in the frequency in cardiac events as the reasons for their decision. In October 2004, the FDA heeded the advisory committee's advice and rejected ximelagatran for all three indications for which it was filed. AstraZeneca then entered long discussions with the FDA on how to proceed.

Ximelagatran was an orally available pro-drug of melagatran, a direct thrombin inhibitor.

Reverse Lipid Transport Pathway Activators

Overview. After wholly acquiring Esperion Therapeutics, Inc. (Ann Arbor, Michigan) in February 2004 for $1.3 billion, Pfizer is developing a series of compounds that mimic the properties of HDL in an effort to modify the reverse lipid transport pathway (RLTP) for the treatment of atherosclerosis in both the acute and chronic setting.

ETC-642, a peptide/phospholipid complex in Phase I development, mimics the structure and function of HDL and is under investigation for reducing atherosclerotic events in patients with acute coronary syndrome (ACS) and those with stable atherosclerosis. ETC-1001 is an orally available small molecule in Phase I development that lowers LDL, TGs, and VLDL while raising HDL and inhibiting the progression of atherosclerosis. This agent is targeted at the chronic treatment of atherosclerosis. ETC-216 and ETC-588, which are in Phase II clinical trials, are discussed in this section.

Mechanism of Action. The RLTP is the HDL-dependent mechanism whereby cholesterol and other lipids are transported out of tissues. HDL first removes excess cholesterol from the walls of arteries, then converts it to a form more closely associated with HDL for transport in the blood to the liver. The final step is the transformation and discarding of cholesterol by the liver. All of the agents in this class stimulate the RLTP by mimicking components of HDL.

ETC-216. Pfizer is developing ETC-216, a recombinant form of apolipoprotein A-I Milano (ApoA-IM), a natural variant of apolipoprotein A-1 (ApoA-I). ETC-216 is currently in U.S. Phase II trials for the treatment of atherosclerosis as a potential short-term treatment to be administered prior to long-term statin therapy.

ApoA-I is the major protein component of HDL, and studies show that levels of this protein are inversely proportional to CHD incidence (Luc G, 2002). Preclinical studies of ETC-216 show that this agent is effective in reducing the lipid and macrophage content of aortic lesions in ApoE knockout mice (Shah PK, 2001). Other studies in rabbits demonstrate that this agent promotes plaque regression in the carotid arteries (Chiesa G, 2002).

The first evidence of the efficacy of HDL mimetics came from a trial of ETC-216 in 57 patients with ACS. Patients were randomly assigned to receive five weekly infusions of ETC-216 (15 mg/kg or 45 mg/kg) or placebo (Nissen SE, 2003). ETC-216 decreased mean percentage atheroma volume, as judged by intravascular ultrasound (IUVS), by 1.06%, while atheroma volume increased by 0.14% in the placebo group. The absolute reduction in atheroma volume in the combined treatment groups was -14.1 mm^3 or a 4.2% decrease from baseline ($p < 0.001$), whereas it decreased in the placebo group by 0.2% ($p = 0.97$). ETC-216 was safe and well tolerated.

These trials bode well for ETC-216, and, if the results are repeated in later clinical trials, this agent should find a place in the initial treatment of PMI patients prior to long-term pharmacotherapy.

ETC-588. Pfizer is developing ETC-588, a large unilamellar vesicle (LUV) formulation of a phospholipid liposome, for the treatment of ACS and atherosclerosis. ETC-588 is currently in Phase II trials in the United States.

ETC-588 activates the RLTP, facilitating the exchange of cholesterol from vascular and peripheral tissues.

Initiation of multicenter, Phase II studies in 2002 followed the completion of a Phase IIa study in 2001. Data from the earlier trial showed that ETC-588 is well tolerated and safe at three dosage strengths (50, 100, and 200 mg/kg) (Esperion, 2001). Patients receiving the 100 and 200 mg/kg doses received 7 doses for either four or six weeks; patients receiving the 50 mg/kg doses received 14 doses for either four or six weeks. Because the study involved only a small number of people (34), the observed changes in vascular function and inflammatory markers were inconclusive. However, all participants showed dose-related cholesterol mobilization and positive vascular changes in the carotid arteries. The ongoing Phase II study will evaluate changes in plaque volume and composition in atherosclerotic patients following eight weekly doses of ETC-588.

Because this drug requires intravenous administration, its use will be limited to the in-hospital setting, possibly for several weeks immediately after an acute myocardial infarction (AMI).

Antioxidants/Vascular Protectants

Overview. The antioxidant probucol (Aventis Pharmaceuticals, Inc. [Bridgewater, New Jersey, now Sanofi-Aventis]/Daiichi's [Tokyo, Japan] sinlestal) was withdrawn in 1995 in the United States and Europe. Although probucol has some major clinical disadvantages—including the potential for causing ventricular arrhythmias in patients with CHD and reductive effects on HDL—it demonstrated impressive plaque stabilization and other antiatherogenic properties (Sawayama Y, 2002; Tardif JC, 2003).

Mechanism of Action. Vascular protectants inhibit vascular inflammation and reduce cholesterol level. They inhibit endothelial expression of vascular cellular adhesion molecule (VCAM)-1 by blocking the oxidant signals that switch on VCAM 1 expression. VCAM-1 is the molecule to which the circulating inflammatory cells attach before they migrate into the artery wall and become components of a newly forming lesion.

AGI-1067. AtheroGenics is developing AGI-1067, a metabolically stable, pharmacologically distinct modification of probucol. The most developmentally advanced member of the composite vascular protectant class of drugs, AGI-1067 is in Phase III trials in the United States and Phase I in the United Kingdom for the treatment of atherosclerosis. Collaboration with Schering-Plough was terminated by mutual agreement in 2001.

AGI-1067 has been shown to inhibit vascular inflammation, reduce total serum cholesterol (TSC), and increase HDL in animal models (Sundell CL, 2003).

In November 2004, AtheroGenics announced the final results from the second Canadian Antioxidant Restenosis Trial (CART-2), a placebo-controlled, Phase IIb trial. This 12-month trial measured the change in atherosclerotic plaque volume, as measured by IUVS, in 500 patients undergoing PCI compared with baseline levels. Initially, results were analyzed at the Montreal Heart Institute, which was conducting the study, but AtheroGenics sent the data to the Cleveland Clinic (renowned for its expertise in IUVS) for reanalysis, where 30% of the data were subsequently discarded. Combined analysis of CART-2 from both laboratories showed that AGI-1067 reduced plaque volume by a statistically significant 3.9 mm^3 (2.3%; $p = 0.0015$) (AtheroGenics, 2004[b]). The group receiving standard of care regressed by a statistically nonsignificant 0.8 mm^3 (0.8%; $p = 0.45$).

When the AGI-1067 treated group was compared with the standard of care-treated group, there was no statistical significance ($p = 0.29$).

CART-1 randomized 305 patients undergoing PCI with or without stenting to treatment with AGI-1067, probucol, or placebo. Treatment started two weeks before angioplasty and continued for four weeks after. The primary end point was minimal luminal area at the site of PCI at six months, as measured by intravascular ultrasound. Minimal lumen area was significantly greater in patients treated with 280 mg/day AGI-1067 and 500 mg twice-daily probucol ($p = 0.046$ and $p = 0.01$, respectively). Restenosis rates in stented patients were lower in the AGI-1067- and probucol-treated patients when compared with placebo, but the reductions were not statistically significant (Tardif JC, 2003).

The Phase III Aggressive Reduction of Inflammation Stops Events (ARISE) trial is ongoing. This large-scale trial will recruit 4,000 patients (or until a minimum of 1,160 primary events occur) with 18 months of follow-up, and is designed to assess the benefit of AGI-1067 in addition to current standard treatment in patients with diagnosed CHD. AtheroGenics has received a positive Special Protocol Assessment from the FDA, stating that ARISE is adequately designed to support an NDA (AtheroGenics, 2003), which the company hopes to submit soon after the study results become available in the first quarter of 2006.

BO-653. Chugai Pharmaceuticals (Tokyo, Japan), now a wholly owned subsidiary of Roche, is developing BO-653 for atherosclerosis and restenosis. The compound is in Phase II studies in the United States and Phase I studies in Japan for restenosis in post-PTCA CHD.

BO-653 is the lead compound in a series of antioxidants specifically designed to be highly reactive against lipoprotein oxidation.

Preclinical results indicate that BO-653 is more potent than other antioxidant agents. It reduces human-macrophage-mediated LDL oxidation (Muller K, 1999) and significantly reduces atherosclerotic lesion size in rabbits and mice, while simultaneously increasing HDL levels (Cynshi O, 1998).

Growth Factor Therapies

Overview. Surgical bypass, angioplasty, and pharmacological therapy have traditionally been used to restore blood flow to hypoperfused tissues (i.e., tissues that have restricted blood flow) after an MI. These therapies all carry risks of complications, particularly angioplasty. Growth factor therapies include agents that promote the development of endogenous collateral vessels in ischemic myocardium. Clinical trials are now showing that growth factor therapies can restore blood flow through hypoperfused tissue following AMI without pharmacological or surgical intervention.

The most advanced agent in this class is GenVec's (Gaithersburg, Maryland) BioBypass (AdGVVEGF121.10), a vascular endothelial growth factor (VEGF) gene therapy. Several other growth factors in development are not discussed here because of their early stage of development or because they are not indicated for

PMI: Hypoxia inducible factor (HIF) triggers VEGF expression, and Genzyme Biosurgery (Cambridge, Massachusetts) is conducting Phase I trials of HIF-1 alpha gene therapy for treatment of CAD in the United Stares and Europe; Corautus has restarted VEGF-2 gene therapy Phase II trials following an FDA-mandated halt in December 2000 (for safety reasons) and the lifting of the ban in November 2002; ViroMed Laboratories, Inc. (Minnetonka, Minnesota) and Dong-A (Seoul, Korea) started Phase I trials in Japan for a plasmid vector carrying a VEGF-165 gene (VMDA-3601) for the treatment of ischemic heart disease in April 2002.

Mechanism of Action. Angiogenesis (the formation of new blood vessels) is a multistep process involving the proliferation, migration, and adhesion of endothelial cells. In healthy tissue, this process is under the control of angiogenic (angiogenesis promoting) and angiostatic (angiogenesis inhibiting) factors. Angiogenic factors include the growth factors VEGF and fibroblast growth factor (FGF). Several efforts are studying the effects of delivering growth factor genes to damaged heart tissue. Local expression of growth factor stimulates new blood vessel formation in and around the damaged myocardium. This collateral vessel development allows bypass of the obstruction, reperfusion of damaged tissue, and improved blood flow in the hypoperfused tissue following an AMI.

BioBypass. GenVec is developing BioBypass (formerly AdGVVEGF121.10, licensed from Scios), a VEGF gene therapy. Phase II trials for the treatment of CAD were completed in 2003. GenVec has subsequently entered into an agreement with Cordis to advance BioBypass into Phase III trials using Cordis's catheter technology.

BioBypass consists of a recombinant form of human $VEGF_{121}$ packaged in an adenovirus vector. The vector is injected into the infarcted myocardium via a cardiac catheter, where the VEGF gene is expressed, stimulating vessel growth and restoring blood flow to ischemic tissue.

The Phase II Randomized Evaluation of VEGF for Angiogenesis in Severe Coronary Disease (REVASC) study was the first trial of a VEGF therapy to induce collateral vessel formation (Stewart DJ, 2002). Patients with severely symptomatic CAD received 30 direct intramyocardial injections of AdGVVEGF121.10 in addition to continuation of standard antianginal agents, nitrates, and antiplatelets. At the six-month follow-up, patients treated with BioBypass exhibited significant improvements in ischemia, as measured by exercise treadmill time to an additional 1-mm ST segment depression using electrocardiogram. These results indicate the therapy could also be of benefit to high-risk PMI patients.

Trials of BioBypass demonstrate the relative safety of targeting VEGF; no differences in adverse events between placebo and AdGVVEGF121.10-treated patients were reported in the REVASC study. Other trial results in patients receiving coronary artery bypass graft (CABG) surgery who were given BioBypass as an adjunct therapy reported no evidence of systemic inflammation in response to adenoviral administration and no cardiac-related adverse events. The most common side effects were sensitivity and swelling at the site of injection

(Basara N, 2001). Because the direct injection procedure may carry some risk, GenVec is planning trials to deliver the growth factor by PCI catheter.

Stem Cell Therapy

Overview. Current PMI therapies limit the damage caused to the heart after an MI, improve blood flow, and prevent further damage from occurring. However, the damage caused by ischemia during the acute event is often irreversible and may lead to progressive heart failure, loss of function, and eventually death. Stem cell therapy offers the possibility of reversing the damage caused by MI through an injection of pluripotent stem cells that can differentiate into functional cardiomyocytes, thus regenerating heart muscle and restoring function.

Although several Phase I studies have been conducted with encouraging results, stem cell therapy in cardiac repair is still in its infancy. Many hurdles must be overcome, including the selection of the most appropriate source of cells. Early data suggest that autologous bone marrow, blood-derived precursors, and skeletal myoblasts are candidates. Infusion of bone marrow or blood-derived precursors in patients receiving a stent after an MI have led to significant improvements in several placebo-controlled trials (Assmus B, 2002; Strauer BE, 2002; Brehm M, 2003; Wollert KC, 2004). However, injection of skeletal myoblasts has, in some cases, been associated with severe ventricular tachycardias (Menasche P, 2003; Smits PC, 2003). This effect is possibly due to ineffective electric coupling of the transplanted cells to existing cardiomyocytes (Makkar RR, 2003). However, this problem may be counteracted with the use of the antiarrhythmic agent amiodarone (Sanofi-Aventis's Cordarone/Cordarex/Carbionax, Merck's Amiodura, generics) as prophylaxis (Siminiak T, 2004).

Another issue is the lack of commercial involvement so far in this technology. Because autologous stem cells are effectively unpatentable, research in this area remains largely confined to the academic sphere. For successful commercialization, companies are likely to rely on developing unique stem-cell isolation and delivery technology.

Mechanism of Action. The precise mechanism by which progenitor cells improve cardiac function is not fully understood. It has been proposed that there is some degree of naturally occurring cardiac repair, where stem cells migrate to the heart and transdifferentiate into active cardiomyocytes. However, studies have shown that progenitor cells do not fully differentiate and instead fuse with local cardiomyocytes. It is also likely that a major contributor to functional improvement is the paracrine effect of the infused cells, which secrete growth factors encouraging new vessel formation and re-establishment of coronary blood flow.

MyoCell. Bioheart, Inc. (Sunrise, Florida) is developing MyoCell, an autologous skeletal muscle-based therapy for CHF and MI, currently in Phase II development in Europe and Phase I in the United States. Bioheart is also developing its own delivery technology for the technique, MyoCath, which allows multiple injections, improved visualization, and reduced procedure time.

MyoCell skeletal myoblasts are isolated from autologous quadriceps muscle biopsies and expanded in culture. Cells are then transferred to the damaged myocardium via a cardiac catheter. Although the precise mechanism of action is unknown, myoblastic cells improve cardiac function by replacing damaged tissue and encouraging new vessel growth in infarcted areas of the heart.

In a Phase I study, five patients with CHF were injected with approximately 296 million autologously derived skeletal myoblasts directly into damaged myocardium as assessed by fluorescence imaging (Smits PC, 2003). Left ventricular ejection fraction (LVEF) measured by angiography increased from a mean of 36% to 41% at three months and 45% at six months ($p = 0.009$ and $p = 0.23$, respectively), although one patient experienced tachycardia and required implantation of a cardioverter-defibrillator.

In line with the theory that stem cell transplantation improves heart function by promoting new vessel growth, Bioheart has entered into an agreement with the University of Florida's Powell Gene Therapy Center to develop a method of delivering controlled-release angiogenic factors with the stem cell injection.

Myoblast Cell Therapy. After acquiring Diacrin, Inc. (Charlestown, Massachusetts) in 2003, GenVec is developing the autologous myoblastic cell transplantation system, currently in Phase I development in the United States for the treatment of CHF and MI.

Similar to Bioheart's MyoCell, GenVec's technology relies on the culture of myoblasts from autologous skeletal muscle, which are then injected into the infarcted area via a cardiac catheter.

Although clinical data on GenVec's myoblast technology are scarce, safety data released at the 2003 American College of Cardiology Annual Scientific Session in Orlando, Florida, were encouraging. A total of 27 patients undergoing heart transplantation or CABG received an infusion of myogenic stem cells with no cases of arrhythmia reported (GenVec, 2003). In a dose-ranging study, 11 patients with CHF were injected with 10 to 300 million autologous skeletal myoblasts. Injections were well tolerated—only one patient experienced transient tachycardia. At nine months' follow-up, LVEF had improved from 23% to 36% (Dib N, 2003). Positive follow-up data on these patients were also presented at the 2004 AHA conference in New Orleans (GenVec, 2004).

REFERENCES

AIRE Study Investigators. Effect of ramipril on mortality and morbidity of survivors of acute myocardial infarction with clinical evidence of heart failure. The Acute Infarction Ramipril Efficacy (AIRE) Study Investigators. *Lancet*. 1993;**342**(8875):821–828.

Alpert JS, et al. Myocardial infarction redefined: A consensus document of the Joint European Society of Cardiology/American College of Cardiology Committee for the redefinition of myocardial infarction. *Journal of the American College of Cardiology*. 2000;**36**:959–969.

Alpert JS, Ariz T. Defining myocardial infarction: "will the real myocardial infarction please stand up?" *American Heart Journal*. 2003;**146**:377–379.

Altmann SW, et al. Niemann-Pick C1 Like 1 protein is critical for intestinal cholesterol absorption. *Science*. 2004;**303**:1201–1204.

American Heart Association. Heart Disease and Stroke Statistics—2003 Update [electronic]. Dallas, TX. American Heart Association; 2002. www.americanheart.org/downloadable/heart/10461207852142003HDSStatsBook.pdf.

AMIS research group. The aspirin myocardial infarction study: final results. The Aspirin Myocardial Infarction Study research group. *Circulation*. 1980;**62**(6 pt 2):V79–V84.

Antiplatelet Trialists' Collaboration. Collaborative overview of randomised trials of antiplatelet therapy, prevention of death, myocardial infarction, and stroke by prolonged antiplatelet therapy in various categories of patients. *British Medical Journal*. 1994;**308**:81–106.

Argmann CA, et al. Transforming growth factor-beta1 inhibits macrophage cholesteryl ester accumulation induced by native and oxidized VLDL remnants. *Arteriosclerosis, Thrombosis, and Vascular Biology*. 2001;**21**(12):2011–2018.

Arnal JF, et al. Omapatrilat, a dual angiotensin-converting enzyme and neutral endopeptidase inhibitor, prevents fatty streak deposit in apolipoprotein E-deficient mice. *Atherosclerosis*. 2001;**155**:291–295.

Aronow WS. Treatment of the elderly post-myocardial infarction patient. *American Journal of Geriatric Cardiology*. 2001;**10**(6):316–322, 376.

Aros F, et al. Management of myocardial infarction in Spain in the year 2000. The PRIAMHO II study. *Revista Española de Cardiologia*. 2003;**56**(12):1165–1173.

Assmus B, et al. Transplantation of progenitor cells and regeneration enhancement in acute myocardial infarction (TOPCARE-AMI). *Circulation*. 2002;**106**(24):3009–3017.

AstraZeneca. New study confirms potential for Exanta (ximelagatran) in prevention of stroke in atrial fibrillation. Press release, November 2003. http://www.astrazeneca.com/pressrelease/694.aspx. Accessed September 2004.

Asztalos BF, et al. High-density lipoprotein subpopulations in pathologic conditions. *American Journal of Cardiology*. 2003;**91**(7A):12E–17E.

Atherogenics. AtheroGenics announces positive interim results from CART-2 study. Press release, September 2004. www.atherogenics.com/press/. Accessed October 2004. [a]

Atherogenics. AtheroGenics reports positive final results from CART-2 clinical trial of AGI-1067. Press release, November 2004. www.atherogenics.com/press/. Accessed December 2004. [b]

Atherogenics. AtheroGenics announces favorable results from special protocol assessment of Phase III clinical trial with AGI-1067. March 2003. www.atherogenics.com/press. Accessed October 2004.

Avant Immunotherapeutics. Avant Immunotherapeutics announces positive Phase II trial results of its experimental cholesterol management vaccine. Press release, November 2003. http://phx.corporate-ir.net/phoenix.zhtml?c=93243&p=irol-news03_NM. Accessed November 2004.

Avanzini F, et al. Gruppo Italiano per lo Studio della Sopravvivenza nell'Infarto miocardico-3 Investigators. Risks and benefits of early treatment of acute myocardial infarction with an angiotensin-converting enzyme inhibitor in patients with a history of arterial hypertension: analysis of the GISSI-3 database. *American Heart Journal*. 2002;**144**(6):1018–1025.

Avkiran M, et al. Rational basis for use of sodium-hydrogen exchange inhibitors in myocardial ischemia. *American Journal of Cardiology*. 1999;**83**(10A):10G–18G.

Ayanian JZ, et al. Use of cholesterol-lowering therapy by elderly adults after myocardial infarction. *Archives of Internal Medicine*. 2002;**162**:1013–1019.

Bajekal M, et al. Bob Erens, Paola Primatesta, eds. *Health Survey of England 1998: cardiovascular disease*. National Centre for Social Research, Department of Epidemiology and Public Health at the Royal Free and University College Medical School. The Department of Health, London; 1998.

Ballantyne CM, et al. Effect of ezetimibe coadministered with atorvastatin in 628 patients with primary hypercholesterolemia: a prospective, randomized, double-blind trial. *Circulation*. 2003;**107**(19):2409–2415.

Ballantyne CM, et al. Efficacy and safety of ezetimibe co-administered with simvastatin compared with atorvastatin in adults with hypercholesterolemia. *American Journal of Cardiology*. 2004;**93**(12):1487–1494.

Barabas EI. Treatment of postmyocardial infarction. *Drug Topics*. 1995;**139**:102.

Barakat K, et al. Acute myocardial infarction in women: contribution of treatment variables to adverse outcome. *American Heart Journal*. 2000;**140**:740–746.

Bardaji A, et al. Applicability of a new definition of myocardial infarction and the opinion of Spanish cardiologists. *Revista Española de Cardologia*. 2003;**56**:23–28.

Baron JH, et al. How do we define myocardial infarction? A survey of the views of consultant physicians and cardiologists. *British Journal of Cardiology*. 2004;**11**(1):34–38.

Barry M. Rosuvastatin-warfarin drug interaction. *Lancet*. 2004;**363**:328.

Basara N. AdGVVEFG121.10 (GenVec). *Current Opinion in Investigational Drugs*. 2001;**2**(6):792–795.

Bates ER. Bivalirudin for percutaneous coronary intervention and in acute coronary syndromes. *Current Cardiology Reports*. 2001;**3**(5):348–354.

Bays HE, et al. Effectiveness and tolerability of ezetimibe in patients with primary hypercholesterolemia: pooled analysis of two Phase II studies. *Clinical Therapeutics*. 2001;**23**(8):1209–1230.

Bays HE, et al. Comparison of once-daily, niacin extended-release/lovastatin with standard doses of atorvastatin and simvastatin (the ADvicor Versus Other Cholesterol-Modulating Agents Trial Evaluation [ADVOCATE]). *American Journal of Cardiology*. 2003;**91**(6):667–672.

Belhassen L, et al. Improved endothelial function by the thromboxane A2 receptor antagonist S 18886 in patients with coronary artery disease treated with aspirin. *Journal of the American College of Cardiology*. 2003;**41**(7):1198–1204.

Bellavance A. Efficacy of ticlopidine and aspirin for prevention of reversible cerebrovascular ischemic events. The Ticlopidine Aspirin Stroke Study. *Stroke*. 1993;**24**(10):1452–1427.

Berger CJ, et al. Prognosis after first myocardial infarction. *Journal of the American Medical Association*. 1992;**268**:1545–1551.

Berlowitz MS, et al. Dose-dependent blockade of the angiotensin II type 1 receptor in normal volunteers: incomplete and transient blockage by losartan 50mg. The 50th Scientific Session of the American College of Cardiology; March 18–21, 2001; Orlando, FL.

Berne C and Siewert-Delle A on behalf of the URANUS study investigators. Use of rosuvastatin versus atorvastatin in type 2 diabetes mellitus subjects: results of the URANUS study. The 74th European Atherosclerosis Society Congress in Seville, Spain, April 2004.

Beswick AD, et al. Provision, uptake and cost of cardiac rehabilitation programmes: improving services to under-represented groups. *Health Technology Assessment*. 2004; **8**(41):1–166.

Betteridge DJ, Gibson M, on behalf of the ANDROMEDA study investigators. Effect of rosuvastatin and atorvastatin on LDL-C and CRP levels in patients with type 2 diabetes: results of the ANDROMEDA study. The 74th European Atherosclerosis Society Congress in Seville, Spain, April 2004.

Bhatt DL, et al. Reduction in the need for hospitalization for recurrent ischemic events and bleeding with clopidogrel instead of aspirin. CAPRIE investigators. *American Heart Journal*. 2000;**140**(1):67–73.

Bittl JA, et al. A randomized comparison of bivalirudin and heparin in patients undergoing coronary angioplasty for postinfarction angina. Hirulog Angioplasty Study Investigators. *American Journal of Cardiology*. 1998;**82**(8B):43P–49P.

Bocan TM, et al. The ACAT inhibitor avasimibe reduces macrophages and matrix metalloproteinase expression in atherosclerotic lesions of hypercholesterolemic rabbits. *Arteriosclerosis Thrombosis and Vascular Biology*. 2000;**20**(1):70–79.

Bocan TM, et al. The combined effect of inhibiting both ACAT and HMG-CoA reductase may directly induce atherosclerotic lesion regression. *Atherosclerosis*. 2001;**157**(1): 97–105.

Boden WE, et al. Diltiazem in acute myocardial infarction treated with thrombolytic agents: a randomised placebo-controlled trial. Incomplete Infarction Trial of European Research Collaborators Evaluating Prognosis post-Thrombolysis (INTERCEPT). *Lancet*. 2000;**355**:1751–1756.

Borghi C, et al. Short- and long-term effects of early fosinopril administration in patients with acute anterior myocardial infarction undergoing intravenous thrombolysis: results from the Fosinopril in Acute Myocardial Infarction Study. FAMIS Working Party. *American Heart Journal*. 1998;Aug;**136**(2):213–225.

Borghi C, et al. Double-blind comparison between zofenopril and lisinopril in patients with acute myocardial infarction: results of the Survival of Myocardial Infarction Long-term Evaluation-2 (SMILE-2) study. *American Heart Journal*. 2003;**145**(1):80–87.

Boyle PJ, et al. Effects of pioglitazone and rosiglitazone on blood lipid levels and glycemic control in patients with type 2 diabetes mellitus: a retrospective review of randomly selected medical records. *Clinical Therapeutics*. 2002;**24**(3):3783–3796.

Braunwald E. Heart Disease: A Textbook of Cardiovascular Medicine, 5th ed. Philadelphia, PA: WB Saunders Company; 1997. [a]

Braunwald, E. Shattuck Lecture: cardiovascular medicine at the turn of the millennium: triumphs, concerns, and opportunities. *New England Journal of Medicine*. 1997;**337**: 1360–1369. [b]

Brehm M, et al. Angiogenesis and myogenesis after intracoronary transplantation of autologous bone marrow cells in patients with acute myocardial infarction. *Circulation*. 2003;**108**:1929. Abstract.

Brewer HB, et al. New insights into the role of the adenosine triphosphate-binding cassette transporters in high-density lipoprotein metabolism and reverse cholesterol transport. *American Journal of Cardiology*. 2003;**91**(7A):3E–11E.

Brousseau ME, et al. Effects of an inhibitor of cholesterol ester transfer protein on HDL cholesterol. *New England Journal of Medicine*. 2004;**350**(15):1505–1515.

Brown WV, et al. Efficacy and safety of rosuvastatin compared with pravastatin and simvastatin in patients with hypercholesterolemia: a randomized, double-blind, 52-week trial. *American Heart Journal*. 2002;**144**(6):1036–1043.

Burnier M, Maillard M. The comparative pharmacology of angiotensin II receptor antagonists. *Blood Pressure*. 2001;**10**(suppl 1):6–11.

Cannon CJ, et al., for the Pravastatin or Atorvastatin Evaluation and Infection Therapy: Thrombolysis in Myocardial Infarction 22 Investigators. Comparison of intensive and moderate lipid lowering with statins after acute coronary syndromes. *New England Journal of Medicine*. 2004. Abstract. Published online before print (April 8 issue). http://content.nejm.org/cgi/content/abstract/NEJMoa040583v1. Accessed September 2004.

Cannon CP, et al. Design of the Pravastatin or Atorvastatin Evaluation and Infection Therapy (PROVE IT)-TIMI 22 trial. *American Journal of Cardiology*. 2002;**89**(7):860–861.

Cannon CP. Pravastatin or Atorvastatin Evaluation and Infection Therapy: Thrombolysis in Myocardial Infarction 22 (PROVE IT-TIMI 22). Program and abstracts from the American College of Cardiology 53rd Annual Scientific Sessions; March 7–10, 2004; New Orleans, LA.

Capewell S, et al. Trends in case-fatality in 117,718 patients admitted with acute myocardial infarction in Scotland. *European Heart Journal*. 2000;**21**:1833–1840.

CAPRIE Steering Committee. A randomised, blinded, trial of clopidogrel versus aspirin in patients at risk of ischaemic events (CAPRIE). *Lancet*. 1996;**348**(9038):1329.

Carney RM, et al. Adherence to a prophylactic medication regimen in patients with symptomatic versus asymptomatic ischemic heart disease. *Behavioral Medicine*. 1998; **24**:35–39.

Casella G, et al. Safety and efficacy evaluation of clopidogrel compared to ticlopidine after stent implantation: an updated meta-analysis. *Italian Heart Journal*. 2003; **4**(10):677–684.

Cayette AJ, et al. The thromboxane receptor antagonist S18886 but not aspirin inhibits atherogenesis in APO-E deficient mice. *Arteriosclerosis, Thrombosis, and Vascular Biology*. 2000;**20**:1724–1728.

Chandra NC, et al. Observations of the treatment of women in the United States with myocardial infarction: a report from the National Registry of Myocardial Infarction-I. *Archives of Internal Medicine*. 1998;**158**:981–988.

Chang WC, et al. Impact of sex on long-term mortality from acute myocardial infarction vs unstable angina. *Archives of Internal Medicine*. 2003;**163**:2476–2484.

Chew DP, et al. Increased mortality with oral platelet glycoprotein IIb/IIIa antagonists: a meta-analysis of Phase III multicenter randomized trials. *Circulation*. 2001;16; **103**(2):201–206.

Chiesa G, et al. Recombinant apolipoprotein A-I (Milano) infusion into rabbit carotid artery rapidly removes lipid from fatty streaks. *Circulation Research*. 2002;**90**(9): 974–980.

Chinetti G, et al. PPAR-alpha and PPAR-gamma activators induce cholesterol removal from human macrophage foam cells through stimulation of the ABCA1 pathway. *Nature Medicine*. 2001;**7**(1):53–58.

Choudhury L. Myocardial infarction in young patients. *American Journal of Medicine*. 1999;**107**:254.

Clark RW, et al. Raising high-density lipoprotein in humans through inhibition of cholesteryl ester transfer protein: an initial multidose study of torcetrapib. *Arteriosclerosis, Thrombosis, and Vascular Biology*. 2004;**24**:490–497.

Cleland JG. Is aspirin "the weakest link" in cardiovascular prophylaxis? The surprising lack of evidence supporting the use of aspirin for cardiovascular disease. *Progress in Cardiovascular Diseases*. 2002;**44**(4):275–292.

Coats AJ. Angiotensin receptor blockers—finally the evidence is coming in: IDNT and RENAAL. *International Journal of Cardiology*. 2001;**79**(2–3):99–102.

Cody RJ. The sympathetic nervous system and the rennin-angiotensis-aldosterone system in cardiovascular disease. *American Journal of Cardiology*. 1997;**80**:9J–14J.

CONSENSUS trial study group. Effects of enalapril on mortality in severe congestive heart failure. Results of the Cooperative North Scandinavian Enalapril Survival Study. *New England Journal of Medicine*. 1987;**316**(23):1429–1435.

Connors KF, et al. Postmyocardial infarction patients: experience from the SAVE trial. *American Journal of Critical Care*. 1995;**4**(1):23–28.

Cooper R, et al. Trends and disparities in coronary heart disease, stroke, and other cardiovascular diseases in the United States: findings of the National Conference on Cardiovascular Disease Prevention. *Circulation*. 2000;**102**:3137–3147.

Cozma LS, et al. Secondary prevention of hypercholesterolaemia: results of an audit conducted in South Wales. *Heart*. 2000;**84**(2):E3.

Crane PB, McSweeney JC. Exploring older women's lifestyle changes after myocardial infarction. *Medsurg Nursing*. 2003;**12**(3):170–176.

CURE Trial Investigators. Effects of Clopidogrel in Addition to Aspirin in Patients with Acute Coronary Syndromes without ST-Segment Elevation. *New England Journal of Medicine*. 2001;**345**:494–502.

Cynshi O, et al. Antiatherogenic effects of the antioxidant BO-653 in three different animal models. *Proceedings of the National Academy of Sciences USA*. 1998;**95**(17): 10123–10128.

Dagenais GR, et al; HOPE Investigators. Effects of ramipril on coronary events in high-risk persons: results of the Heart Outcomes Prevention Evaluation Study. *Circulation*. 2001;**104**(5):522–526.

Dargie HJ. Effect of carvedilol on outcome after myocardial infarction in patients with left-ventricular dysfunction: the CAPRICORN randomised trial. *Lancet*. 2001;**357**(9266): 1385–1390.

Davidson MH, et al. Ezetimibe coadministered with simvastatin inpatients with primary hypercholesterolemia. *Journal of the American College of Cardiology*. 2002;**40**(12): 2125–2134.

Davidson MH, et al. ZD4522 (rosuvastatin) is superior to atorvastatin in decreasing low-density lipoprotein cholesterol and increasing high-density lipoprotein cholesterol in patients with type IIa or IIb hypercholesterolemia. The 50th Scientific Session of the American College of Cardiology; March 18–21, 2001; Orlando, FL.

de Grooth GJ, et al. Efficacy and safety of a novel cholesteryl ester transfer protein inhibitor, JTT-705, in humans: a randomized phase II dose-response study. *Circulation*. 2002;**105**(18):2159–2165.

de Lemos JA, et al. Early intensive vs. a delayed conservative simvastatin strategy in patients with acute coronary syndromes: phase Z of the A to Z trial. *Journal of the American Medical Association*. 2004;**292**(11):1307–16.

De Luca G. Comparison between ticlopidine and clopidogrel in patients with ST-segment elevation myocardial infarction treated with coronary stenting. *Thrombosis and Haemostasis*. 2004;**91**(6):1084–1089.

Deedwania PC, et al. Evidence-based, cost-effective risk stratification and management after myocardial infarction. *Archives of Internal Medicine*. 1997;**157**:273–280.

Delahaye F, et al. French Society of Cardiology recommendations regarding the management of post-myocardial infarction. *Archives des Maladies du Couer et des Vaisseux*. 2001;**94**(7):697–738.

Delsing DJM, et al. Acyl-coA:cholesterol acyltransferase inhibitor avasimibe reduces atherosclerosis in addition to its cholesterol-lowering effect in ApoE*3-Leiden mice. *Circulation*. 2000;**103**(13):1778–1786.

Department of Health. Use of aspirin, beta blockers, statins and ACE inhibitors on discharge from hospital after a heart attack, January-December 2003, England and Wales. www.heartstats.org/datapage.asp?id=846. Accessed September 2004. [a]

Department of Health. British Association Cardiac Rehabilitation Database (2003). www.heartstats.org/temp/TABsp3.10spweb04.xls. Accessed August 2004. [b]

DeStefano F, et al. Trends in nonfatal coronary heart disease in the United States, 1980 through 1989. *Archives of Internal Medicine*. 1993;**153**(21):2489–2494.

Dib N, et al. Safety and feasibility of autologous myoblast transplantation in patients undergoing CABG: Results from United States experience. *Journal of the American College of Cardiology*. 2003;**41**(6) suppl A.

Di Cecco, et al. Is there a clinically significant gender bias in post-myocardial infarction pharmacological management in the older (>60) population of a primary care practice? *BMC Family Practice*. 2002;**3**(1):8.

Dickstein K, et al. Comparison of baseline data, initial course, and management: losartan versus captopril following acute myocardial infarction (The OPTIMAAL Trial). OPTIMAAL Trial Steering Committee and Investigators. Optimal Trial in Myocardial Infarction with the Angiotensin II Antagonist Losartan. *American Journal of Cardiology*. 2001;**87**(6):766–771, A7.

Dickstein K, Kjekshus J; OPTIMAAL Steering Committee of the OPTIMAAL Study Group. Effects of losartan and captopril on mortality and morbidity in high-risk patients after acute myocardial infarction: the OPTIMAAL randomised trial. Optimal Trial in Myocardial Infarction with Angiotensin II Antagonist Losartan. *Lancet*. 2002;**360**(9335):752–760.

Dornelas EA, et al. A randomised controlled trial of smoking cessation counseling after myocardial infarction. *Preventative Medicine*. 2000;**4**:261–268.

Downs JR, et al. Primary prevention of acute coronary events with lovastatin in men and women with average cholesterol levels. *Journal of the American Medical Association*. 1998;**279**:1615–1622.

Ducimetière P, et al. Why mortality from heart disease is low in France. *British Medical Journal*. 2000;**320**:249–250.

Duez H, et al. Fenofibrate treatment reduces lesion size and aortic cholesterol content in human APOA1-transgenic x APO-E-deficient mice and APO-E-deficient mice *Circulation*. 2001;**104**(17):A1129.

Dujovne CA, et al. Randomized comparison of the efficacy and safety of cerivastatin and pravastatin in 1,030 hypercholesterolemic patients. The Cerivastatin Study Group. *Mayo Clinic Proceedings*. 2000;**75**(11):1124–1132.

Einhorn D, et al. Pioglitazone hydrochloride in combination with metformin in the treatment of type 2 diabetes mellitus: a randomized, placebo-controlled study. The Pioglitazone 027 Study Group. *Clinical Therapeutics*. 2000;**22**(12):1395–1409.

Etgen GJ, et al. A tailored therapy for the metabolic syndrome: the dual peroxisome proliferators-activated receptor-alpha/gamma agonist LY465608 ameliorates insulin resistance and diabetic hyperglycemia while improving cardiovascular risk factors in preclinical models. *Diabetes*. 2002;**51**(4):1083–1087.

ESC/AHA. Myocardial infarction redefined--a consensus document of The Joint European Society of Cardiology/American College of Cardiology Committee for the redefinition of myocardial infarction. *European Heart Journal*. 2000;**21**(18):1502–1513.

Esperion Therapeutics. ETC-588 mobilizes unesterified cholesterol in a dose-dependent fashion in healthy volunteers. Press release, September 2001. www.esperion.com. Accessed September 2004.

European Society of Cardiology. Lifestyle and risk factor management and use of drug therapies in coronary patients from 15 countries. Principal results from EUROASPIRE II Euro Heart Survey Programme. *European Heart Journal*. 2001;**22**(7):554–572.

Ezzati TM, et al. Sample design: Third National Health and Nutrition Examination Survey. *Vital Health Statistics*. 1992; 1–35.

Farnier M, et al. Current and future treatment of hyperlipidemia: the role of statins. *American Journal of Cardiology*. 1998;**82**:3J–10J.

FDA. FDA Public Health Advisory for Crestor (rosuvastatin). www.fda.gov/cder/drug/advisory/crestor.htm. Accessed September 2004.

Feldman T, et al. Treatment of high-risk patients with ezetimibe plus simvastatin co-administration versus simvastatin alone to attain National Cholesterol Education Program Adult Treatment Panel III low-density lipoprotein cholesterol goals. *American Journal of Cardiology*. 2004;**93**(12):1481–1486.

Fiore LD, et al. Department of Veterans Affairs Cooperative Studies Program Clinical Trial comparing combined warfarin and aspirin with aspirin alone in survivors of acute myocardial infarction: primary results of the CHAMP study. *Circulation*. 2002;**105**(5):557–563.

Fiorucci S, et al. Gastrointestinal safety of NO-aspirin (NCX-4016) in healthy human volunteers: a proof of concept endoscopic study. *Gastroenterology*. 2003;**124**(3):600–607.

Fiorucci S, et al. Cooperation between aspirin-triggered lipoxin and nitric oxide (NO) mediates antiadhesive properties of 2-(acetyloxy)benzoic acid 3-(nitrooxymethyl) phenyl ester (NCX-4016) (NO-aspirin) on neutrophil-endothelial cell adherence. *Journal of Pharmacology and Experimental Therapeutics*. 2004;**309**(3):1174–1182.

Flather MD, et al. Long-term ACE-inhibitor therapy in patients with heart failure or left-ventricular dysfunction: a systematic overview of data from individual patients. *Lancet*. 2000;**355**:1575–1581.

Flores-Runk P, Raasch RH. Ticlopidine and antiplatelet therapy. *Annals of Pharmacotherapy*. 1993;**27**(9):1090–1098.

Folsom AR, et al. Association of C-reactive protein with markers of prevalent atherosclerotic disease. *American Journal of Cardiology*. 2001;**88**(2):112–117

Fonarow GC, et al. Use of lipid lowering medications at discharge in patients with acute myocardial infarction. *Circulation*. 2001;**103**:38–44.

Ford ES, et al. Prevalence of nonfatal coronary heart disease among American adults. *American Heart Journal*. 2000;**139**:371–377.

Foy SG, et al. Placebo-controlled, randomized, ACE inhibitor, comparative trial in cardiac infarction and LV function. *American Journal of Cardiology*. 1994;**73**:1180–1186.

Franzosi MG, et al. Ten-year follow-up of the first megatrial testing thrombolytic therapy in patients with acute myocardial infarction. Results of GISSI-1 study. *Circulation*. 1998;**98**:2659–2665.

Freemantle N, et al. Beta blockade after myocardial infarction: systematic review and meta regression analysis. *British Medical Journal*. 1999;**318**(7200):1730–1737.

Fukiyama K, et al. Incidence and long-term prognosis of initial stroke and acute myocardial infarction in Okinawa, Japan. *Hypertension Research*. 2000;**23**:127–135.

Furman MI, et al. Twenty-two year (1975–1997) trends in the incidence, in-hospital and long-term case fatality rates from initial Q-wave and non-Q-wave myocardial infarction: a multi-hospital, community-wide perspective. *Journal of the American College of Cardiology*. 2001;**37**:1571–1580.

Gagne C, et al. Efficacy and safety of ezetimibe added to ongoing statin therapy for treatment of patients with primary hypercholesterolemia. *American Journal of Cardiology*. 2002;**90**(10):1084–1091. [a]

Gagne C, Efficacy and safety of ezetimibe coadministered with atorvastatin or simvastatin in patients with homozygous familial hypercholesterolemia. *Circulation*. 2002;**105**(21): 2469–2475. [b]

Galatius S, et al. 5993 survivors of suspected myocardial infarction: 10 year incidence of later myocardial infarction and subsequent mortality. *European Heart Journal*. 1998;**19**:564–569.

Gent M. The Canadian American Ticlopidine Study (CATS) in thromboembolic stroke. *Lancet*. 1989;**1**(8649):1215–1220.

GenVec. GenVec presents Phase 1 safety results in myoblast cell transplantation program. Press release, November 2003. www.genvec.com. Accessed October 2004.

GenVec. GenVec's myoblast cell transplantation program highlighted at American College of Cardiology Scientific Sessions. Press release, March 2004. www.genvec.com. Accessed October 2004.

Gersh BJ. The changing late prognosis of acute myocardial infarction: implications and mechanisms. *European Heart Journal*. 1995;**16**:50–53.

Gheorghiade M, et al. Natural history of the first non-Q wave myocardial infarction in the placebo arm of the Beta-Blocker Heart Attack Trial. *American Heart Journal*. 1991;**122**:1548–1553.

Gheorghiade M. Decline in the rate of hospital mortality from acute myocardial infarction: impact of changing management strategies. *American Heart Journal*. 1996;**131**:250.

Ghidh-Jain M, et al. Alterations in cardiac gene expression during ventricular remodeling following experimental myocardial infarction. *Journal of Molecular and Cellular Cardiology*. 1998;**30**:627–637.

Giampaoli S, et al. Estimating population-based incidence and prevalence of major coronary events. *International Journal of Epidemiology*. 2001;**30**(suppl 1):S5–S10.

Gilpin EA, et al. Periods of differing mortality distribution during the first year after acute myocardial infarction. *American Journal of Cardiology*. 1983;**52**:240–244.

Goldberg RJ, et al. Age-related trends in short and long-term survival after acute myocardial infarction: a 20-year population-based perspective (1975–1995). *American Journal of Cardiology*. 1998;**82**:1311–1317.

Goldberg RJ. A two-decades (1975 to 1995) long experience in the incidence, in-hospital and long-term case-fatality rates of acute myocardial infarction: A community-wide perspective. *Journal of the American College of Cardiology*. 1999;**33**:1533–1539.

Gorkin L, et al. Quality of life among patients post-myocardial infarction at baseline in the Survival and Ventricular Enlargement (SAVE) trial. *Quality of Life Research*. 1994;**3**(2):111–119.

Gottlieb SS, et al. Comparative effects of three beta blockers (atenolol, metoprolol and propranolol) on survival after acute myocardial infarction. *American Journal of Cardiology*. 2001;**87**(7):823–826.

Gradman AH, et al. A randomized, placebo-controlled, double-blind, parallel study of various doses of losartan potassium compared with enalapril maleate in patients with essential hypertension. *Hypertension*. 1995;(6):1345–1350.

Grundy SM. Statin trials and goals of cholesterol-lowering therapy. *Circulation*. 1998;**97**: 1436–1439.

Grundy SM, et al. Implications of recent clinical trials for the National Cholesterol Education Program Adult Treatment Panel III guidelines. *Circulation*. 2004;**110**(2):227–239.

Gruppo Italiano per lo Studio della Sopravvivenza nell'Infarto Miocardico (GISSI). GISSI-3: effects of lisinopril and transdermal glyceryl trinitrate singly and together on 6-week mortality and ventricular function after acute myocardial infarction. *Lancet*. 1994;**343**:1115–1122.

Gunter N, et al. Cooperative cardiovascular project. *Journal of the South Carolina Medical Association*. 1997;**93**(5):177–179.

Gustafsson D, et al. The direct thrombin inhibitor melagatran and its oral prodrug H 376/95: intestinal absorption properties, biochemical and pharmacodynamic effects. *Thrombosis Research*. 2001;**101**(3):171–181.

Gutstein DE. Pathophysiologic bases for adjunctive therapies in the treatment and secondary prevention of acute myocardial infarction. *Clinical Cardiology*. 1998;**21**: 161–168.

Haffner SM, et al. Mortality from coronary artery disease in subjects with type 2 diabetes and in nondiabetic subjects with and without prior myocardial infarction. *New England Journal of Medicine*. 1998;**339**:229–234.

Haffner SM, et al. Effect of rosiglitazone treatment on nontraditional markers of cardiovascular disease in patients with type II diabetes mellitus. *Circulation*. 2003;**107**(15): 1954–1957.

Haim M, et al. The prognosis of a first Q-wave versus non-Q wave myocardial infarction in the reperfusion era. *American Journal of Medicine*. 2000;**108**:381–386.

Hall AS, et al. Follow-up study of patients randomly allocated ramipril or placebo for heart failure after acute myocardial infarction: AIRE Extension (AIREX) Study. *Lancet*. 1997;**349**(9064):1493–1497.

Harder S, et al. Lipid-lowering treatment in coronary artery disease: a survey in an ambulatory outpatient clinic. *International Journal of Clinical Pharmacology and Therapeutics*. 2001;**39**(12):534–538.

Heart Protection Study (HPS) Collaborative Group. Heart Protection Study of cholesterol lowering with simvastatin in 20,536 high-risk individuals: a randomized placebo-controlled trial. *Lancet*. 2002;**360**:7–22.

Heidenreich PA, McClellan M. Trends in treatment and outcomes for acute myocardial infarction: 1975–1995. *American Journal of Medicine*. 2001;**110**:165–174.

Hennekens CH, et al. Additive benefits of pravastatin and aspirin to decrease risks of cardiovascular disease: randomized and observational comparisons of secondary prevention trials and their meta-analyses. *Archives of Internal Medicine*. 2004;**164**(1):40–44.

Herlitz J, et al. Long-term mortality after acute myocardial infarction in relation to prescribed dosages of beta blocker at hospital discharge. *Cardiovascular Drugs and Therapy*. 2001;**14**:589–595.

Herlitz J, et al. Effect of fixed low-dose warfarin added to aspirin in the long term after acute myocardial infarction; the LoWASA Study. *European Heart Journal*. 2004;**25**(3): 232–239.

Hillert B, et al. Improving patient outcomes by pooling resources. (The Texas Heart Care Partnership experience). *American Journal of Cardiology*. 2000;**85**(3A):43A–51A.

Hooper L, et al. Dietary fat intake and prevention of cardiovascular disease: systematic review. *British Medical Journal*. 2001;**322**:757–763.

HOPE Study Investigators. Effects of an angiotensin-converting-enzyme inhibitor, ramipril, on cardiovascular events in high-risk patients *New England Journal of Medicine*. 2000,**342**:145–153.

Hosoda S, et al. Follow-up of 2,733 patients with myocardial infarction. *Japanese Circulation Journal*. 1995;**59**:121–129.

Houghton T, et al. Are beta-blockers effective in patients who develop heart failure soon after myocardial infarction? A meta-regression analysis of randomised trials. *European Journal of Heart Failure*. 2000;(3):333–340.

Huang, Z et al. Cholesteryl ester transfer protein inhibitor (JTT-705) and the development of atherosclerosis in rabbits with severe hypercholesterolaemia. *Clinical Science (London)*. 2002;**103**(6):587–594.

Insull W, et al. Efficacy and short-term safety of a new ACAT inhibitor, avasimibe, on lipids, lipoproteins, and apolipoproteins in patients with combined hyperlipidemia. *Atherosclerosis*. 2001;**157**(1):137–144.

Ishikawa K, et al. Retrospective analysis showing less cardiac events in post myocardial patients treated with metoprolol. *Japanese Circulation Journal*. 2000;**64**:358–364.

ISIS-4 Collaborative Group. A randomized factorial trial assessing early oral captopril, oral mononitrate and intravenous magnesium sulphate in 58,050 patients with suspected acute myocardial infarction. *Lancet*. 1995;**345**:669–685.

Jackevecius CA, et al. Adherence with statin therapy in elderly patients with and without acute coronary syndromes. *Journal of the American Medical Association*. 2002;**288**(4): 462–467.

Jarvis GE, et al. The P2T antagonist AR-C69931MX is a more effective inhibitor of ADP-induced platelet aggregation than clopidogrel. *Blood*. 1999;**94**(10 pt 1). Abstract no. 81.

Jneid H, et al. Aspirin and clopidogrel in acute coronary syndromes: therapeutic insights from the CURE study. *Archives of Internal Medicine*. 2003;**163**(10):1145–1153.

Johnson PH. Hirudin: clinical potential of a thrombin inhibitor. *Annual Review of Medicine*. 1994;**45**:165–177.

Jokhadar M, et al. Sudden death and recurrent ischemic events after myocardial infarction in the community. *American Journal of Epidemiology*. 2004;**159**(11):1040–1046.

Jolly K, et al. Randomised controlled trial of follow-up care in general practice of patients with myocardial infarction and angina: final results of the Southampton heart integrated care project (SHIP). The SHIP Collaborative Group. *British Medical Journal*. 1999;**318**(7185):706–711.

Jones PH, for the STELLAR study group. Statin therapies for elevated lipid levels compared across dose ranges to rosuvastatin: low-density lipoprotein cholesterol and high density lipoprotein cholesterol results. *Journal of the American College of Cardiology*. 2003;**41**(6 suppl A):876–872.

Kajinami K, et al. Pitavastatin efficacy and safety profiles of a novel synthetic HMG-CoA reductase inhibitor. *Cardiovascular Drug Review*. 2003;**21**:199–215.

Kannel WB. Hazards, risks, and threats of heart disease from the early stages to symptomatic coronary heart disease and cardiac failure. *Cardiovascular Drugs and Therapy*. 1997;**11**:199–212.

Kannel WB. The Framingham Study: historical insight on the impact of cardiovascular risk factors in men versus women. *Journal of Gender Specific Medicine*. 2002;**5**(2):27–37.

Keavney B, et al. Large-scale test of hypothesised associations between the angiotensin-converting enzyme insertion/deletion polymorphism and myocardial infarction in about 5000 cases and 6000 controls. *Lancet*. 2000;**355**:434–442.

Kenchaiah S, et al. Effect of antecedent systemic hypertension on subsequent left ventricular dilation after acute myocardial infarction (from the Survival and Ventricular Enlargement trial). *American Journal of Cardiology*. 2004;**94**(1):1–8.

Kerzner B, et al. Efficacy and safety of ezetimibe coadministered with lovastatin in primary hypercholesterolemia. *American Journal of Cardiology*. 2003;**91**(4):418–424.

Kimura Y, et al. Demographic study of first-ever stroke and acute myocardial infarction on Okinawa, Japan. *Internal Medicine*. 1998;**37**:736–745.

Kinoshita M, et al. Guidelines for secondary prevention of myocardial infarction. *Japan Circulation Journal*. 2000;**64**(suppl IV):1081–1127.

Klimt CR, et al. Persantine-Aspirin Reinfarction Study. Part II. Secondary coronary prevention with persantine and aspirin. *Journal of the American College of Cardiology*. 1986;**7**(2):251–269.

Knopp RH, et al. Ezetimibe reduces low-density lipoprotein cholesterol: results of a phase III, randomised, double-blind, placebo-controlled trial. *Atherosclerosis*. 2001;**2**(suppl): 38. Abstract.

Kober L, et al. Changes in absolute and relative importance in the prognostic value of left ventricular systolic function and congestive heart failure after acute myocardial infarction. TRACE Study Group. Trandolapril Cardiac Evaluation. *American Journal of Cardiology*. 1998;**81**(11):1292–1297.

Kontos MC, et al. Where do you draw the line? Implications of the new troponin standard on the prevalence of myocardial infarction. Program and abstracts from the American Heart Association Scientific Sessions; November 11–14, 2001; Anaheim, California. Abstract 112088.

Kontos MC, et al. Impact of the troponin standard on the prevalence of acute myocardial infarction. *American Heart Journal*. 2003;**146**:446–452.

Koren MJ, et al. Clinical outcomes in managed-care patients with coronary heart disease treated aggressively in lipid-lowering disease management clinics: the alliance study. *Journal of the American College of Cardiology*. 2004;**44**(9):1772–1779.

Kosoglou T, et al. Pharmacodynamic interaction between ezetimibe and rosuvastatin. *Current Medical Research and Opinion*. 2004;**20**(8):1185–1195.

Kos Pharmaceuticals. Kos reports achievement of new research and development milestones. Press release, August 2004. www.kospharm.com/data/files/8312004.pdf. Accessed November 2004.

Krauss RM, et al. AHA Dietary Guidelines, Revision 2000: a statement for healthcare professionals from the Nutrition Committee of the American Heart Association. *Circulation*. 2000;**102**:2208–2299.

Kris-Etherton P, et al. Benefits of a mediterranean-style, National Cholesterol Education Program/American Heart Association step I dietary pattern on cardiovascular disease. *Circulation*. 2001;**103**:1823–1825.

Kunsch C, Medford RM. Oxidative stress as a regulator of gene expression in the vasculature. *Circulation Research*. 1999;**85**(8):753–766.

Kurata C, et al. Syncope caused by nonsteroidal anti-inflammatory drugs and angiotensin-converting enzyme inhibitors. *Japanese Circulation Journal*. 1999;**63**(12):1002–1003.

LaCivita KA, et al. Differences in lipid profiles of patients given rosiglitazone followed by pioglitazone. *Current Medical Research and Opinion*. 2002;**18**(6):363–370.

Lampe FC, et al. The natural history of prevalent ischaemic heart disease in middle-aged men. *European Heart Journal*. 2000;**21**:1052–1062.

Latini R, et al; GISSI-3 Investigators. Aspirin does not interact with ACE inhibitors when both are given early after acute myocardial infarction: results of the GISSI-3 Trial. *Heart Disease*. 2000 May–Jun;**2**(3):185–190.

Law M, Wald N. Why heart disease mortality is low in France: the time lag explanation. *British Medical Journal*. 1999;**318**:1471–1480.

Leon MB. A clinical trial comparing three antithrombotic-drug regimens after coronary-artery stenting. Stent Anticoagulation Restenosis Study Investigators. *New England Journal of Medicine*. 1998;**339**(23):1665–1671.

Liao JK. Role of statin pleiotropism in acute coronary syndromes and stroke. *International Journal of Clinical Practice supplement*. 2003;(134):51–57.

Liebson PR, et al. The non-Q wave myocardial infarction revisited: 10 years later. *Progress in Cardiovascular Diseases*. 1997;**39**:399–444.

Liem AH, et al. Fluvastatin On Risk Diminishment after Acute myocardial infarction study group. Effect of fluvastatin on ischaemia following acute myocardial infarction: a randomized trial. *European Heart Journal*. 2002;**23**(24):1931–1937.

Lipka LJ, et al. Reduction of LDL-cholesterol and elevation of HDL-cholesterol in subjects with primary hypercholesterolemia by SCH 58235: Pooled analysis of two phase II studies. *Journal of the American College of Cardiology*. 2000;**35**(2 suppl A):257A. Abstract 1046-21.

Lonn EM, Yusuf S. Emerging approaches in the prevention of atherosclerotic cardiovascular diseases. *International Journal of Clinical Practice*. 1998;**94**(suppl):7–19.

Luc G, et al. Value of HDL cholesterol, apolipoprotein A-I, and lipoprotein A-I/A-II in prediction of coronary heart disease: the PRIME Study. Prospective Epidemiological Study of Myocardial Infarction. *Arteriosclerosis, Thrombosis, and Vascular Biology*. 2002;**22**(7):1155.

Maggioni AP, et al. Epidemiology of post-infarction risk stratification strategies in a country with a low volume of revascularization procedures: the GISSI Prognosis Registry. *European Heart Journal*. 1998;**19**:1784–1794.

Makkar RR, et al. Stem cell therapy for myocardial repair: is it arrhythmogenic? *Journal of the American College of Cardiology*. 2003;**42**(12):2070–2072.

Mark DB, et al. Use of medical resources and quality of life after acute myocardial infarction in Canada and the United States. *New England Journal of Medicine*. 1994;**331**: 1130–1135.

Marques-Vidal P, et al. Trends in myocardial infarction treatment in subjects aged 35–64 in Southwestern France, 1986–93. *International Journal of Cardiology*. 2003;**88**:239–245.

Marrugat J, et al. Epidemiology of ischaemic heart disease in Spain: Estimation of the number of cases and trends from 1997 to 2005. *Revista Española de Cardiologia*. 2002;**55**(4):337–346.

Marx N, et al. Effect of rosiglitazone treatment on soluble CD40L in patients with type II diabetes and coronary artery disease. *Circulation*. 2003;**107**(15):1954–1957.

Matsuno H, et al. Pharmacokinetic and pharmacodynamic properties of a new thromboxane receptor antagonist (Z-355) after single and multiple oral administration to healthy volunteers. *Journal of Clinical Pharmacology*. 2002;**42**(7):782–790.

Mazzolai L, Burnier M. Comparative safety and tolerability of angiotensin II receptor antagonists. *Drug Safety*. 1999;**21**(1):23–33.

McCarty MF. ACE inhibition may decrease diabetes risk by boosting the impact of bradykinin on adipocytes. *Medical Hypotheses*. 2003;**60**(6):779–783.

Mehta RH, et al. Current concepts in secondary prevention after acute myocardial infarction. *Herz*. 2000;**25**:47–60.

Mehta RH, et al. Secondary prevention in acute myocardial infarction. *British Medical Journal*. 1998;**316**:838–842.

Meier MA. The new definition of myocardial infarction: what does it mean clinically? The 50th Scientific Session of the American College of Cardiology; March 18–21, 2001; Orlando, FL.

Meier MA, et al. The new definition of myocardial infarction. Diagnostic and prognostic implications in patients with acute coronary syndromes. *Archives of Internal Medicine*. 2002;**162**:1585–1589.

Melville M, et al. Outcome and use of health services four years after admission for acute myocardial infarction: case record follow-up study. *British Medical Journal*. 1999;**319**:230–231.

Menasche P, et al. Autologous skeletal myoblast transplantation for severe postinfarction left ventricular dysfunction. *Journal of the American College of Cardiology*. 2003;**41**(7): 1078–1083.

Meune C, et al. Interaction between angiotensin-converting enzyme inhibitors and aspirin: a review. *European Journal of Clinical Pharmacology*. 2000;**56**:609–620.

Milliat F, et al. Overexpression of SR-BI in hamsters treated with a novel ACAT inhibitor (F12511). *Comptes rendus de l'Academie des sciences. Serie III, Sciences de la vie.* 2001;**324**(3):229–234.

Miura T, et al. Infarct size limitation by a new Na(+)-H + exchange inhibitor, Hoe 642: difference from preconditioning in the role of protein kinase C. *Journal of the American College of Cardiology.* 1997;**29**(3):693–701.

Muhlestein JB. Post-hospitalization management of high-risk coronary patients. *American Journal of Cardiology.* 2000;**85**:13B–20B.

Mulder HJ, et al. Improvement of serum oxidation by pravastatin might be one of the mechanisms by which endothelial function in dilated coronary artery segments is ameliorated. *Atherosclerosis.* 2003;**169**:309–315.

Muller K, et al. Antioxidant BO-653 and human macrophage-mediated LDL oxidation. *Free Radical Research.* 1999;**30**(1):59–71.

Myerburg RJ, et al. Frequency of sudden cardiac death and profiles of risk. *American Journal of Cardiology.* 1997;**80**(5B):10F–19F.

Nakamura Y, et al. Comparison between Japan and North America in the post-hospital course after recovery from an acute coronary event. *International Journal of Cardiology.* 1996;**55**:245–254.

Napoli C, et al. Effects of nitric oxide-releasing aspirin versus aspirin on restenosis in hypercholesterolemic mice. *Proceedings of the National Academy of Sciences USA.* 2001;**98**(5):2860–2864.

Nappi G, et al. Postinfarction ventricular septal defect in a patient without coronary lesions. *Annals of Thoracic Surgery.* 2003;**75**(4):1315–1317.

National Center for Health Statistics. National Health and Nutrition Examination Survey, 1999–2000 and 2001–2002. Public-use data file and documentation. www.cdc.gov/nchs/about/major/nhanes/datalink.htm. 2004.

National Centre for Social Research. Health Survey of England 1998: Cardiovascular Disease. Department of Epidemiology and Public Health, Royal Free and University College Medical School. The Stationary Office, London. 1998.

National Heart, Lung and Blood Institute (NHLBI). *Morbidity and Mortality: 2000 Chartbook on Cardiovascular, Lung, and Blood Diseases.* Bethesda, MD: Public Health Service, National Institutes of Health; 2000:17–35.

National Heart Lung and Blood Institute. *Morbidity and Mortality: 2002 Chartbook on Cardiovascular, Lung, and Blood Diseases.* Public Health Service, National Institutes of Health. 2002; 29.

NCEP (National Cholesterol Education Program) Expert Panel on Detection, Evaluation, and Treatment of High Blood Cholesterol in Adults (Adult Treatment Panel III). Third Report of the National Cholesterol Education Program (NCEP) Expert Panel on Detection, Evaluation, and Treatment of High Blood Cholesterol in Adults (Adult Treatment Panel III) final report. *Circulation.* 2002;**106**(25):3143–3421.

Nissen SE. (REVERSAL) A prospective, randomized, double blind, multi-center study comparing the effects of atorvastatin vs. pravastatin on the progression of coronary atherosclerotic lesions as measured by intravascular ultrasound. American Heart Association Scientific Sessions 2003; November 9–12, 2003; Orlando, FL. Plenary Session XI: Late Breaking Clinical Trials.

Noji Y, et al. Long-term treatment with pitavastatin (NK-104), a new HMG-CoA reductase inhibitor, of patients with heterozygous familial hypercholesterolemia. *Atherosclerosis*. 2002;**163**(1):157–164.

O'Connor CM, et al. Comparison of two aspirin doses on ischemic stroke in post-myocardial infarction patients in the warfarin (Coumadin) Aspirin Reinfarction Study (CARS). *American Journal of Cardiology*. 2001;**88**(5):541–546.

O'Keefe JH, et al. Should an angiotensin-converting enzyme inhibitor be standard therapy for patients with atherosclerotic disease? *Journal of the American College of Cardiology*. 2001;**37**(1):1–8.

Ohno J, et al. Risk stratification and survival in post myocardial infarction patients: a large prospective and multicenter study in Japan. *International Journal of Cardiology*. 2004;Feb;**93**(2–3):263–268.

Oliver WR, et al. A selective peroxisome proliferators-activated receptor delta agonist promotes reverse cholesterol transport. *Proceedings of the National Academy of Sciences USA*. 2001;**98**(9):5306–5311.

Olsson AG, et al. Long-term efficacy and safety of rosuvastatin: results of a 52-week comparator-controlled trial versus atorvastatin [abstract]. *European Heart Journal* 2001;**22**(suppl):253. [a]

Olsson AG, et al. MIRACL (Myocardial Ischemia Reduction with Aggressive Cholesterol Lowering). *Clinical Cardiology*. 2001;**24**(1):85–86. [b]

Olsson AG, et al. Effects of rosuvastatin and atorvastatin compared over 52 weeks of treatment in patients with hypercholesterolemia. *American Heart Journal*. 2002;**144**(6): 1044–1051.

Olsson G, et al. Long-term treatment with metoprolol after myocardial infarction: effect on 3 year mortality and morbidity. *Journal of the American College of Cardiology*. 1985;**5**(6):1428–1437.

Olsson L, et al. Validity of a postal questionnaire with regard to the prevalence of myocardial infarction in a general population sample. *European Heart Journal*. 1989;**10**: 1011–1016.

Olsson SB, et al. Stroke prevention with the oral direct thrombin inhibitor ximelagatran compared with warfarin in patients with non-valvular atrial fibrillation (SPORTIF III): randomised controlled trial. *Lancet*. 2003;**362**(9397):1691–1698.

Osende JI, et al. Antithrombotic effects of S 18886, a novel orally active thromboxane A2 receptor antagonist. *Journal of Thrombosis and Haemostasis*. 2004;**3**:492–498.

Otterstad JE, Ford I. The effect of carvedilol in patients with impaired left ventricular systolic function following an acute myocardial infarction. How do the treatment effects on total mortality and recurrent myocardial infarction in CAPRICORN compare with previous beta-blocker trials? *European Journal of Heart Failure*. 2002;**4**(4):501–506.

Paoletti R, et al. ZD4522 (rosuvastatin) is superior to pravastatin and simvastatin in reducing low density lipoprotein cholesterol, enabling more hypercholesterolemic patients to achieve target low density lipoprotein cholesterol guidelines. The 50th Scientific Session of the American College of Cardiology; March 18–21, 2001; Orlando, FL.

PARIS investigators. The Persantine-aspirin reinfarction study. The Persantine-aspirin Reinfarction Study (PARIS) research group. *Circulation*. 1980 (6 Pt 2):V85–V88.

Park SW, et al. Comparison of cilostazol versus ticlopidine therapy after stent implantation. *American Journal of Cardiology*. 1999;**84**(5):511–514.

Pedersen TR, et al. Safety and tolerability of cholesterol lowering with simvastatin during 5 years in the Scandinavian Simvastatin Survival Study. *Archives of Internal Medicine*. 1996;**156**:2085–2092.

Pepine CI, et al. Changing myocardial infarction population characteristics: reasons and implications. *American Heart Journal*. 1997;**134**:S1.

Pepine CJ. Optimizing lipid management in patients with acute coronary syndromes. *American Journal of Cardiology*. 2003;**91**(4A):30B–35B.

Pereira EC, et al. Effects of simvastatin and L-arginine on vasodilation, nitric oxide metabolites and endogenous NOS inhibitors in hypercholstrolemic subjects. *Free Radical Research*. 2003;**37**:529–536.

Pérez G, et al. Myocardial infarction in Girona, Spain: attack rate, mortality rate and 28-day case fatality in 1988. *Journal of Clinical Epidemiology*. 1993;**46**:1173.

Peterson ED, et al. Clinical guideline part II. Risk stratification after myocardial infarction. *Annals of Internal Medicine*. 1997; **126**:561–582.

Pfeffer MA, et al. Effect of captopril on mortality and morbidity in patients with left ventricular dysfunction after myocardial infarction. Results of the survival and ventricular enlargement trial. *New England Journal of Medicine*. 1992;**327**:669–677.

Pfeffer MA, et al. Cholesterol and Recurrent Events: a secondary prevention trial for normolipidemic patients. CARE Investigators. *American Journal of Cardiology*. 1995; **76**(9):98C–106C.

Pfeffer MA, et al. Valsartan in acute myocardial infarction trial (VALIANT): rationale and design. *American Heart Journal*. 2000;**140**(5):727–750.

Pfeffer MA, et al. Valsartan, captopril, or both in myocardial infarction complicated by heart failure, left ventricular dysfunction, or both. *New England Journal of Medicine*. 2003;**349**(20):1893–1906.

Pfisterer M, et al. Atenolol use and clinical outcomes after thrombolysis for acute myocardial infarction: the GUSTO I experience. Global Utilization of Streptokinase and TPA (alteplase) for Occluded Coronary Arteries. *Journal of the American College of Cardiology*. 1998;**32**(3):634–640.

Phibbs B, et al. Q-wave and non-Q wave myocardial infarction: a meaningless distinction. *Journal of the American College of Cardiology*. 1999;**33**:576–582.

Pitt B. Natural history of myocardial infarction and its prodromal syndromes. *Circulation*. 1976;**53**(3 suppl):I132–I135.

Pitt B, et al. Effect of losartan compared with captopril on mortality in patients with symptomatic heart failure: randomised trial—the Losartan Heart Failure Survival Study ELITE II. *Lancet*. 2000;**355**(9215):1582–1587.

Pitt B, et al. Eplerenone, a selective aldosterone blocker in patients with left ventricular dysfunction after myocardial infarction. *New England Journal of Medicine*. 2003; **348**(4):1309–1321.

Population Division of the Department of Economic and Social Affairs of the United Nations Secretariat. *World Population Prospects: The 2002 Revision*, vol. I, *Comprehensive Tables* (United Nations publication, Sales No. E.03.XIII.6); and *World Population Prospects: The 2002 Revision*, vol. II, *The Sex and Age Distribution of Populations* (United Nations publication, Sales No. E.03.XIII.7), 2003.

Post SM, et al. Fibrates suppress bile acid synthesis via peroxisome proliferator-activated receptor-alpha-mediated downregulation of cholesterol 7alpha-hydroxylase and sterol

27-hydroxylase expression. *Arteriosclerosis, Thrombosis, and Vascular Biology*. 2001; **21**(11):1840–1845.

Rajagopalan S, et al. A phase I study of intramuscular administration of CI-1023 (ADGVVEGF121.10) in patients with peripheral vascular disease. *Circulation*. 2001; **104**:A262.

Rapaport E, et al. Pharmacologic therapies after myocardial infarction. *American Journal of Medicine*. 1996;**101**(suppl 4A):61S–70S.

Reynolds G, et al. What have the ACE-inhibitor trials in postmyocardial patients with left ventricular dysfunction taught us? *European Journal of Clinical Pharmacology*. 1996;**49**(suppl 1):S35–S39.

Rezaie-Majid A, et al. Simvastatin reduces the expression of adhesion molecules in circulating monocytes from hypercholestrolemic patients. *Arteriosclerosis, Thrombosis, and Vascular Biology*. 2003;**23**:397–403.

Richards AM, et al. Antecedent hypertension and heart failure after myocardial infarction. *Journal of the American College of Cardiology*. 2002;**39**:1182–1188.

Rickards L, et al. Living in Britain—the 2002 General Household Survey. www.statistics. gov.uk. Published March 2004. Accessed August 17, 2004.

Rival Y, et al. Anti-atherosclerotic properties of the acyl-coenzyme A:cholesterol acyltransferase inhibitor F 12511 in casein-fed New Zealand rabbits. *Journal of Cardiovascular Pharmacology*. 2002;**39**(2):181–191.

Robertson RM, Smaha L. Can a Mediterranean-style diet reduce heart disease? *Circulation*. 2001;**103**:1821–1822.

Rochon PA, et al. Rate of heart failure and 1-year survival for older people receiving low-dose beta-blocker therapy after myocardial infarction. *Lancet*. 2000;**356**(9230):639–644.

Rosamond WD, et al. Trends in the incidence of myocardial infarction and in mortality due to coronary heart disease, 1987–1994. *New England Journal of Medicine*. 1998;**339**:861–867.

Rosenblatt S, et al. The impact of pioglitazone on glycemic control and atherogenic dyslipidemia in patients with type 2 diabetes mellitus. *Coronary Artery Disease*. 2001; **12**(5):413–423.

Rosengart TK, et al. Angiogenesis gene therapy: Phase I assessment of direct intramyocardial administration of an adenovirus vector expressing VEGF121 cDNA to individuals with clinically significant severe coronary artery disease. *Circulation*. 1999;**100**(5): 468–474.

Rosengren A, et al. Natural history of myocardial infarction and angina pectoris in the general population sample of middle-aged men: a 16-year follow-up of the Primary Prevention Study, Goteborg, Sweden. *Journal of Internal Medicine*. 1998;**244**:495–505.

Ross R. Atherosclerosis—an inflammatory disease. *New England Journal of Medicine*. 1999;**340**(2):115–126.

Rossoni G, et al. The nitroderivative of aspirin, ncx 4016, reduces infarct size caused by myocardial ischemia-reperfusion in the anesthetized rat. *Journal of Pharmacological Experimental Therapy*. 2001;**7**(1):380–387.

Rouleau JL, et al. Comparison of vasopeptidase inhibitor, omapatrilat, and lisinopril on exercise tolerance and morbidity in patients with heart failure: IMPRESS randomised trial. *Lancet*. 2000;19;**356**(9230):615–620.

Ruggeri ZM. Von Willebrand factor. *Current Opinion in Hematology*. 2003;**10**(2): 142–149.

Ryan TJ, et al. 1999 update: ACC/AHA guidelines for the management of patients with acute myocardial infarction: executive summary and recommendations: a report of the American College of Cardiology/American Heart Association Task Force on Practice Guidelines (Committee on Management of Acute Myocardial Infarction). *Circulation*. 1999;**100**:1016–1030.

Ryan TJ, Melduni RM. Highlights of latest American College of Cardiology and American Heart Association Guidelines for Management of Patients with Acute Myocardial Infarction. *Cardiology Review*. 2002 Jan–Feb;**10**(1):35–43.

St. John Sutton M, et al. Cardiovascular death and left ventricular remodelling 2 years after myocardial infarction. Baseline predictors and impact of long-term use of captopril: information from the survival and ventricular enlargement trial. *Circulation*. 1997;**96**:3294–3299.

Saito D, et al. Risk factors indicating recurrent myocardial infarction after recovery from acute myocardial infarction. *Circulation Journal*. 2002;**66**(10):877–880.

Saito M, et al. Long-term prognosis of patients with acute myocardial infarction: is mortality and morbidity as low as the incidence of ischemic heart disease in Japan? *American Heart Journal*. 1987;**113**(4):891–897.

Saito Y, et al. A randomized, double-blind trial comparing the efficacy of pitavastatin versus pravastatin in patients with primary hypercholesterolemia. *Atherosclerosis*. 2002; **162**(2):373–379.

Sala J, et al. Improvement in survival after myocardial infarction between 1978–1985 and 1986–1988 in the REGICOR Study. *European Heart Journal*. 1995;**16**:779–784.

Sanchez RG, et al. Survey of cardiovascular acute myocardial infarction and stroke and its risk factors in the elderly population of Spain: the EPICARDIAN study—methods and demographics findings. *CVD Prevention*. 1999;**2**:290–300.

Sawayama Y, et al. Effects of probucol and paravastatin on common carotid atherosclerosis in patients with asymptomatic hypercholesterolemia. Fukuoka Atherosclerosis Trial (FAST). *Journal of the American College of Cardiology*. 2002;**39**(4):610–616.

Scandinavian Simvastatin Survival Study Group. Randomised trial of cholesterol lowering in 444 patients with coronary heart disease: the Scandinavian Simvastatin Survival Study (4S). *Lancet*. 1994;**344**:1383–1389.

Schaefer E. HDL raising: the next frontier in heart disease prevention. The Knowledge Foundation's 4th Annual International Conference: HDL Cholesterol—Metabolic Pathways and Drug Developments; March 2–4, 2003; Cambridge, MA.

Schlant RC, et al. The natural history of coronary heart disease: prognostic factors after recovery from myocardial infarction in 2,789 men. The 5-year findings of the Coronary Drug Project. *Circulation*. 1982;**66**:401–414.

Schuster H, for the MERCURY I study group. Effects of switching to rosuvastatin from atorvastatin or other statins on achievement of international low-density lipoprotein cholesterol goals: MERCURY I trial. *Journal of the American College of Cardiology*. 2003;**416** (suppl A):1010–1149.

Schwartz GG, et al. Effects of atorvastatin on early recurrent ischemic events in acute coronary syndromes: the MIRACL study: a randomized controlled trial. *Journal of the American Medical Association*. 2001;**285**(13):1711–1718.

Scrip. Late-stage U.S. licensing opportunities. *Scrip*. 2003;**2902**:22.

Scrutino D, et al. Ticlopidine versus aspirin after myocardial infarction (STAMI) trial. *Journal of the American College of Cardiology*. 2001;**37**:1259–1265.

Shah PK, et al. High-dose recombinant apolipoprotein A-I(milano) mobilizes tissue cholesterol and rapidly reduces plaque lipid and macrophage content in apolipoprotein e-deficient mice. Potential implications for acute plaque stabilization. *Circulation*. 2001;**103**(25):3047–3050.

Shepherd J. The West of Scotland Coronary Prevention Study: a trial of cholesterol reduction in Scottish men. *American Journal of Cardiology*. 1995;**76**(9):113C–117C.

Shepherd J. A review of the safety profile of rosuvastatin in an international phase II/III clinical trial program. *XIV International Symposium on Drugs Affecting Lipid Metabolism*. September 9–12, 2001; New York, NY.

Shepherd J, et al. From best evidence to best practice: What are the obstacles? *Atherosclerosis*. 1999;**147**(suppl 1):S45–S51.

Sica DA. Class effects of angiotensin-converting enzyme inhibitors. *American Journal of Managed Care*. 2000;**6**:S85–S108.

Sidhu JS, et al. The PPAR-gamma agonist rosiglitazone reduces endothelial activation in non-diabetic coronary artery disease patients. *European Heart Journal*. 2002;**4**(suppl):492.

Sigurdsson E, et al. Unrecognized myocardial infarction: epidemiology, clinical characteristics, and the prognostic role of angina pectoris. *Annals of Internal Medicine*. 1995;**122**:103–106.

Siminiak T, et al. Autologous skeletal myoblast transplantation for the treatment of postinfarction myocardial injury: phase I clinical study with 12 months of follow-up. *American Heart Journal*. 2004;**148**(3):531–537.

Smits PC, et al. Catheter-based intramyocardial injection of autologous skeletal myoblasts as a primary treatment of ischemic heart failure: clinical experience with six-month follow-up. *Journal of the American College of Cardiology*. 2003;**42**(12):2063–2069.

Snowden M. Redefining acute MI: the potential impact on rehabilitation services. *British Journal of Cardiology*. 2004;**11**(1):39–41.

SOLVD Investigators. Effect of enalapril on survival in patients with reduced left ventricular ejection fractions and congestive heart failure. *New England Journal Medicine*. 1991;**325**(5):293–302.

Sowers JR. Hypertension, angiotensin II, and oxidative stress. *New England Journal Medicine*. 2002;**346**(25):1999–2001.

Spijkers JA, et al. ABCA1 but not SR-BI is regulated by PPAR-α,-δ and -γ in cultured rat hepatocytes. *Circulation*. 2001;**104**:II–713.

Spyrou N, et al. Myocardial beta-adrenoreceptor density one month after acute myocardial infarction predicts left ventricular volumes at six months. *Journal of the American College of Cardiology*. 2000;**36**:2072–2080.

Stalenhoef AFH, et al. A comparative study with rosuvastatin in subjects with metabolic syndrome: results of the COMETS study. The 40th Annual Meeting of the European Association for the Study of Diabetes, Munich, Germany. 2004.

Stein EA, et al. ZD4522 (rosuvastatin) compared with diet and maximal lipid therapy in patients with heterozygous familial hyper-cholesterolemia. *Journal of the American College of Cardiology*. 2001;**37**(suppl):291A. Abstract. [a]

Stein EA, et al. ZD4522 is superior to atorvastatin in the treatment of patients with heterozygous familial hypercholesterolemia. *Journal of the American College of Cardiology*. 2001;**37**(suppl):292A. Abstract. [b]

Steinhubl SR, et al. CREDO Investigators. Clopidogrel for the Reduction of Events During Observation. Early and sustained dual oral antiplatelet therapy following percutaneous coronary intervention: a randomized controlled trial. *Journal of the American Medical Association*. 2002;**288**(19):2411–2420.

Stephens WB. Post-myocardial infarction pain in a series of male patients in the Albury-Wodonga District. *Medical Journal of Australia*. 1970;**2**:492–494.

Stewart DJ. A Phase 2, randomized, multicenter, 26-week study to assess the efficacy and safety of BioBypass (AdgvVEFG121.10) delivered through invasive surgery versus maximum medical treatment in patients with severe angina, advanced coronary artery disease (CAD), and no options for revascularization. Presented at the American Heart Association Scientific Sessions 2002. November 17–20, 2002. Chicago, IL.

Storey RF, et al. The central role of the P(2T) receptor in amplification of human platelet activation, aggregation, secretion and procoagulant activity. *British Journal of Haematology*. 2000;**110**(4):925–934.

Strauer BE, et al. Repair of infarcted myocardium by autologous intracoronary mononuclear bone marrow cell transplantation in humans. *Circulation*. 2002;**106**(15): 1913–1918.

Sugidachi A, et al. Antiplatelet action of R-99224, and active metabolite of a novel thienopyridine-type G9i0-linked P2T antagonist, CS-747. *British Journal of Pharmacology*. 2001;**132**:47–54.

Sundell CL, et al. AGI-1067: a multifunctional phenolic antioxidant, lipid modulator, anti-inflammatory and antiatherosclerotic agent. *Journal of Pharmacologic Experimental Therapeutics*. 2003.

Swedberg K, et al. Cooperative new Scandinavian enalapril survival study II. *New England Journal of Medicine*. 1992;**327**:678–684. [a]

Swedberg K, et al. Effects of the early administration of enalapril on mortality in patients with acute myocardial infarction. Results of the Cooperative New Scandinavian Enalapril Survival Study II (CONSENSUS II). *New England Journal of Medicine*. 1992;**327**(10):6786–6784. [b]

Tanabe M, et al. Epidemiology of acute coronary syndrome. *Nippon Rinsho*. 1998;**56**: 2681–2685.

Tanabe N, et al. Event rates of acute myocardial infarction and coronary deaths in Niigata and Nagaoka cities in Japan. *Circulation Journal*. 2003;**67**:40–45.

Tardif JC, et al. Design features of the Avasimibe and Progression of coronary Lesions assessed by intravascular UltraSound (A-PLUS) clinical trial. *American Heart Journal*. 2002;**144**(4):589–596.

Tardif JC. Clinical results with AGI-1067: a novel antioxidant vascular protectant. *American Journal of Cardiology*. 2003;**91**(3A):41A–49A.

Tom B, et al. Bradykinin, angiotensin-(1–7), and ACE inhibitors: how do they interact? *International Journal of Biochemistry and Cell Biology*. 2003;**35**(6):792–801.

Tonkin AM, et al. Effects of pravastatin in 3260 patients with unstable angina: results from the lipid study. *Lancet*. 2000;**355**:1871–1875.

Trippodo NC, et al. Effects of omapatrilat in low, normal, and high renin experimental hypertension. *American Journal of Hypertension*. 1998;**11**(3 Pt 1):363–372.

Trippodo NC, et al. Vasopeptidase inhibition with omapatrilat improves cardiac geometry and survival in cardiomyopathic hamsters more than does ACE inhibition with captopril. *Journal of Cardiovascular Pharmacology*. 1999;**34**(6):782–790.

Tunstall-Pedoe H, et al. Contribution of trends in survival and coronary event rates to changes in coronary heart disease mortality: 10-year results from 37 WHO MONICA Project populations. *Lancet*. 1999;**353**:1547–1557.

Ulvenstam G, et al. Recurrent myocardial infarction. 1. Natural history of fatal and non-fatal events. *European Heart Journal*. 1985;**6**:294–302.

United Nations Population Division, Department of Economics and Social Affairs. *Sex and age quinquennial 1950–2050*. 1998 revision. New York, NY. 1998.

Vaccarino V, et al. Long-term outcome of myocardial infarction in women and men: a population perspective. *American Journal of Epidemiology*. 2000;**152**:965–973.

Vaccarino V, et al. Sex differences in 2-year mortality after hospital discharge for myocardial infarction. *Annals of Internal Medicine*. 2001;**134**:173–181.

van der Pal-de Bruin KM, et al. The incidence of suspected myocardial infarction in Dutch general practice in the period 1978–1994. *European Heart Journal*. 1998;**19**:429–434.

Volmink JA. Coronary event and case fatality rates in an English population: results of the Oxford Myocardial Infarction Incidence Study. *Heart*. 1998;**80**:40

Volpi A, et al. Incidence and prognosis of early primary ventricular fibrillation in acute myocardial infarction—results of the Gruppo Italiano per lo Studio della Sopravvivenza nell'Infarto Miocardico (GISSI-2) database. *American Journal of Cardiology*. 1998;**82**(3):265–271.

Volpi A, et al. Incidence and short-term prognosis of late sustained ventricular tachycardia after myocardial infarction: results of the Gruppo Italiano per lo Studio della Sopravvivenza nell'Infarto Miocardico (GISSI-3) database. *American Heart Journal*. 2001;**142**(1):87–92

Wainwright CL, et al. NCX4016 (NO-aspirin) reduces infarct size and suppresses arrhythmias following myocardial ischaemia/reperfusion in pigs. *British Journal of Pharmacology*. 2002;**135**(8):1882–1888.

Wallentin L, et al. Oral ximelagatran for secondary prophylaxis after myocardial infarction: the ESTEEM randomised controlled trial. *Lancet*. 2003;**362**(9386):789–797.

Wassmann S, et al. HMG-CoA reductase inhibitors improve endothelial dysfunction in normocholesterolemic hypertension via reduced production of reactive oxygen species. *Hypertension*. 2001;**37**(6):1450–1457.

Weinberg SL. Natural history six years after acute myocardial infarction: is there a low-risk group? *Chest*. 1976;**69**:23–28.

White CM. A review of the pharmacologic and pharmacokinetic aspects of rosuvastatin. *Journal of Clinical Pharmacology*. 2002;**42**:963–970.

White HD, et al. Left ventricular end-systolic volume as the major determinant of survival after recovery from myocardial infarction. *Circulation*. 1987;**76**:44–51.

Wiesner G, et al. Note on the myocardial infarction scene in the Federal Republic of Germany: prevalence, incidence, trends, comparison between Eastern and Western Germany [Zum Herzinfarktgeschehen in der Bundesrepublik Deutschland: Prävalenz, Inzidenz, Trend, Ost-West-Vergleich]. *Gesundheitswesen*. 1999;**61**:S72–S78.

Wilhelmsen L, et al. Risk factors for a major coronary event after myocardial infarction in the Scandinavian Simvastatin Survival Study (4S). Impact of predicted risk on the benefit of cholesterol-lowering treatment. *European Heart Journal*. 2001;**22**(13):1119–1127.

Wolffenbuttel BHR, et al., on behalf of the Dutch CORALL study group. Cholesterol-lowering effects of rosuvastatin compared with atorvastatin in patients with type 2 diabetes. The 74th European Atherosclerosis Society Congress. Seville, Spain, April 2004.

Wollert KC. Intracoronary autologous bone-marrow cell transfer after myocardial infarction: the BOOST randomised controlled clinical trial. *Lancet*. 2004;**364**(9429): 121–122.

Wright RS, et al. Statin lipid-lowering therapy for acute myocardial infarction and unstable angina: efficacy and mechanism of benefit. *Mayo Clinic Proceedings*. 2002;**77**(10): 1085–1092.

Yoshitomi Y, et al. Antiplatelet treatment with cilostazol after stent implantation. *Heart*. 1998;**80**(4):393–396.

Yusuf S, et al. Beta blockade during and after myocardial infarction: an overview of the randomized trials. *Progress in Cardiovascular Diseases*. 1985;**27**:335–371.

Yusuf S, et al. Clopidogrel in Unstable Angina to Prevent Recurrent Events (CURE) Trial Investigators. Effects of clopidogrel in addition to aspirin in patients with acute coronary syndromes without ST-segment elevation. *New England Journal of Medicine*. 2001;**345**:494–502.

Zhang L, et al. Adventitial expression of VCAM-1 and its regulation by peroxisome proliferators activated receptor gamma. *Circulation*. 2001;**104**(17):A250.

Pulmonary Hypertension

ETIOLOGY AND PATHOPHYSIOLOGY

Introduction

Pulmonary hypertension (PH) is a very complex condition characterized by non-specific signs and symptoms that results from multiple causes, making diagnosis extremely difficult (Nauser TD, 2001). In a healthy individual, the mean pulmonary artery pressure, at sea level, lies between 12 and 16 mm Hg. PH is generally defined as a mean pulmonary artery pressure higher than 25 mm Hg at rest or 30 mm Hg during exercise (Strange JW, 2002).

Until the late 1990s, PH was classified either as primary (idiopathic) or secondary (associated with cardiopulmonary and systemic diseases). Then, in 1998, the World Health Organization (WHO) held a symposium in Evian, France, where a new classification system for PH was introduced. This classification system was based on current knowledge of the clinical and pathological features of the condition. These guidelines were revised at the Third World Symposium on Pulmonary Arterial Hypertension in Venice in 2003 to reflect further scientific understanding. The Venice classification for PH outlines five classes of disease: pulmonary arterial hypertension (PAH), PH with left-heart disease, PH associated with lung diseases and/or hypoxemia, PH due to chronic thrombotic and/or embolic disease, and miscellaneous forms of PH (Simonneau G, 2004). Table 1 provides further detail on the Venice classification. Physicians assess the severity of the disease

Wiley Handbook of Current and Emerging Drug Therapies, Volumes 5–8
Copyright © 2007 Decision Resources, Inc. Published by John Wiley & Sons, Inc.

TABLE 1. Summary of Revised Classification for Pulmonary Hypertension (Venice 2003)

Pulmonary arterial hypertension (PAH)	Idiopathic pulmonary arterial hypertension (IPAH)
	Familial pulmonary arterial hypertension (FPAH)
	Associated pulmonary arterial hypertension (APAH): collagen vascular disease, congenital systemic-to-pulmonary shunts, portal hypertension, HIV infection, drugs and toxins, other (thyroid disorders, glycogen storage disease, Gaucher's disease, hereditary hemorrhagic telangiectasia, hemoglobinopathies, myoproliferative disorders and splenectomy)
	Associated with significant venous or capillary involvement: pulmonary veno-occlusive disease (PVOD), pulmonary capillary hemangiomatosis (PCH)
	Persistent pulmonary hypertension of the newborn
Pulmonary hypertension with left-heart disease	Left-sided atrial or ventricular heart disease
	Left-sided valvular heart disease
Pulmonary hypertension associated with lung diseases and/or hypoxemia	Chronic obstructive pulmonary disease (COPD)
	Interstitial lung disease
	Sleep-disordered breathing
	Alveolar hypoventilation disorders
	Chronic exposure to high altitude
	Developmental abnormalities
Pulmonary hypertension due to chronic thrombo and/or embolic disease	Thromboembolic obstruction of the proximal pulmonary arteries
	Thromboembolic obstruction of the distal pulmonary arteries
	Nonthrombotic pulmonary embolism (tumor, parasite, infection)
Pulmonary hypertension — miscellaneous	Sarcoidosis
	Histiocytosis X
	Lymphangiomatosis
	Pulmonary artery compression

Source: Based on Simonneau G, et al. Clinical classification of pulmonary hypertension. Journal of the American College of Cardiology. 2004;43(12 suppl S):5 S–12 S.

TABLE 2. New York Heart Association (NYHA) Functional Class: Pulmonary Hypertension

NYHA Functional Class	Criteria
Class I	Patients have pulmonary hypertension but without limits on physical activity.
	Ordinary physical activity does not cause undue dyspnea or fatigue, chest pain, or near syncope.
Class II	Patients with pulmonary hypertension resulting in some limitation of physical activity.
	Patients are comfortable at rest, but ordinary physical activity causes dyspnea or fatigue, chest pain, or near syncope.
Class III	Patients with pulmonary hypertension resulting in marked limitation of physical activity.
	Patients are comfortable at rest but less than ordinary physical activity causes dyspnea, fatigue, chest pain, or near syncope.
Class IV	Patients with pulmonary hypertension resulting in inability to perform any physical activity.
	Patients show signs of right-heart failure.
	Dyspnea and/or fatigue may be present at rest.
	Discomfort is increased by any physical activity.

Source: Based on Humbert M, et al. Treatment of pulmonary arterial hypertension. New England Journal of Medicine. 2004;351(14):1425–1436.

and assign treatment based on New York Heart Association (NYHA) functional class. Table 2 summarizes the NYHA classification system.

This section focuses on the PAH class because agents currently approved and in development for pulmonary hypertension target this patient group. PAH encompasses idiopathic pulmonary arterial hypertension (IPAH), familial pulmonary arterial hypertension (FPAH), and PAH related to various conditions (known as associated pulmonary arterial hypertension [APAH]). Examples of associated conditions include collagen vascular disease, portal hypertension, and human immunodeficiency virus (HIV) (Table 1). All patients within the PAH group share comparable clinical management, and the outcome of the disease is generally associated with an increase in pulmonary vascular resistance leading to right-ventricular failure (Galié N, 2003).

Anatomy

The Pulmonary Circulation. The pulmonary circulation performs an extremely important function (Figure 1): It brings blood into close proximity to alveolar air sacs within the lungs to allow gaseous exchanges (transfer of oxygen and carbon dioxide). Oxygen-deficient blood (dark red in color) is pumped from the right ventricle of the heart into the pulmonary trunk, which branches into the right and left pulmonary arteries. Within the lungs, the pulmonary arteries subdivide further into the lobar arteries, three supplying the right lung and two supplying the left lung. These lobar arteries accompany the main bronchi

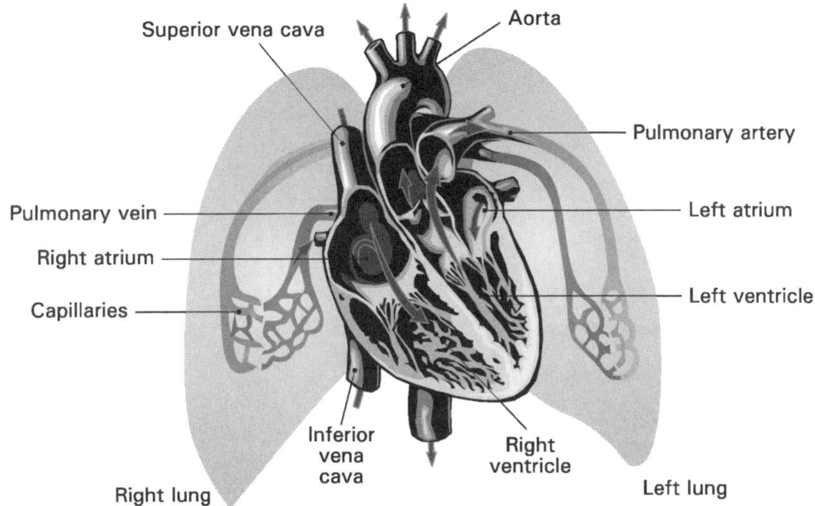

FIGURE 1. *Anatomy of the pulmonary circulatory system.*

into the lungs and then branch into arterioles and finally into a dense network of capillaries surrounding the alveolar air sacs, where an exchange of oxygen and carbon dioxide occurs. As gas exchange occurs, there is an increase in the oxygen content of the blood, which in turn becomes bright red in color. Blood drains from the pulmonary capillaries into venules, which supply the pulmonary veins and are responsible for delivering oxygenated blood to the left atrium of the heart, where it enters the systemic circulation. The pulmonary circulation is very compliant because it has few muscle fibers, allowing the system to function as a high-flow, low-pressure circuit (Gaine SP, 1998). Figure 2 depicts the structure of a pulmonary artery.

Pulmonary Vascular Remodeling. In patients with chronic PH, structural changes occur to the pulmonary vasculature, leading to a narrowing of the arteries and negatively affecting pulmonary vascular function. The narrowing of the arteries in the pulmonary circulation increases pulmonary vascular resistance, which, in turn, increases the workload of the right ventricle of the heart. The right ventricle becomes enlarged to compensate for the increased pressure; this process eventually culminates in right-heart failure (Figure 3).

The changes in vascular structure that occur are commonly referred to as vascular remodeling. The remodeling process comprises dilation and atheroma formation (thickening and fatty degeneration of the inner coat of the artery) in the elastic arteries, medial hypertrophy, muscularization of arterioles, and intimal proliferation. These lesions occur in all forms of PH (Voelkel NF, 2004). However, additional features of remodeling—for example, plexiform lesions (disorganized

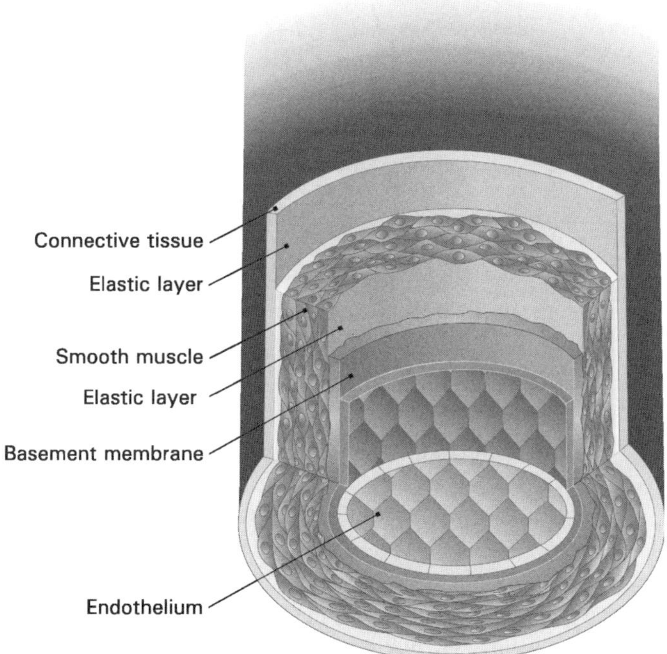

FIGURE 2. *Cell layers of a pulmonary artery.*

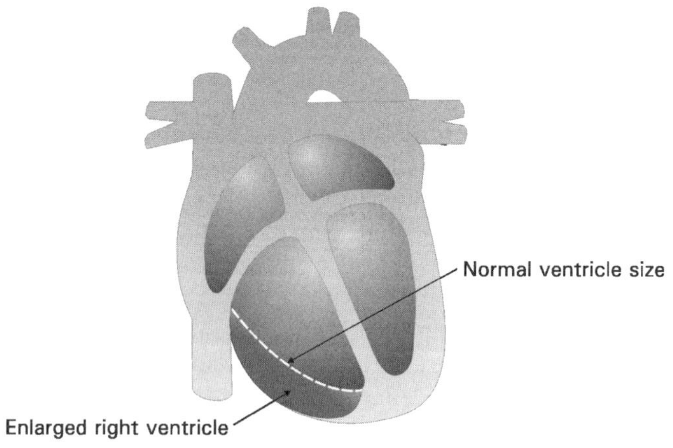

FIGURE 3. *Enlargement of the right ventricle.*

endothelial cell proliferation), intimal fibrosis, fibrinoid (fibrin-like protein) necrosis, organized thrombus, and inflammation of the pulmonary artery—are characteristic of PAH. Plexiform lesions have been identified in IPAH, FPAH, and APAH (Hoeper MM, 2002). Analysis of these additional lesions in PAH suggests they represent a more advanced stage of the remodeling process, and evidence suggests that their presence is associated with a worse prognosis (Humbert M, 2004[a]; Strange JW, 2002).

Pathophysiology

The underlying pathophysiology of PH and, in particular, PAH is very complex and not entirely understood. Scientific research to date has identified a range of factors contributing to abnormal pulmonary vascular response (vasoconstriction and altered cellular proliferation) leading to the altered vascular structure characteristic of PAH. Figure 4, which shows the cellular activity involved in the pathogenesis of PAH, summarizes these factors, which are discussed in more detail in the following sections.

BMPR2 and ALK/Endoglin Mutations. Recent analysis of the genetic profiles of patients with PAH has led to significant breakthroughs in the understanding of the pathogenesis of this complex disease, particularly with regard

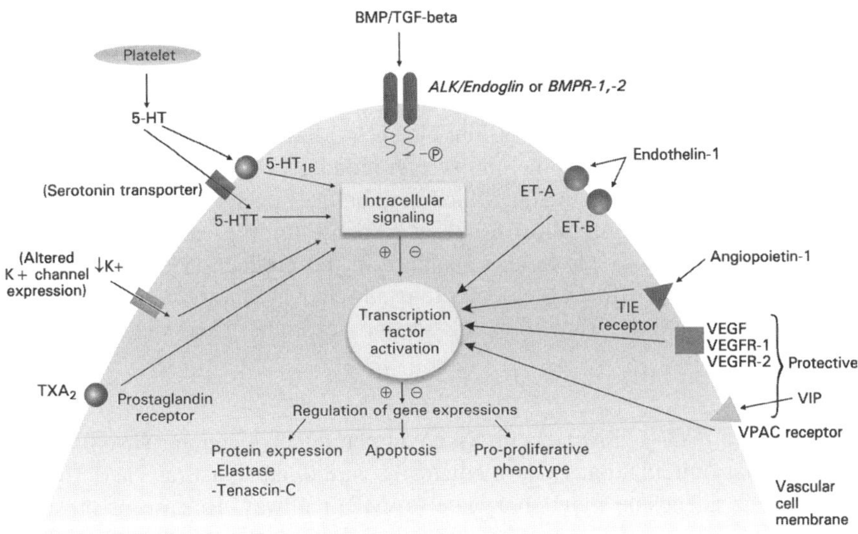

FIGURE 4. *Cellular activity involved in the pathogenesis of pulmonary arterial hypertension.*

to the FPAH and IPAH patient groups. The presence of specific genetic mutations appears to result in increased susceptibility to the disease. For example, linkage studies in families in which multiple members suffered PAH mapped the disease locus to a 3 cm section of chromosome 2q31–32. Scientists examined candidate genes within this section and identified mutations in the *BMPR2* gene, which encodes the protein for the bone morphogenetic (BMP) receptor BMPR2. BMP is a member of the transforming growth factor-beta (TGF-β) superfamily. This superfamily performs diverse roles in an array of physiological processes (Humbert M, 2004[a]; Strange JW, 2002). Activation of the TGF-β-BMPR2 axis leads to cell signaling through a pathway of highly tissue-specific regulatory proteins, known as Smads, which culminates in gene transcription that leads to suppression of cell proliferation and activation of apoptosis (regulated cell death). Hence, the consequence of such loss-of-function mutations in *BMPR2* is that cells in the pulmonary vasculature have an increased tendency to proliferate (Newman JH, 2004).

Mutations of *BMPR2* have been identified in 60% of FPAH cases and 10–30% of IPAH cases (Runo JR, 2003). Because such mutations are absent in some cases of FPAH, investigators began to consider the possibility of other TGF-β receptor mutations. Alterations in the *ALK-1* and *endoglin* receptor genes have since been identified in PAH patients (Humbert M, 2004[a]; Newman JH, 2004). However, phenotypic disease is seen in only 10–20% of individuals with the *BMPR2* mutation; scientists stress the importance of modifier genes and environmental conditions in the manifestation of the disease in these individuals (Runo JR, 2003). Further research is under way into this issue.

Endothelial Dysfunction. An early component of the PAH disease process is vasoconstriction. Excessive constriction of the pulmonary vessels in PAH patients is associated with abnormal potassium channels (discussed further on) and dysfunction of the vascular endothelium (a thin monolayer of cells lining the blood vessels). Endothelial dysfunction, which may be due to such factors as hypoxia, inflammation, shear stress (shear flow), or response to drugs or toxins on top of genetic susceptibility, leads to an imbalance in the production of vasoconstrictors and vasodilators affecting vascular tone and the vascular remodeling process (Humbert M, 2004[a]). The following sections examine these vasoconstrictors and vasodilators.

Prostacyclin (PGI$_2$). Prostacyclin is an important endogenous vasodilator in the pulmonary circulation. PGI$_2$ mediates its vasodilatory action via activation of the cyclic adenosine monophosphate (cAMP) pathway. Release of prostacyclin also inhibits platelet aggregation and vascular smooth-muscle cell (VSMC) proliferation. Lower levels of prostacyclin metabolites can be measured in the urine of PAH patients, and reduced expression of prostacyclin synthase has been observed in studies of endothelial cells from this patient group (Runo JR, 2003; Humbert M, 2004[a]).

Nitric Oxide. Levels of the potent pulmonary vasodilator nitric oxide (NO) are low in the exhaled breath of patients with PAH. NO stimulates dilation of VSMC through activation of the cyclic guanosine monophosphate (cGMP) pathway. Studies have demonstrated that the severity of disease inversely correlates with the NO levels (Ghamra ZW, 2003). Reduced levels of expression of the enzyme responsible for the production of NO, nitric oxide synthase (NOS), have been observed in the endothelial cells of PAH patients (Humbert M, 2004[a]). Researchers are investigating whether preventing the breakdown of cGMP (released in response to NO activity) by targeting phosphodiesterase (PDE)-5 in PAH patients is a potential treatment for this disease.

Vasoactive Intestinal Peptide. Researchers have also observed plasma concentrations of the less well-characterized vasodilator vasoactive intestinal peptide (VIP) in PAH patients. VIP acts at the vasoactive intestinal peptide and pituitary adenylate cyclase-activating peptide (VPAC) receptors on VSMCs that are mediating vasodilation and reduced VSMC proliferation. Increased VIP-receptor expression and -receptor binding activity has been observed in tissue from IPAH in response to the deficiency. Members of the scientific community consider the VIP pathway an interesting potential drug target due to its vasodilatory and antiproliferative actions (Channick RN, 2003; Humbert M, 2004[a], [b]).

Endothelin-1. Endothelin-1 (ET-1) is a 21 amino acid peptide produced by cells of the vascular endothelium. ET-1 has powerful vasoconstrictive, mitogenic, and fibrogenic actions in the pulmonary vasculature. It mediates its actions via two cell surface receptors, ET-A and ET-B. The ET-B receptor, which is located primarily on vascular endothelial cells, favors ET-1 clearance and induces vasodilator production; this negative feedback system prevents excessive activity of the ET-1. Vasoconstrictor effects, largely ET-A-mediated, are due to activation of calcium channels and calcium influx, while the mitogenic and fibrogenic effects are mediated via activation of mitogen-activated protein (MAP) kinase signaling cascades (Galié N, 2003; Newman JH, 2004). Elevated plasma ET-1 has been observed in PAH patients and PAH animal models. Increased expression of ET-1 has also been observed on endothelial cell preparations from the pulmonary arteries of PAH patients (Ghamra ZW, 2003). Currently available therapies for PAH target this important pathway.

Thromboxane A_2. An increased 24-hour excretion of thromboxane A_2, another potent vasoconstrictor with proliferative activity, has also been identified in patients with PAH, further contributing to the imbalance between vasoconstrictors and vasodilators in this complex disease process. Such observations suggest interesting future drug targets (Galié N, 2003).

Role of Potassium Channels. Increased intracellular calcium concentration leads to contraction of pulmonary VSMCs and ultimately promotes pulmonary VSMC hypertrophy. Voltage-gated potassium channels are responsible for the control of the cell membrane potential and the release of intracellular calcium (Runo JR, 2003). The mechanism observed in the pulmonary vascular response to hypoxia (lack of oxygen) may be highly relevant to the PAH disease process. Hypoxia has been shown to inhibit more than one type of potassium channel in pulmonary VSMCs; it opens voltage-gated calcium channels and raises the intracellular calcium concentration, an action that results in contraction. Researchers have observed that Kv1.5 and Kv1.2 voltage-gated potassium channels are down-regulated (reduced channel expression) in pulmonary VSMCs from PAH patients. Loss of these channels from the cell leads to depolarization of the cell membrane, vasoconstriction, and cell proliferation (Humbert M, 2004[a]; Newman JH, 2004; Sims JM, 2003).

Role of Serotonin. Serotonin (5-HT) has been implicated in the pathogenesis of PAH for several years (Nicod LP, 2003). 5-HT is thought to have both vasoconstrictive (primarily through stimulation of 5-HT_{1B} receptors, although other 5-HT receptors may have a role) and mitogenic actions (MacLean MR, 2000; Newman JH, 2004). Plasma levels of 5-HT are higher in patients with PAH than in controls; in contrast, the levels of 5-HT in platelets (primary storage site for 5-HT in the periphery) are low (Hervé P, 1995). Appetite suppressants that can cause PH (see the "Etiology" section) result in the release of 5-HT from platelets and have been shown to interfere with 5-HT metabolism by monoamine oxidase (MOA). Recent investigations have also shown these drugs can interfere with 5-HT reuptake by the serotonin transporter (5-HTT). Expression and/or activity of the 5-HTT in pulmonary VSMCs is thought to contribute to the vascular remodeling process. The gene for the transporter is located on chromosome 17q11.2; a variant in the upstream promoter region has been described (Humbert M, 2004). This gene polymorphism (variant) has been identified in 65% of patients with IPAH and only 27% of controls (Eddahibi S, 2001). Hence, researchers propose that the presence of this polymorphism increases the susceptibility of an individual to develop PAH. The polymorphism is associated with 5-HTT overexpression and increased pulmonary VSMC growth (Newman JH, 2004).

Figure 5 summarizes the contribution of 5-HT to the disease process in PAH.

Elastase Activity. Studies carried out in rat models of pulmonary hypertension reveal that increased elastase activity occurs very soon after the disease-inducing stimuli (either hypoxia or monocrotaline) (Rabinovitch M, 1998). The breakdown of the extracellular matrix by elastases and matrix metalloproteinases increases pulmonary VSMC proliferation due to the release of matrix-bound mitogens and by induction of tenascin C (a substance responsible for increasing the response of VSMCs to growth factors) (Cowan KN, 2000[a]). Further rat studies demonstrate that an inhibitor of serine elastase suppresses the disease process (Cowan KN, 2000[b]). The presence of NO also reduces the activity of elastases in smooth muscle (Mitani Y, 2000).

Role of Vascular Endothelial Growth Factor. Expression of vascular endothelial growth factor (VEGF) is abundant in normal lung tissue. VEGF is an

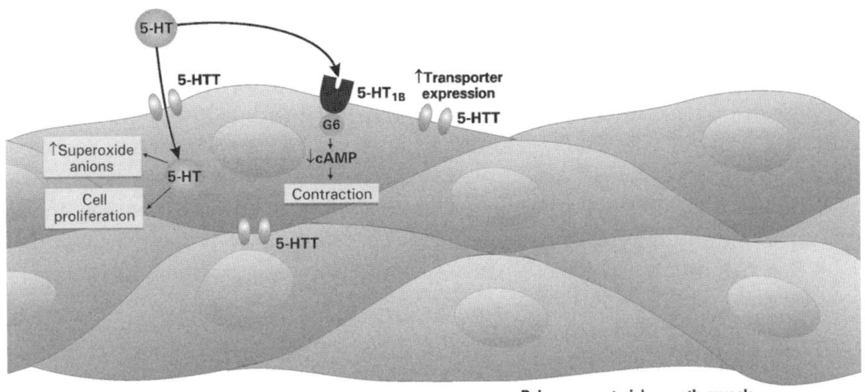

FIGURE 5. *Overview of serotonin (5-HT) in the pathogenesis of pulmonary arterial hypertension — actions on pulmonary arterial smooth muscle.*

endothelial-cell-specific angiogenic mitogen that acts at two cell surface receptors known as vascular endothelial growth factor receptors-1 and -2 (VEGFR-1 and VEGFR-2). The exact role of VEGF in the pathogenesis PAH is unknown, though it has been suggested that the growth factor may have a protective effect by promoting pulmonary endothelial survival (Humbert M, 2004[a]). Evidence of this protective role stems from studies in rat models. In the rat model of hypoxia-induced PH, blockade of the VEGFR-2 increased the severity of the disease, allowing cell death and the selection of an apoptosis-resistant endothelial cell phenotype. The researchers deemed this altered endothelial cell phenotype significant with regard to endothelial cell proliferation and the PAH disease process (Taraseviciene-Stewart L, 2001). Plasma levels of VEGF have been shown to be elevated in PAH patients (Voelkel NF, 2004). An increased expression of VEGF has also been shown in plexiform lesions in the pulmonary arteries of PAH patients (Runo JR, 2003). Several other growth factors, including platelet-derived growth factor, fibroblast growth factor, insulin-like growth factor-1, and epidermal growth factor, have been implicated in the pathophysiology of PAH, but further studies are needed to determine their role.

Role of Angiopoietin-1. The angiogenic factor angiopoietin-1 has an important role in pulmonary vascular development. Angiopoietin-1 is secreted by VSMCs and acts on TIE2 receptors present on the vascular endothelium. Activation of TIE2 receptors induces the proliferation of VSMCs around the endothelium during fetal development. Following development, levels of angiopoietin-1 are low. There is considerable discussion regarding the role of angiopoietin-1 in the pathogenesis of PAH. One study suggested that all forms of PAH, with the exception of FPAH, are characterized by an upregulation in angiopoietin-1 and activated TIE2 receptors; the latter are, in turn, are linked to disease severity (Du L, 2003). Then, a role for angiopoietin-1 in FPAH was supported by the observation that angiopoietin inactivates proteins associated with the *BMPR2* pathway. Animal studies have demonstrated medial thickening, resulting from VSMC hyperplasia in response to treatment with angiopoietin. Relationships have also been described between the angiopoietin/TIE2 pathway and the 5-HT pathway (Sullivan CC, 2003). However, some investigators propose a protective role for angiopoietin-1 based on work carried out in the monocrotaline rat model (Zhao YD, 2003). Further investigations are needed to resolve the confusion regarding the role of angiogenic factors in this disease process, particularly given that manipulation of these pathways may provide interesting drug targets.

Etiology

An extensive amount of scientific research in recent years has led to the identification of a collection of risk factors and associated conditions for PAH. They include a relationship between the development of PAH and gender, the presence of underlying medical conditions or disease, and an association between PAH and the ingestion of specific drugs or toxins. Figure 6 summarizes these risk factors and associated conditions; the most important ones are discussed in the following sections.

Female Gender and Ethnicity. Studies examining the gender ratio for IPAH and FPAH revealed that in childhood, the ratio of females to males with the condition is 1:1. In adulthood, the ratio is 1.7:1 (Brenot F, 1994). Females appear to be at greater risk of developing PAH in general. Analysis of the United States' National Institutes of Health registry also points to a greater incidence of PAH in African-American females, with a female to male ratio of 3:1.

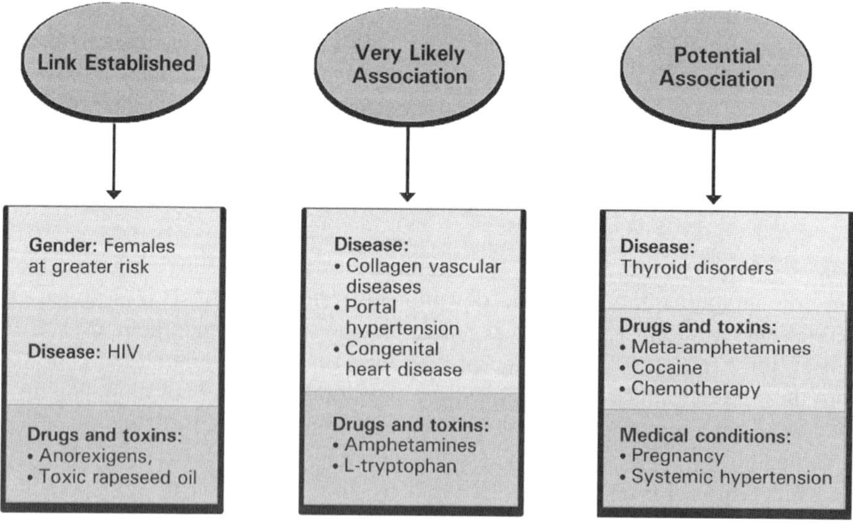

FIGURE 6. *Risk factors for pulmonary arterial hypertension.*

Researchers speculate this ethnic group may be more susceptible than Caucasians to autoimmune-like disorders (Humbert M, 2001).

Disease

Human Immunodeficiency Virus. Infection with HIV has been associated with the development of pulmonary vascular diseases. The presence of PAH associated with HIV infection was first reported in 1987 in a patient with hemophilia with membrane proliferative glomerulonephritis (inflammation of the capillary loops in the kidney nephron). Subsequent reports in HIV-infected hemophiliacs followed; then came reports of cases of PAH in nonhemophiliacs, highlighting a direct association between PAH and HIV. The nature of the association between HIV and PAH remains unknown, but the medical community stresses the interaction between genetic and environmental factors. There appears to be no link to the stage of HIV infection and the prevalence or severity of PAH. In light of improvements in drug therapy for HIV and the increasing prevalence of HIV worldwide, the number of HIV-related PAH cases will likely increase (Seone L, 2001).

Connective Tissue Diseases. PAH has been linked with a range of connective tissue disease, including systemic sclerosis (scleroderma) and systemic lupus erythematosus (SLE). Associations have also been made between PAH and rheumatoid arthritis, dermatopolymyositis, and primary Sjögren's syndrome, but to a lesser extent (McLaughlin VV, 2004[a]). Within the population with connective tissue disease, PAH is most frequently observed in patients with scleroderma-related disease, often referred to as CREST (calcinosis, Raynaud's phenomenon, esophageal dysmotility, sclerodactyly [thickening or tightening of the skin], and telangiectasia [permanent dilation of the blood vessels causing small red lesions in the skin or mucosal membranes]) syndrome (Humbert M, 2001). Histopathological changes observed in this group are similar to those in IPAH, although there is often a greater degree of thickening of the adventitia (connective tissue covering) (McLaughlin VV, 2004[a]; Voelkel NF, 2004).

Early studies using the echocardiogram to investigate the presence of PAH estimated the incidence of PAH in association with scleroderma at 30–50%. However, a new study involving 722 scleroderma patients performed right-heart catheterization (a more accurate assessment of the presence of PAH) to determine the presence of PAH, which the researchers identified in only 12% of patients. This value may be a more realistic marker (McLaughlin VV, 2004[a]; Mukerjee D, 2003). The mechanisms responsible for PAH in patients with connective tissue disease remain unknown. An immunological mechanism has been suggested due to the presence of an anticentromere antibody, rheumatoid factor, immunoglobulin-G, and complement fragments (the complement system has an important role in the immune response) (Humbert M, 2001). Patients with connective tissue disease and PAH are primarily female and older (mean age of 66 years). They generally have a worse prognosis than IPAH patients because they tend to respond poorly to available PAH therapies and they have underlying disease (Hoeper MM, 2002[a]; Humbert M, 2001).

Portal Hypertension. An association between PAH and hepatic dysfunction was first reported in 1951 (Krowka M, 2004). The presence of portal hypertension resulting from hepatic abnormality rather than the hepatic disorder itself appears to be the key to the development of PAH. PAH associated with portal hypertension is also histopathologically similar to IPAH. The exact mechanism by which the presence of portal hypertension leads to the development of PAH remains unknown. Researchers have suggested that the presence of a portal-systemic shunt (abnormal vascular connections between the hepatic vein and the systemic circulation) may facilitate the delivery of vasoconstrictors and inflammatory mediators, including 5-HT, into the pulmonary circulation (McLaughlin VV, 2004[a]); in healthy individuals, the vasoconstrictors and inflammatory mediators would be cleared by the liver. Liver transplant centers report the frequency of portopulmonary hypertension is 4–15% (Krowka M, 2004).

Congenital Heart Disease (Eisenmenger's Syndrome). Pulmonary vascular disease due to the presence of an altered systemic-pulmonary connection such as an atrial septal defect, a ventricular septal defect, patent ductus arteriosis (failure of key fetal blood vessel to close after birth), or an aortopulmonary window (a hole between the main pulmonary artery and the aorta) is collectively referred to as Eisenmenger's syndrome. PAH resulting from Eisenmenger's syndrome is histologically similar to IPAH. The condition generally occurs following a period of reduced pulmonary vascular resistance and high pulmonary blood flow that occurs after left-to-right shunt (movement of the blood from the left-heart circulation to the right-heart circulation). Morphologic changes occur in the pulmonary vessels, and when pulmonary vascular resistance exceeds systemic vascular resistance, the movement of blood reverses. The development of PAH is related to the size and type of defect. Patients with PAH associated with congenital heart disease generally have a better prognosis than do patients with IPAH (McLaughlin VV, 2004[a]).

Drugs and Toxins

Appetite Suppressants. The use of appetite suppressants including aminorex fumarate and fenfluramine derivatives for more than three months is associated with a 30 times greater risk of developing PAH (Nauser TD, 2001). The relationship between appetite suppressants and PAH was identified in the 1960s when a 20-fold increase in PH was reported in Switzerland, Austria, and the former West Germany following the introduction of aminorex fumarate to the marketplace. The increase in the number of cases subsided when the substance was banned (Humbert M, 2001). Fenfluramine derivatives have also been used as anorexic agents since the 1960s. In a study of 73 IPAH/FPAH patients, 25% of the patient group was found to have been exposed to fenfluramines (Brenot F, 1993). This observation followed the introduction of the fenfluramine derivative dexfluramine and extensive increases in fenfluramine sales in France over the period 1985–1992. The Surveillance of North American Pulmonary Hypertension Study investigated 579 patients with PH and found a strong association between the use of fenfluramine derivatives and the development of primary pulmonary hypertension (PPH, now classified as IPAH and FPAH) (Rich S, 2000). The association was stronger with longer duration of use and more pronounced in recent users when compared with remote users. Both fenfluramine and dexfluramine were withdrawn from the U.S. market in 1997, only 18 months after they launched.

These agents may initiate the disease process by several mechanisms. Aminorex and dexfenfluramine have been shown to directly inhibit the voltage-gated potassium channels Kv1.5 and Kv2.1. Aminorex has been shown to induce 5-HT release from platelets and inhibit 5-HT metabolism, while fenfluramine derivatives have been shown to interact with the 5-HTT (Humbert M, 2004[a]). The WHO states that other appetite suppressants such as amphetamines are "very likely" to have a causative role in PH as well (Nauser TD, 2001).

L-Tryptophan. The food supplement L-tryptophan is commonly used to treat premenstrual syndrome, insomnia, depression, and drug detoxification. In the late 1980s, L-tryptophan was linked with a newly characterized disease—eosinophilia-myalgia syndrome (EMS), of which 1,500 cases have been reported in the United States. In severe cases of the disease, the pulmonary circulation is affected, and in some individuals PAH has been reported (Humbert M, 2001). The FDA continues to express its concern about products containing the food supplement L-tryptophan but has not prohibited the marketing of such products.

Toxic Rapeseed Oil. So-called toxic oil syndrome was first recognized in Spain in 1981 and is an interesting example of how PH can develop following exposure to chemicals. A total of 20,688 cases of the toxic oil syndrome were reported, and the WHO determined the cause of the condition to be related to the consumption of contaminated rapeseed oil. One study following 322 patients with toxic oil syndrome found that 8.1% of the group developed PH (Humbert M, 2001). After an eight-year follow-up period, severe PH had developed in 2% of PH sufferers. It was estimated that PH was the cause of death in 1.6% of toxic oil syndrome sufferers. Histopathological changes—characterized by the presence of plexiform lesions—observed on examining the lungs of the patient population were similar to those seen in PAH.

CURRENT THERAPIES

Greater understanding of the etiology and pathophysiology of pulmonary arterial hypertension (PAH) has led to significant advances in therapy for this disease. In addition, the publication of the American College of Chest Physicians' (ACCP's) evidence-based treatment guidelines in *Chest* in 2004 has aided physicians somewhat in treatment decisions. Nevertheless, treatment remains very complicated because patients respond differently to available therapies. Treatment protocols are generally tailored to suit the individual and are devised in pulmonary hypertension (PH) specialist centers. As mentioned previously, PAH is one class of conditions under PH. Table 3 summarizes the therapies currently used for PAH.

The major drug classes used in the treatment of PAH are vasodilators, such as the prostacyclin analogues (e.g., epoprostenol sodium [GlaxoSmithKline's (Brentford, Middlesex, United Kingdom) Flolan]); endothelin-receptor antagonists (ERAs); calcium-channel blockers (CCBs); vitamin K antagonists; diuretics; and cardiac glycosides. The aim of pharmacotherapy is to reduce pulmonary vascular resistance, temper pulmonary vascular remodeling, prevent thrombus formation, reduce volume overload, and maintain cardiac output. A series of lifestyle modifications—most importantly reduced physical activity—is often recommended in addition to drug therapy. In the more advanced stages of disease, patients may become candidates for surgical interventions, including lung transplantation (Nauser TD, 2001; Rubin LJ, 2002[a]).

Prostacyclin Analogues

Overview. Prostacyclin (PGI_2) is a metabolite of arachidonic acid and is endogenously produced by vascular endothelial cells. PGI_2 is a potent vasodilator in both the systemic and pulmonary circulations and strongly inhibits platelet activation. A reduction in levels of PGI_2 is thought to contribute to the pathogenesis of PAH (see "Etiology and Pathophysiology"). Clinical studies over the last two decades have investigated the possibility of using analogues of endogenous PGI_2 for the long-term treatment of PAH. Various compounds and methods of administration have been investigated, leading to a range of marketed products that remain the mainstay therapies for this complex disease (Badesch DB, 2004[a]; Runo JR, 2003).

Mechanism of Action. PGI_2 analogues mediate their effects (vasodilation and antiplatelet activity) by activating G-protein-coupled receptors, known as IP receptors, on target cells. These IP receptors are coupled to the adenyl cyclase intracellular signaling cascade, and activation triggers the production of intracellular cyclic adenosine monophosphate (cAMP), culminating in cellular responses (Harker LA, 1986; Samuelsson B, 1975).

Formulation. The short half-life and lack of bioavailability of PGI_2 (three to five minutes) create problems in terms of drug delivery. A range of formulations of PGI_2 analogues are available, including intravenous, subcutaneous, inhaled, and oral preparations. The choice of formulation depends on the severity of the disease and the patient's circumstances (Badesch DB, 2004[a]; Galié N, 2003).

Epoprostenol Sodium. Epoprostenol sodium (GlaxoSmithKline's Flolan) (Figure 7) has been available in the United States for the treatment of PAH (idiopathic PAH [IPAH], familial PAH [FPAH], and associated PAH [APAH]) since 1995; the agent is also available in most of Europe and in Japan. Epoprostenol has

TABLE 3. Current Therapies Used for Pulmonary Arterial Hypertension

Agent	Company/Brand	Daily Dose	Availability
Prostacyclin analogues			
Epoprostenol sodium	GlaxoSmithKline's Flolan	Initial dose: 2 ng /kg/min. Dose increased in increments of 2 ng/kg/min every 15 mins or longer as needed until dose-limiting pharmacologic effects/tolerance limit reached	US, F, I, S, UK, J
Treprostinil (subcutaneous and intravenous preparations)	United Therapeutics' Remodulin	Adjusted according to weight. Initial dose: 0.625–1.25 ng/kg/min. Dose increased as needed until dose-limiting pharmacologic effects/tolerance limit reached	US
Iloprost (inhaled preparation)	Schering AG/Cotherix's Ventavis	2.5–5.0 µg six to nine times	US, F, G, I, S, UK
Iloprost (intravenous preparation)	Schering AG's Ilomedin/Ilomedine	Initial dose: 0.5 ng/kg/min. Dose increased as needed until dose-limiting pharmacologic effects/tolerance limit reached	G
Beraprost	Yamanouchi's Dorner, Kaken's Procylin	60–180 µg	J
Endothelin-receptor antagonists			
Bosentan	Actelion's Tracleer	125–250 mg	US, F, G, I, S, UK
Calcium-channel blockers			
Nifedipine	Bayer's Adalat/Adalat CC, Pfizer's Procardia/Procardia XL, generics	90–480 mg	US, F, G, I, S, UK, J
Diltiazem	Sanofi-Aventis's Cardizem, generics	360–720 mg	US, F, G, I, S, UK, J
Vitamin K antagonists			
Warfarin	Bristol-Myers Squibb's Coumadin, Sanofi-Aventis's Coumadine, generics	Adjusted dose to achieve INR 2.5, range 2.0–3.0 (in Japan, target INR of 1.8–2.0)	US, F, G, I, S, UK, J

(*continued overleaf*)

TABLE 3. (*continued*)

Agent	Company/Brand	Daily Dose	Availability
Diuretics			
Furosemide	Sanofi-Aventis's Lasix, generics	40–120 mg	US, F, G, I, S, UK, J
Spironolactone	Pfizer's Aldactone, generics	25–100 mg	US, F, G, I, S, UK, J
Cardiac glycosides			
Digoxin	GlaxoSmithKline's Lanoxin/Lanoxicaps, generics	0.0625–0.25 mg qd	US, F, G, I, S, UK, J

bid = Twice daily; INR = International normalized ratio; qd = Once daily.

US = United States; F = France; G = Germany; I = Italy; S = Spain; UK = United Kingdom; J = Japan.

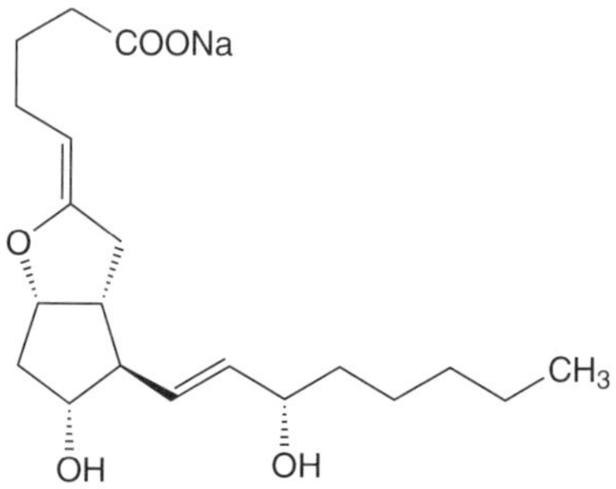

FIGURE 7. *Structure of epoprostenol sodium.*

an extremely short half-life of two to seven minutes; hence, it is administered as a continuous IV infusion through a central-line catheter. Medication must be kept cold for reasons of stability, a requirement that makes administration somewhat problematic.

Epoprostenol's mechanism of action follows that outlined for the prostacyclin analogues in general. Treatment causes direct vasodilation of pulmonary and systemic vascular beds via activation of prostanoid receptors. It also inhibits platelet activation.

Several clinical trials have assessed the benefits of epoprostenol therapy in PAH. A 12-week, multicenter, open-label trial compared the effects of epoprostenol plus standard symptom-relieving therapy (oral vasodilators, anticoagulation, and diuretics) with standard symptom-relieving therapy alone in 81 patients with PAH (IPAH/FPAH) who were New York Heart Association (NYHA) classes III and IV (Barst RJ, 1996). Results demonstrated a statistically significant ($p < 0.002$) improvement in exercise capacity as measured by the six-minute walk test—the distance an individual can walk in six minutes (6MWD)—in 41 patients treated with continuous-infusion epoprostenol (362 meters at 12 weeks compared with 315 meters at baseline); the 6MWD actually declined in the group treated with conventional therapy. Improvements were also observed in quality of life ($p < 0.01$) and hemodynamics (pulmonary artery pressure and pulmonary vascular resistance).

Several studies have assessed the long-term effect of continuous-infusion epoprostenol. One large study investigated 162 patients diagnosed with PAH (IPAH/FPAH) treated with continuous-infusion epoprostenol for a mean of 36.1 months (McLaughlin VV, 2002). The one-, two-, and three-year survival rates for the epoprostenol group were 87.8%, 76.3%, and 62.8%, respectively, compared with survival rates of 58.9%, 46.3%, and 35.4% based on historical data. The authors reported that baseline predictors of survival included tolerance to exercise, NYHA functional class, right atrial pressure, and acute vasodilator response to adenosine.

Researchers have evaluated continuous infusion of IV epoprostenol in patients with APAH related to connective tissue disease. A randomized, open-label, controlled study included 111 patients with moderate-to-severe PAH with scleroderma-associated disease (Badesch DB, 2000). Patients received continuous-infusion epoprostenol or conventional therapy for PAH; the follow-up period was 12 weeks. Results showed an improvement in exercise capacity, as measured by the 6MWD, in the epoprostenol-treated group compared with the conventional treatment group. The difference between treatment groups in median walk distance at week 12 was 108 m (95% confidence interval = 52.5–180 m; $p < 0.001$). Hemodynamics also improved in those treated with epoprostenol. Twenty-one patients in the epoprostenol-treated group and no patients in the conventional therapy group showed improvements in terms of NYHA functional class. Borg dyspnea index scores (a common method of measuring breathlessness) and dyspnea-fatigue ratings dropped in the epoprostenol group, and there was a trend toward an improvement in the severity of Raynaud's syndrome—fewer new digital ulcers formed. The researchers did not observe a survival difference in this population during the study period, but the study's design meant it was not significantly powered to detect such a difference (Badesch DB, 2004[a]).

One study revealed that continuous-infusion epoprostenol improved exercise capacity, hemodynamics, and quality of life in patients with PAH associated with a congenital heart defect who had failed conventional therapy (digitalis, diuretics, oxygen, warfarin, calcium-channel blockade, and surgery if operable) (Rosenzweig EB, 1999).

Side effects commonly associated with epoprostenol therapy include flushing, headache, jaw pain, diarrhea, nausea, blotchy erythematous rash, and musculoskeletal pain in the feet and legs. These side effects are generally dose-related and usually respond to a reduction in dose. Because the agent is administered via continuous IV infusion, complications, including line-related infections (exit-site reactions, tunnel infections and cellulitis, bacteremia, sepsis), catheter-associated venous thrombosis, thrombocytopenia, and ascites (fluid in the peritoneal cavity, a common symptom of hepatic disease) may occur (Badesch DB, 2004[a]).

Treprostinil. The prostacyclin analogue treprostinil has two key advantages over epoprostenol: It is stable at room temperature and its half-life is longer (three to four hours), permitting its administration as a subcutaneous infusion. In May 2002, the FDA approved the subcutaneous form of treprostinil (United Therapeutics Corporation's [Silver Spring, Maryland] Remodulin) for the treatment of PAH patients in NYHA functional classes II, III and IV. An IV preparation of the agent (to be used in patients unable to tolerate the subcutaneous formulation) was approved by the FDA in November 2004, following studies showing bioequivalence with the subcutaneous formulation in patients with PAH.

Treprostinil's mechanism of action follows that outlined for prostacyclin analogues in general, and the agent's vasodilatory, platelet inhibitory, and hemodynamic actions mirror those of epoprostenol (Horn EM, 2002).

A small pilot study investigated subcutaneous treprostinil versus placebo (2:1) in 26 IPAH patients who were NYHA functional classes III and IV (Badesch DB, 2004[a]; Horn EM, 2002). The follow-up period was eight weeks. An improvement in the 6MWD of $37 \pm 17\,\mathrm{m}$ was seen in the treprostinil-treated group compared with $6 \pm 28\,\mathrm{m}$ in the placebo group (results were not statistically significant). There was also a trend toward an improvement in hemodynamics (20% reduction in pulmonary vascular resistance over eight weeks) in the treprostinil group.

A 12-week, multicenter, randomized, placebo-controlled study investigated the actions of treprostinil (maximum dose 22.5 ng/kg/min) in 470 PAH patients (IPAH or patients with PAH associated with connective tissue disease or congenital heart defects) (Simonneau G, 2002). The study's primary end point was the 6MWD. Results showed an improvement in the treprostinil group and no improvement in the placebo group. The median difference in the 6MWD between the two groups was $16\,\mathrm{m}$ ($p = 0.006$), and improvements were shown to be dose-dependent. Those patients receiving doses greater than 13.8 ng/kg/min experienced an improvement of 36 m. The treprostinil group also experienced improvements in indices of dyspnea, signs and symptoms of PH, and hemodynamics. The effect of treprostinil on the 6MWD was rather modest compared with trials investigating epoprostenol, but researchers have suggested that entry criteria for this study were much broader than those for the epoprostenol studies (Badesch DB, 2004[a]). Patients who entered the study as NYHA functional class IV showed an improvement in the 6MWD of 54 m, which is comparable to that of other clinical investigations (Horn EM, 2002). Long-term efficacy (more than 12 weeks) was not included in this study; however, open-label studies suggest that improvements in exercise capacity are maintained (Horn EM, 2002).

In October 2003, the results of a small study of treprostinil were presented at the 54th Annual Meeting of the American Association for the Study of Liver Diseases in Boston (Benza RL, 2003). The study, which involved 37 patients, demonstrated that treprostinil is safe in patients with PAH associated with portal hypertension/liver disease. The drug also maintained or improved the hemodynamics in the majority of the patients in the study group. The safety profile followed that of the studies outlined in the following paragraph.

Clinical studies evaluating the IV preparation of treprostinil are limited. One multicenter, open-label, acute trial compared the effects of IV epoprostenol with IV treprostinil (McLaughlin VV, 2003). Fourteen PAH patients were enrolled in the study. Following right-heart catheterization, epoprostenol was administered by IV infusion at 2 ng/kg/min and increased at 15- to 30-minute intervals by 2 ng/kg/min intervals to a maximum-tolerated dose; hemodynamic measurements were taken along the way. Epoprostenol was then washed out, and after a 90-minute rest period, 5 ng/kg/min of treprostinil was administered for 30 minutes and increased every 30 minutes to 10, 20, 30, 40, and 60 ng/kg/min. Dose ranging was carried out until dose side effects warranted a dose reduction or discontinuation of therapy (nontolerated dose). A 90-minute maintenance dose was continued at 10–20 ng/kg/min below the nontolerated dose; it was followed by a 120-minute washout period. Results showed the maximum-tolerated dose of IV epoprostenol was 6.4 ± 0.8 ng/kg/min and that of treprostinil was 24 ± 4.0 ng/kg/min. Adverse events were similar in both groups and included jaw pain, headache, nausea, chest pain, backache, and restlessness. Similar reductions in pulmonary artery pressure also occurred. There was a 22% reduction in pulmonary vascular resistance for epoprostenol compared with a 20% reduction in pulmonary vascular resistance for treprostinil (differences were not statistically significant). One patient experienced a serious adverse event during the maintenance infusion due to a documented foramen ovale (atrial septal defect); the patient recovered after the infusion was terminated.

A randomized crossover study design compared the bioequivalence and comparative pharmacokinetics of subcutaneous and IV treprostinil in 51 healthy volunteers (Laliberte K, 2003). Results showed that IV and subcutaneous treprostinil were bioequivalent at a steady state. Treprostinil's elimination half-life was 4.4 and 4.6 hours following IV and subcutaneous administration, respectively.

Common side effects associated with treprostinil therapy in clinical trials include headache, diarrhea, nausea, rash, and jaw pain. More importantly, infusion-site pain was commonly reported in studies of the subcutaneous preparation; 85% of patients in the large multicenter study of subcutaneous treprostinil complained of pain around the site of infusion, and 83% reported erythema (redness of the skin) or induration of the infusion site (Badesch DB, 2004[a]). United Therapeutics is working closely with health care professionals in the PAH field to address the issue of infusion-site pain. The company also provides a free telephone advisory service for treprostinil patients, known as the Remodulin Therapy Assistance Program. This problem of infusion site pain was the driving force behind the company's investigation of an IV formulation. A smaller pump size makes the IV formulation of treprostinil potentially more attractive than IV epoprostenol to physicians.

Iloprost. Iloprost (Figure 8) is a stable analogue of epoprostenol (prostacyclin; PGI_2). In contrast to epoprostenol, which must be dissolved, continuously cooled, and protected from light to ensure maximal activity, iloprost is stable at room temperature and in normal light. It has a half-life of 20–25 minutes.

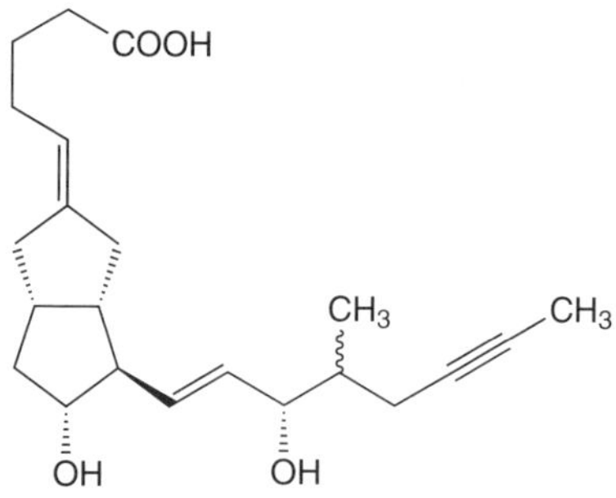

FIGURE 8. *Structure of iloprost.*

Iloprost can be administered intravenously (Schering AG's [Berlin, Germany] Ilomedin/Ilomedine, marketed only in Germany) as an alternative to epoprostenol, but more interestingly, it is available as an inhaled preparation (Schering AG's Ventavis, available in Europe) that is administered six to nine times daily. Each inhalation requires 10–15 minutes; some devices can reduce the inhalation time to 4 minutes. The use of an inhaled prostacyclin analogue is particularly attractive to patients who often experience variations in systemic blood pressure—for example, those with portopulmonary hypertension (Badesch DB, 2004[a]).

In December 2004, CoTherix, Inc. (Brisbane, California) the company developing inhaled iloprost for the U.S. market, received FDA approval for the agent. Reports suggest the U.S. label for inhaled iloprost will permit the agent to be used to treat a much wider PH population compared with that specified on the European label. Administration of the agent will also be less cumbersome in the United States because CoTherix has an agreement with Profile Drug Delivery that will enable iloprost to be delivered via a handheld nebulizer system.

Iloprost's mechanism of action follows that outlined for the prostacyclin analogues in general. Treatment causes direct vasodilation of pulmonary and systemic vascular beds via activation of prostanoid receptors. Like all prostacyclin analogues, iloprost inhibits platelet activation.

A large-scale, randomized, placebo-controlled trial performed in Europe investigated the effects of inhaled iloprost (average daily dose of 30 micrograms over six to nine inhalations) (Olschewski H, 2002). The study involved 203 patients in NYHA functional classes III and IV with IPAH or PAH associated with appetite suppressant use, collagen vascular disease, or inoperable thromboembolic disease. The initial follow-up period was 12 weeks. The primary end point was an improvement in NYHA functional class, at least a 10% improvement in the 6MWD, and no deterioration or death. Results showed that 16.8% of patients in the inhaled iloprost group compared with 4.9% in the placebo arm ($p = 0.007$) met the combined clinical end point. Increases in the 6MWD were 36.4 m in the iloprost group ($p = 0.004$); in the subgroup of patients with IPAH, the increases were 58.8 m. Hemodynamics deteriorated in the placebo group but not in the iloprost group. The number of patients remaining on medication, a proxy for event-free survival, was significantly higher in the iloprost group.

An open-label, multicenter study investigated the long-term treatment benefits of inhaled iloprost in 63 PAH patients (40 with IPAH and 23 with APAH) over a two-year period, which included a three-month randomized phase (Badesch DB, 2004[a]). The mean daily dose administered was 100 micrograms (over an average of six inhalations). During the course of the investigation, 5 patients switched from inhaled iloprost to alternative therapy (primarily IV iloprost) but remained in the study; 13 patients discontinued the therapy altogether. After the two-year follow-up, 37 patients were receiving therapy with inhaled iloprost. Eight patients died during the study period—three with IPAH and five with APAH (two patients before receiving iloprost treatment). The survival rate measured by Kaplan-Meier analysis was 0.850 for all PAH patients and 0.914 for those with IPAH for the two-year period. The predicted survival rate for IPAH patients (taken from previous studies) was 0.631, which corresponds to about 14.8 deaths. Given that only three IPAH patients died, treatment with iloprost appears to result in substantial improvement.

Clinical studies have shown inhaled iloprost to be well tolerated. Side effects more frequently encountered in the iloprost group compared with placebo include headache, cough, and flushing. A more serious side effect associated with iloprost is syncope; indeed, there were signs of clinical deterioration due to this adverse effect (Badesch DB, 2004[a]).

A small comparative study compared IV epoprostenol with IV iloprost in eight patients with severe pulmonary hypertension (five with IPAH and three with thromboembolic pulmonary hypertension) (Higgenbottam TW, 1998). A continuous infusion of either drug was given during the first phase (three to six weeks), and patients were then crossed over to receive the alternative agent for an equivalent period. Both epoprostenol and iloprost treatment significantly improved exercise tolerance. The results suggest IV iloprost is a suitable alternative to epoprostenol therapy in this extremely vulnerable patient group.

Beraprost. Beraprost (Kaken Pharmaceuticals's [Tokyo, Japan] Procylin, Yamanouchi Pharmaceutical Co., Ltd's [Tokyo, Japan] Dorner) (Figure 9) was the first orally active prostacyclin analogue to reach the market. It has been used to treat PAH in Japan since 1995, but it is not licensed in the United States or Europe. Toray manufactures the agent under the brand name Dorner to treat peripheral arterial disease (PAD). Beraprost is rapidly absorbed and has a half-life of 35–40 minutes (Badesch DB, 2004[a]; Melian EB, 2002). It mediates vasodilation and inhibition of platelet activation via the mechanism of action previously outlined for prostacyclin analogues.

Two large, randomized, double-blind, placebo-controlled studies investigated the effects of beraprost therapy in PAH patients. The first involved 130 PAH patients randomized to receive beraprost (80 micrograms four times daily) or placebo for 12 weeks (Galié N, 2002). The primary end point was the 6MWD. Results showed that patients treated with beraprost demonstrated an improvement

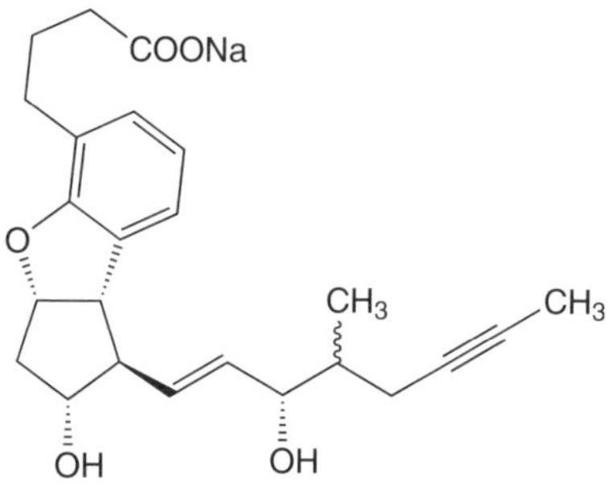

FIGURE 9. *Structure of beraprost.*

in exercise capacity and symptoms. The difference in the 6MWD was 25.1 m between the beraprost and placebo groups (95% confidence interval = 1.8–48.3; $p = 0.036$) and 45 m for the patients with IPAH. Hemodynamics showed no statistically significant change, and there was no change in survival benefit in either group.

The second study involved 116 PAH (IPAH and PAH associated with connective tissue disease or congenital heart defects) patients considered NYHA classes III and IV (Barst RJ, 2003). The median dose of beraprost was 120 micrograms four times daily, and the follow-up period was 12 months. This study's primary end point was disease progression (death, need for transplantation, epoprostenol rescue, or a greater than 25% reduction in peak oxygen consumption). Results showed that patients treated with beraprost exhibited less evidence of disease progression at six months ($p = 0.002$), although this effect was not evident at either shorter or longer follow-up intervals. The 6MWD improved at 3 months (22 m improvement) and 6 months (31 m improvement) when compared with placebo but not at 9 or 12 months.

These results are disappointing given that an earlier, small study involving 24 IPAH patients showed an improvement in three-year survival on treatment with beraprost (76% survived) compared with patients receiving conventional therapy for PAH (44% survived) (Nagaya N, 1999).

Side effects experienced with beraprost were related to systemic vasodilation; they were particularly frequent during the study's dose-finding stage (Badesch DB, 2004[a]).

Endothelin-Receptor Antagonists

Overview. The potent vasoconstrictor and mitogen endothelin-1 (ET-1) has been implicated in the pathogenesis of PAH (see "Etiology and Pathophysiology"). Increased plasma levels of ET-1 have been reported in both experimental models and human PAH. ET-1 binds to cell surface receptors known as endothelin-A (ET-A) and endothelin-B (ET-B) receptors; both ET-A and ET-B are members of the G-protein-coupled receptor (GPCR) superfamily. Antagonists acting at these receptors have been shown to reverse the pathologic and hemodynamic changes in hypoxia- and monocrotaline-induced PH animal models, and more recently, such agents have demonstrated beneficial effects in clinical trials (Galié N, 2003). The dual ET-A/ET-B antagonist, bosentan (Actelion Ltd's [Allschwil, Switzerland] Tracleer), was the first endothelin-receptor antagonist (ERA) to reach the marketplace. The agent is approved for the treatment of PAH patients in NYHA functional classes III and IV.

Mechanism of Action. Binding of ET-1 to its receptors activates signal transduction via the phospholipase C (PLC) second messenger system, ultimately generating mitogenesis and vasoconstriction. ET-A receptors are expressed in vascular smooth muscle, the heart, the kidney, and the lung. ET-B receptors are located on vascular smooth muscle as well, where activation elicits responses similar to those of ET-A receptors. However, ET-B receptors are also expressed in the endothelium, where activation leads to vasodilation through stimulation of the nitric oxide pathway. Small-molecule ERAs antagonize ET-1 action by binding endothelin receptors and inhibiting ligand (ET-1) interaction (Rang HP, 1999).

Bosentan. Bosentan (Actelion's Tracleer) is an orally active nonpeptide dual ERA. The agent, which was first in class, received full marketing approval from the FDA in November 2001 for the treatment of all subpopulations within the PAH patient group considered NYHA functional classes III or IV. Bosentan also received approval in Canada and Europe. The agent was finally approved and launched in June 2005

Bosentan blocks the actions of ET at both ET-A and ET-B receptors, inhibiting the vasoconstrictor, proliferative, and profibrotic effects of ET-1 (Rubin LJ, 2002[a]).

The FDA's approval of bosentan was based on the results of two randomized, double-blind, placebo-controlled clinical trials. The first, referred to as Study 351, compared bosentan therapy with placebo (Channick RN, 2001). The study's primary end point was a change in exercise capacity from baseline as measured by the 6MWD. A number of secondary end points were also considered, including cardiopulmonary hemodynamics, Borg dyspnea index, NYHA functional class, withdrawal due to clinical worsening, safety, and tolerability. The study enrolled 32 patients with PAH who were NYHA functional class III. Patients from all subpopulations within the PAH category were included in the study, although those with primary PAH (IPAH, FPAH) were more prevalent. Subjects were randomized to receive 62.5 mg of bosentan twice daily for 4 weeks followed by 125 mg twice daily for a minimum of 12 weeks or placebo. Results showed a significant improvement in the 6MWD from baseline for patients receiving bosentan compared with placebo, with a mean change of 76 m ($p = 0.021$). The length of treatment varied from 83 to 202 days; in the bosentan arm, a statistically significant ($p = 0.0097$) change in exercise capacity was seen at least until week 20. Improvements were also observed with respect to the secondary end points (cardiopulmonary hemodynamics, Borg dyspnea index, NYHA functional class, withdrawal due to clinical worsening, safety, and tolerability).

The Bosentan in Pulmonary Arterial Hypertension (BREATHE-1) study was a larger investigation (Rubin LJ, 2002[b]). This randomized, double-blind, placebo-controlled study involved 213 patients with PAH (IPAH, FPAH, and PAH associated with connective tissue disease), of whom 144 received bosentan (74 patients were assigned to 125 mg and 70 patients to 250 mg) and 69 received placebo. The mean duration of treatment was 124 days. The study's primary end point was the degree of change in exercise capacity, as measured by the 6MWD. Secondary end points included change in Borg dyspnea index, change in NYHA functional class, and time to clinical worsening. At 16 weeks, patients in the bosentan arm demonstrated an improved 6MWD; the mean difference between the placebo group and the bosentan group was 44 m ($p < 0.001$). Effects observed were greater in patients with IPAH and FPAH than in those with PAH associated with connective tissue disease. The changes in the Borg dyspnea index mirrored those reported for exercise capacity; bosentan-treated patients demonstrated a mean reduction from baseline. At baseline, 90% of patients in both groups were NYHA functional class III. By week 16, 38% of patients receiving 125 mg and 34% of patients receiving 250 mg of bosentan had improved to functional class II, and 3% and 1%, respectively, had improved to class I. In contrast, 28% of placebo-treated patients improved to class II. During the course of the study, treatment with bosentan also significantly delayed the time to clinical worsening compared with placebo ($p = 0.002$).

Data presented in May 2004 at the American Thoracic Society meeting in Orlando, Florida, suggest an improvement in quality of life in PAH patients treated with bosentan. The VITAL study (Study 359) surveyed a group of PAH patients for one year (Gabbay E, 2004). Following six months of bosentan therapy, patients experienced a statistically significant improvement in quality of life compared with baseline ($p < 0.0001$), particularly with regard to their ability to perform physical and social tasks. At one year, patients reported significantly improved general health when compared with baseline ($p < 0.001$).

An open-label study, an extension of Study 351, investigated bosentan's long-term efficacy (Sitbon O, 2003[a]). Twenty-nine of the original 32 patients received bosentan—62.5 mg twice daily for four weeks and 125 mg twice daily for an additional year. Study end points included change in exercise capacity as measured by the 6MWD, improvement in NYHA functional class, and withdrawal due to clinical worsening. At six months, patients continuing bosentan treatment from the previous study maintained their improvement in walk distance (60 ± 11 m), while patients starting bosentan treatment (these patients had previously being receiving placebo) improved their walk distance by 45 ± 13 m. Long-term bosentan treatment (more than one year) was also associated with an improvement in hemodynamic parameters and NYHA functional class.

Mortality data for 169 patients treated with bosentan were recently reported (Channick RN, 2004). Three-year survival was 86% for those treated with bosentan, compared with a predicted survival of 48% for these individuals based on a validated NIH survival equation. In this patient group, 70% of patients were maintained on bosentan therapy alone.

As discussed in the "Etiology and Pathophysiology" section, the number of patients with HIV is increasing, and patients with HIV are living longer due to improvements in medications, thus making PAH associated with HIV an important target subpopulation. The BREATHE-4 study investigated bosentan in 16 patients with PAH associated with HIV (NYHA functional classes III and IV) (Sitbon O, 2003[b]; Sitbon O, 2003[c]). Treatment with the drug significantly improved this patient group's exercise capacity, NYHA functional class, hemodynamics, and quality of life without interfering with the control of HIV itself.

The BREATHE-2 study investigated bosentan in combination with IV epoprostenol (Humbert M, 2003). The study involved 33 patients in NYHA functional classes III and IV. All patients received epoprostenol therapy (2 ng/kg/min) for two days; the dose was then titrated up to a target dose of 14 ± 2 ng/kg/min. After the initial two days, patients were randomized to receive placebo or bosentan (62.5 mg twice daily for four weeks, increasing to 125 mg twice daily). The follow-up period was 12 weeks. Researchers did not observe a statistically significant reduction in total pulmonary resistance (the primary end point) in the bosentan group, although they noted a trend toward a reduction. They also noted a trend in terms of improvement in hemodynamic parameters in the bosentan group. A greater percentage of patients in the bosentan group did demonstrate an improvement in NYHA functional class (59% compared with 46% in the placebo group).

Other studies investigating combinations of bosentan and prostacyclins have shown more favorable outcomes. Studies have also demonstrated the successful transition of patients from IV epoprostenol or subcutaneous treprostinil to oral bosentan therapy (Suleman N, 2004).

Unfortunately, bosentan therapy has some drawbacks, including adverse drug-drug interactions. The most serious adverse effects are the potential for altered hepatic (liver) function and major birth defects. Data from clinical pharmacology and efficacy studies show elevations of the liver enzymes aspartate aminotransferase and alanine aminotransferase levels by more than three times the upper limit of normal in 11% of treated patients compared with 2% receiving placebo (Kenyon KW, 2003). In the BREATHE-1 study, abnormal liver function was greater in the bosentan arm (9%) than in the placebo arm (3%), and effects were found to be dose-dependent. However, the dose-related elevations in this study were usually transient in nature and returned to normal in all patients upon dose-reduction or discontinuation (Rubin LJ, 2002[b]). Studies in animal models treated with bosentan have resulted in stillbirths, fetal abnormalities, and dose-dependent teratogenic effects. There are no data on the use of bosentan in pregnant women. Minor side effects associated with bosentan therapy include headache, flushing, nasopharyngitis, and lower extremity edema (Kenyon KW, 2003).

Bosentan is metabolized via the cytochrome P450 system, hence the potential for drug interactions. The agent has been shown to induce CYP2C9 and CYP3A4, the primary metabolism pathways for warfarin; this action can reduce warfarin levels and so require an increase in the dose of the anticoagulant (Murphy L, 2003). Physicians are advised to carefully monitor the internal normalized ratio

(INR) of patients receiving both bosentan and warfarin. Hormonal contraceptives are also metabolized by CYP3A4; thus, coadministration of bosentan may reduce the effectiveness of contraception, an action that could have serious consequences given the potential adverse effects of bosentan in pregnancy.

The potential for serious adverse events prompted the FDA to instruct Actelion to include a warning on the package labeling and restrict access to bosentan through the Tracleer Access Program (TAP). Physicians planning to prescribe the agent must request a patient enrollment form, which details patient information, including patient insurance coverage, physician's information, prescription requirements, and an explanation of why the therapy is needed. Following confirmation of the patient benefits, the drug can then be distributed via one of four specialist pharmacies in the United States (Caremark [Northbrook, Illinois], Gentiva Health Services [Melville, New York], Procare Pharmacy [Duluth, Georgia], and Nova Factor, Inc. [Memphis, Tennessee]). Physicians must send a statement with the enrollment form expressing their commitment to perform blood testing to monitor liver function and pregnancy testing in female patients of childbearing age (Kenyon KW, 2003).

Calcium-Channel Blockers

Overview. CCBs have been used to treat PH, including PAH, for many years. Randomized, controlled studies examining these agents in the treatment of PH and chronic obstructive pulmonary disease (COPD) have had positive outcomes. However, robust data highlighting the beneficial effects of this treatment approach for PAH (the focus of this study) are lacking (Channick RN, 2003; Sajkov D, 1997).

Indeed, not all patients with PAH respond to CCB therapy, and it is not possible at the outset to determine who will benefit without intervention. Acute vasodilator testing is normally performed during right-heart catheterization (a procedure required to confirm the diagnosis of PAH) with short-acting agents such as adenosine, prostacyclin, or nitric oxide; those who respond positively to such a test are candidates for long-term CCB therapy as outlined in the ACCP evidence-based guidelines for PAH. The proposed definition of a positive acute vasoreactive response is a reduction of mean pulmonary artery pressure of ≥ 10 mm Hg to reach a pulmonary artery pressure of ≤ 40 mm Hg with an increased or unchanged cardiac output (Galié N, 2004). Recent studies suggest only a small percentage of patients are responders. In a retrospective analysis of more than 500 patients, 12% were found to be acutely vasoreactive. This group was placed on CCB therapy, but less than 50% were reported to experience a long-term benefit.

Treatment with CCBs can trigger adverse side effects, including symptomatic leg edema and hypotension, which may exacerbate existing manifestations of PAH; hence, patients should always be carefully assessed (Channick RN, 2003).

Nifedipine (Bayer Pharmaceuticals Corporation's [West Haven, Connecticut] Adalat, Pfizer's [New York, New York] Procardia, generics), diltiazem (Sanofi-Aventis's [Bridgewater, New Jersey] Cardizem, generics), and amlodipine (Pfizer's Norvasc/Amlor) are the most frequently used CCBs for PH. The choice of agent generally depends on the patient's heart rate at baseline (i.e., if a patient has bradycardia, nifedipine is favored; in the case of tachycardia, diltiazem is the agent of choice) (Rubin LJ, 2004[a]). The following sections discuss nifedipine and diltiazem because of the availability of clinical data for the PAH population.

Mechanism of Action. CCBs induce vasodilation by inhibiting the entry of calcium ions, which mediate cellular contraction via L-type calcium channels, into vascular smooth muscle cells (VSMCs); this process, in turn, lowers pulmonary artery pressure and pulmonary vascular resistance.

Nifedipine. Nifedipine (Bayer's Adalat, Pfizer's Procardia, generics) (Figure 10) has been available in the United States since 1986; it is also available in Europe and Japan. The agent is a long-acting dihydropyridine that inhibits entry of calcium ions that mediate contraction into VSMCs, thereby reducing pulmonary artery pressure and pulmonary vascular resistance in patients who are acutely vasoreactive.

There is a distinct lack of robust clinical data assessing the benefits of CCB therapy for PAH. Researchers examined long-term therapy with CCBs in 64 PAH patients considered vasoreactive (defined as a reduction in pulmonary vascular resistance of 20% or more on challenge with vasodilators) (Rich S, 1992). This patient group's survival was compared with that of patients considered non-vasoreactive who were enrolled in the NIH registry. Seventeen (26%) of the patients in the study responded to CCB treatment (39% drop in pulmonary artery pressure and a 53% drop in pulmonary vascular resistance index, $p < 0.001$). Thirteen patients in this group received nifedipine (172 $\pm$ 41 mg), while four received diltiazem (720 $\pm$ 208 mg). After a five-year follow-up, 94% of patients who responded to treatment survived compared with 55% of nonresponders. The survival of this responding group was also significantly better than that of the aforementioned NIH patients ($p = 0.002$). This study clearly demonstrates that long-term CCB therapy benefits vasoreactive patients.

An open-label study investigated the effects of vasodilators—including nifedipine—in combination with the anticoagulant warfarin in 20 patients with IPAH (Ogata M, 1993). Seven patients received treatment (vasodilator plus warfarin), while 13 patients acted as the control group, receiving no treatment. Five-year survival was significantly higher in the treated group (57%) than in the untreated group (15%).

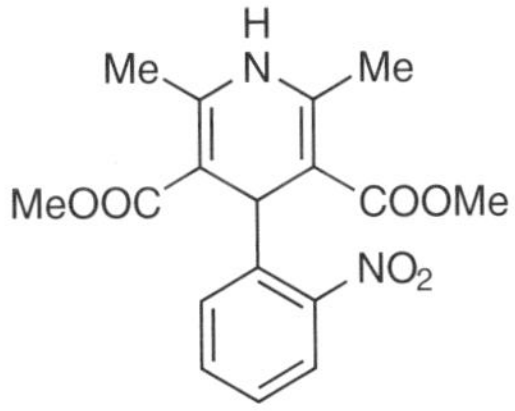

FIGURE 10. *Structure of nifedipine.*

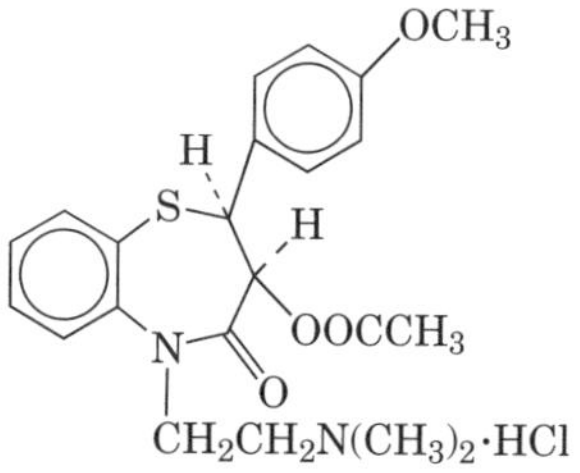

FIGURE 11. *Structure of diltiazem.*

Diltiazem. Diltiazem (Sanofi-Aventis's Cardizem, generics) (Figure 11) is a popular nondihydropyridine CCB that was approved in the United States in 1982; it is also available in Europe and Japan. Like all CCBs, this agent prevents calcium entry into VSMCs, disturbing smooth-muscle contraction in vasoreactive individuals with PH.

Clinical studies investigating the outcome of diltiazem therapy in individuals with PAH are scarce. The "Nifedipine" section discussed a study in which the agent was used, along with nifedipine, to treat 64 PAH patients considered vasoreactive (defined as a reduction in pulmonary vascular resistance of 20% or more on challenge with vasodilators) (Rich S, 1992). In this study, the five-year survival for PAH patients who responded to diltiazem was significantly greater than for those who failed to respond to CCB therapy.

Vitamin K Antagonists

Overview. For many years, experts in the PH field have strongly recommended anticoagulant therapy to treat PAH patients, particularly those without associated diseases for which contraindications may exist. This recommendation is based on the fact there is an increased risk of thrombosis and thromboembolism as a result of the sluggish pulmonary blood flow, dilation of the right-heart chambers, venous stasis, and limitations on physical activity associated with the disease (Rubin LJ, 1997). The recent publication of the American College of Chest Physicians (ACCP) evidence-based guidelines for the diagnosis and management of PAH supports this recommendation (Badesch DB, 2004[b]). These guidelines also emphasize that anticoagulant therapy is of prime importance in patients receiving long-term IV prostaglandin therapy because of the increased risk of catheter-induced thrombosis. The vitamin K antagonist warfarin (Bristol-Myers Squibb's [North Billerica, Massachusetts] Coumadin, Sanofi-Aventis's Coumadine, generics) is the anticoagulant of choice for PAH patients. Physicians adjust the dose to achieve an internal normalized ratio of approximately 2.0, and they carefully monitor patients for side effects associated with the drug.

Mechanism of Action. Vitamin K is an essential component in the activation of several clotting factors in the coagulation cascade, including prothrombin

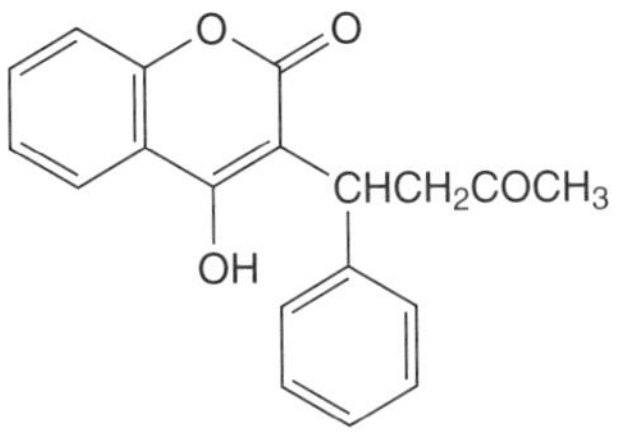

FIGURE 12. Structure of warfarin.

(factor II [FII]), FVII, factor IX (FIX), and factor X (FX). Vitamin K antagonists produce their anticoagulant effect by inhibiting this process.

Warfarin. The FDA first approved warfarin (Bristol-Myers Squibb's Coumadin, Sanofi-Aventis's Coumadine, generics) (Figure 12) in 1955 for the prevention of thrombosis and thromboembolism. It is also available in Europe and Japan. The agent's anticoagulant action stems from its inhibition of vitamin K, an essential component in the activation of several clotting factors.

Although the medical community recommends warfarin therapy and widely uses it for the prevention of thrombosis and thromboembolism in PAH, evidence supporting its use in this patient population does not come from rigorous or well-designed clinical trials. In a long-term retrospective study, researchers investigated 120 patients with PAH (Fuster V, 1984). The mean age of disease onset was 34 years; after a five-year follow-up, only 21% of the patients remained alive. Of the factors tested for prognostic importance in the study, two proved significant: oxygen saturation ($p < 0.00001$) and treatment with anticoagulant therapy ($p = 0.01$). The study's authors suggested the use of anticoagulants for this patient group.

Another study involving warfarin and PAH was previously discussed in the "Nifedipine" section (Rich S, 1992). In that study, the researchers investigated 64 PAH patients, of whom 55% received warfarin therapy on the basis of a lung scan demonstrating non-uniformity of pulmonary blood flow. Results demonstrated that warfarin significantly improved survival ($p = 0.025$), particularly for patients who did not respond to treatment with CCBs (nifedipine and diltiazem).

Unfortunately, many physiological and pharmacological factors can affect warfarin's therapeutic efficacy, and patient response is variable. The most serious risks associated with vitamin K antagonist therapy are hemorrhage in any tissue or organ and, less frequently ($<0.1\%$), necrosis and/or gangrene of skin and other tissues. Studies show that major bleeding occurs in up to 9% of patients treated with vitamin K antagonists (So L, 2001; Stern SH, 2000). Vitamin K antagonists are also contraindicated in pregnancy; this is not such an issue in the case of the treatment of PAH, where physicians stress that pregnancy should be avoided.

Clinicians should consider several important factors when deciding whether to use warfarin to treat patients with PAH and associated diseases (APAH). Patients with connective tissue disease or portopulmonary hypertension are at greater risk of a gastrointestinal (GI) bleed, while those with congenital heart disease are prone to hemoptysis (discharge of blood from the lungs by coughing). The ACCP guidelines stress that physicians must weigh the potential benefits of this therapy against the risks for this patient group (Badesch DB, 2004[b]).

Diuretics

Overview. Diuretics are commonly used to treat PAH patients with right-ventricular failure (e.g., those suffering from peripheral edema and/or ascites). The ACCP guidelines emphasize that the long-term management of PAH patients requires the maintenance of near-normal intravascular volume via the use of diuretics in addition to reduced dietary salt intake. However, the guidelines also stress that rapid and excessive diuresis may exacerbate patient symptoms, leading to systemic hypotension, renal problems, and syncope (Badesch DB, 2004[b]). As a result, patients receiving diuretic therapy should be carefully monitored.

The choice of diuretic is tailored to suit the individual, taking into account the severity of the disease and any potential contraindications. If only mild diuresis is required or the physician has concerns about electrolytes, a potassium-sparing diuretic such as spironolactone (Pfizer's Aldactone, generics) is the agent of choice. If a greater diuretic effect is needed, loop diuretics such as furosemide (Sanofi-Aventis's Lasix, generics) and torsemide (Roche's Demadex, generics) are recommended. If a thiazide is needed, hydrochlorothiazide (Merck's Hydrodi-uril, Novartis's Esidrex, generics) is the agent of choice.

Mechanism of Action. All diuretics increase the excretion of sodium and water, thereby reducing plasma volume, cardiac output, and peripheral resistance. Thiazide diuretics increase sodium and water excretion via inhibition of the sodium/chloride cotransporter in the distal convoluted tubule of the kidney nephron. Loop diuretics are more potent than thiazides, causing up to 15–20% of filtered sodium to be excreted. These agents act on the sodium-potassium-2-chloride cotransporter located in the ascending loop of Henle. Potassium-sparing diuretics are generally weak diuretics that act on aldosterone-sensitive sites in the nephron; they are associated with fewer side effects than the other subclasses (Rang HP, 1999).

Furosemide. First approved by the FDA in 1968 for the treatment of systemic hypertension, furosemide (Sanofi-Aventis's Lasix, generics) (Figure 13) is a popular treatment option for reducing fluid volume in PAH patients. It is available in Europe and Japan as well. Furosemide is a loop diuretic that exerts its effects on sodium and chloride reabsorption in the proximal and distal tubules and in the ascending loop of Henle. The diuretic effects of furosemide therapy are observed after one hour and last six to eight hours. Because furosemide is a highly potent agent, patients must be monitored for side effects, such as systemic hypotension and syncope, although these problems are generally experienced at high doses—180 mg per day or more. Clinical trials assessing the benefits of furosemide in the treatment of PAH are not available.

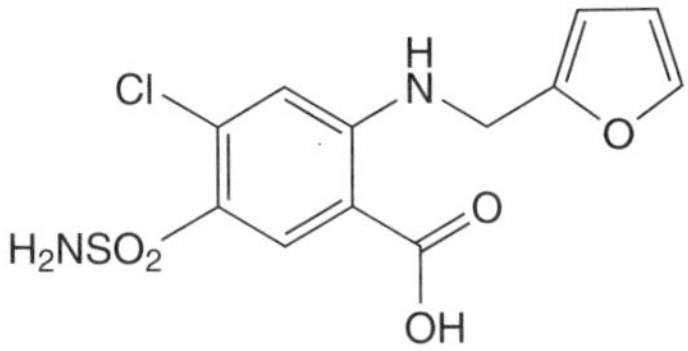

FIGURE 13. Structure of furosemide.

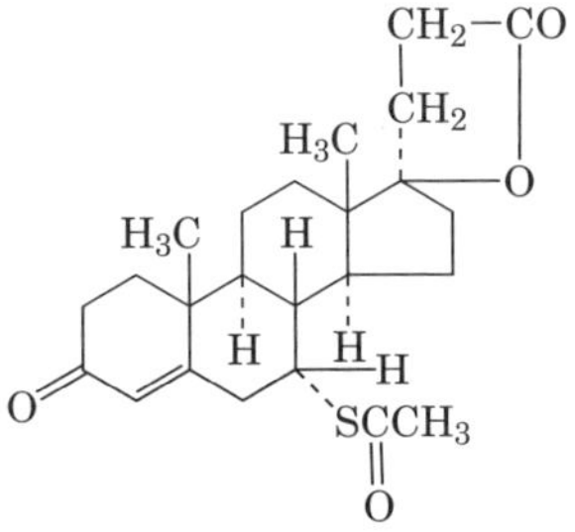

FIGURE 14. Structure of spironolactone.

Spironolactone. Spironolactone (Pfizer's Aldactone, generics) (Figure 14) has been available in the United States since 1982. The potassium-sparing diuretic promotes diuresis via inhibition of mineralocorticoid receptors. Spironolactone is used to treat PAH when other diuretic agents are inappropriate or not sufficient (i.e., it may be used in combination with other diuretic agents). Spironolactone is often a popular choice in the presence of ascites. The agent may have unwanted side effects, including gynecomastia due to the agent's activity on androgen receptors, and hyperkalemia, which may lead to cardiac abnormalities. The presence of such side effects may require that treatment be discontinued. No clinical studies have evaluated spironolactone in the treatment of PAH.

Cardiac Glycosides

Overview. Cardiac glycosides—namely, digoxin (GlaxoSmithKline's Lanoxin/ Lanoxicaps, generics)—may be part of a treatment regimen for patients with right-ventricular failure and/or atrial arrhythmias. As with diuretics, the ACCP guidelines emphasize that physicians must carefully monitor PAH patients on digoxin, especially if they already have impaired renal function.

Mechanism of Action. Cardiac glycosides inhibit sodium/potassium adenosine triphosphatase (ATPase) in cardiac cells, resulting in stronger heart contractions. New data also demonstrated that some of the benefits of cardiac glycosides are due to their effect on noncardiac tissue. For instance, inhibiting sodium/potassium ATPase in vagal nerves can sensitize cardiac baroreceptors

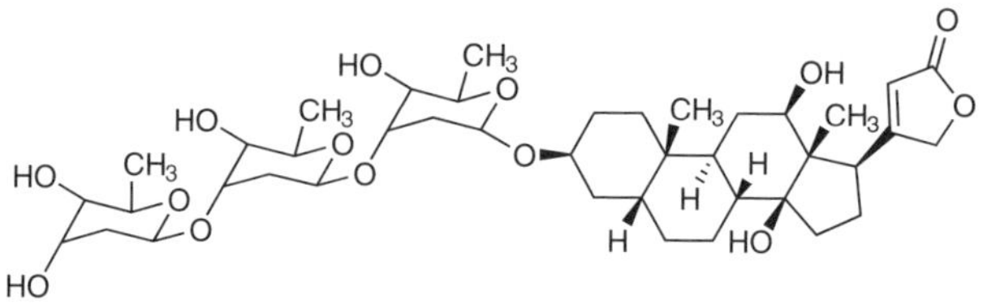

FIGURE 15. *Structure of digoxin.*

(pressure receptors), which in turn can reduce sympathetic tone of the heart. Inhibiting sodium/potassium ATPase in the kidney reduces sodium reabsorption, resulting in more sodium being delivered to the distal tubules and suppression of renin secretion. Some researchers have suggested that cardiac glycosides' modification of the neurohormonal system is more beneficial than their positive inotropic effects (Gheorghiade M, 1991).

Digoxin. Digoxin (GlaxoSmithKline's Lanoxin/Lanoxicaps, generics) (Figure 15) has been used as a treatment for the failing heart for many years. The agent acts on the sodium/potassium ATPase, strengthening cardiac contraction. Increased strength and efficiency of the heart improve the circulation and reduce the symptoms associated with right-heart failure in PAH, including peripheral edema. The major side effects of digoxin occur at high doses and include cardiac arrhythmias, anorexia, nausea, vomiting, and neurological disturbances. The concomitant use of quinidine, verapamil, spironolactone, flecainide, propafenone, or amiodarone can increase serum digoxin levels and may increase the risk of digoxin toxicity. Researchers have determined that the risk of death increases above a digoxin level of 1.0 ng/mL (Gheorghiade M, 1997), thus the need to monitor patients' digoxin level. To date, no clinical studies have directly evaluated digoxin therapy in patients with PAH.

Nonpharmacological Approaches

Lifestyle Modifications. Lifestyle modifications are essential following the diagnosis of PAH. Patients are advised to eat a low-salt diet and avoid participation in strenuous physical activities.

Supplemental Oxygen. Oxygen supplementation is common practice in the treatment of PAH. Some patients experience arterial oxygen desaturation during physical activity resulting from increased oxygen extraction; in such cases, ambulatory supplemental oxygen is recommended. Oxygen desaturation during sleep (without evidence of sleep apnea) may also occur. Patients may benefit from supplemental oxygen during the night. For patients with severe right-heart failure and resulting hypoxemia due to elevated oxygen extraction, continuous oxygen supplementation is common practice (Barst RJ, 2001).

Atrial Septostomy. Following reports that patients with IPAH and FPAH with a patent foramen ovale (anatomical interatrial communication) had a better survival than those without the condition, a surgical procedure known as atrial septostomy (creation of a small perforation in the atrial septum) has been performed in select PAH patients with severe right-heart failure. Performing this procedure may reduce mean right-atrial pressure and increase left-ventricular preload, leading to right-ventricle unloading and improved cardiac output. Patients who underwent the procedure have reported a reduced incidence of syncope and improved exercise capacity. However, the recently published ACCP guidelines recommend that this procedure be performed only in institutions with an established record of surgery in PAH patients because the procedure is associated with high levels of mortality (Ramona L, 2004; Runo JR, 2003).

Lung Transplantation. The first lung transplantation procedure for PAH was performed in 1982 (Runo JR, 2003). Since then, both single- and double-lung transplantations have been performed when all other methods have failed. For some highly select patients, lung transplantation may offer the chance of improved survival and NYHA functional class. It remains unclear whether single- or double-lung transplantation should be standard therapy. Single-lung transplants are less surgically invasive, and they allow two recipients to benefit from one donor. However, recent data from the International Society for Heart and Lung Transplantation (ISHLT) show a slight advantage for patients receiving double-lung transplants, although observations were not statistically significant (Orens JB, 2004).

Candidates for lung transplantation must have end-stage disease and must not possess any other diseases (e.g., HIV, which may affect survival post-transplantation). The World Health Organization has put in place criteria to aid with candidate selection; these criteria are outlined in Table 4. The overall success of lung transplantation is 77.4% at one year and 42.5% at five years, according

TABLE 4. Summary of WHO Criteria for Lung Transplantation in PAH

New York Heart Association functional class III or IV.
Mean right arterial pressure $\geq$10 mm Hg.
Mean pulmonary arterial pressure $\geq$50 mm Hg.
Cardiac index $\leq$2.0 L/min/m^2.
Failure of medical therapy in the following settings:

- WHO class III or IV symptoms.
- Mean right arterial pressure $\geq$10 mm Hg.
- Mean pulmonary arterial pressure $\geq$50 mm Hg.
- Cardiac index $\leq$2.0 L/min/m^2.

PAH = Pulmonary arterial hypertension.
WHO = World Health Organization.
Source: Based on Orens JB. Listing the patient: deciding when transplantation is the only viable life-sustaining option. Advances in Pulmonary Hypertension. 2004;3(1):4–8.

to the ISHLT. However, patients with PAH fare less well; their one-year survival rate is 72%, and their five-year survival rate is 37%. Early mortality in patients who have undergone a lung transplant may be due to factors such as infection, primary graft failure, acute tissue rejection, cardiovascular factors, or bronchiolitis. Factors responsible for late mortality in lung transplant patients differ and include chronic allograft rejection or obliterative bronchiolitis (occurs in 40% of patients at two years and approximately 70% of patients at five years) (Orens JB, 2004; Runo JR, 2003).

EMERGING THERAPIES

R&D for pulmonary hypertension (PH) is currently limited to the development of agents for pulmonary arterial hypertension (PAH), thus leaving considerable untapped opportunity for the pharmaceutical industry with respect to investigation of potential therapies for other classifications of PH. (The "Etiology and Pathophysiology" section describes the Venice classification system.) Not surprisingly, drug development pipelines for PAH itself generally reflect this indication's status as a rare disease. However, commercial interest in the disease has increased in the last year due to the presence of three compounds in late-stage development: sildenafil (Pfizer's Revatio), sitaxsentan (Encysive Pharmaceuticals's [Houston, Texas] Thelin), and Myogen's (Westminster, Colorado) ambrisentan.

New delivery methods for existing compounds—namely, treprostinil (United Therapeutics Corporation's [Silver Spring, Maryland] Remodulin), which has been plagued by problems associated with infusion-site pain—are also under development. Physicians and PAH patients attending the Sixth Annual Conference of the Pulmonary Hypertension Association in Miami in June 2004 were very excited about the prospect of inhaled and even oral preparations of this agent.

Other compounds and treatment approaches for PAH, including gene therapy, remain at early stages in the development process. For example, the exact role of serotonin (5-HT [5-hydroxytryptamine]) in the pathophysiology of PAH is a matter of debate; however, elevated 5-HT—as seen in PAH patients—has been associated with vasoconstriction and mitogenesis. The receptors involved in the actions of 5-HT in this disease remain to be determined, although 5-HT_{1B}, 5-HT_{2A}, and 5-HT_{2B} have all been implicated (Humbert M, 2004[a]). Two companies are investigating compounds that target the 5-HT_{2B} receptor. Biofrontera's BF1 is a 5-HT_{2B} receptor antagonist in preclinical development; studies in mice demonstrated the agent has a good pharmacokinetic profile and is not associated with any notable side effects, including sedation. Predix Pharmaceuticals has a similar R&D program.

Atrial natriuretic peptide (ANP) clearance receptor antagonists are an avenue of preclinical research that AstraZeneca (Wilmington, Delaware) is pursuing for this indication. Produced endogenously, ANPs are important vasodilators; preventing their clearance may have therapeutic implications by increasing their availability. Meanwhile, Australia-based Cytopia Limited (Melbourne, Australia) and U.S.-based Myomatrix Therapeutics (Albany, New York) have signed a collaborative agreement to evaluate the therapeutic potential of several kinase targets for cardiovascular diseases, including PH.

Therapeutic avenues for this indication being pursued in an academic, rather than commercial, setting include L-arginine supplementation. Inhaled nitric oxide (NO) is an effective treatment for acute PH and can improve exercise capacity in patients with the chronic condition; unfortunately, continuous treatment requires constant use of an inhalation device and so is very inconvenient. Researchers therefore investigated supplementation with L-arginine, the amino acid from which NO is synthesized. In one study, intravenous (IV) L-arginine reduced pulmonary vascular resistance and increased endogenous NO production, but these results could not be reproduced (Hoeper MM, 2002). In another investigation, supplementation of PAH patients for one week with oral L-arginine improved exercise capacity and hemodynamics (Nagaya N, 2001). Some researchers propose that a possible alternative to L-arginine supplementation, in terms of the delivery of NO, is inhaled diazeniumdiolates (NONOates), but further basic research is needed (Lam CF, 2002).

Table 5 lists agents in commercial development for PAH.

Phosphodiesterase Inhibitors

Overview. Vasodilators such as prostacyclin analogues have been the mainstay therapy for PAH for some time. Unfortunately, current agents are dogged by problems associated with drug delivery (e.g., injection-site pain), and in the case of currently marketed oral agents, there is a need for improved efficacy. Phosphodiesterase (PDE) inhibitors are also vasodilators. Sildenafil, which is approved for erectile dysfunction, is the most advanced agent in this class in development for PAH. It has demonstrated both potency and a degree of pulmonary selectivity in initial clinical investigations. PDE inhibitors can be administered orally, a clear advantage to patients in terms of convenience.

In addition to sildenafil, several other PDE inhibitors are being researched for potential use in PAH. Dong-A Pharmaceutical Co., Ltd. (Yongin, Korea) is conducting preclinical studies for its PDE-5 inhibitor, DA-8159. This compound is also in Phase II development for erectile dysfunction. Other agents under investigation for PAH include Pfizer's sildenafil analogue UK-343664, Tanabe's PDE-5 inhibitor T-1032, and Altana's PDE-3/4 inhibitor tolafentrine. Because of their early stage of development, these agents are not discussed in detail here.

If sildenafil (a PDE-5 inhibitor [see "Mechanism of Action" further on]) continues to demonstrate therapeutic potential in PAH, it would create an opportunity for other already-commercialized PDE-5 inhibitors such as vardenafil (Bayer's Levitra) and tadalafil (Eli Lilly and Company's [Indianapolis, Indiana]/ICOS Corporation's [Bothell, Washington] Cialis) to capitalize on the needs in the PAH market that remain underserved. Both of these agents have longer half-lives than sildenafil, a characteristic that could translate to a more convenient once-daily dosing regimen. Thus far, clinical studies using sildenafil to treat PAH have, on

TABLE 5. Emerging Therapies in Development for Pulmonary Arterial Hypertension

Compound	Development Phase	Marketing Company
Sildenafil (Revatio)		
United States	PR	Pfizer
Europe	PR	Pfizer
Japan	—	—
Sitaxsentan (Thelin)		
United States	III	Encysive Pharmaceuticals
Europe	—	—
Japan	—	—
Ambrisentan		
United States	III	Myogen
Europe	III	Myogen
Japan	—	—
Treprostinil (inhaled preparation)		
United States	II	United Therapeutics
Europe	II	United Therapeutics
Japan	—	—
Treprostinil (oral preparation)		
United States	PC	United Therapeutics
Europe	—	—
Japan	—	—
Aviptadil		
United States	—	—
Europe	II	Mondobiotech
Japan	—	—
Coxagen		
United States	PC	Aradigm/GeneRx+
Europe	—	—
Japan	—	—

PC = Preclinical (including discovery).
PR = Preregistered.

average, used a thrice-daily dosing schedule. It must be noted, however, that although both vardenafil and tadalafil are PDE-5 inhibitors, rigorous efficacy and safety studies will be necessary to guarantee approval for PAH, assuming sildenafil itself gains marketing authorization for this indication. Furthermore, sildenafil has been granted orphan drug status in Europe for PAH and chronic thromboembolic pulmonary hypertension (CTEPH), a designation that could, in the near term, prevent the addition of PAH to vardenafil's and tadalafil's labels. Orphan drug exclusivity afforded to sildenafil in Europe extends to December 2013, although off-label use of available PDE inhibitors during this time cannot be discounted.

Mechanism of Action. Of the family of PDE isozymes identified, types 1, 3, 4, and 5 are involved in controlling pulmonary arterial resistance. Under normal circumstances, PDE regulates the production of NO by metabolizing cyclic guanosine monophosphate (cGMP), the signaling molecule that promotes

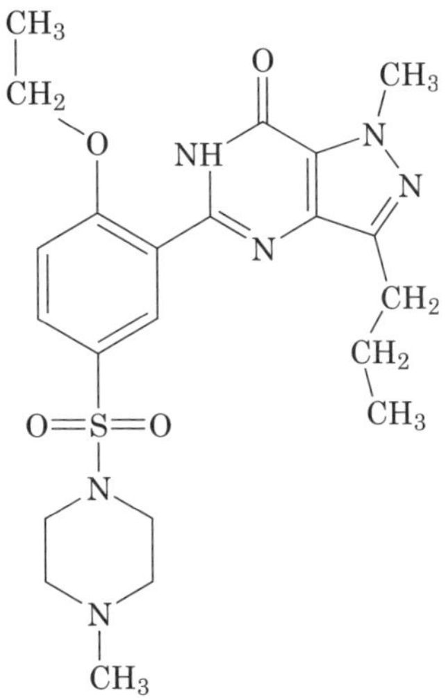

FIGURE 16. *Structure of sildenafil.*

NO production. Inhibition of PDE in the lung yields higher cGMP concentrations in vascular smooth muscle, thereby enhancing NO activity and vasodilation and reducing pulmonary artery pressure. Inhibition of PDE-5 is also believed to reduce platelet aggregation action of NO and inhibit thrombus formation.

Sildenafil. Sildenafil (Pfizer's Revatio) (Figure 16) is a potent, selective inhibitor of PDE-5 that is approved for the treatment of erectile dysfunction. Under pressure from PH patient support groups, Pfizer initiated Phase III trials in the United States and Europe for PAH and submitted regulatory filings in the United States and Europe in November 2004. In January 2004, the European Medicines Agency granted sildenafil orphan drug status for PAH and CTEPH. Data presented here focus primarily on the use of the drug for PAH.

Sildenafil inhibits the enzyme PDE-5, an isoform that is abundant in the pulmonary vasculature and inactivates cGMP, a second messenger involved in NO-mediated vasodilation. Sildenafil promotes NO-induced pulmonary vasodilation in the lung by blocking catabolization of cGMP by PDE-5.

Many studies to date on the effectiveness of sildenafil in treating PAH are limited by inconsistent trial design, small patient sample sizes, or the short-term administration of the agent. One nonrandomized trial evaluated the functional and symptomatic benefits of sildenafil therapy for five PAH patients over a period of 12 weeks (Michelakis ED, 2003). Treatment (50 mg sildenafil twice daily) improved NYHA disease class in all patients and significantly increased the patients' exercise capacity as measured by the six-minute walk distance (6MWD).

A randomized, double-blind, crossover study of 22 patients with idiopathic PAH (IPAH) in NYHA class II or III compared sildenafil (25, 50, or 100 mg three times a day) with placebo for six weeks (Sastry BK, 2004). Patients on sildenafil exhibited a 44% improvement in exercise tolerance, based on treadmill exercise times, and a reduction in both dyspnea and fatigue, based on patient-assessed quality of life (QoL) questionnaires. Patients did not suffer any major adverse effects.

Besides IPAH, sildenafil therapy has been shown to reduce pulmonary vascular resistance in patients suffering from HIV-associated PAH (Carlsen J, 2002). Moreover, in an open-label trial involving 16 patients with PH secondary to lung fibrosis, oral sildenafil (50 mg, $n = 8$) compared favorably with infused epoprostenol (GlaxoSmithKline's Flolan) ($n = 8$) (Ghofrani HA, 2002[a]). At the conclusion of the study, patients demonstrated significant improvements in gas exchange and pulmonary vasodilation.

At the October 2004 meeting of the American College of Chest Physicians (ACCP), Pfizer unveiled the most recent data from a Phase III placebo-controlled multicenter trial. The Sildenafil Use in Pulmonary Arterial Hypertension (SUPER-1) study randomized 278 patients (mean age 49, 75% women) to placebo ($n = 70$) or to 20 mg ($n = 69$), 40 mg ($n = 68$), or 80 mg ($n = 71$) of sildenafil three times a day for 12 weeks (Ghofrani HA, 2004). Of the total patient pool, 38% were NYHA functional class II and 58% class III. After 12 weeks, patients on the 80 mg dose demonstrated an increase in the 6MWD of up to 50 m, while those on 40 mg and 20 mg showed improvements in the 6MWD of 46 m and 45 m, respectively ($p < 0.001$). Overall, 35% of the sildenafil patient group improved by one functional class compared with 7% of the placebo group. The most common adverse event reported was headache (46 patients on sildenafil, 39 on placebo). Pfizer has extended the trial for patients on the 80 mg sildenafil dose; results are expected by mid to late 2005.

Several investigations have shown the synergistic benefit of adding sildenafil to an existing therapy, particularly prostacyclin analogues. In one study involving 73 patients on long-term inhaled iloprost (Schering AG [Berlin, Germany]/CoTherix's Ventavis), sildenafil was added to the regimen in 14 patients unresponsive to iloprost monotherapy (Ghofrani HA, 2003). Adjunct sildenafil therapy after 9–12 months improved exercise capacity and pulmonary hemodynamics. A prior open-label, randomized trial, conducted by the same group, found that a regimen of sildenafil plus inhaled iloprost improved pulmonary vasodilation better than the administration of either agent alone (Ghofrani HA, 2002[b]). Another group of researchers published similar results, finding sildenafil increased iloprost's vasodilatory effect (Wilkens H, 2001). Numerous case reports have also identified favorable effects on pulmonary artery pressure when sildenafil is combined with inhaled NO, primarily in an acute setting (Lepore JJ, 2002; Michelakis ED, 2002).

Despite sildenafil's potential benefit, the agent does pose a risk of adverse effects. Because it is not specific to the pulmonary circulation, it could trigger a systemic vasodilatory response, resulting in hypotension, headache, nausea, and syncope. In clinical studies assessing sildenafil's efficacy for treating erectile dysfunction, researchers reported low levels of visual disturbance (Goldstein I, 1998; Gonzalez CM, 1999) that correlated to the indirect inhibition of PDE-6 in the retina. However, in trials conducted so far in patients with PAH, there have been no recorded cases of any serious side effects or drug interactions with agents such as digoxin (GlaxoSmithKline's Lanoxin/Lanoxicaps, generics) and warfarin (Bristol-Myers Squibb's Coumadin, Sanofi-Aventis's Coumadine, generics).

Endothelin-Receptor Antagonists

Overview. The launch of bosentan (Actelion Pharmaceuticals's [South San Francisco, California] Tracleer) in both the United States and Europe established a clear role for endothelin-receptor antagonists (ERAs) in the treatment of PAH. However, bosentan inhibits both the endothelin-A (ET-A) and endothelin-B (ET-B) receptors, is associated with a high incidence of liver toxicity, and requires twice-daily dosing. These issues have prompted several pharmaceutical companies to pursue the development of novel agents in the ERA class. These novel agents are all selective for the ET-A-receptor subtype. In theory, ET-A-selective agents could block the vasoconstrictor effects of ET-A while maintaining the vasodilator and clearance effects of ET-B (Humbert M, 2004[b]).

ET-A antagonists in the later stages of development include sitaxsentan (Encysive Pharmaceuticals' Thelin) and Myogen's ambrisentan. Other compounds in early development include Tanabe Seiyaku Company's (Osaka, Japan) TA-0201 in Phase I, Abbott Laboratories's (Abbott Park, Illinois) ABT-306552 in preclinical development, and two derivatives of sitaxsentan being developed by Encysive—namely, TBC-3711 in Phase I and TBC-3214 at the preclinical stage. The lack of published data precludes further discussion of these earlier-stage molecules.

Mechanism of Action. Binding of ET-1 to its receptors activates signal transduction via the phospholipase C (PLC) intracellular signaling pathway, ultimately resulting in mitogenesis and vasoconstriction. ET-A receptors are expressed in vascular smooth muscle, the heart, the kidney, and the lung. ET-B receptors are also located on vascular smooth muscle, where activation elicits responses similar to those of ET-A receptors. However, ET-B receptors are also expressed in the endothelium, where activation leads to vasodilation through stimulation of the NO pathway. Small-molecule endothelin antagonists inhibit ET-1 action by binding endothelin receptors and inhibiting ligand (ET-1) interaction (Rang HP, 1999).

Sitaxsentan. Sitaxsentan (Thelin) is an orally active ET-A-selective ERA being developed by Encysive Pharmaceuticals (formerly Texas Biotechnology, Houston, Texas) for the treatment of cardiovascular diseases, including PAH and chronic congestive heart failure (CHF). The FDA granted sitaxsentan orphan drug designation for the treatment of PAH in November 2004, an action that ensures seven years of marketing exclusivity for PAH and confers tax and procedural advantages. Phase III studies for PAH are under way.

Sitaxsentan is 6500-fold more selective for the ET-A receptor than the ET-B receptor. Selective inhibition of ET-A counteracts the vasoconstrictive and mitogenic actions of endothelin in PAH. Animal investigations showed the agent had a half-life of six to seven hours and good oral bioavailability. Human studies determined a similar pharmacokinetic profile (half-life of five to seven hours) (Wu-Wong JR, 2001).

Clinical studies assessing the actions of sitaxsentan in PAH are available. The Sitaxsentan to Relieve Impaired Exercise (STRIDE-1) study, a randomized, double-blind, placebo-controlled Phase IIb/IIII trial, examined the effects of two doses of sitaxsentan (100 mg and 300 mg) administered orally, once daily to 178 PAH patients (Barst RJ, 2004[b]). The study lasted 12 weeks. Patients were NYHA functional class II, III, or IV and had IPAH, PAH associated with connective tissue disease, or PAH associated with congenital pulmonary shunts. The primary end point of maximum oxygen consumption was not reached, but those in the drug-treated arm did show improvements in the 6MWD and NHYA functional class. Sitaxsentan-treated patients experienced an improvement in the 6MWD of 35 m ($p < 0.01$) for those receiving the 100 mg dose and 33 m ($p < 0.01$) for those receiving 300 mg. NYHA functional class improved in 29% (16 out of 55) of the 100 mg group and in 30% (19 out of 63) of the 300 mg group. In the placebo group, 15% (9 out of 60) of patients demonstrated an improvement in NYHA functional class. Hemodynamic improvements were also observed on treatment with sitaxsentan.

A post hoc analysis of data from the STRIDE-1 study presented at the November 2004 meeting of the American Heart Association (AHA) in New Orleans revealed that sitaxsentan improved the 6MWD, NYHA functional class, and hemodynamics in PAH patients with connective tissue disease (McLaughlin VV, 2004[b]).

A blinded, follow-up study examined the effects of chronic sitaxsentan in patients who had taken part in STRIDE-1 (Horn EM, 2004). Seventy-nine patients received the 100 mg dose while 91 received 300 mg. The median length of treatment was 26 weeks, although some patients received therapy for up to 59 weeks. The study's end point was the effect of sitaxsentan on NYHA functional class. The researchers also analyzed the time to first improvement and the rate at which patients deteriorated. Results demonstrated that 53% of the patients in the 100 mg group had an improvement of one NYHA functional class, while 44% in the 300 mg group showed a similar improvement. During the study, 5% of patients in the 100 mg group and 8% in the 300 mg group deteriorated.

Based on data collected from bosentan studies, liver enzyme abnormalities are of prime concern when treating patients with ERAs, and indeed, elevated liver transaminases appear to be a problem with sitaxsentan. In the STRIDE-1 study, 10% of patients receiving 300 mg sitaxsentan experienced liver function abnormalities. In the follow-up study, no liver enzyme abnormalities (three times above normal levels) were reported in the first 12 weeks of the investigation, although over the entire course of therapy, overall rates were 5% for the 100 mg dose and 21% for the 300 mg dose. It should also be noted that in a pilot study of sitaxsentan, higher doses were associated with fatal hepatitis (Channick RN, 2004; Horn EM, 2004).

Other commonly experienced adverse events reported in STRIDE-1 were headache, peripheral edema, nausea, and nasal congestion. These effects have been reported with other ERAs. Treatment with sitaxsentan also appears to increase the international normalized ratio (INR) in patients treated with warfarin. Interactions with warfarin are due to sitaxsentan's inhibition of the CYP2 C9 P450 enzyme, which is the principal hepatic enzyme involved in warfarin metabolism (Channick RN, 2004).

Further Phase III trials for sitaxsentan are under way. In September 2004, Encysive announced it had completed enrolling 240 PAH patients in the company's multicenter pivotal study, STRIDE-2. STRIDE-2 is a randomized, double-blind, placebo-controlled study of sitaxsentan with a blinded bosentan arm. Patients will be randomized to receive one of four treatments: 50 mg sitaxsentan once daily, 100 mg sitaxsentan once daily, placebo once daily, or bosentan twice daily according to the package insert. STRIDE-2 will last 18 weeks. Data from STRIDE-2 were announced in February 2005, and the NDA officially filed in May 2005.

Following data from STRIDE-4 (a small trial designed to test whether the 50 mg dose was equivalent to the 100 mg dose) presented at an Encysive Pharmaceuticals press conference, the company is not hopeful about the results for the 50 mg dose in STRIDE-2. In STRIDE-4, the 50 mg dose demonstrated no meaningful efficacy trends on any of the parameters tested.

The company also recently reported data from a small study of 24 healthy volunteers conducted to examine potential drug interactions between sitaxsentan and sildenafil. Results demonstrated that the addition of sildenafil to a sitaxsentan treatment regimen did not appear to alter sitaxsentan levels. In the presence of sitaxsentan, the maximum concentration (C_{max}) of sildenafil increased by 18%. The minor effects on sildenafil pharmacokinetics are thought to be due to weak cytochrome P450 inhibition seen in earlier studies in cultured hepatocyte studies. Nevertheless, Encysive does not expect an adjustment to sildenafil's label will be required (Encysive Pharmaceuticals, press release, August 26, 2004).

Ambrisentan. Ambrisentan is an orally active ET-A selective antagonist being developed by Myogen under license from Abbott (formerly BASF Pharma) for the treatment of PAH. The compound is also under investigation for cardiovascular disease and renal failure. Phase III trials for PAH are under way. In July 2004, the FDA awarded ambrisentan orphan drug status for PAH and in March 2006 gave the product fast track status. Myogen has exclusive marketing rights to the compound. GSK has commercialization rights outside of the United States.

Inhibition of ET-A by ambrisentan counteracts the vasoconstrictive and mitogenic actions of endothelin in PAH. Myogen reports the compound has a half-life of 9–15 hours and may therefore be suitable for once-daily dosing.

In May 2004, the results of a Phase II study of ambrisentan were presented at the American Thoracic Society conference in Orlando, Florida. Researchers randomized 64 patients (61% had primary PAH [idiopathic or familial] and 39% had PAH associated with scleroderma, HIV, or anorexigen use) for a 12-week, blinded period to receive doses of 1, 2.5, 5, or 10 mg once daily (Rubin L, 2004[c]) A placebo arm was not included. The majority of the patients (64%) were NYHA functional class III, although some patients (36%) were class II. The initial blinded period was followed by a 12-week, open-label, dose-adjustment period. The study's primary end point was a change in the 6MWD at week 12.

The study found that ambrisentan improved the 6MWD at all doses tested (1, 2.5, 5, and 10 mg daily) (33.9 m ± 9.6, [$p = 0.003$], 37 m ± 8.6 [$p = 0.0004$], 38.1 m ± 13.2 [$p = 0.011$], and 35.1 m ± 11.1, respectively) at week 12. At week 16, the mean increase in the 6MWD was 48.4 m for all groups. In patients with primary PAH, a dose-dependent increase in the 6MWD was observed at week 12 ranging from 31.2 m to 54.1 m. NYHA functional class improved by one in 31% of patients in the study and by two in 5.2% of patients. A worsening in functional class was experienced by 3.5% of patients. Improvements in Borg dyspnea index and hemodynamic parameters were also observed. Adverse events experienced were not dose-related. Four patients experienced elevations in liver transaminases three times above normal levels. One patient had to discontinue therapy, and one patient had to reduce the dose of the agent; the other two patients' elevations were not confirmed on retesting. At the conclusion of the study, 48% of the patients were receiving the 10 mg/day dose of ambrisentan, and none experienced any liver abnormalities. No drug interactions were observed. This finding is extremely positive considering other ERAs appear to interact with warfarin (Rubin L, 2004[c]). Myogen reports that 60–70% of the patients were receiving anticoagulant therapy.

Randomized, controlled Phase III studies for ambrisentan, which include a placebo arm, are under way. The Ambrisentan in Patients with Moderate-to-Severe Pulmonary Arterial Hypertension (ARIES) I trial is investigating 5 and 10 mg/day doses of ambrisentan for 12 weeks in the United States and Canada, while ARIES II is evaluating the 2.5 and 5 mg/day doses over 12 weeks in Europe and South America. The primary efficacy end point is improvement in the 6MWD. The company completed these trials in August 2005.

Prostacyclin Analogues

Overview. Prostacyclin analogues' short half-lives have historically presented problems in respect to drug delivery. An important step forward in improving patient convenience while maintaining efficacy in this drug class was the development of treprostinil (United Therapeutics' Remodulin). This compound is more stable than epoprostenol (GlaxoSmithKline's Flolan) and has a longer half-life, thus permitting its delivery by subcutaneous infusion. However, clinical studies revealed that subcutaneous treprostinil caused infusion-site pain in 85% of patients, leading to the discontinuation of therapy in 8%. An open-label study revealed that the pain persisted for up to 18 months (Hoeper MM, 2002). The issue of infusion-site pain prompted United Therapeutics to investigate other formulations of this highly effective agent with a view to maximizing patient care. This section discusses two formulations (inhaled and oral) of treprostinil under development.

Mechanism of Action. Prostacyclin analogues mediate their effects (vasodilation and antiplatelet activity) through activation of G-protein-coupled receptors, known as IP receptors, on target cells. These IP receptors are coupled to the adenyl cyclase intracellular signaling cascade, and activation triggers the production of intracellular cyclic adenosine monophosphate (cAMP), culminating in cellular responses (Harker LA, 1986; Samuelsson B, 1975).

Treprostinil (Inhaled Preparation). United Therapeutics is developing an inhaled preparation of treprostinil as a potential first-line therapy for PAH. Phase II studies are under way in the United States and Europe. Inhaled treprostinil's mechanism of action follows that outlined for the prostacyclin analogues in general.

The development program is known as the TRIUMPH project. The goal of TRIUMPH is to develop a portable prostacyclin therapy that can be inhaled for not more than one to two minutes and administered no more than three to four times per day. United Therapeutics reports that approximately 180 patients have already been dosed with the agent acutely and 10 patients are receiving the agent chronically; the key centers involved are Giessen, Germany, and the University of California in San Diego.

In one open-label study, presented at the AHA meeting in 2004, treprostinil administered via a nebulizer (three inhalations) was given to 17 patients in the acute setting, during catheterization (Voswinckel R, 2004). Two patients continued to receive this therapy (four inhalations per day) on a compassionate-use basis for more than three months following acute testing. Both patients improved their NYHA functional class, and one patient's 6MWD increased from 0 m (bedridden) to 143 m and the other patient's increased by 176 m from baseline. The treatment was well tolerated, and no side effects were observed.

United Therapeutics is employing several measures to reduce this product's time to market. For example, it is using an off-the-shelf nebulizer, which has reduced the device R&D time. The company expects to submit an NDA to the FDA and the European Medicines Agency in 2007.

Treprostinil (Oral Preparation). United Therapeutics is developing an oral, sustained-release formulation of treprostinil for the treatment PAH and peripheral arterial disease. Phase I studies for peripheral arterial disease have begun, but the compound remains in the preclinical phase of development for PAH. Oral treprostinil's mechanism of action is as described for the prostacyclin class in general.

Studies investigating the actions of oral treprostinil in animal models of PAH and in PAH patients are not available in the public domain.

Vasoactive Intestinal Peptide Derivatives

Overview. Vasoactive intestinal peptide (VIP) and derivative VIP appear to be promising new ways to treat PAH. A study conducted at the University of Vienna involved eight patients with IPAH (Petkov V, 2003). Inhalation of VIP increased 6MWD from 296 m $\pm$ 138 m at baseline to 409 m $\pm$ 102 m in three months, reduced mean pulmonary artery pressure, increased cardiac output, and increased mixed venous oxygen saturation. The following paragraphs discuss Mondobiotech's VIP derivative aviptadil.

Mechanism of Action. VIP inhibits platelet activation and smooth-muscle-cell proliferation and dilates pulmonary vascular smooth muscle through activation of adenylate cyclase (Humbert M, 2004[b]).

Aviptadil. Mondobiotech is developing an inhaled formulation of aviptadil for PAH. The company recently signed an agreement with Bachem, which will produce and supply the agent. The European Medicines Agency has granted aviptadil orphan drug status for PAH and chronic thromboembolic PH. Company literature states the product is based on VIP and belongs to the glucagon-secretin superfamily. Aviptadil consists of 28 amino acids and is synthetically produced. Its mechanism, although not fully defined, follows the general mechanism of action outlined for VIPs. Phase II trials for PAH are under way in Europe.

Gene Therapies

Overview. For many years, researchers have envisioned using gene-based medicines—which introduce a new gene or block the expression of a gene—to cure or slow the progression of disease. A major advance in gene-based medicine occurred in June 2000 when a working draft of the human genome was announced to the scientific community. Researchers in the field of genomics have continued to make rapid progress identifying genes involved in human diseases and determining their function. Although this progress has generated much hope for gene-based medicines, several hurdles remain, including the limited efficacy of gene transfer, immune responses to vectors, and problems with vector specificity.

Two gene therapy programs are under way for PAH: a collaboration between Aradigm Corporation (Hayward, California) and geneRx+, Inc. (Nashville, Tennessee), which is discussed in further detail in the following section; and a discovery program at Northern Therapeutics (Montreal, Quebec, Canada) directed by Duncan Stewart of the University of Toronto. Northern Therapeutics initiated the Pulmonary Hypertension: Assessment of Cell Therapy (PHACeT) single-center trial in January 2005. This 18-patient study will establish the safety and tolerability of the therapeutic injection of endothelial precursor cells to regenerate the small pulmonary arteries of the lung. The precursor cells, which are initially collected from the patient's bloodstream prior to undergoing genetic modification, are delivered to the pulmonary artery via a catheter.

Mechanism of Action. Gene therapy involves the replacement, removal, or introduction of genes or other manipulation of genetic material. Gene therapies contain large DNA molecules that make up an entire gene and may include part of a vector or other delivery vehicle.

Coxagen. U.S.-based companies Aradigm and GeneRx+ are collaborating on the development of the pulmonary delivery of one of GeneRx+'s lead gene drug candidates, coxagen, to treat PH. Aradigm specializes in pulmonary drug delivery, while GeneRx + is involved in protein and gene-based technologies. Coxagen is a cyclooxygenase gene encoded in a plasmid vector formulated with a cationic lipid. This particular gene therapy involves delivering the gene to the lungs via aerosol administration. It is at the preclinical stage.

GeneRx+ reports that in both large and small animal studies, coxagen has been shown to increase specifically endogenous generation of protective prostanoids in the lungs, to prevent PH produced by administration of endotoxin, and to reduce pulmonary vascular reactivity. Investigations of lung structure and function demonstrate no adverse effects of aerosol administration. The company also states the product's therapeutic effects last for approximately a week following a single administration. GeneRx+ is hoping this product will qualify for orphan drug status from the FDA.

REFERENCES

Appelbaum L, et al. Primary pulmonary hypertension in Israel: a national survey. *Chest*. 2001;**119**:1801–1806.

Badesch DB, et al. Continuous intravenous epoprostenol for pulmonary hypertension due to the scleroderma spectrum of disease. A randomized, controlled trial. *Annals of Internal Medicine*. 2000;**132**(6):425–434.

Badesch DB, et al. Prostanoid therapy for pulmonary arterial hypertension. *Journal of the American College of Cardiology*. 2004;**43**(12 suppl S):56S–61S. [a]

Badesch DB, et al. Medical therapy for pulmonary arterial hypertension (ACCP evidence-based clinical practice guidelines). *Chest*. 2004;**126**:35S–62S. [b]

Barbera JA, et al. Pulmonary hypertension in chronic obstructive pulmonary disease. *European Respiratory Journal*. 2003;**21**(5):892–905.

Barst RJ. A comparison of continuous intravenous epoprostenol (prostacyclin) with conventional therapy for primary pulmonary hypertension. The Primary Pulmonary Hypertension Study Group. *New England Journal of Medicine*. 1996;**334**(5):296–302.

Barst RJ. Medical therapy for pulmonary hypertension. *Clinics in Chest Medicine*. 2001;**22**(3):509–515.

Barst RJ. Beraprost therapy for pulmonary hypertension. *Journal of the American College of Cardiology*. 2003;**41**:2119–2125.

Barst RJ, et al. Diagnosis and differential assessment of pulmonary arterial hypertension. *Journal of the American College of Cardiology*. 2004;**16**;**43**(12 suppl S):40S–47S. [a]

Barst RJ, et al. Sitaxsentan therapy for pulmonary arterial hypertension. *American Journal of Respiratory and Critical Care Medicine*. 2004;**169**(4):441–447. [b]

Benza RL, et al. Safety and efficacy of treprostinil in cirrhosis-related pulmonary arterial hypertension. Abstract presented at the 54th Annual Meeting of the American Association for the Study of Liver Diseases (AASLD); October 2003; Boston, MA.

Bjornsson J, Edwards WD. Primary pulmonary hypertension: a histopathologic study of 80 cases. *Mayo Clinic Proceedings*. 1985;**60**(1):16–25.

Brenot F, et al. Primary pulmonary hypertension and fenfluramine use. *British Heart Journal*. 1993;**70**:537–541.

Brenot F. Primary pulmonary hypertension: case series from France. *Chest*. 1994;**105**(2 suppl):33S–36S.

British Cardiac Society Guidelines. Recommendations on the management of pulmonary hypertension in clinical practice. *Heart*. 2001;**86**(suppl 1):i1–i13.

Budev MM, et al. Diagnosis and evaluation of pulmonary hypertension. *Cleveland Clinic Journal of Medicine*. 2003;**70**(suppl 1):S9–S17.

Carlsen J, et al. Sildenafil as a successful treatment of otherwise fatal HIV-related pulmonary hypertension. *AIDS*. 2002;**16**(11):1568–1569.

Channick RN, et al. Effects of the dual endothelin-receptor antagonist bosentan in patients with pulmonary hypertension: a randomized, placebo-controlled study. *Lancet*. 2001;**358**(9288):1119–1123.

Channick RN. What's on the horizon in therapy, from current approaches to experimental agents. *Advances in Pulmonary Hypertension*. 2003;**2**(4):9–16.

Channick RN, et al. Endothelin-receptor antagonists in pulmonary arterial hypertension. *Journal of the American College of Cardiology*. 2004;**43**(12 suppl S):62S–67S.

Corden ZM, et al. Home nebulized therapy for patients with COPD: patient compliance with treatment and its relation to quality of life. *Chest*. 1997;**112**(5):1278–1282.

Cowan KN, et al. Elastase and matrix metalloproteinase inhibitors induce regression, and tenascin-C antisense prevents progression, of vascular disease. *Journal of Clinical Investigation*. 2000;**105**(1):21–34. [a]

Cowan KN, et al. Complete reversal of fatal pulmonary hypertension in rats by a serine elastase inhibitor. *Nature Medicine*. 2000;**6**(6):698–702. [b]

D'Alonzo GE, et al. Survival in patients with primary pulmonary hypertension. Results from a national prospective registry. *Annals of Internal Medicine*. 1991;**115**(5):343–349.

Date H, et al. Lung transplantation for primary pulmonary hypertension. *Heart View*. 2004;**18**(8):92–95.

de la Calzada CS, et al. Clinical practice guidelines of the Spanish Society of Cardiology for pulmonary thromboembolism and hypertension. *Revista Española de Cardiologia*. 2001;**54**(2):194–210.

Du L, et al. Signaling molecules in nonfamilial pulmonary hypertension. *New England Journal of Medicine*. 2003;**348**:500–509.

Eddahibi S, et al. Serotonin transporter overexpression is responsible for pulmonary artery smooth-muscle hyperplasia in primary pulmonary hypertension. *Journal of Clinical Investigation*. 2001;**108**(8):1141–1150.

European Society of Cardiology Guidelines. The task force on diagnosis and treatment of pulmonary arterial hypertension of the European Society of Cardiology. Guidelines on diagnosis and treatyent of pulmonary arterial hypertension. *European Heart Journal*. 2004;**25**:2243–2278.

Evans TW, et al. A national pulmonary hypertension service for England and Wales: an orphan disease is adopted? *Thorax*. 2002;**57**:471–472.

Fuster V, et al. Primary pulmonary hypertension: natural history and importance of thrombosis. *Circulation*. 1984;**70**(4):580–587.

Gabbay E, et al. Tracleer (bosentan) therapy in patients with pulmonary arterial hypertension (PAH): the relationship between improvements in six-minute walk test (6MWT) and quality of life (Qol). 100th International Conference of the American Thoracic Society; May 2004; Orlando, FL. Abstract 56.

Gaine SP, Rubin LJ. Primary pulmonary hypertension. *Lancet*. 1998;**352**:719–725.

Galié N, et al. Primary pulmonary hypertension: insights into pathogenesis from epidemiology. *Chest*. 1998;**114**:184S–S194.

Galié N, et al. Effects of beraprost sodium, an oral prostacyclin analogue in patients with pulmonary arterial hypertension: a randomized, double-blind, placebo-controlled trial. *Journal of the American College of Cardiology*. 2002;**39**(9):1496–1502.

Galié N, et al. Advances in treatment of pulmonary hypertension. *Business Briefing-European Pharmacotherapy*. 2003:1–9.

Galié N, et al. Comparative analysis of clinical trials and evidence-based treatment algorithm in pulmonary arterial hypertension. *Journal of the American College of Cardiology*. 2004;**43**(12 suppl S):81S–88S.

Ghamra ZW, Dweik RA. Primary pulmonary hypertension: an overview of epidemiology and pathogenesis. *Cleveland Clinic Journal of Medicine*. 2003;**70**(suppl 1):S2–S8.

Gheorghiade M, et al. Digoxin. A neurohormonal modulator in heart failure? *Circulation*. 1991;**84**(5):2181–2186.

Gheorghiade M. Digoxin therapy in chronic heart failure. *Cardiovascular Drugs and Therapy*. 1997;**11**(suppl 1):279–283.

Ghofrani HA, et al. Sildenafil for treatment of lung fibrosis and pulmonary hypertension: a randomised controlled trial. *Lancet*. 2002;**360**(9337):895–900. [a]

Ghofrani HA, et al. Combination therapy with oral sildenafil and inhaled iloprost for severe pulmonary hypertension. *Annals of Internal Medicine*. 2002;**136**(7):515–522. [b]

Ghofrani HA, et al. Oral sildenafil as long-term adjunct therapy to inhaled iloprost in severe pulmonary arterial hypertension. *Journal of the American College of Cardiology*. 2003;**42**(1):158–164.

Ghofrani HA, et al. Late-breaking clinical trial session. 70th Annual Meeting of the American College of Chest Physicians; October 2004; Seattle, WA.

Giuliano F, et al. Randomized trial of sildenafil for the treatment of erectile dysfunction in spinal cord injury. *Annals of Neurology*. 1999;**46**(1):15–21.

Goldstein I, et al. Oral sildenafil in the treatment of erectile dysfunction. Sildenafil Study Group. *New England Journal of Medicine*. 1998;**338**(20):1397–1404.

Gomez-Varela S, et al. Stenting in primary pulmonary hypertension with compression of the left main coronary artery. *Revista Española de Cardiología*. 2004;**57**(7):695–698. Abstract.

Gonzalez CM, et al. Sildenafil causes a dose- and time-dependent downregulation of phosphodiesterase type 6 expression in the rat retina. *International Journal of Impotence Research*. 1999;**11**(suppl 1):S9–S14.

Hachulla E, et al. Pulmonary arterial hypertension in systemic sclerosis: definition of a screening algorithm for early detection (the ItinerAIR-Sclerodermie Study). *Revue de Médecine Interne*. 2004;**25**(5):340–347. English abstract.

Harker LA, et al. Pharmacology of platelet inhibitors. *Journal of the American College of Cardiology*. 1986;**8**(6 suppl B):21B–32B.

HCUPnet, Healthcare Cost and Utilization Project. Agency for Healthcare Research and Quality, Rockville, MD, 2003. www.ahrq.gov/data/hcup/hcupnet.htm. Accessed January 20, 2004.

Hervé P, et al. Increased plasma serotonin in primary pulmonary hypertension. *American Journal of Medicine*. 1995;**99**(3):249–254.

Higgenbottam TW, et al. Treatment of pulmonary hypertension with continuous infusion of prostacyclin analogue iloprost. *Heart*. 1998;**79**(2):175–179.

Hoeper MM. Pulmonary hypertension in collagen vascular disease. *European Respiratory Journal*. 2002;**19**:571–576. [a]

Hoeper MM, et al. New treatments for pulmonary arterial hypertension. *American Journal of Critical Care Medicine*. 2002;**65**:1209–1216. [b]

Horn EM, Barst RJ. Treprostinil therapy for pulmonary hypertension. *Expert Opinion in Investigational Drugs*. 2002;**11**(11):1615–1622.

Horn EM, et al. Sitaxsentan, a selective endothelin-A receptor antagonist for the treatment of pulmonary arterial hypertension. *Expert Opinion in Investigational Drugs*. 2004;**13**(11):1483–1492.

Humbert M, et al. Short-term and long-term (prostacyclin) therapy in pulmonary hypertension secondary to connective diseases: results of a pilot study. *European Respiratory Journal*. 1999;**13**:1351–1356.

Humbert M, et al. Risk factors for pulmonary hypertension. *Clinics in Chest Medicine*. 2001;**22**(3):459–475.

Humbert M, et al. Safety and efficacy of bosentan combined with epoprostenol in patients with severe pulmonary arterial hypertension. *American Journal of Respiratory and Critical Care Medicine*. 2003;**16**(7):Abstract 441.

Humbert M. Cellular and molecular pathophysiology of pulmonary arterial hypertension. *Journal of the American College of Cardiology*. 2004;**43**(12 suppl S):13S–24S. [a]

Humbert M, et al. Treatment of pulmonary arterial hypertension. *New England Journal of Medicine*. 2004;**351**:1525–1436. [b]

Japanese Intractable Disease Information Center (JIDIC). www.nanbyou.or.jp. Accessed August 4, 2004.

Kenyon KW, Nappi JM. Bosentan for the treatment of pulmonary arterial hypertension. *Annals of Pharmacotherapy*. 2003;**37**:1055–1062.

Keogh AM, et al. Pulmonary arterial hypertension: a new era in management. *Medical Journal of Australia*. 2003;**78**:564–567.

Kim NHS. Diagnosis and evaluation of the patient with pulmonary hypertension. *Cardiology Clinics*. 2004;**22**(3):367–373.

Kozak LJ, et al. National Hospital Discharge Survey: 2001 annual summary with detailed diagnosis and procedure data. National Center for Health Statistics. *Vital Health Statistics*. 2004;**13**(156):1–198.

Krowka M. Portopulmonary hypertension: understanding pulmonary hypertension in the setting of liver disease. *Advances in Pulmonary Hypertension*. 2004;**3**(2):4–8.

Kuhn KP, et al. Outcome in 91 consecutive patients with pulmonary arterial hypertension receiving epoprostenol. *American Journal of Respiratory and Critical Care Medicine*. 2003;**167**(4):580–586.

Laliberte K, et al. Pharmacokinetics and steady-state bioequivalence of treprostinil sodium (Remodulin) administered by the intravenous, subcutaneous route to normal volunteers. *Journal of Cardiovascular Pharmacology*. 2003;**60**(9):916–922.

Lam CF, et al. Inhaled diazeniumdiolates (NONOates) as selective pulmonary vasodilators. *Expert Opinion in Investigational Drugs*. 2002;**11**(7):897–909.

Lepore JJ, et al. Effect of sildenafil on the acute pulmonary vasodilator response to inhaled nitric oxide in adults with primary pulmonary hypertension. *American Journal of Cardiology*. 2002;**90**(6):677–680.

MacLean MR, et al. 5-hydroxytryptamine and the pulmonary circulation: receptors, transporters, and relevance to pulmonary arterial hypertension. *British Journal of Pharmacology*. 2000;**131**(2):161–168.

Martin-Morales A, et al. Clinical safety of oral sildenafil citrate (Viagra) in the treatment of erectile dysfunction. *International Journal of Impotence Research*. 1998;**10**(2):69–74.

McDonnell P, et al. Primary pulmonary hypertension and cirrhosis: are they related? *American Review of Respiratory Diseases*. 1983;**127**:437–441.

McLaughlin VV, et al. Survival in primary pulmonary hypertension: the impact of epoprostenol therapy. *Circulation*. 2002;**106**(12):1477–1482.

McLaughlin VV, et al. Efficacy and safety of treprostinil: an epoprostenol analogue for primary pulmonary hypertension. *Journal of Cardiovascular Pharmacology*. 2003;**41**:293–299.

McLaughlin VV. Classification and epidemiology of pulmonary hypertension. *Cardiology Clinics*. 2004;**22**(3):327–341. [a]

McLaughlin VV. Sitaxsentan improves 6MW and hemodynamics in patients with pulmonary arterial hypertension (PAH) related to connective tissue disease. *Circulation*. 2004;**110**(17). Abstract 2602. [b]

Melian EB, Goa KL. Beraprost: a review of its pharmacology and therapeutic efficacy in the treatment of peripheral arterial disease and pulmonary arterial hypertension. *Drugs*. 2002;**62**(1):107–133.

Mesquita SM, et al. Likelihood of left main coronary artery compression based on pulmonary trunk diameter in patients with pulmonary hypertension. *American Journal of Medicine*. 2004;**116**(6):369–374.

Michelakis E, et al. Oral sildenafil is an effective and specific pulmonary vasodilator in patients with pulmonary arterial hypertension: comparison with inhaled nitric oxide. *Circulation*. 2002;**105**(20):2398–2403.

Michelakis ED, et al. Long-term treatment with oral sildenafil is safe and improves functional capacity and hemodynamics in patients with pulmonary arterial hypertension. *Circulation*. 2003;**108**(17):2066–2069.

Ministry of Health, Labor, and Welfare Guidelines. *Japanese Circulation Journal*. 2001;**65**(suppl V):1077–1126.

Mitani Y, et al. Nitric oxide reduces vascular smooth muscle cell elastase activity through cGMP-mediated suppression of ERK phosphorylation and AM1B nuclear partitioning. *FASEB Journal*. 2000;**14**:805–814.

Miyamoto S, et al. Clinical correlates and prognostic significance of six-minute walk test in patients with primary pulmonary hypertension. Comparison with cardiopulmonary exercise testing. *American Journal of Respiratory and Critical Care Medicine*. 2000;**161**(2 Pt 1):487–492.

Montorsi F, et al. Efficacy and safety of fixed-dose oral sildenafil in the treatment of erectile dysfunction of various etiologies. *Urology*. 1999;**53**(5):1011–1018.

Mukerjee D, et al. Prevalence and outcome in systemic sclerosis associated with pulmonary arterial hypertension: application of a registry approach. *Annals of Rheumatic Disease*. 2003;**62**(11):1088–1093.

Murphy L, Hood E. Bosentan and warfarin interaction. *Annals of Pharmacotherapy*. 2003;**37**:1029–1031.

Nagaya N, et al. Effect of orally active prostacyclin analogue on survival of outpatients with primary pulmonary hypertension. *Journal of the American College of Cardiology*. 1999;**34**(4):1188–1192.

Nagaya N, et al. Short-term oral administration of L-arginine improves hemodynamics and exercise capacity in patients with precapillary pulmonary hypertension. *American Journal of Critical Care Medicine*. 2001;**163**:887–891.

Nauser TD, Stites SW. Diagnosis and treatment of pulmonary hypertension. *American Family Physician*. 2001;**63**(9):1789–1797.

Newman JH, et al. Pulmonary arterial hypertension–future directions. *Circulation*. 2004;**109**:2947–2952.

Nicod LP. Pulmonary hypertension. *Swiss Medicine Weekly*. 2003;**133**:103–110.

Ogata M, et al. Effects of a combination therapy of anticoagulant and vasodilator on the long-term prognosis of primary pulmonary hypertension. *Japanese Circulation Journal*. 1993;**57**(1):63–69.

Okada O, et al. Collaborated research to establish treatment guidelines for primary pulmonary hypertension. Research report 2000 from the study group of respiratory diseases in the Ministry of Health, Labor and Welfare. 2001:205–208. [a]

Okada O, et al. Analysis of clinical survey sheet for primary pulmonary hypertension. Research Report 2000 from the study group of respiratory diseases in the Ministry of Health, Labor and Welfare. 2001:196–199. [b]

Olschewski H, et al. Inhaled iloprost for severe pulmonary hypertension. *New England Journal of Medicine*. 2002;**347**(5):322–329.

Opitz CF, et al. Assessment of the vasodilator response in primary pulmonary hypertension. Comparing prostacyclin and iloprost administered by either infusion or inhalation. *European Heart Journal*. 2003;**24**(4):356–365.

Orens JB. Listing the patient: deciding when transplantation is the only viable life-sustaining option. *Advances in Pulmonary Hypertension*. 2004;**3**(1):4–8.

Oudiz RJ. Primary pulmonary hypertension. September 4, 2004. www.emedicine.com/MED/topic1962.htm. Accessed October 15, 2004.

Peacock AJ. Treatment of pulmonary hypertension: several options exist, but they are expensive and necessitate specialist care. *BMJ*. 2003;**326**:835–836.

Pelio D. Secondary pulmonary hypertension and the development of *cor pulmonale*. *Physician Assistant*. 2002;**26**(6):21–31.

Petrov V, et al. Vasoactive intestinal peptide as a new drug for the treatment of primary pulmonary hypertension. *Journal of Clinical Investigation*. 2003;**111**(9):1339–1346.

Population Division of the Department of Economic and Social Affairs of the United Nations Secretariat. *World Population Prospects: The 2002 Revision*, vol. I, *Comprehensive Tables* (United Nations publication, Sales No. E.03.XIII.6); and *World*

Population Prospects: The 2002 Revision, vol. II, *The Sex and Age Distribution of Populations* (United Nations publication, Sales No. E.03.XIII.7), 2003.

Rabinovitch M. Elastase and the pathobiology of unexplained pulmonary hypertension. *Chest*. 1998;**114**(3 suppl):213S–224S.

Ralph D. Best practice of medicine. Pulmonary hypertension, 2001. http://merck.micromedex.com/index.asp?page=bpm_brief&article_id=BPM01CA11.   Accessed October 16, 2004.

Ramona L, et al. Surgical treatments and interventions for pulmonary arterial hypertension. ACCP evidence-based clinical practice guidelines. *Chest*. 2004;**126**:63S–92S.

Rang HP, et al. Pharmacology. Fourth Ed. New York, NY: Churchill and Livingstone; 1999:250–309.

Rich S, et al. Primary pulmonary hypertension. A national prospective study. *Annals of Internal Medicine*. 1987;**107**(2):216–223.

Rich S, et al. The prevalence of pulmonary hypertension in the United States. Adult population estimates obtained from measurements of chest roentgenograms from the NHANES II Survey. *Chest*. 1989;**96**:236–241.

Rich S, et al. The effect of high-dose calcium-channel blockers on survival in primary pulmonary hypertension. *New England Journal of Medicine*. 1992;**327**(2):76–81.

Rich S, et al. Anorexigens and pulmonary hypertension in the United States: results of the surveillance of North American pulmonary hypertension. *Chest*. 2000;**117**(3):870–874.

Rosenzweig EB, et al. Long-term prostacyclin for pulmonary hypertension with associated congenital heart disease. *Circulation*. 1999;**99**(14):1858–1865.

Rothman A. Pulmonary hypertension. www.vascularbiosciences.com/html/pulmonary_hypertension.html. Accessed January 16, 2004.

Rubin LJ. Primary pulmonary hypertension. *New England Journal of Medicine*. 1997;**336**(2):111–117.

Rubin LJ, et al. Bosetan therapy for pulmonary arterial hypertension. *New England Journal of Medicine*. 2002;**346**:896–903. [a]

Rubin LJ, Roux S. Bosentan: a dual endothelin-receptor antagonist. *Expert Opinion in Investigational Drugs*. 2002;**11**(7):991–1002. [b]

Rubin LJ. Diagnosis and management of pulmonary arterial hypertension: ACCP evidence-based clinical practice guidelines. *Chest*. 2004;**126**:7S–34S. [a]

Rubin LJ, Galié N. Pulmonary arterial hypertension: a look to the future. *Journal of the American College of Cardiology*. 2004;**43**(12 suppl S):S89–S90. [b]

Rubin LJ. Ambrisentan improves exercise capacity and clinical measures in pulmonary arterial hypertension. American Thoracic Society—100th International Conference; Orlando, FL; May 21–26, 2004. Abstract 352958. [c]

Runo JR, Lloyd JE. Primary pulmonary hypertension. *Lancet*. 2003;**361**:1533–1544.

Sajkov D, et al. A comparison of two long-acting vasoselective calcium antagonists in pulmonary hypertension secondary to COPD. *Chest*. 1997;**111**(6):1622–1630.

Samuelsson B, et al. Prostaglandins. *Annual Review of Biochemistry*. 1975;**44**:669–695.

Sastry BK, et al. Clinical efficacy of sildenafil in primary pulmonary hypertension: a randomized, placebo-controlled, double-blind, crossover study. *Journal of the American College of Cardiology*. 2004;**43**(7):1149–1153.

Seone L, et al. Pulmonary hypertension associated with HIV infection. *Southern Medical Journal*. 2001;**94**(6):635–639.

Shah MR, et al. Hemodynamics as surrogate end points for survival in advanced heart failure: an analysis from FIRST. *American Heart Journal*. 2001;**141**(6):908–914.

Simonneau G, et al. Continuous subcutaneous infusion of treprostinil, a prostacyclin analogue in patients with pulmonary arterial hypertension: a double-blind, randomized, placebo-controlled trial. *American Journal of Critical Care Medicine*. 2002;**165**(6):800–804.

Simonneau G, et al. Clinical classification of pulmonary hypertension. *Journal of the American College of Cardiology*. 2004;**43**(12 suppl S):5S–12S.

Sims JM. What's new in pulmonary artery hypertension? *Dimensions in Critical Care Nursing*. 2003;**22**(4):167–170.

Sitbon O, et al. Long-term intravenous epoprostenol infusion in primary pulmonary hypertension: prognostic factors and survival. *Journal of the American College of Cardiology*. 2002;**40**:780–788.

Sitbon O, et al. Effects of dual endothelin-receptor antagonist bosentan in patients with pulmonary arterial hypertension: a one-year follow-up study. *Chest*. 2003;**124**(1):247–254. [a]

Sitbon O, et al. Haemodynamic and clinical improvement with bosentan in patients with pulmonary hypertension associated with HIV infection. European Society of Cardiology; August 30–September 3, 2003; Vienna, Austria. Abstract 2568. [b]

Sitbon O, et al. Bosentan in pulmonary arterial hypertension associated with HIV infection. 13th Congress of the European Respiratory Society; September 27–October 1, 2003; Vienna, Austria. Abstract 3538. [c]

So L. Oral direct thrombin inhibition. International Society of Thrombosis and Haemostasis—XVII Congress Report; July 6–12, 2001; Paris, France.

Stern SH. Evaluation of the safety and efficacy of enoxaparin and warfarin for prevention of deep vein thrombosis after total knee arthroplasty. *Journal of Arthroplasty*. 2000;**15**(2):153–158.

Strange JW, et al. Recent insights into the pathogenesis and therapeutics of pulmonary hypertension. *Clinical Science*. 2002;**102**:253–268.

Stricker H, et al. Severe pulmonary hypertension: data from the Swiss Registry. *Swiss Medical Weekly*. 2001;**131**:345–350.

Suleman N, Frost AE. Transition from epoprostenol and treprostinil to oral endothelin receptor-antagonist bosentan in patients with pulmonary hypertension. Pulmonary Hypertension Association–Sixth Annual Conference; 2004; Miami, FL. Abstract 1042.

Sullivan CC, et al. Induction of pulmonary hypertension by angiopoietin 1/TIE2/serotonin pathway. *Proceedings of the National Academy of Sciences, USA*. 2003;**100**:122331–122336.

Taraseviciene-Stewart L, et al. Inhibition of the VEGF receptor 2 combined with chronic hypoxia causes cell death-dependent pulmonary endothelial cell proliferation and severe pulmonary hypertension. *FASEB Journal*. 2001;**15**:367–374.

Vachiery JL, et al. Transitioning from IV epoprostenol to subcutaneous treprostinil in pulmonary arterial hypertension. *Chest*. 2002;**121**(5):1561–1565.

Voelkel NF, Cool C. Pathology of pulmonary hypertension. *Cardiology Clinics*. 2004;**22**(3):343–351.

Voswinckel R, et al. Inhaled treprostinil sodium (TRE) for the treatment of pulmonary hypertension. *Circulation: Abstracts from Scientific Sessions*. 2004;**110**(17):III–295. Abstract 1414.

Wilkens H, et al. Effect of inhaled iloprost plus oral sildenafil in patients with primary pulmonary hypertension. *Circulation*. 2001;**104**(11):1218–1222.

Wu-Wong JR. Sitaxsentan (Icos-Texas Biotechnology). *Current Opinion in Investigational Drugs*. 2001;**2**(4):531–536.

Zhao YD, et al. Protective role of angipoietin-1 in experimental pulmonary hypertension. *Circulation Research*. 2003;**92**:984–991.

Venous Thromboembolism

ETIOLOGY AND PATHOPHYSIOLOGY

Introduction

Deep vein thrombosis (DVT) and pulmonary embolism (PE) are two distinct conditions of the same dynamic process known as venous thromboembolism (VTE). In medical practice, prophylaxis of VTE is administered to at-risk patients. When discussing prophylaxis, this section refers to VTE. To reflect medical practice and approved drug indications, treatment of DVT and of PE are discussed as separate entities.

DVT occurs when a blood clot, or thrombus, develops in the deep outflow veins (the femoral, popliteal, and tibial) of the legs. In contrast to thrombi that develop in other parts of the body, a thrombus in the deep veins is significantly more likely to embolize (detach from the vessel wall) and be carried via the heart to the pulmonary circulation. Once the embolus has entered the pulmonary circulation, it may become lodged in a pulmonary artery, where it will interrupt blood supply to areas of the lung and cause infarction of the lung tissue, or PE. Up to 50% of symptomatic DVT may result in subclinical pulmonary emboli (Meignan M, 2000), and up to 95% of cases of PE originate from clots in the deep venous system of the lower limbs (Saeger W, 1994).

Wiley Handbook of Current and Emerging Drug Therapies, Volumes 5–8
Copyright © 2007 Decision Resources, Inc. Published by John Wiley & Sons, Inc.

Anatomy of the Lower Extremities

The venous system of the lower extremities consists of deep and superficial veins, connected by perforator veins. The deep veins, which parallel the flow of the associated arteries, provide the greatest contribution to the draining of the blood from the leg (Figure 1). These veins are the most clinically relevant in DVT and PE. The deep venous system begins at the common iliac veins in the abdomen, which continue downward to connect to the femoral veins. After blood is received by the deep femoral vein, it descends to the thigh, passing through the adductor canal to the popliteal vein located behind the knee. The popliteal vein in turn extends into the calf, first dividing into the anterior tibial veins and the tibioperoneal trunk. The latter branches to form the posterior tibial veins, which drain the back of the calf, and the peroneal veins of the lower calf. The anterior tibial veins drain the front part of the calf. Crucial to the mechanics of the venous system are the one-way bicuspid valves, which prevent blood from flowing backward within veins, and the contraction of muscles surrounding the deep veins that propel blood upward. Thrombus formation often originates in the cusp of valves of the deep calf veins.

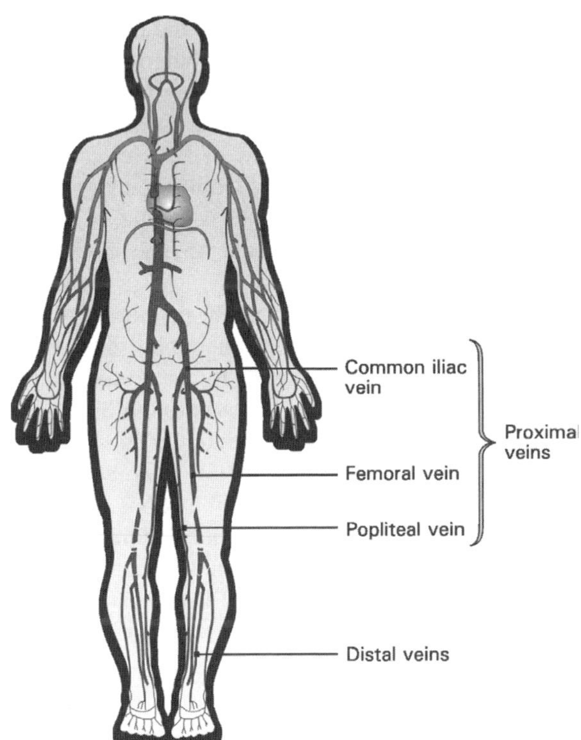

FIGURE 1. *Veins of the lower extremities involved in deep vein thrombosis.*

Etiology

DVT and associated PE are caused by a triad of factors (originally postulated in 1856 by Rudolf Virchow) that upset the normal hemostatic process responsible for minimizing blood loss from injured vessels and promote inappropriate clotting of venous blood:

- Vascular injury, which initiates the coagulation cascade.
- Venous stasis, which impairs the clearance of activated coagulation factors and limits the accessibility of thrombin present in the veins to thrombomodulin, which is concentrated primarily in the capillaries.
- Hypercoagulation, or the prothrombotic state, which occurs when coagulation overrides fibrinolysis as a result of hereditary factors or illness.

The first two conditions are usually acquired, while hypercoagulation may be inherited or acquired. Most commonly, a combination of these factors predisposes a patient to DVT. Underpinning these elements are a number of local or general risk factors, which are discussed in more detail later in this section; the presence of more than one risk factor increases the probability of an event.

Risk Factors. DVT is associated with a number of risk factors, each of which may be viewed as contributing to at least one of the three factors of Virchow's triad (vascular injury, venous stasis, hypercoagulation). In several cases, a risk factor may contribute to more than one aspect of the triad. For example, hip replacement surgery not only damages the vessels of the lower limbs (vascular injury), but is also associated with a period of bed rest (venous stasis). Risk factors are loosely grouped among the three components of the triad, based on their areas of greatest impact, and are outlined in Figure 2. Table 1 lists the risk factors for DVT and PE pertaining to vascular injury or venous stasis and the corresponding incidence of events.

Table 2 lists the risk factors for DVT and PE pertaining to hypercoagulation and estimates the prevalence of genetic thrombophilic defects in patients with confirmed DVT or PE. Deficiencies in any of the naturally occurring anticoagulants, such as antithrombin (AT), protein C, and protein S, can increase the risk of DVT and PE (see the "Pathophysiology" section). These deficiencies are rare but carry a high risk of thrombosis when they do occur, so lifelong anticoagulation is usually prescribed. Recently discovered mutations, such as those of factor V Leiden, prothrombin, and factor VIII, are much more prevalent genetic risk factors. There is significant incidence of patients with confirmed DVT who show no readily recognizable risk factors (idiopathic DVT). Studies have reported up to 50% of patients presenting with first-time DVT who fall into this category (Cushman M, 2001).

Combined Risk Factors.
Advancing Age. Numerous studies demonstrate the correlation between advancing age and the incidence of DVT or PE. For example, one study estimated that

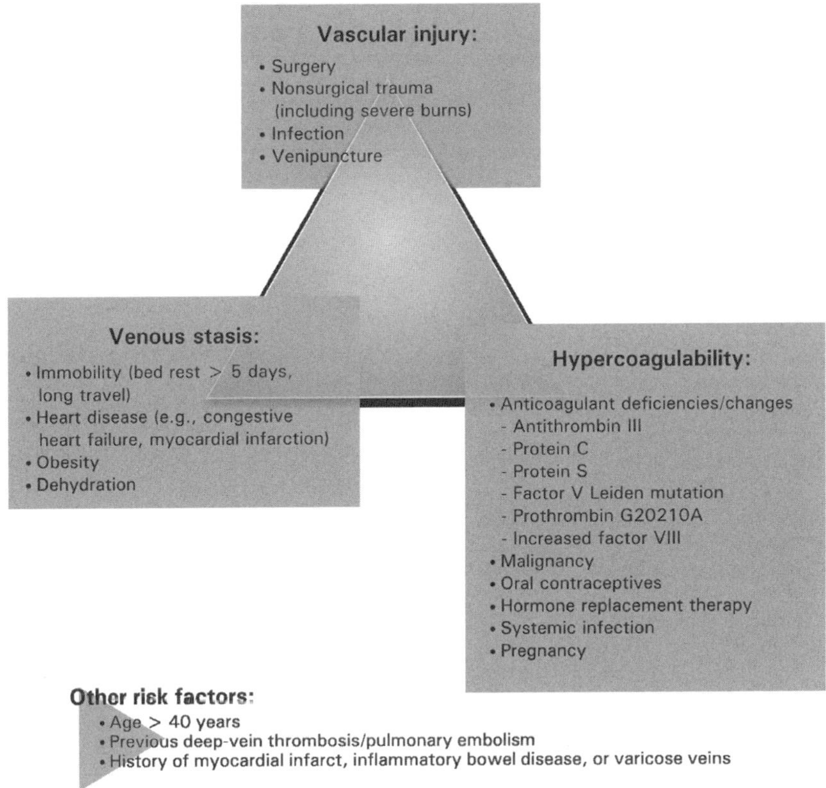

FIGURE 2. *Virchow's triad and associated risk factors.*

the incidence of thrombosis increases from 1 per 100,000 people per year during childhood to 1 per 100 people per year in old age (Rosendaal FR, 1995). A patient's increasing age may reduce veins' elasticity and cause dilatation and stasis. In addition, muscle mass generally declines, and the venous return system becomes less effective. Prothrombotic changes (increased in vitro platelet sensitivity to aggregating agents; increased circulating concentrations of fibrinogen, coagulation factors VII and VIII, fibrinopeptide A, and PAI-1) and clinical conditions that predispose the person to the activation of the hemostatic system (obesity, diabetes mellitus, high-density lipid [HDL] cholesterol, prolonged immobilization) often occur in association (Di Minno G, 2001). Lastly, the elderly have a higher incidence of congestive heart failure, malignancy, hyperlipidemia, and varicose veins, all of which may potentiate the primary factors (Circlincione AS, 2000).

Prior Deep Vein Thrombosis. A clinical history of DVT is considered a risk factor for subsequent DVT and is an especially important consideration in combination with other DVT and PE risk factors. The tendency of certain patients

TABLE 1. Risk Factors for Deep Vein Thrombosis and Pulmonary Embolism Pertaining to Vascular Injury or Venous Stasis and Corresponding Incidence of Events

Event	Incidence of DVT Following Event (%)[a]	Incidence of PE Following Event (%)[a]	Reference
Vascular injury			
Orthopedic surgery	>50		
Knee	84	7	Colwell CW, 2001
Hip	35–60	16	Hirsh J, 1996; Mizel MS, 1998
Foot/ankle	0.2	0.15	
Obstetric/gynecological surgery	30	—	Cardosi RJ, 2000
Neurosurgery	22–35	0.38	Attia J, 2001; Page RB, 2004
General surgery	20–30	—	Clagett GP, 1998
Trauma	38–60	19	Venet C, 2000; Attia J, 2001
Acute spinal cord injury	50–80	—	Attia J, 2001
Peripherally inserted central catheters	2.47	0.001	Chemaly RF, 2002
Venous stasis			
Immobility			
General (e.g., bed rest)	1–3		Giannadakis K, 2000; Heit JA, 2000
Air travel (including one other risk factor, such as taking oral contraceptives)	4–10		Belcaro G, 2001; Scurr JH, 2001
Obesity (waist circumference >100 cm compared with >100 cm)	Increased relative risk of 3.92	—	Hansson PO, 1997
Heart disease			
Stroke	25	—	THRIFT II Consensus Group, 1998
Atrial fibrillation	21	—	Wood KA, 1997

[a]Without prophylaxis unless otherwise stated.
THRIFT = Thromboembolic Risk Factors Trial.
Note: Full source citations appear in "References."

to have recurrent DVT or PE is known as thrombophilia. Recurrence is most common in patients with a deficiency of AT, protein C, or protein S; in those with more than one inherited thrombophilia; and in those who are homozygous for factor V Leiden (Seligsohn U, 2001). Of those people who have experienced an episode of DVT, up to 30% may have a recurrence within a year (Kearon C, 1999). Studies have also indicated that a higher risk of recurrence is more likely for patients suffering from idiopathic DVT when compared with those with transient risk factors such as recent surgery (Pinide L, 2000).

Pregnancy. DVT and PE are the most frequent causes of death associated with childbirth. During pregnancy, all three of Virchow's factors occur. Hypercoagulability results from the combination of increased procoagulant factors (VWF,

TABLE 2. Estimated Prevalence of Genetic Thrombophilic Defects in Patients with Confirmed Deep Vein Thrombosis or Pulmonary Embolism and in the General Population

Risk Factor	Notes	Deep Vein Thrombosis (DVT) (%)	General Population (%)	Increased Risk of Developing DVT over General Population	Reference
Antithrombin deficiency		1–2	0.1–0.3	Tenfold	Lensing AWA, 1999
Protein C or protein S deficiency		2–3	0.2–0.5	Tenfold	Rosendaal FR, 1999
Antiphospholipid antibodies (lupus anticoagulant or anticardiolopin type)	Most common acquired hypercoaguable disorder; anticardiolupin antibody five times more common than lupus type.	28	6–8	16- to 25-fold	Berube C, 1998; Thomas RH, 2001; Bick RL, 1993
Factor V Leiden (activated protein C resistance)	Most common genetic hypercoaguable disorder; leads to excess thrombin generation.	15–25; rare among Asians and Africans	3–7	Threefold (heterozygous); 80-fold (homozygous)	Rosendaal FR, 1998; Thomas RH, 2001; Faioni EM, 1997; Dalen JE, 2002
Prothrombin G20210A		5–6; rare among Asians and Africans	1–3	Threefold	Margaglione M, 1998; Thomas RH, 2001; Baglin T, 2003
High factor VIII concentrations	Controlled primarily by genes determining blood group; pregnancy and oral contraceptive use raise levels.	15–25	6–8	Sixfold	Thomas RH, 2001; van der Meer FJM, 1997
Hyperhomocysteinemia	Usually caused by insufficient folic acid, vitamin B6, or B12.	10–20	2–6	2.4–4%	Cattaneo M, 2001; Thomas RH, 2001; Dalen JE, 2002
Malignancy	Second most common acquired cause of hypercoaguability; thrombosis is the result of overexuberant host response to tumor growth.	15% cancer patients have clinical thromboses	—	Four- to sevenfold	Rickles FR, 2001; Sallah S, 2000

(continued overleaf)

TABLE 2. (continued)

Risk Factor	Notes	Deep Vein Thrombosis (DVT) (%)	General Population (%)	Increased Risk of Developing DVT over General Population	Reference
Oral contraceptives (OC)	Third-generation pills pose greater risk than second-generation pills; presence of genetic risk factors increases risk (e.g., factor V Leiden).	25/100,000 (third-generation pills)	—	Tenfold increased risk for combined OCs; 35-fold increased risk if also heterozygous for factor Leiden	Parkin L, 2000; Vandenbroucke JP, 1994
Hormone replacement therapy (HRT)	Increased risk may not be relevant after first year; guidelines for screening of DVT/PE with HRT are available.	—	—	Threefold increased risk	Varas-Lorenzo C, 1998; Royal College of Obstetricians and Gynecologists, 1999
Pregnancy	Combined risk factors: hypercoaguability, venous stasis, and venous injury (caesarean).	0.11% (20% occur during pregnancy, 80% after caesarean), all have severe thrombophilia	0.04%		Adachi T, 2001

Note: Full source citations appear in "References."

clotting factors V and VIII, and fibrinogen) and increased plasminogen activator inhibitors (reducing fibrinolysis). In addition, venous stasis occurs by the end of the first trimester. Finally, vaginal or abdominal (caesarean) delivery causes vascular trauma to the pelvic and abdominal region. The postpartum period is also associated with increased risk of DVT and PE because of the accompanying tissue breakdown and traumatic/surgical factors (e.g., prolonged labor, cesarean section, infection).

Pathophysiology

Vascular Injury. When a vessel is injured as a result of surgery, trauma, or infection, a number of processes—collectively termed *hemostasis*—act to prevent further blood loss. First, a platelet plug is formed; then a clot, consisting of a network of fibrin strands, develops via the coagulation cascade; and finally the clot dissolves after vessel repair is complete.

TABLE 3. Current Therapies Used in the Treatment of Deep Vein Thrombosis and Pulmonary Embolism

Agent	Company/Brand	Dose	Availability
Heparins			
Unfractionated heparin	Various, generics	5,000 units IV loading dose, then 15–25 units/kg/h continuous infusion	US, F, G, I, S, UK, J
Enoxaparin	Sanofi-Aventis's Clexane/Lovenox	150 IU/kg once daily (or 100 IU/kg bid)	US, F, I, UK
Nadroparin	Formerly Sanofi-Synthélabo's, now GlaxoSmithKline's Fraxiparine	86 IU/kg bid or 171 IU/kg daily	F, G, I, S
Dalteparin	Pfizer's Fragmin	100 IU/kg bid or 200 IU/kg daily	F, S, UK
Danaparoid sodium	Organon's Orgaran	2,500 IU followed by 400 IU/h for 2 hours, then 300 units/h for 2 hours then 200 IU/h for 5 days	US, G
Vitamin K antagonists			
Warfarin	Bristol-Myers Squibb's Coumadin, Sanofi-Aventis's Coumadine, generics	Adjusted dose to achieve INR 2.5, range 2.0–3.0 (in Japan, target INR of 1.8–2.0)	US, F, G, I, S, UK, J
Direct thrombin inhibitors			
Lepirudin	Schering's Refludan	400 μg/kg followed by IV 150 μg/kg/h adjusted according to aPTT	US, F, G, I, S, UK
Argatroban	Mitsubishi Tokyo's Novastan, Daiichi Seiyaku's Slonnon, Encysive/Glaxo-SmithKline's Acova	2 μg/kg/min adjusted according to aPTT	US
Synthetic pentasaccharides			
Fondaparinux	Formerly Sanofi-Synthélabo's, now GlaxoSmithKline's Arixtra	5 mg SC (body weight less than 50 kg), 7.5 mg SC (body weight: 50–100 kg), or 10 mg SC (body weight greater than 100 kg) once daily	US
Thrombolytics			
Alteplase (recombinant tissue plasminogen activator [rt-PA])	Genentech's Activase, Boehringer Ingelheim's Actilyse, Mitsubishi-Tokyo's Activacin	100 mg over 2 hours	US, F, G, I, S, UK, J

(*continued overleaf*)

TABLE 3. (*continued*)

Agent	Company/Brand	Dose	Availability
Streptokinase	Sanofi-Aventis/ AstraZeneca's Streptase	250,000 IU over 30 minutes followed by 100,000 IU every hour for 24 hrs (PE) or 72 hrs (DVT)	US, F, G, I, S, UK
Urokinase	Abbott's Abbokinase, generics	4,400 IU/kg IV loading dose over 10 minutes, then 4,400 IU/kg/h	F, G, I, S, J

aPTT = Activated partial thromboplastin time.
bid = Twice daily.
INR = International normalized ratio.
IU = International units.
SC = Subcutaneous.
US = United States; F = France; G = Germany; I = Italy; S = Spain; UK = United Kingdom; J = Japan.

The coagulation cascade consists of a chain of reactions that activate circulating clotting factors, such as factors V, VIII, IX, X, XI, and XII, to generate insoluble fibrin strands that strengthen the already established hemostatic plug. Figure 3 illustrates how the coagulation cascade can be initiated by the intrinsic or extrinsic pathway, depending on whether platelets releasing phospholipid PF3 or damaged tissues releasing tissue factor are responsible for converting factor X to its activated form, factor Xa. Essentially, the intrinsic pathway requires only components present in the blood rather than tissue factor, as is the case for the extrinsic pathway. Both pathways culminate in the production of factor Xa. Factor Xa converts prothrombin to thrombin, a protease that plays multiple roles in the hemostatic process, including activating factors V, VIII, and XIII, and binding to and activating platelets and endothelial cells. Thrombin also plays a critical role in converting fibrinogen, a soluble plasma protein, into fibrin, the insoluble fibrous protein that integrates itself within the mass of aggregated platelets to form a stable blood clot. Also, endothelial cell activation via tissue damage causes progressive transcription of many genes, including cytokines (interleukin-1 [IL-1], IL-6, IL-8) and tissue factor, all of which are involved in initiating coagulation.

In addition to activating coagulation, tissue damage can impair fibrinolysis, the process by which plasmin breaks down fibrin and dissolves thrombi so that blood flow within the obstructed blood vessel is restored. Plasmin is produced when plasminogen (a protein that is selectively incorporated into fibrin thrombi at the time of thrombus formation) is activated by plasminogen activators such as urokinase-type plasminogen activators and tissue plasminogen activator (tPA). These plasminogen activators are secreted by endothelial cells in response to a variety of stimuli, such as oxygen deprivation, fibrin deposition, and/or stasis. Tissue damage affects fibrinolysis because inflammatory cytokines induce endothelial cell synthesis of plasminogen activator inhibitor, thereby preventing the production of plasmin.

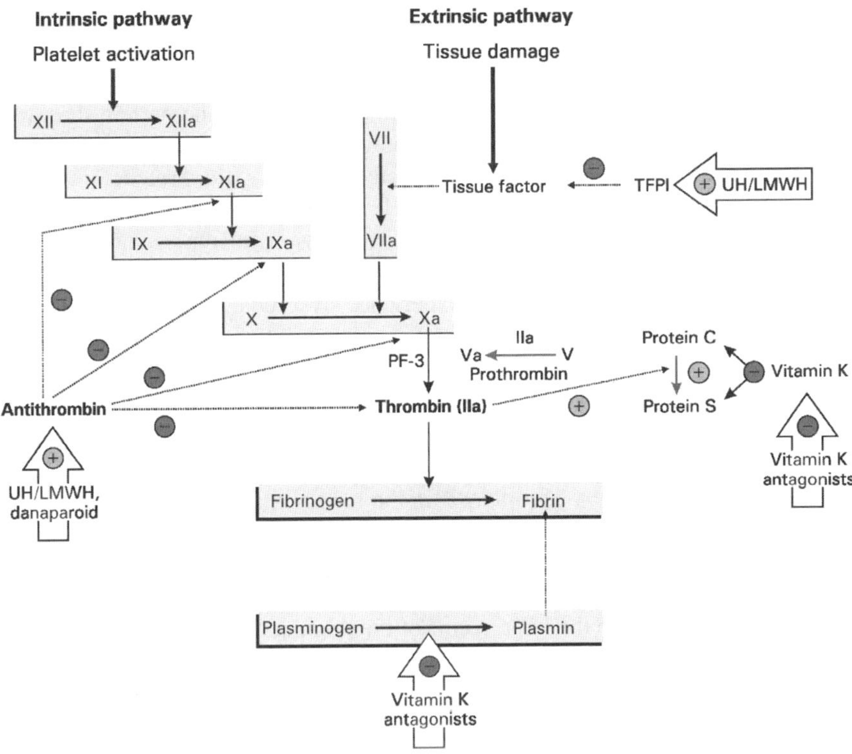

LMWH = Low-molecular-weight heparin.
rtPA = Recombinant tissue plasminogen activator.
TFPI = Tissue factor pathway inhibitor.
UH = Unfractionated heparin.

FIGURE 3. *Major reactions of the coagulation cascade.*

Venous Stasis. Venous stasis essentially results from conditions that enhance low blood pressure, which promotes thrombus formation by failing to clear activated coagulation factors quickly from the site of platelet aggregation. Because blood pressure in the venous setting is already relatively low, the slower-moving blood cells easily become entangled in the clot. Stasis is most obviously the result of physical immobility, which can be caused by illness or obesity, but it may also stem from increased venous pressure (heart failure), venous dilation (anesthesia, pregnancy, hormone replacement therapy), venous obstruction (pelvic tumors), and increased blood viscosity (polycythemia vera, hypergammaglobulinemia, chronic inflammatory disorders).

Hypercoagulation (Prothrombotic State). Natural anticoagulants and the fibrinolytic system allow coagulation to proceed locally in response to injury without progressing to the point of a systematic and potentially dangerous process, thereby balancing the process of thrombus formation. The three most important natural anticoagulants are antithrombin III (ATIII), protein C, and protein S. AT III interacts primarily with thrombin, but it also inactivates factors IXa, Xa, XIa, and XIIa. Protein C, when bound to the endothelial membrane protein thrombomodulin, is converted to an active serine protease by thrombin and, in its activated form, inhibits coagulation by inactivating factors Va and VIIIa. Protein S increases the rate of proteolysis of factors Va and VIIIa by protein C. Deficiencies in any of these naturally occurring anticoagulants may result in hypercoagulation and predispose the patient to DVT and PE. Patients with deficiencies in plasminogen or plasminogen activators may also experience hypercoagulation and are again predisposed to DVT and PE because of the central role these factors play in fibrinolysis.

Disease Progression. The location and extent of the thrombus will affect prognosis and treatment modality and may relate to the risk of disease recurrence (Douketis JD, 2001). Thrombosis in the lower extremities is categorized as either proximal (encompassing the popliteal, femoral, and iliofemoral veins) or distal (calf) vein thrombosis (Figure 1). The vast majority of thrombi originate in the distal veins. Symptoms are typically observed only when the thrombus is extended proximally into the larger veins of the thigh and pelvis (Ouriel K, 2000). Approximately 25% of symptomatic calf DVT cases propagate to the proximal veins, thereby increasing the risk of resultant PE (Meignan M, 2000). About 20% of venous thrombi develop in the proximal vein without prior calf involvement (Kroegel C, 2003).

Pathophysiological Consequences of DVT and PE. Acute PE can lead to death within an hour after the onset of symptoms, depending on the number and size of emboli in the pulmonary circuit (Stein PD, 1995). However, hemodynamic instability and abnormalities in gas exchange as a result of submassive and nonfatal massive PE are sometimes precursors to bronchoconstriction, pulmonary hypertension, and arterial hypoxemia.

A rise in pulmonary artery pressure can be expected following arterial occlusion, and the risk of pulmonary hypertension increases accordingly. It has been estimated that 5% of patients suffering from PE develop chronic thromboembolic pulmonary hypertension (Ribeiro A, 1999). If this vascular resistance does not diminish, the right ventricle must compensate in an attempt to maintain cardiac output. Over time, excess ventricular strain can lead to right ventricular dysfunction and the development of hypotension.

Aside from PE, the other symptoms and signs of DVT are caused by obstruction to venous outflow and vascular inflammation. However, up to 50% of patients may be asymptomatic (Aschwanden M, 2001), and about 70% of patients referred for clinically suspected venous thrombosis do not have the diagnosis confirmed by objective testing (Prandoni P, 2001).

Patients who survive an initial DVT episode are prone to chronic leg pain, swelling, and even venous ulceration as a result of the damage to the veins that occurs as part of the thrombotic process. This chronic condition, known as *post-thrombotic syndrome*, displays some of the same symptoms as recurrent DVT, thus often complicating diagnosis of the latter condition.

CURRENT THERAPIES

Deep vein thrombosis (DVT) and pulmonary embolism (PE) are two distinct conditions of the same dynamic process known as venous thromboembolism (VTE). In medical practice, prophylaxis of VTE is administered to at-risk patients; when discussing prophylaxis, this section refers to VTE. To reflect medical practice and approved drug indications, the treatment of DVT and of PE are discussed as separate entities. Anticoagulation therapies—including heparins, vitamin K antagonists, and direct thrombin inhibitors—are the mainstay of both DVT and PE treatment and VTE prophylaxis. However, well-established agents such as unfractionated heparin and vitamin K antagonists are associated with unpredictable drug response, narrow therapeutic range (maintaining adequate anticoagulation while minimizing bleeding risk), and inconvenient administration. Newer agents, including low-molecular-weight heparin and synthetic pentasaccharides, resolve some of these issues. Thrombolytics are reserved for patients having massive PE. Tables 3, 4, and 5 list the leading therapies for DVT and PE treatment and VTE prophylaxis, respectively.

Heparins

Overview. Derived from beef lung or pork intestinal mucosa, heparins are a mixture of glycosaminoglycans of varying lengths and thus varying molecular weights. Heparin is available in two forms: unfractionated (UH) and low-molecular-weight heparin (LMWH). Parenteral UH (generics) is a mixture of glycosaminoglycans (straight-chain anionic polysaccharides) of varying lengths. UH's molecular weight ranges from approximately 3000 to 30,000 daltons, and this heterogeneity is a primary cause of the variable anticoagulant activity of UH, resulting in the need for extensive patient monitoring. Some of the problems associated with UH were overcome following the introduction of LMWH. LMWH's major advantage is its more reliable pharmacokinetic profile compared with that of UH, resulting from a more homogenous molecular-weight profile, ranging from 4000 to 5000 daltons. LMWHs have a longer plasma half-life and better bioavailability following subcutaneous (SC) administration; subsequently, LMWHs do not require extensive laboratory monitoring, making this therapy an attractive option for home use and conferring a significant advantage for these agents over UH.

Reviews of trials comparing different LMWHs suggest they are equivalent on clinical grounds, with a similar incidence of bleeding (Janni W, 2001; Lopez LM, 2001; Lassen MR, 2000; Planes A, 2000; Morris TA, 2000). Of the eight marketed LMWH agents, three are in common usage: enoxaparin (Sanofi-Aventis's [Tokyo, Japan] Clexane/Lovenox), nadroparin (formerly Sanofi-Synthélabo's [New York, New York], now GlaxoSmithKline's [Brentford, Middlesex, United Kingdom]

TABLE 4. Current Therapies Used in the Prophylaxis of Venous Thromboembolism

Agent	Company/Brand	Dose	Availability
Heparins			
Unfractionated heparin	Various, generics	High risk/moderate risk: 5,000 IU SC q12 h starting 1–2 hours preop	US, F, G, I, S, UK, J
Enoxaparin	Sanofi-Aventis's Clexane/Lovenox	High risk: 40 mg SC q12 h starting 12–24 hours postop; 40 mg SC once daily starting 10–12 hours preop Moderate/low risk: 20–30 mg SC, 1–2 hours preop and once daily postop Medical prophylaxis: 40 mg SC once daily	US, F, G, I, S, UK
Nadroparin	Formerly Sanofi-Synthélabo's, now GlaxoSmithKline's Fraxiparine	High risk: 38 IU/kg SC 12 hours preop, 12 hours postop, once daily on postop days 1, 2, and 3, then 57 IU/kg SC once daily Moderate risk: 2,850 IU SC 2–4 hours peop and once daily postop Medical prophylaxis: 2,850 IU SC once daily	F, G, I, S
Dalteparin	Pfizer's Fragmin	High risk: 5,000 IU SC 8–12 hours preop and once daily postop Moderate risk: 2,500 IU SC 1–2 hours preop and once daily postop Medical prophylaxis: 2,500 IU SC once daily	US, F, G, I, S, UK
Danaparoid sodium	Organon's Orgaran	High risk: 750 IU SC 1–4 hours preop and q12 h postop Medical prophylaxis:750 IU SC q12 h	US, F, G, UK
Synthetic pentasaccharides			
Fondaparinux	Formerly Sanofi-Synthélabo's, now GlaxoSmithKline's Arixtra	High risk: 2.5 mg SC once daily 6–8 hours postop	US, F, G, I, S, UK

TABLE 4. (*continued*)

Agent	Company/Brand	Dose	Availability
Vitamin K antagonists			
Warfarin	Bristol-Myers Squibb's Coumadin, Sanofi-Aventis's Coumadine, generics	5–10 mg day of or day after surgery and adjust to target INR 2–3, (in Japan, 3–6 mg/day for INR of 1.8–2)	US, F, G, I, S, UK, J
Direct thrombin inhibitors			
Lepirudin	Schering's Refludan	0.1 mg/kg/h infusion adjusted according to aPTT	G
Argatroban	Mitsubishi Tokyo's Novastan, Daiichi Seiyaku's Slonnon, Ency-sive/GlaxoSmithKline's Acova	2 μg/kg/min infusion adjusted according to aPTT	US

aPTT = Activated partial thromboplastin time; bid = Twice daily; INR = International normalized ratio; IU = International units; O.L. = Off-label; preop = Preoperative; postop = Postoperative; q12h = Every 12 hours; SC = Subcutaneous; tid = Three times a day.
US = United States; F = France; G = Germany; I = Italy; S = Spain; UK = United Kingdom; J = Japan.

Fraxiparine), and dalteparin (Pfizer's [New York, New York] Fragmin). Other currently marketed LMWHs are reviparin (Abbott Laboratories's [Abbott Park, Illinois] Clivarin; Mitsui & Co.'s [Tokyo, Japan] Lowmorin), tinzaparin (Novo Nordisk's [Mainz, Germany] Logiparin; Leo's Innohep), certoparin (Novartis's Troparin; Alpha Therapeutics' Monoembolex), ardeparin (Celsus's Centaxarin), and parnaparin (Alfa Wasserman's [Woerden, The Netherlands] Flaxum).

Mechanism of Action. Heparin acts indirectly at multiple sites in the coagulation cascade, potentiating the inhibitory action of antithrombin III (ATIII). Heparin and ATIII form a complex that changes ATIII from a slow, progressive clotting factor inhibitor to a very rapid thrombin, factor Xa (FXa) , factor IXa (FIXa), and factor XIa (FXIa) inactivator. Thrombin and FXa are the coagulant proteins most responsive to inhibition, and thrombin is ten times more sensitive to inhibition than FXa. By inactivating thrombin, heparin not only prevents fibrin formation but also inhibits thrombin-induced activation of factor V (FV) and factor VII (FVII). Heparins also induce secretion of tissue factor pathway inhibitor (TFPI) from the endothelium, reducing the procoagulant activity of the TF/FXIIa complex. Some researchers believe this TFPI stimulation may also contribute to heparin's antithrombotic action (Lupu C, 1999; Altman R, 1998; Gori AM, 1999) and estimate that released TFPI contributes one third of heparin's anticoagulant effect (Sandset PM, 2000).

In contrast to UH, which generates an ATIII/UH complex with an FXa to thrombin binding ratio of 1:1, the ATIII/LMWH complex exhibits a two- to

TABLE 5. Emerging Therapies in Development for Deep Vein Thrombosis, Pulmonary Embolism, and Venous Thromboembolism

Compound	Development Phase	Marketing Company
Direct thrombin inhibitors		
Melagatran (Exanta, SC formulation)		
United States	W	AstraZeneca
Europe	W	AstraZeneca
Japan	—	—
Ximelagatran		
United States	W	AstraZeneca
Europe	W	AstraZeneca
Japan	—	—
BIBR-1048		
United States	—	—
Europe	III	Boehringer Ingelheim
Japan	—	—
ART-123		
United States	II	Asahi Kasei
Europe	—	—
Japan	III	Asahi Kasei
Synthetic pentasaccharides		
Idraparinux sodium		
United States	III	Sanofi-Aventis
Europe	III	Sanofi-Aventis
Japan	—	—
Thrombolytics		
V-10153		
United States	II	Vernalis
Europe	I	Vernalis
Japan	—	—
Direct factor Xa inhibitors		
Razaxaban		
United States	II	Bristol-Myers Squibb
Europe	—	—
Japan	—	—
DX-9065a		
United States	I	Daiichi Seiyaku
Europe	I	Daiichi Seiyaku
Japan	II	Daiichi Seiyaku
BAY-59-7939 oral		
United States	II	Bayer
Europe	II	Bayer
Japan	II	Bayer
Oral heparins		
Solid oral unfractionated heparin		
United States	I	Emisphere Technologies
Europe	—	—
Japan	—	—

PR = Preregistered; R = Registered; M = Marketed; W = Withdrawn.

fourfold greater affinity for FXa than for thrombin. As a result, LMWHs can inhibit coagulation (through effects on FXa) while not disrupting normal hemostatic processes as much (because of its lesser effect on thrombin activity). Like UH, LMWH also potentiates the actions of TFPI, but unlike UH, which is associated with a strong rebound activation of coagulation after treatment is stopped, LMWHs do not have the progressively depletive effects on TFPI that trigger this rebound (Sandset PM, 2000).

Unfractionated Heparin. Available generically, parenteral UH is historically the standard of care for VTE prophylaxis and is indicated for anticoagulant therapy in the treatment of DVT and PE. LMWHs are replacing UH in the major pharmaceutical markets (United States, France, Germany, Italy, Spain, United Kingdom, and Japan). A low-dose regimen is indicated for the prevention of postoperative VTE in patients undergoing major abdomino-thoracic surgery. Other indications treatable with LMWHs include the following:

- Patients at risk of developing thromboembolic disease.
- Atrial fibrillation with embolization.
- Diagnosis and treatment of acute and chronic consumption coagulopathies (disseminated intravascular coagulation [DIC]).
- Prevention of clotting in arterial and heart surgery.
- Prophylaxis and treatment of peripheral arterial embolism.
- Use as an anticoagulant in blood transfusions, extracorporeal circulation and dialysis procedures, and blood samples for laboratory purposes.

The first randomized prospective trial of UH therapy for acute DVT and PE took place in 1960 (Barritt DW, 1960). Researchers compared adjusted-dose IV UH with placebo in patients with acute DVT or PE. Only the placebo group experienced nonfatal PE and death from PE. As a result, treatment of DVT and PE patients with adjusted-dose IV UH became standard practice.

Later data confirmed the importance of continuous IV UH in achieving a therapeutic anticoagulant response compared with intermittent SC UH in the treatment of proximal DVT (Hull RD, 1986). In this double-blind trial, 115 patients were randomly assigned to either IV or SC heparin. The SC regimen induced an anticoagulant response below therapeutic range, resulting in a recurrent VTE rate of 19.3% compared with 5.2% in patients with IV heparin; the majority of IV-treated patients achieved a therapeutic anticoagulant response.

Additionally, adjusted low-dose UH is a safe and efficacious method for VTE prophylaxis. Seventy-nine patients undergoing elective hip arthoplasty were randomly assigned to either a fixed dose of UH (3500 IU) SC over eight hours or dose-adjusted UH over eight days. Thirteen percent of the dose-adjusted arm developed DVT compared with 39% in the fixed-dose arm (Leyvraz PF, 1983).

The main side effect of UH is bleeding, the risk of which increases with the dose and length of therapy. In recent trials, the level of bleeding was 2.5–5%

in UH-treated patients (Siragusa S, 1996; Merli GJ, 2000). Increased bleeding is also associated with risk factors such as renal failure, age, and use of concomitant aspirin therapy. In addition, approximately 1–5% of UH-treated patients develop the serious condition heparin-induced thrombocytopenia (HIT), in which an antibody-mediated response causes a precipitous drop in platelet count (Boneu B, 2000). Contraindications for UH are active bleeding, active ulcer disease, thrombocytopenia, central nervous system (CNS) anatomic lesion, uncontrolled hypertension, bleeding diathesis, subacute bacterial endocarditis, and pericarditis (Davis JD, 2001).

Enoxaparin. Enoxaparin (Sanofi-Aventis's Lovenox) is the most extensively indicated LMWH for both the treatment of DVT and PE and prophylaxis of VTE; it is approved in the United States, France, Italy, and the United Kingdom for the treatment of DVT and PE and is used off-label in Germany and Spain for these indications. Enoxaparin is licensed in all major markets except Japan for prophylaxis following knee and hip replacement, general surgery, and major trauma. Enoxaparin is also licensed for VTE prophylaxis in patients hospitalized for general medical conditions and for the treatment of acute coronary syndromes (ACS), including unstable angina and myocardial infarction.

The clinical equivalency of enoxaparin and UH in the acute treatment of DVT is well established. In one study, 198 patients with symptomatic DVT were randomly assigned to dose-adjusted IV UH or fixed-dose enoxaparin administered at home (Koopman MM, 1996). No significant differences were found between groups in the primary outcome of recurrent DVT, nor were there differences in major bleeding between the two groups. Quality of life as measured by physical activity and social functioning were better in the enoxaparin arm.

Although UH is the standard treatment for PE, data suggest that LMWHs provide comparable results. One randomized, controlled, partially blinded trial of 900 patients (74 hospitals, 16 countries) established the equivalence of SC enoxaparin once daily (1.5 mg/kg) or twice daily (1.0 mg/kg) with dose-adjusted IV UH in the acute treatment of VTE (32% PE) (Merli GJ, 2001[a]). Regimens were continued for five days and warfarin therapy initiated within 72 hours; symptomatic VTE reoccurred in 4.1%, 4.4%, and 2.9% of patients receiving UH and once- or twice-daily enoxaparin, respectively. The incidence of major hemorrhage was also equivalent between groups: 2.1%, 1.7%, and 1.3% of patients receiving UH and once- or twice-daily enoxaparin, respectively.

Other trials support the use of enoxaparin compared with warfarin in the secondary prevention of VTE. In one such trial, 165 patients were randomized to treatment with enoxaparin (40 mg twice daily for seven days followed by 40 mg once daily for three months) or to treatment with standard IV UH followed by warfarin for three months (Gonzalez-Fajardo JA, 1999). Patients assigned to the enoxaparin treatment group showed a significant improvement in the primary end point of rate of thrombus regression compared with the warfarin-treated group. Additionally, patients in the enoxaparin-treated arm demonstrated a significantly lower incidence of bleeding compared with patients treated with warfarin.

Trials have also established the efficacy of both short- and long-term regimens of enoxaparin in VTE prophylaxis. In one short-term, open-label trial, 453 patients were randomized to treatment with either 30 mg of enoxaparin every 12 hours or 5000 units of UH every 8 hours (Colwell CW, 1995). Treatment commenced on the first day after elective knee arthroplasty and continued for a maximum of seven days. The incidence of the primary efficacy outcome of distal DVT was 24.6% in the enoxaparin arm and 34.2% in patients treated with UH. The incidence of the primary safety outcome of major bleeding episodes was equivalent in both treatment groups.

Enoxaparin's efficacy has also been established in instances when prophylaxis treatment is extended for a total of four weeks postoperatively (Comp PC, 2001). Following elective hip or knee replacement, 968 patients received 30 mg enoxaparin (twice daily) for seven to ten days; 873 patients (435 elective hip replacement; 438 elective total knee replacement) were then randomized to receive three weeks of double-blind 40 mg enoxaparin once daily or placebo. Following hip replacement, prolonging enoxaparin therapy proved superior to placebo in the primary efficacy outcome of prevalence of VTE; 8% of patients treated with extended enoxaparin suffered a DVT or PE, compared with 23.2% in the placebo arm. However, no significant benefit of extending enoxaparin use was noted in patients undergoing knee replacement; 17.5% of patients treated with extended enoxaparin suffered a DVT or PE, compared with 20.8% in the placebo arm. Researchers also noted no significant difference in hemorrhagic events between the placebo and extended-treatment arms.

As discussed in the "Overview" section, LMWHs can be administered at home because they have a predictable pharmacokinetic profile. Another benefit is a lower risk of HIT with LMWH (0–0.9%) than with UH (1–5%) (Boneu B, 2000). However, contraindications do exist with LMWHs. Patients with renal insufficiency show delayed elimination of LMWH, hence this agent should be used only at a lower dose—if at all—in this group. Epidural or spinal hematomas are a rare occurrence following spinal or epidural anesthesia when LMWH is used as thromboprophylaxis (Horlocker TT, 1997).

Nadroparin. The LMWH nadroparin (Fraxiparine) was sold to GlaxoSmithKline as part of the regulatory requirement for the Sanofi-Aventis merger with. Nadroparin is licensed for the prophylaxis of VTE in patients undergoing orthopedic surgery and moderate-risk general surgery; it is also used off-label in high-risk general surgery and major trauma. Nadroparin is not available in the United States, United Kingdom, or Japan.

The clinical equivalency of nadroparin with UH in the acute treatment of DVT is well established. One randomized trial of 170 symptomatic patients with proximal DVT established the equivalence of SC nadroparin with dose-adjusted IV UH (Prandoni P, 1992). The LMWH regimen was continued for ten days with warfarin therapy initiated within 72 hours and continued for three months. At a six-month follow-up, the recurrence of DVT or PE did not differ significantly between the nadroparin (7%) and UH (14%) arms. The incidence of clinically important bleeding was infrequent in both groups.

Although UH is the standard method of treating PE, studies of nadroparin show equivalent efficacy with UH. One dose-ranging study randomly assigned 101 patients with submassive PE to one of four groups: continuous IV infusion of UH or SC nadroparin at 400, 600, or 900 units/kg (Thery C, 1992). Improvement in pulmonary vascular obstruction and a decrease in incidence of major bleeds were similar in the IV UH group and the 400 unit/kg nadroparin group; the 600 and 900 units/kg nadroparin groups were stopped prematurely due to a high incidence of major bleeds.

The efficacy of both short- and long-term regimens of nadroparin in VTE prophylaxis has been established, illustrated by one trial of 1,190 patients undergoing various elective and emergency operations randomized to treatment with either a daily fixed dose of weight-adapted nadroparin or 3000 units of UH (Egger B, 2000). Treatment commenced 2.5–6 hours preoperatively and continued until discharge. Incidence of the primary efficacy and safety outcomes—clinically evident DVT and PE and LMWH-related complications, respectively—was not significantly different between groups.

Wound- and injection-site hematomas are the most frequently reported adverse effects in clinical studies, although LMWHs are generally well tolerated (Egger B, 2000; Charbonnier BA, 1998). Compared with UH in elderly patients, prophylactic nadroparin is associated with fewer treatment withdrawals (Davis R, 1997). More recent data from a retrospective study of 1,954 patients undergoing spinal surgery show that postoperative prophylactic nadroparin does not increase the risk of hemorrhage (Gerlach R, 2004).

Dalteparin. Dalteparin (Pfizer's Fragmin) is used in both Europe and the United States for the prophylaxis of VTE. Although approved for the treatment of DVT only in France, Spain, and the United Kingdom, dalteparin is used off-label for this indication in Germany and the United States. Dalteparin is also used in the following instances:

- Prophylaxis of DVT following high-risk general surgery and in patients with major trauma.
- Treatment of acute DVT, PE, or stroke.
- Long-term DVT prophylaxis in warfarin-failure cancer patients.
- Outpatient perioperative anticoagulation.
- Anticoagulation during hemodialysis.
- Prophylaxis of complications in unstable angina and myocardial infarction.

The clinical equivalency of dalteparin and UH in the acute treatment of DVT is well established. One randomized, controlled, partially blinded trial of 204 patients with venographically confirmed DVT established the equivalence of SC dalteparin (200 IU/kg) with continuous dose-adjusted IV UH (Lindmarker P, 1994). Warfarin therapy was concomitantly started. Therapy with UH or dalteparin was continued for a minimum of five days until an international normalized ratio (INR) between 2.0 and 3.0 was established with warfarin therapy. No major bleeding events, symptomatic PE, thrombus progression, or death occurred during hospitalization. At a six-month follow-up, only five and three VTE events occurred in the dalteparin and UH arms, respectively.

Although UH is the standard method of treating PE, studies of dalteparin show that it provides efficacy equivalent to that provided by UH (Meyer G, 1995). One study randomly assigned 60 patients with submassive PE to receive either continuous IV infusion of UH or 120 IU/kg of SC dalteparin twice daily. Improvement in pulmonary vascular obstruction was 17% in the dalteparin group and 16% in the UH group. No major bleeds or PE recurrence were noted in either group.

Studies evaluating dalteparin have helped promote the extended use of LMWH in the prophylaxis of VTE. The double-blind North American Fragmin Trial (NAFT) evaluated 569 hip arthroplasty patients randomly assigned to either dalteparin—preoperatively or postoperatively extended to 35 days of treatment—or a combination of warfarin in the hospital and placebo after discharge (Hull RD, 2000). The primary outcome of all DVT was achieved by 19.7% of patients receiving dalteparin compared with 36.7% in the warfarin/placebo group. No major bleeding events occurred in the extended prophylaxis interval.

In line with other LMWH agents, the risk of developing an epidural/spinal hematoma increases with the administration of dalteparin in patients undergoing neuraxial anesthesia. The probability of such an event is raised further with the use of in-dwelling catheters or concomitant therapies that affect hemostasis, such as platelet inhibitors, and patients subject to these procedures must be monitored carefully (PDR, 2004).

Danaparoid Sodium. Danaparoid sodium (Organon's [Roseland, New Jersey] Orgaran) is a low-molecular-weight heparinoid consisting of a mixture of heparin sulfate (84%), dermatan sulfate (12%), and chondroitin sulfate (4%). First approved in the United Kingdom for DVT prophylaxis following orthopedic surgery, it is now available in the United States, France, and Germany for prophylaxis in orthopedic surgery and in Germany and the United States for the treatment of DVT and PE.

Theoretically, danaparoid is a more potent thrombin inhibitor than either UH or LMWH because it inhibits FXa and factor IIa (FIIa) at a greater ratio than either UH or LMWH.

A study comparing the thromboprophylactic effect of enoxaparin, dalteparin, and danaparoid on patients with hip fracture found no statistically significant differences in the frequency of DVT, in blood loss, or in bleeding complications between the three groups (TIFDED [Thromboprophylaxis In Hip Fracture Surgery: A Pilot Study Comparing Danaparoid, Enoxaparin, and Dalteparin] Study Group, 1999). Compared with lepirudin, however, danaparoid had a lower incidence of bleeding (2.5% versus 10.4%) (Farner B, 2001). In addition, danaparoid's minimal effect on platelet function suggests that it is safer than UH, LMWH, or warfarin because it presents a reduced risk of bleeding complications (Comp PC, 1998).

Vitamin K Antagonists

Overview. Until the recent launch of ximelagatran (AstraZeneca's [Wilmington, Delaware] Exanta), vitamin K antagonists were the only available oral anticoagulant treatment for the secondary prevention of DVT and PE. Warfarin (DUPont's [Philadelphia, Pennsylvania] Coumadin; Sanofi-Aventis Pharmaceuticals, Inc.'s [Bridgewater, New Jersey] Coumadine; generics) is the most commonly used vitamin K antagonist for DVT and PE treatment and VTE prophylaxis. Other vitamin K antagonists, including phenprocoumon (Roche's Marcumar) and fluindione (Procter & Gamble's [Cincinnati, Ohio] Previscan), are used in some European countries but are not discussed here.

Mechanism of Action. Vitamin K is an essential component in the activation of several clotting factors in the coagulation cascade, including prothrombin (factor II [FII]), FVII, factor IX (FIX), and factor X (FX), and vitamin K antagonists produce their anticoagulant effect by inhibiting this process. Conversely, these agonists also have a procoagulant action because vitamin K is required for the activation of the natural anticoagulant proteins C and S.

Warfarin. Warfarin (DuPont's Coumadin; Aventis's Coumadine; generics) (Figure 4) is indicated for the following uses:

- Prophylaxis of VTE and treatment of DVT and PE.
- Prophylaxis and treatment of thromboembolic complications associated with atrial fibrillation and/or cardiac valve replacement.
- Reduction of the risk of death, recurrent myocardial infarction, and thromboembolic events such as stroke or systemic embolization after myocardial infarction.

Warfarin's efficacy in the treatment of acute DVT and PE is well established, largely by anecdotal evidence (Wessler S, 1984). Debate regarding the optimal length of treatment with oral anticoagulation—three or six months or chronic therapy—to prevent recurrent VTE, however, is ongoing in the medical community. The recent publication of the Prevention of Recurrent Venous Thromboembolism (PREVENT) trial establishes the benefits of extending treatment with oral anticoagulation beyond six months (Ridker PM, 2003).

In the PREVENT trial, 508 patients with idiopathic recurrent VTE who had received full-dose anticoagulation for a median of 6.5 months were randomized to

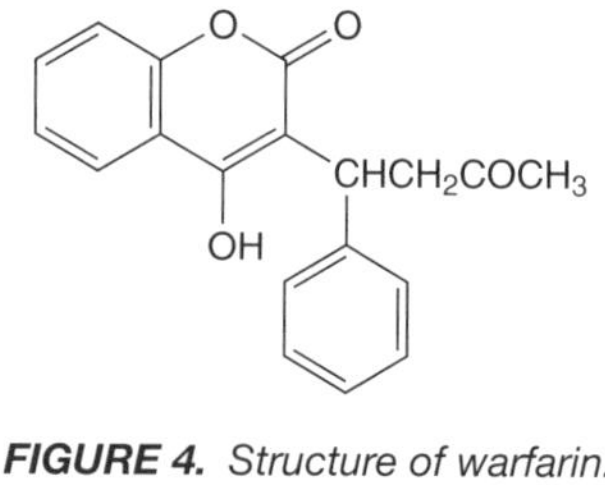

FIGURE 4. *Structure of warfarin.*

placebo or low-dose warfarin (target INR of 1.5–2.0, dose not exceeding 10 mg). Patients were monitored for recurrent VTE, major hemorrhage, and death. The trial was terminated early after 14 of the 255 patients in the warfarin-treated arm experienced a recurrent VTE, compared with 37 of 253 in the placebo arm, representing a risk reduction for recurrent VTE of 64% in the treated arm. Overall, low-dose warfarin was associated with a 48% reduction in the combined primary end point of recurrent VTE, major hemorrhage, and death.

Other studies, however, dispute the continuing benefits of long-term oral warfarin therapy versus discontinuation of treatment. One study of 267 patients with a first incidence of idiopathic DVT found no significant difference at 37 months follow-up in patients who had completed just three months of oral anticoagulant therapy (97% warfarin, 3% acenocoumarol [Novartis's Sintrom]) or those who had completed an additional nine months (Agnelli G, 2001). Following randomization to either patient group, 1 patient (0.7%) in the continuing therapy group had a recurrent DVT event, compared with 11 patients (8.3%) in the discontinuation arm. After 37 months follow-up, the rate of DVT recurrence in the continuation and discontinuation treatment arms was 15.7% and 15.8%, respectively.

Warfarin is also used for VTE prophylaxis, and in the United States, it is preferred to heparins. One randomized, double-blind trial comparing warfarin with LMWH in 1,436 patients who had just undergone hip or knee replacement found that the benefit conferred by LMWH was offset by an increase in bleeding complications. The incidence of major bleeding was 1.2% in the warfarin group compared with 2.8% in the LMWH-treated arm (Hull RD, 1993).

Many physiological and pharmacological factors influence the therapeutic effectiveness of warfarin, and patient response is variable. Other disadvantages include a slow onset of action—anticoagulation is delayed with warfarin until newly synthesized dysfunctional vitamin K-dependent clotting factors replace the normal clotting factors. The most serious risks associated with vitamin K antagonist therapy are hemorrhage in any tissue or organ and, less frequently (<0.1%), necrosis and/or gangrene of skin and other tissues. Studies show that major bleeding occurs in up to 9% of patients treated with vitamin K antagonists (Stern SH, 2000; So L, 2001). These agents can increase the risk of systemic atheroemboli and cholesterol microemboli, both of which present as "purple toe syndrome," rash, and severe pain in the limbs and which can progress to involve visceral organs. Vitamin K antagonists are also contraindicated in pregnancy.

Direct Thrombin Inhibitors

Overview. Direct thrombin inhibitors (DTIs) are the most recent entrants to the anticoagulant drug class and are used in the treatment of DVT and PE and in prophylaxis of VTE. They are used for maintaining anticoagulation during an episode of HIT and for patients with known HIT. DTIs produce a more predictable anticoagulant effect than the indirect mechanism of action of the heparins, thereby eliminating the need for continual monitoring and titration. However, some marketed DTIs bind irreversibly to both the anionic and catalytic site of thrombin, thus generating the potential for significant bleeding. To date—despite efficacy that has been proven superior to both UH and LMWH in the prophylaxis of DVT prior to surgery—the main application of DTIs has been in patients with HIT. DTIs that are used in the treatment of DVT and PE and prophylaxis of VTE but are not discussed in the following sections include desirudin (Aventis/Novartis's Revasc) and bivalirudin (The Medicines Company's [Parsippany, New Jersey] Angiomax).

Mechanism of Action. DTIs do not require the cofactor ATIII for antithrombotic activity. They exert their anticoagulant effect by selectively inhibiting free-circulating and clot-bound thrombin. Thrombin's critical role in coagulation is the conversion of fibrinogen, a soluble plasma protein, into fibrin monomers. The fibrin monomers are cross-linked by factor XIIIa (FXIIIa), and the insoluble fibrous protein integrates itself within a mass of aggregated platelets to form a stable blood clot. In addition to the procoagulant activities of thrombin, this clotting factor also regulates the coagulation cascade by activating the natural anticoagulant protein C; the clotting factors FV, factor VIII (FVIII), FXI, and factor XIII (FXIII); and platelets.

Lepirudin. Schering AG (Berlin, Germany) inlicensed lepirudin (Refludan) from Aventis in November 2001 for the treatment of DVT and PE and prophylaxis of VTE. Lepirudin is now available in the United States and Europe for the treatment of HIT and DVT but is approved only in Germany for prophylaxis; it is used off-label in the United States and Spain for prophylaxis in cases where HIT contraindicates the use of heparins.

Lepirudin is a selective irreversible inhibitor of free-circulating and clot-bound thrombin. Thrombin's critical role in coagulation is the conversion of fibrinogen, a soluble plasma protein, into fibrin monomers. The fibrin monomers are cross-linked by FXIIIa, and the insoluble fibrous protein integrates itself within a mass of aggregated platelets to form a stable blood clot. In addition to the procoagulant activities of thrombin, this clotting factor also regulates the coagulation cascade by activating the natural anticoagulant protein C; the clotting factors FV, FVIII, FXI, and FXIII; and platelets. One molecule of lepirudin binds irreversibly to one molecule of thrombin and so blocks the latter's thrombogenic activity.

Data to support lepirudin's use in DVT treatment are scarce. One multicenter, randomized, dose-ranging study involving 155 DVT patients compared three lepirudin doses (0.75, 1.25, and 2.00 mg/kg every 12 hours) with adjusted-dose UH for acute treatment of DVT (Schiele F, 1997). All four groups demonstrated similar regression of thrombi, although the lowest dose lepirudin regimen achieved regression in the highest percentage of patients (38%). The lepirudin groups also demonstrated a significantly lower number of ventilation/perfusion scan abnormalities (indicating fewer thrombotic events) after five days of treatment than did the heparin group (3–9% versus 27%). There were no significant differences in bleeding complications among the four groups.

Two studies demonstrated the utility of lepirudin in VTE prophylaxis; the number of thrombotic events fell from 52% (control group) to 31% (lepirudin group) (Greinacher A, 1997).

Bleeding complications mandate careful monitoring of lepirudin therapy, especially in patients with weakened renal function. Hemorrhagic events are the most common adverse effect encountered in patients treated with lepirudin. Data from the Heparin Associated Thrombocytopenia-1 (HAT-1) and HAT-2 studies show the rate of major bleeding in HIT patients with thrombosis is 18.8% compared with 14.4% in patients with isolated HIT (Greinacher A, 1995). However, bleeding was attributed to the high activated partial thromboplastin time (aPTT) ratios used (>2.5). Improvements in dosing and monitoring protocols have led to a lower incidence of hemorrhage (Lubenow N, 2002[b]). Additionally, because lepirudin is almost entirely excreted in the kidney, the manufacturer recommends renally impaired patients receive a reduced bolus infusion rate to prevent overdose.

Argatroban. Argatroban (Mitsubishi Tokyo's [Tokyo, Japan] Novastan, comarketed by Daiichi Sankyo's [Tokyo, Japan] as Slonnon; Encysive Pharmaceuticals [Houston, Texas]/GlaxoSmithKline's Acova) is a DTI approved for anticoagulation in patients with HIT in the United States; in July 2005 it was also approved in Germany for this indication. The drug is approved in Japan for acute cerebral thrombosis (atherothrombosis in cerebral brain tissue, not embolic or lacunar strokes) and is used off-label in this country for patients with contraindications to heparin.

Argatroban is a DTI that reversibly binds to the thrombin active site. It does not require the cofactor antithrombin III for antithrombotic activity. Argatroban exerts its anticoagulant effects by inhibiting thrombin-catalyzed or thrombin-induced reactions, including fibrin formation; activation of coagulation factors V, VIII, and XIII; protein C; and platelet aggregation.

In one study, clinical outcomes from patients with HIT (160 patients) or HIT with thrombosis syndrome (HITTS) (144 patients) were compared with 193 historical control subjects (76% with HIT, 24% with HITTS) (Lewis BE, 2001). The incidence of the primary outcome of combined all-cause death, all-cause amputation, or new thrombosis was significantly reduced in the argatroban-treated HIT group (25.6%) compared with control (38.8%). No significant difference was noted in the HITTS group between argatroban-treated patients and the control group. Major bleeding events were not significantly increased in either the HIT or HITTS group compared with control.

Unlike lepirudin, argatroban is eliminated hepatically and can therefore be used in patients with renal dysfunction. As with other anticoagulant therapy, however, argatroban can induce hemorrhagic events. A recent study in HIT patients with associated thrombotic complications showed major bleeding episodes in 11.1% of argatroban-treated patients compared with 2.2% of historical control patients (Lewis BE, 2001).

Synthetic Pentasaccharides

Overview. Synthetic pentasaccharides are heparin derivatives and represent the unique pentasaccharide sequence found in heparin that binds to ATIII. Because this class is produced synthetically, all problems associated with the heterogeneity of the molecular weight of heparin are eliminated, there is no batch-to-batch variability in biological activity, and there is less potential for the pathogenic contamination that is associated with the production of compounds of biological origin, like UH and LMWH.

Mechanism of Action. Synthetic pentasaccharides potentiate the inhibitory action of ATIII. Because the pentasaccharide represents the unique sequence of a heparin chain that binds to ATIII, the resulting pentasaccharide/ATIII complex inhibits factor Xa clotting factor alone, conferring a more targeted mechanism of action: Only one third of UH molecules contain this unique pentasaccharide sequence.

Fondaparinux. Parenteral fondaparinux (GlaxoSmithKline's Arixtra) (Figure 5) is at various stages of development in the major markets for a range of indications, including DVT and PE treatment, VTE prophylaxis, unstable angina, and myocardial infarction. Sanofi-Synthélabo was previously marketing fondaparinux after acquiring all rights from Organon, but the franchise was sold to GlaxoSmithKline as a condition of the Sanofi-Aventis merger. Fondaparinux is registered for VTE prophylaxis in patients undergoing hip and knee replacement and hip fracture in Europe and the United States and is in Phase III trials for VTE prophylaxis in Japan in patients undergoing orthopedic surgery. Submissions for VTE prophylaxis in high-risk surgery and medical patients were made in 2003. In June 2004, the FDA approved fondaparinux for the treatment of DVT and PE in the United States; the compound is in Phase III development for these indications in Japan and Europe.

Synthetic pentasaccharides selectively potentiate the inhibitory action of ATIII to factor Xa only. Because the pentasaccharide represents the unique sequence of a heparin chain that binds to ATIII, the resulting pentasaccharide/ATIII complex inhibits factor Xa clotting factor alone, conferring a more targeted mechanism of action: Only one third of UH molecules contain this unique pentasaccharide sequence.

Two multicenter, randomized studies—MATISSE PE and MATISSE DVT—established the noninferiority of fondaparinux to standard therapy in the treatment of acute DVT and PE. In the double-blind MATISSE DVT trial, 2,205 patients were randomized to fondaparinux (7.5 mg daily) or enoxaparin (1 mg/kg

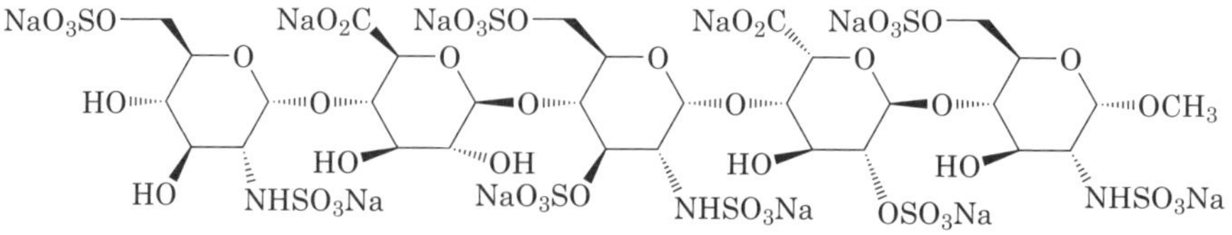

FIGURE 5. *Structure of fondaparinux.*

twice daily) (Büller HR, 2003). Of the fondaparinux-treated patients, 3.9% suffered a recurrent DVT compared with 4.1% in the heparin-treated group, meeting the study's primary end point of noninferiority. The incidence of major bleeding was low and comparable in both groups.

In the open-label MATISSE PE study, 2203 patients were randomized to fondaparinux (5.0, 7.5, or 10 mg) once daily or dose-adjusted IV UH (1 mg/kg twice daily) (Büller HR, 2003). Of the fondaparinux-treated patients, 3.8% reached the combined primary end point of three-month incidence of symptomatic recurrent PE and new or recurrent DVT compared with 5% in the heparin-treated group. Major bleeding occurred in 1.3% and 1.1% of the fondaparinux- and heparin-treated patients, respectively. This trial establishes fondaparinux as equally efficacious as UH, which is widely regarded as the standard treatment for acute PE (Büller HR, 2003).

In trials thus far, fondaparinux has proved more efficacious than LMWH in the prevention of VTE, and it has a good safety profile. Four large Phase III trials—the 1711-patient European Pentasaccharide in Hip Fracture (PentHiFra) trial (Eriksson BI, 2001); the 2275-patient U.S. Pentasaccharide in Total Hip Replacement (Pentathlon) trial (Turpie AGG, 2001[b]); the 2309-patient European Pentasaccharide in Hip Surgery (Ephesus) trial (Lassen MR, 2002); and the 1049-patient U.S. Pentasaccharide in Major Knee Surgery (PentaMaks) trial (Bauer K, 2002)—examined the use of fondaparinux following orthopedic surgery.

Designed to be the subject of a meta-analysis, these four Phase III trials show that administration of fondaparinux (2.5 mg once-daily postoperatively for five to ten days) provides an overall 55.2% decline in DVT and PE events, an outcome that is greater than the decline in events observed with preoperative 30 mg twice-daily or 40 mg once-daily administration of the LMWH enoxaparin (Turpie AGG, 2002). Furthermore, the incidence of bleeding events was low and did not differ significantly between treatment arms.

The European Pentasaccharide in Hip Fracture (PentHiFra PLUS) investigated the benefits of extending prophylaxis with fondaparinux treatment to four weeks (Eriksson BI, 2003[a]). In this double-blind, placebo-controlled trial, 656 patients undergoing hip fracture surgery were randomly assigned to receive prophylaxis with a once-daily SC injection of fondaparinux (2.5 mg) or placebo for 19–23 days. Prior to randomization, all patients received fondaparinux for six to eight days. The primary efficacy outcome of VTE—detected by venograph—was used as a surrogate end point for symptomatic events. Treatment with fondaparinux significantly reduced the incidence of VTE from 35% in the placebo arm to 1.4%. The incidence of symptomatic events also fell, from 2.7% to 0.3% in the placebo- and fondaparinux-treated arms, respectively. A trend toward more major bleeding was observed in the fondaparinux group, although no significant difference in clinically relevant bleeding was noted.

To extend the use of fondaparinux to populations beyond orthopedic surgery, the Pentasaccharide in General Surgery Study (PEGASUS) compared fondaparinux and dalteparin in the prevention of VTE following major abdominal surgery. Reports from Sanofi-Synthélabo of this study state that fondaparinux exhibits efficacy and safety at least comparable to that of LMWH (Sanofi-Synthélabo, press release, 2003). Overall incidence of VTE was 4.6% in the fondaparinux group and 6.1% in the LMWH arm. However, in those patients undergoing surgery for cancer, the incidence of VTE was significantly reduced in the fondaparinux group (4.7%) compared with dalteparin (7.7%).

Further clinical investigations were undertaken to evaluate fondaparinux in the prevention of VTE in medical patients. Although the general medical population at risk of VTE is not covered in this section, these results are discussed here because the Arixtra for Thromboembolism Prevention in Medical Indications Study (ARTEMIS) showed a significant benefit of fondaparinux in reducing the risk of VTE compared with placebo (Cohen AT, 2003).

Fondaparinux has some potential drawbacks. Although its long half-life (18 hours) is an advantage in terms of once-daily dosing, this feature may present problems, particularly when it is used in surgical environments where the risk of major bleeding increases; currently, there is no reversal agent available. Additionally, fondaparinux contains a black box warning stating it should not be used in patients undertaking spinal anesthesia or spinal puncture because of the risk of developing a blood clot in the spine. The FDA also warns that this product should not be taken by patients with seriously impaired kidney function or those weighing less than 110 pounds—due to the increased risk of bleeding—and should be used with caution in patients aged 73 or older (because of the lack of trial data in this population).

Thrombolytics

Overview. Unlike the anticoagulant therapies discussed previously that prevent clot formation, thrombolytic agents promote the dissolution of blood clots once they have formed and thus are used only in the treatment of DVT and PE. The selection of appropriate candidates for thrombolytic therapy is under debate; there are few large clinical trials with survival end points in populations other than those defined as having massive PE (Goldhaber SZ, 2002). Establishing large clinical trials to extend indications to other types of PEs is difficult because PE is difficult to detect, and its treatment and detection require a multidisciplinary approach. In addition, massive PE is a minor indication compared with acute coronary syndromes (ACS)—the treatment of which is the primary use of thrombolytics—so pharmaceutical companies have been reluctant to invest in these trials. However, there are many contraindications to thrombolytic therapy, so its use is limited to patients who do not have or have not had active internal bleeding, recent surgery, or a cerebral vascular incident within two months. Patients with DVT or PE who receive thrombolytic therapy have a 3% risk of intracranial bleeding (Goldhaber SZ, 1999). Because of their potential to increase the risk of bleeding, thrombolytics are reserved for patients with massive or hemodynamically unstable PE or massive, extensive iliofemoral DVT.

Mechanism of Action. Thrombolytic agents are plasminogen activators that convert plasminogen to plasmin, which dissolves the fibrin of a blood clot into soluble peptides—an action called fibrinolysis. In addition to lysing the clot to prevent subsequent PE, thrombolytics can also reduce pain, swelling, and loss of venous valves, thus lowering the incidence of post-thrombotic syndrome.

Alteplase (Recombinant Tissue Plasminogen Activator [rt-PA]). Rt-PA (Genentech's Activase) is approved for the treatment of acute PE and myocardial infarction. Genentech markets the agent in the United States; Boehringer Ingelheim markets it as Actilyse throughout Europe for PE; and Mitsubishi-Tokyo Pharmaceuticals, Tanabe Seiyaku (Osaka, Japan), and Kyowa Hakko Kogyo (Tokyo, Japan) all market the drug in Japan for DVT and PE.

Endothelial cells produce endogenous tPA, a natural thrombolytic agent. This agent binds specifically to fibrin in organized thrombi (not to circulating plasminogen) and facilitates the conversion of plasminogen to the proteolytic enzyme plasmin, which then dissolves the tPA-bound fibrin—an action called fibrinolysis. Rt-PA is a sterile, 527-amino-acid glycoprotein synthesized using the complementary DNA for natural human tPA obtained from a human melanoma cell line, and it can bind to fibrin with 400 times greater affinity than can endogenous tPA.

Early trial data show the benefits of alteplase compared with urokinase (Goldhaber SZ, 1988). In a comparative randomized trial of 45 patients with angiographically documented PE, 82% of patients treated with rt-PA met the primary end point of moderate or marked lysis of pulmonary emboli when assessed by perfusion lung scanning two hours after treatment initiation. In contrast, only 48% of urokinase-treated patients ($p = 0.008$) experienced moderate or marked lysis, although improvement in lung scanning perfusion at 24 hours was identical in both groups. All patients received the full dose of rt-PA, but urokinase infusions were terminated early in nine patients because of allergy in one and uncontrolled bleeding in eight.

In the largest trial of thrombolytics to date, Konstantinides and others were the first researchers to establish the benefits of alteplase treatment beyond the traditional definition of massive PE (Konstantinides S, 2002). In this trial, 256 patients with acute PE and pulmonary hypertension or right-ventricular dysfunction but without arterial hypotension or cardiogenic shock were randomly assigned to receive either heparin plus alteplase or heparin plus placebo. The incidence of the combined primary end point—in-hospital death or clinical deterioration requiring escalation of treatment—was significantly higher in the placebo arm compared with the patients treated with heparin and alteplase. Analysis of mortality data alone reveals no significant difference in mortality between groups; all benefits of the alteplase/heparin regimen were due to the higher incidence of treatment escalation in the placebo arm. Because no benefits were seen in mortality, the validity of these results in advocating the extension of alteplase treatment options to patients without traditionally defined massive PE will be debated.

A systematic review of the clinical safety and efficacy of rt-PA for DVT shows that although rt-PA is effective in lysing thrombi, bleeding complications preclude its use from DVT patients (Forster A, 2001).

Streptokinase. Streptokinase (Sanofi-Aventis/AstraZeneca's Streptase) is the only thrombolytic approved in the United States for both DVT and PE treatment.

Streptokinase is a protein produced by several strains of hemolytic *Streptococcus* that consists of a single polypeptide chain and acts with plasminogen to form an "activator complex" that converts plasminogen to plasmin. The plasmin then dissolves the fibrin of a blood clot into soluble degradation products—an action called fibrinolysis.

High-dose, short-term streptokinase infusion has been shown to improve survival in the treatment of massive PE (Jerjes-Sanchez C, 2001). Forty patients were treated with 1.5 MU in one hour of streptokinase infusion. In the acute phase, 5 patients died and 35 experienced reversed acute pulmonary arterial hypertension, right-ventricular dysfunction, or improved pulmonary infusion; no increase in hemorrhagic complications was noted. At a seven-year follow-up, 33 patients were alive without recurrence of chronic pulmonary arterial hypertension.

Streptokinase is manufactured from bacterial cells, so complications including the risk of allergy and febrile reactions can arise as a direct result of antistreptococcal antibodies circulating in the blood stream. In addition, high titers of neutralizing antibodies generated by the initial administration of streptokinase preclude readministration of the drug. However, few cases of streptokinase-associated allergy have been reported, and severe antigenicity during therapy is rare (Pilger E, 1996). Bleeding is the most problematic adverse effect of treatment, most commonly occurring at the site of vascular puncture (Wells PS, 2001). When compared with other thrombolytic agents, streptokinase shares a similar safety profile with regard to severe hemorrhage, including intracranial bleeding (Arcasoy SM, 1999).

Urokinase. In addition to treating PE, urokinase (Abbott's Abbokinase, generics) is used to lyse thrombi in myocardial infarction, coronary artery thrombosis, and intravenous catheter occlusion.

Endogenous urokinase (a thrombolytic enzyme) is present in plasma and various tissues, including endothelial cells, and it directly activates the conversion of plasminogen to the proteolytic enzyme plasmin. Plasmin then dissolves fibrin, initiating fibrinolysis. It is presumed to be less effective than rt-PA because urokinase has no activity specific to fibrin, instead activating both fibrin-bound and circulating plasminogen.

Several early trials demonstrated urokinase's efficacy in PE (Urokinase PE Trial Coordinators, 1973; Goldman I, 1973; Research Group on Urokinase and PE, 1984). However, comparative efficacy data with other thrombolytics are mixed. Continuous infusion of urokinase compared with alteplase is both less efficacious and less safe (Goldhaber SZ, 1988), while later data established a comparable efficacy between streptokinase and urokinase when urokinase is delivered over a short-time course (3 MU over two hours, with the initial 1 MU given as a bolus injection over ten minutes) (Goldhaber SZ, 1992).

Contraindications for urokinase include documented hypersensitivity, internal bleeding, and intracranial or intraspinal surgery or trauma. Bleeding is the primary safety concern when using urokinase for PE. In the first urokinase clinical studies for the treatment of PE—the Urokinase Pulmonary Embolism Trial (UPET) (Sasahara AA, 1973) and the Urokinase-Streptokinase Pulmonary Embolism Trial (USPET) (Sasahara AA, 1975) trials—bleeding resulting in at least a 5% decline in hematocrit was observed in 52 of 141 treated patients. However, trials comparing urokinase with other thrombolytics for the treatment of PE have indicated a similar risk of suffering hematomas or intracranial bleeding (Schweizer J, 1998; Goldhaber SZ, 1988).

Nonpharmacological Prophylaxis

In addition to pharmacological therapy, mechanical therapy can play an important role in the prevention of primary and secondary DVT and PE. Early ambulation, graded elastic compression stockings (GECS), and intermittent pneumatic compression (IPC) all reduce the incidence of VTE (Partsch H, 2001; Wells PS, 1994; Clagett GP, 1998). These therapies have proved cost-effective and lack side effects. They will likely continue to support other therapies in VTE.

Surgical intervention to treat DVT or PE is unusual because of the effectiveness of pharmacological and mechanical therapies and the potential for surgical complications. Nevertheless, thrombectomy (direct surgical removal of a thrombus by way of the common femoral veins), pulmonary embolectomy, and the insertion of a vena cava filter are used in certain situations.

Thrombectomy is usually reserved for venous obstruction in patients with impending venous gangrene. Pulmonary embolectomy is reserved for patients with acute massive PE in whom thrombolytic therapy is contraindicated or is failing. Insertion of an inferior vena cava filter is a more common procedure that may be used to protect patients with DVT or PE from recurrent episodes, in combination with anticoagulant therapy or after failure of anticoagulant therapy. Filters are also used in patients in whom anticoagulant therapy is contraindicated. Although vena cava filters show an initial benefit comparable to that of LMWH in preventing recurrent VTE, this benefit becomes obsolete at two years (Decousus H, 1998), demonstrating that anticoagulation should be resumed as soon as possible after insertion of the filter.

EMERGING THERAPIES

Although modern anticoagulants—namely, low-molecular-weight heparins (LMWHs)—offer safe and effective treatment of deep vein thrombosis (DVT) and pulmonary embolism (PE) and prophylaxis of venous thromboembolism (VTE), considerable opportunity remains for drugs that have predictable mechanisms of action and better side-effect profiles. Furthermore, the widely used oral anticoagulant warfarin, which requires dose titration and monitoring and has many drug interactions, is universally viewed as far from ideal. Hence, there is a clear need for safe, effective, and predictable oral anticoagulants. Several drugs in development should fulfill these criteria and are likely to improve patient care and boost the value of both the VTE prophylaxis and DVT and PE treatment markets. Of note are the direct thrombin inhibitors, long-acting synthetic pentasaccharides, and direct factor Xa inhibitors.

Table 5 summarizes the drug therapies in development for the treatment of DVT and PE and the prophylaxis of VTE.

Direct Thrombin Inhibitors

Overview. Current anticoagulants have several shortcomings. Warfarin, a vitamin K antagonist and the most commonly used oral anticoagulant in the major markets, has an unpredictable response that requires close monitoring, a narrow therapeutic window, and serious side effects such as hemorrhage. Heparins, which are also frequently used, have an unpredictable response, leading to serious side effects such as heparin-induced thrombocytopenia (HIT).

Thrombin activity is regulated by antithrombin, which irreversibly binds to the active site of thrombin, thereby inhibiting its activity. Glycosaminoglycans such as heparin and LMWHs may alter the conformation of antithrombin, enhancing its ability to bind to thrombin. As such, these medications act as indirect thrombin inhibitors. Although they are effective inhibitors of circulating thrombin, heparins do not possess the ability to inhibit thrombin that is bound to a fibrin clot, a potential limitation to their use in antithrombotic treatment.

Unlike heparin, direct thrombin inhibitors (DTIs) do not require an intermediate such as antithrombin to exert their effects. Several DTIs—such as argatroban (Mitsubishi-Tokyo's Novastan), bivalirudin, and lepirudin (Schering's Refludan)—are available, but they must be administered intravenously and so are not practical for long-term use. A DTI with good anticoagulant efficacy after oral administration would represent a potentially significant therapeutic advance.

Several DTIs are in development for the prophylaxis of VTE and treatment of DVT and PE, the most advanced being ximelagatran (AstraZeneca's oral formulation of Exanta).

Mechanism of Action. Thrombin plays a central role in modulating the coagulation cascade, primarily by catalyzing the formation of fibrinogen from fibrin (see Figure 3) Thrombin possesses three major substrate binding sites: exosites 1 and 2 and the active site. The active site mediates the enzymatic activity of the molecule, catalyzing the conversion of fibrin from fibrinogen. By blocking this site, DTIs inhibit the enzymatic activity of thrombin and prevent coagulation.

Currently available agents such as bivalirudin and lepirudin have the ability to both inhibit fibrin binding to exosite 1 and interact with the thrombin active site, thereby inhibiting thrombin activity even in the presence of bound fibrin. Molecules such as the emerging agent melagatran (see the following discussion) bind competitively but reversibly to the active site.

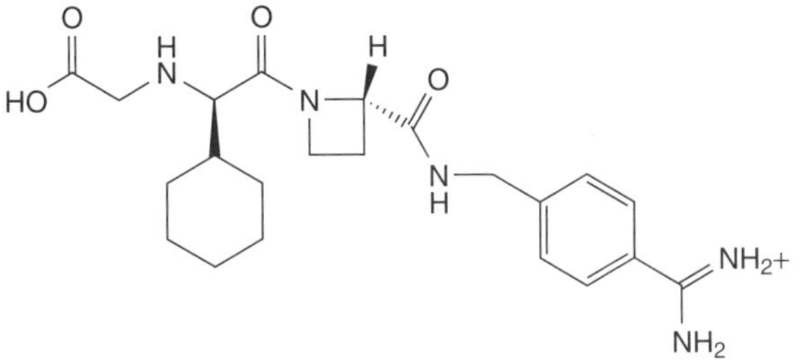

FIGURE 6. *Structure of melagatran.*

Melagatran. AstraZeneca's low-molecular-weight DTI melagatran (Figure 6) (the company's subcutaneous formulation of Exanta and the active metabolite of ximelagatran) was approved for the prevention of VTE during hip or knee surgery in France, which was acting as the reference member state for the European Union mutual recognition process in May 2004. However, the FDA rejected the NDA in October 2004, following advice from the Cardiovascular and Renal Drugs Advisory Committee that current data did not support approval of Exanta for any indication. One of the major areas of concern was the risk of liver toxicity. After further data revealed an increased risk of liver toxicity in patients receiving VTE prophylaxis up to 35 days post-operatively, AstraZeneca withdrew ximelagatran from the market in Europe and terminated its development for all indications in February 2006.

Ximelagatran. AstraZeneca's ximelagatran (Exanta) (Figure 7), the orally active pro-drug of melagatran, was the first oral DTI to be approved for the prophylaxis of VTE and the first new orally active anticoagulant to be licensed since warfarin debuted nearly 60 years ago. Ximelagatran was approved for the prevention of VTE during hip or knee surgery in France, which acted as the reference member state for the European Union mutual recognition process. However,

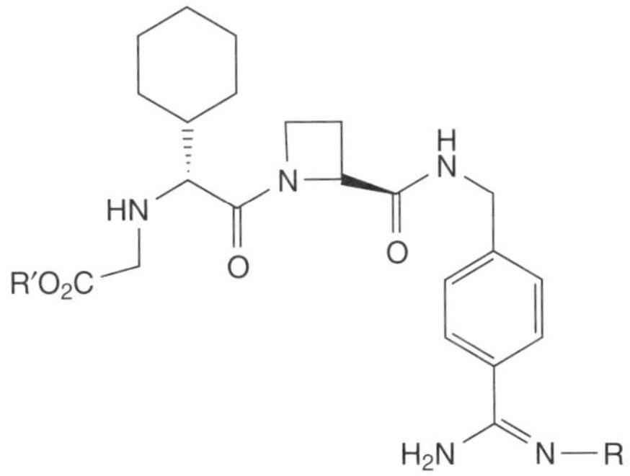

FIGURE 7. *Structure of ximelagatran (R = OH, R_1 = CH$_2$CH$_3$).*

the FDA rejected the NDA in October 2004, following advice from the Cardio-vascular and Renal Drugs Advisory Committee that current data did not support approval of Exanta for any indication. One of the major areas of concern was the risk of liver toxicity. After further data revealed an increased risk of liver toxicity in patients receiving VTE prophylaxis up to 35 days postoperatively, AstraZeneca withdrew ximelagatran from the market in Europe and terminated its development for all indications in February 2006. Ximelagatran has been withdrawn.

BIBR-1048. Boehringer Ingelheim's (Ingelheim, Germany) nonpeptidic, orally active, low-molecular-weight thrombin inhibitor BIBR-1048 (dabigatran etexi-late) (Figure 8) is in Phase IIb/III trials for the prevention of VTE in Europe.

The pharmacodynamically active component of BIBR-1048 is BIBR-953ZW, which has a half-life of 15 hours and has been shown to positively interfere with the coagulation cascade in preclinical trials (Stassen JM, 2001[a]). BIBR-1048 has also demonstrated a dose-dependent prolongation of activated partial thromboplastin time (aPTT; a measure of the anticoagulation efficacy of thrombin inhibitors) in a rodent model of thrombosis, an action that reduces coagulation levels (Wienen W, 2001). However, BIBR-1048's oral bioavailability is lower than that of ximelagatran (Gustafsson D, 2003 [a]).

Phase I and II placebo-controlled trials demonstrated that BIBR-1048 is well tolerated: A Phase I trial found that single oral doses up to 400 mg are well tolerated in healthy male volunteers (Stassen JM, 2001[b]), and a Phase II trial demonstrated that multiple oral doses of BIBR-1048 are well tolerated up to 200 mg. However, hematoma and bleeding—of mild severity—occurred in two of eight subjects administered 200 mg three times daily and six of eight subjects administered 400 mg three times daily (Stassen JM, 2001[a]).

In the dose-escalation safety study BISTRO I (Boehringer Ingelheim Study in Thrombosis), 289 patients undergoing THR surgery were treated with 12.5–300 mg oral BIBR-1048 twice daily or 150 and 300 mg four times daily for six to ten days, with the first dose administered four to eight hours after surgery.

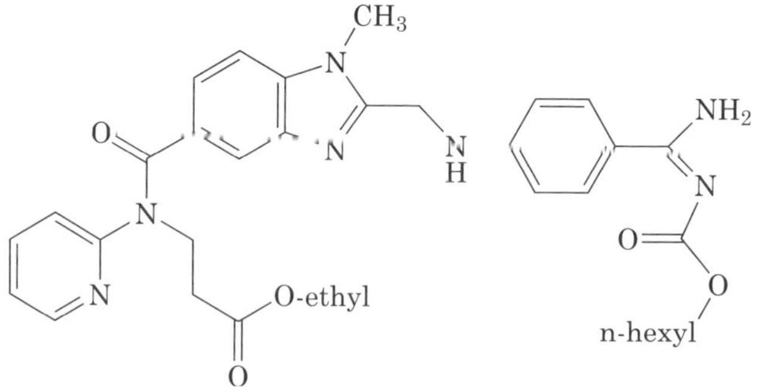

FIGURE 8. *Structure of dabigatran etexilate (BIBR-1048).*

Plasma concentrations of the active metabolite BIBR-953ZW increased rapidly after oral doses of BIBR-1048 and reached steady state on day 2 or day 3 of treatment. As the dose increased, investigators noted a declining rate of DVT but increased bleeding (Stangier J, 2003[a]).

A further Phase II single-dose study (BISTRO Ib) investigated the absorption of BIBR-1048 administered orally after surgery. When single oral doses of 150 mg BIBR-1048 were administered one to three hours after THR surgery to 59 patients, peak plasma concentrations of BIBR-953ZW were attained at approximately six hours. Mean maximum plasma concentrations of 61 ng/mL were lower than at steady state in BISTRO I, but the area under the plasma concentration curve was not significantly reduced. Two of the 59 patients vomited after drug intake (Stangier J, 2003[a]).

The BISTRO II trial was a multicenter, parallel-group, double-blind study, in patients undergoing THR or TKR. Patients were randomized to 6–10 days of BIBR-1048 (50, 150 mg bid, 300 mg qd, or 225 mg bid), starting 14 h after surgery, or subcutaneous enoxaparin (40 mg qd) starting 12 h prior to surgery. Of the 1464 patients included in the evaluation, there was a significant dose-dependent decrease in events; DVT occurred in 28.5%, 17.4%, 16.6%, 13.1% and 24% of patients assigned to BIBR-1048 50, 150 mg bid, 300 mg qd, 225 mg bid and enoxaparin, respectively. Compared with enoxaparin, DVT was significantly lower in patients receiving 150 mg bid ($p = 0.02$) and 225 mg bid ($p = 0.0007$). Bleeding rates were higher with BIBR-1048 at doses higher than 50 mg compared with enoxaparin.

ART-123. Asahi Kasei Corporation (Tokyo, Japan) is developing a recombinant thrombomodulin (ART-123), a human protein with both thrombin-inhibiting and protein-C-stimulating activities, for the potential treatment of thromboembolism and blood-clotting disorders. ART-123 is in Phase II trials in the United States and Phase III in Japan for the treatment of DVT and PE.

Thrombomodulin is an endothelial cell membrane glycoprotein that neutralizes thrombin procoagulant activity and accelerates the thrombin-catalyzed activation of anticoagulant protein C. Asahi Kasei's ART-123 reversibly blocks an exosite of thrombin, which is necessary for interaction with fibrinogen. Because of its activation of protein C and subsequent inactivation of factor V, ART-123 reduces thrombin generation and inhibits clot growth.

In a Phase I study, 55 healthy subjects received doses of between 0.02 and 0.06 mg/kg intravenously and between 0.02 and 0.45 mg/kg subcutaneously. After SC administration, the half-life of ART-123 was 63 hours and the bioavailability was 67%. Eighty percent prothrombinase inhibition was achieved eight hours after an SC dose of 0.3 and 0.45 mg/kg. The effective concentration was maintained for 6 days with a single SC dose of 0.45 mg/kg and for 12 days with two SC 0.3 mg/kg doses of ART-123. There were no severe adverse events (Moll S, 2003).

In a multicenter, open-label Phase II study in the prevention of VTE after unilateral hip replacement, patients received a single 0.3 mg/kg or 0.45 mg/kg injection and a repeat injection five days later. Some patients also received intermittent pneumatic compression (IPC). Of the 223 patients who completed the primary efficacy evaluation, patients receiving the two 0.3 mg/kg doses of ART-123 plus IPC had no VTE or DVT events, though 3.2% reported major bleeds. No patients in the 0.45 mg/kg single-dose group reported any VTE or DVT episodes, though 5.7% reported major bleeds (Kearon C, 2003).

Synthetic Pentasaccharides

Overview. The molecules in this class are synthetic derivatives of heparin. The specific pentasaccharide sequence is the portion of heparin that binds to antithrombin III (ATIII). Because this class is produced synthetically, problems associated with the heterogeneity of the molecular weight of heparin are eliminated; there is no batch-to-batch variability in biological activity, and there is less potential for the pathogenic contamination associated with the production of compounds of biological origin, like UH and LMWH. The first agent in this class (fondaparinux) was launched in 2002 (see "Current Therapies") for VTE prophylaxis in hip or knee surgery. The follow-up compound to this agent (idraparinux, examined here) is in late-stage clinical trials.

Mechanism of Action. Synthetic pentasaccharides potentiate the inhibitory action ATIII. Because the pentasaccharide represents the unique sequence of a heparin chain that binds to ATIII, the resulting pentasaccharide and ATIII complex inhibits factor Xa clotting factor alone, conferring a more targeted mechanism of action: Only one third of UH molecules contain this unique pentasaccharide sequence.

Idraparinux Sodium. After Sanofi-Synthélabo acquired all rights from Organon in 2004, Sanofi (now part of Sanofi-Aventis) is developing idraparinux sodium (SanOrg-34006), a long-acting pentasaccharide and follow-up molecule to fondaparinux sodium. The compound is in Phase III clinical trials in the United States and Europe for the prevention of VTE and the treatment of DVT and PE.

Idraparinux selectively binds to ATIII, thus potentiating the innate neutralization of factor Xa by ATIII, with no effect on thrombin. Neutralization of factor Xa interrupts the blood coagulation cascade and inhibits thrombin formation and thrombus development.

In addition to its longer half-life (120 hours), idraparinux has a higher affinity than fondaparinux for human antithrombin and so may prove more efficacious. Phase I trials show this drug to be well tolerated, with no significant adverse events (Faaij RA, 1999).

A Phase II study (PERSIST) compared 12 weeks' treatment with idraparinux (2.5, 5.0, 7.5, and 10 mg subcutaneously) with warfarin in 37 patients with confirmed symptomatic proximal DVT. Patients were initially treated with weight-adjusted enoxaparin for four to seven days and then randomized to either idraparinux (2.5, 5.0, 7.5, or 10 mg) or warfarin. Results showed that a dose of 2.5 mg idraparinux was at least as effective as warfarin in VTE prevention and was not associated with major bleeding (PERSIST Investigators, 2002). Idraparinux also did not appear to significantly affect liver enzymes (Reiter M, 2003).

Owing to its long half-life, idraparinux can be administered as a weekly subcutaneous injection, giving it an advantage over fondaparinux (which must be administered daily) both in short-term prophylaxis and in the long-term prevention of DVT and PE events after symptomatic DVT or PE. However, idraparinux's long half-life may present problems should bleeding require that its action be reversed.

Recently, recombinant factor VIIa (rFVIIa) was shown to reverse the anticoagulation caused by idraparinux (Bijsterveld NR, 2004). These results suggest that rFVIIa may be useful in serious bleeding complications in idraparinux-treated patients.

The development of idraparinux is being supported by an extensive Phase III program in the treatment of DVT and PE. The Van Gogh PE trial aims to recruit 2,200 patients with PE to a treatment regimen of idraparinux (2.5 mg), UH, or LMWH for 13 or 26 weeks. The Van Gogh DVT trial is seeking to recruit a similar number of patients with DVT to the same regimen, while the Van Gogh Ext trial will treat 1,200 DVT or PE patients (who have previously completed six months of treatment) to a further six months of idraparinux or placebo.

Another ongoing trial is the Phase III AMADEUS (AF Monitored Adjusted Dose VKA Comparing Efficacy and Safety with Unadjusted SanOrg-34006/Idraparinux), designed to demonstrate that idraparinux is at least as effective as dose-adjusted warfarin but provides superior safety in the long-term prevention of thromboembolic events associated with atrial fibrillation.

Thrombolytics

Overview. Thrombolytic agents promote the dissolution of blood clots once they have formed and thus have the potential to reduce pain, swelling, and loss of venous valves due to DVT or PE. However, the use of thrombolytics is usually reserved for patients with massive or hemodynamically unstable PE or extensive iliofemoral DVT (discussed in the "Current Therapies" section). This practice is primarily due to the high rates of complications associated with thrombolytic therapy (patients with DVT or PE receiving thrombolytic therapy have a 3% risk of intracranial bleeding). Thrombolytics in development seek to improve on the safety of currently available agents by employing a more specific mechanism of action.

Mechanism of Action. Current thrombolytic agents are tissue plasminogen activators (tPAs; see Figure 3) that convert plasminogen into its active form, plasmin. Plasmin catalyzes the breakdown of insoluble fibrin in a blood clot into soluble peptides. The blood clot is thus dissolved in a process known as fibrinolysis. In addition to lysing the clot to prevent subsequent PE, thrombolytics can reduce the incidence of post-thrombotic syndrome.

V-10153. V-10153 (BB-10153, TAPgen) is a recombinant plasminogen under development by Vernalis (Oxford, United Kingdom; formerly British Biotech). The compound is in Phase II clinical trials for thrombosis and thrombolysis after acute myocardial infarction (AMI) in the United States and in Phase I trials in Europe. A Phase II trial has also been initiated for stroke in the United States and Canada; Vernalis is seeking a partner to develop the molecule for this indication.

V-10153 is a recombinant plasminogen. Whereas endogenous plasminogen is converted to the active plasmin through cleavage of a bond by tPA, in V-10153 the tPA-sensitive site has been replaced with a site that is cleaved by thrombin. Because thrombin is found only at sites of ongoing clotting, V-10153 exists as an inactive pro-drug that is selectively activated at the site of a fresh or forming thrombus. Researchers hope this specific mechanism of action will reduce the bleeding risk involved in fibrinolysis and enable the drug to prevent the formation of new clots.

Data regarding this molecule are limited, but in a rabbit model of arterial thrombosis, V-10153 (10 mg/kg IV) produced sustained reperfusion in four out of four animals for up to four hours. In contrast, alteplase (3 mg/kg) was associated with prolonged periods of flow in three out of four animals, with reocclusion occurring in two of these animals. In addition, the effects of V-10153 were not associated with any changes in concentrations of circulating fibrinogen and alpha2-antiplasmin. Alteplase increased bleeding time from 3.7 minutes at baseline to 24.8 minutes at 30 minutes after administration, while bleeding time was not significantly affected by V-10153 (Cackett KS, 1995).

The safety and tolerability of V-10153 were determined in a Phase I clinical study in which 32 healthy volunteers were given eight doses of V-10153 (ranging from 0.08 to 4.8 mg/kg). A plasma half-life of three to four hours was observed. The potential thrombolytic activity of V-10153 was demonstrated by a dose-dependent increase in fibrin D-dimers and by the drug's efficacy in an ex vivo clot lysis assay. There was no effect on either prothrombin time or thrombin time (Curtis LD, 2002).

A Phase IIb study of increasing doses of V-10153 (1–5 mg/kg) in 28 patients with acute myocardial infarction (AMI) led to full coronary blood flow restoration in three out of seven patients at the 5 mg/kg dose. No bleeding events were observed (Vernalis, press release, 2003). A follow-up study evaluated doses up to 10 mg/kg in 35 patients with AMI. The drug was well tolerated at all doses, and blood flow was fully restored in approximately 40% of the patients one hour after they received 5 mg/kg or greater. This outcome is comparable to the efficacy of other marketed thrombolytics (Vernalis, press release, 2004).

Direct Factor Xa Inhibitors

Overview. Based on its position at the start of the common pathway of the extrinsic and intrinsic coagulation systems, factor X plays a central role in thrombin generation. As such, there has been much interest in developing anticoagulants that are specific inhibitors of factor X or activated factor X (factor Xa). Several orally active direct factor Xa inhibitors are in clinical development. Other compounds in this class that are in Phase II clinical trials but not specifically covered here are Yamanouchi Pharmaceutical's (Tokyo, Japan) YM-150, Eli Lily's LY-517717, and Sanofi-Aventis's SR-123781. These agents are not discussed in detail here due to a lack of available information.

Mechanism of Action. Neutralization of factor Xa interrupts the blood coagulation cascade and inhibits thrombin formation and thrombus development. Direct factor Xa inhibitors bind directly to factor Xa without a requirement for ATIII. Once activated by either the extrinsic or intrinsic pathway, factor Xa becomes an essential component of the prothrombinase complex (together with factor Va, prothrombin, phospholipid, and calcium). Because assembly of the prothrombinase complex represents the penultimate step in thrombin generation, interference with factor Xa activity directly affects the amount of active thrombin generated and, therefore, the amount of fibrin formed (Figure 3).

Razaxaban. After acquiring the rights to this molecule from DuPont Pharmaceuticals in 2001, Bristol-Myers Squibb is developing razaxaban hydrochloride, an oral direct factor-Xa-inhibiting agent. It is in Phase II clinical trials for the prophylaxis of VTE in the United States. This molecule may also have potential in the treatment of DVT and PE.

As a direct factor Xa inhibitor, razaxaban binds directly to factor Xa without a requirement for ATIII. Interference with factor Xa activity directly affects the amount of active thrombin generated and, therefore, the amount of fibrin formed.

Preclinical studies have shown that razaxaban is a potent selective factor Xa inhibitor. In a rabbit model of thrombosis, IV razaxaban was compared with melagatran and fondaparinux. Reduction in thrombus weight in experimentally induced arterio-venous shunt thrombosis (AVST) gave ID_{50} values of 1.6, 0.09, and 0.03 µM/kg/hour following administration of melagatran, razaxaban hydrochloride, and fondaparinux, respectively. In an electrically induced carotid arterial thrombosis (ECAT) model, razaxaban increased blood flow to 601% of control (Wong PC, 2003).

A Phase II trial compared the efficacy of razaxaban in the prevention of VTE after surgery with that of enoxaparin. In the trial, 656 patients undergoing TKR surgery were treated with razaxaban (25, 50, 75, or 100 mg, twice daily, started eight hours after the end of surgery) or enoxaparin (30 mg twice daily given SC, started 12–24 hours after the end of surgery). Treatment continued for ten days. An 8.6% venous VTE rate was observed with the 25 mg razaxaban dose compared with a 15.9% VTE rate with enoxaparin. Major bleeding was observed in 0.7% patients treated with the 25 mg razaxaban dose, while no cases were observed in the enoxaparin-treated arm. The three highest doses were stopped before the intended per-group sample size of 150 patients was reached due to increased reports of bleeding (Lassen MR, 2003).

DX-9065a. Daiichi Seiyaku is developing DX-9065a, a selective direct factor Xa inhibitor. An IV formulation is in Phase II trials in the United States, Japan, and Europe for the treatment of unstable angina. An oral formulation is in Phase I trials in the United States; Phase I and II trials of an injectable formulation have been conducted in Europe and Japan, respectively, for the prophylaxis of VTE.

DX-9065a is a direct, competitive inhibitor of factor Xa. The compound inactivates both free and fibrin-bound factor Xa and, as such, affects the clot-associated procoagulant activity that might be responsible for the propagation of intravascular thrombi as well as for recurrent thrombosis and thrombotic reocclusion after lysis.

DX-9065a's plasma half-life is reportedly 120–138 hours in patients with moderate or severe renal impairment and 84 hours in healthy subjects (Depasse F, 2003).

Phase I clinical trial data indicate that DX-9065a is safe and well tolerated and exhibits linear pharmacokinetics (Murayama N, 1999; 2000). Phase Ib studies of a 72-hour infusion of DX-9065a in 73 patients with clinically stable coronary artery disease (CAD) found that the drug effectively inhibits factor Xa and does not adversely affect renal or hepatic function, platelet count, or hemoglobin (Dyke CK, 2002). Importantly, no major bleeding complications occurred in this trial. Only a nonsignificant, dose-related increase in minor bleeding took place in the highest-dose group (200 ng/mL) compared with placebo recipients.

Another Phase II trial, the Xa Neutralization for Atherosclerotic Disease Understanding study (XANADU-PCI), compared DX-9065a with UH in 175 patients undergoing percutaneous coronary intervention (PCI). Results demonstrated that DX-9065a provides a measurable anticoagulant effect. However, the incidence of major and minor bleeding was higher in the DX-9065a arm than in the UH arm. The researchers did not comment on the significance of these data (Alexander JH, 2002).

In a dose-escalation study of DX-9065a versus enoxaparin, six patients were treated with enoxaparin plus aspirin, escalating doses of DX-9065a (bolus followed by 0.25–1.25 mg/hour), or the same doses of DX-9065a plus aspirin pretreatment (three days). DX-9065a (alone or with aspirin pretreatment) significantly inhibited thrombus formation at high and low shear rate conditions, while enoxaparin did not have a significant effect. Standard coagulation parameters were not as prolonged in the DX-9065a treatment groups as those induced by enoxaparin (Shimbo D, 2002).

Trials of DX-9065a are ongoing in patients with acute coronary syndromes (ACS) and for VTE prophylaxis.

BAY-59-7939. Bayer Pharmaceuticals (West Haven, Connecticut) is developing the oral factor Xa inhibitor BAY-59-7939 for the potential treatment of cardiovascular disease. The compound is in Phase III trials for cardiovascular disease including thrombosis in the United States, and Phase II in Europe and Japan.

In a Phase I placebo-controlled, randomized, crossover study, 12 subjects received a single dose of BAY-59-7939 (5 or 30 mg). The drug exhibited dose-dependent inhibition of thrombin generation both in platelets and plasma. Maximum inhibition (observed two hours following drug administration) was 28% and 56% for the 5 and 30 mg doses, respectively (Kubitza D, 2003[a]).

Results from a Phase I single-dose escalation study demonstrate that BAY-59-7939 has predictable, dose-dependent pharmacodynamics and pharmacokinetics. The compound has a rapid onset of action, with maximal effects being observed after two hours. At the highest dose (80 mg), maximal factor Xa inhibition was 60% (Kubitza D, 2003[b]). In a further dose-escalation study, 64 subjects were treated with 5–60 mg/day BAY-59-7939 for five days. Factor Xa was inhibited in a dose-dependent manner, with no increase in bleeding time (Harder S, 2003).

Oral Heparins

Overview. Oral heparins were once thought to hold great promise for the prophylaxis of VTE and treatment of DVT and PE, but development has been slow and clinical trial results disappointing. Nonetheless, several oral formulations of heparin remain in development. Emisphere Technologies's (Tarrytown, New York) solid oral UH is the agent for which the most information is available. Also in development but not specifically addressed here are Emisphere's solid oral LMWH and Generex Biotechnology Corporation's (Toronto, Ontario, Canada) buccal heparin.

Mechanism of Action. Heparin binds to ATIII to form a complex that changes ATIII from a slow, progressive clotting factor inhibitor to a very rapid thrombin, factor Xa, factor IXa, and factor XIa inactivator (see "Heparins" in the "Current Therapies" section). However, because of their anionic nature and high molecular weight, heparins are very poorly absorbed after oral administration. Oral heparins are combined with a carrier molecule in order to potentiate the absorption of heparin from the gastrointestinal tract (Leone Bay A, 1998).

Solid Oral Unfractionated Heparin. Emisphere Technologies is investigating a solid oral formulation of UH with a sodium-N-amino decanoate (SNAD) delivery agent. The formulation is in Phase I trials in the United States for the potential treatment of thrombotic disorders, including VTE prophylaxis.

As noted in the "Mechanism of Action" for the class as a whole, heparin binds to ATIII to form a complex that changes ATIII from a slow, progressive clotting factor inhibitor to a very rapid thrombin, factor Xa, factor IXa, and factor XIa inactivator.

Emisphere has evaluated the use of carrier molecules for the oral delivery of LMWH in primates. One study used two carriers—SNAC (sodium N-[8(2-hydroxybenzoyl)amino] caprylate) and SNAD (sodium-N-amino decanoate)—and showed that a combination of LMWH and SNAD could be delivered orally with a bioavailability of 38% relative to SC injection. Emisphere reports that SNAD is four times more effective than SNAC for oral heparin delivery.

Liquid oral forms of UH and LMWH complexed to a SNAD carrier showed promise and had progressed to Phase III trials. In May 2002, however, liquid oral heparin failed to meet its primary end point of superiority over enoxaparin in the Prophylaxis with Oral SNAC/Heparin Against Thromboembolic Complications Following Total Hip Replacement Surgery (PROTECT) trial. This Phase III study compared liquid oral heparin (in a 30-day treatment regimen) with enoxaparin (in a 10-day treatment regimen) for the prevention of VTE in 2,292 THR surgery patients. The investigators attributed its failure to dosing limitations imposed to ensure patient compliance. Although the data did demonstrate comparable efficacy and a significant reduction in adverse events compared with the high dose of liquid heparin, Emisphere discontinued development of liquid heparins and has refocused its heparin program efforts on a solid-dosage formulation.

Emisphere has reported results from a human Phase I study evaluating solid oral heparin in tablet and capsule form. The data demonstrate that following oral administration, resultant plasma concentrations of heparin are sufficient to lower blood coagulation to a level acceptable for the prevention of VTE, without any tolerability issues. In addition, the total volume of delivery material was significantly reduced in both the tablet and capsule compared with previous solid formulations and liquid oral heparin solutions.

On the one hand, the solid oral UH is likely to require monitoring and multiple daily doses and must be taken with food. On the other hand, solid oral UH may be able to exploit the wealth of long-term trials supporting the use of UH in DVT and PE treatment and VTE prophylaxis (Hirsh J, 1991; Hirsh J, 1989).

REFERENCES

Acostamadiedo JM, et al. Danaparoid sodium expert opinion. *Pharmacotherapy*. 2000;**1**[4]:803–814.

Adachi T, et al. Clinical study of venous thromboembolism during pregnancy and puerperium. *Seminars in Thrombosis and Hemostasis*. 2001;**27**[2]:149–153.

Adolf J, et al. Comparison of 3,000 IU aXa of the low-molecular-weight heparin certoparin with 5,000 IU aXa in prevention of deep vein thrombosis after total hip replacement. German Thrombosis Study Group. *International Journal of Angiology*. 1999;**18**(2):122–126.

Agnelli G, et al. Three months versus one year of oral anticoagulant therapy for idiopathic deep venous thrombosis. Warfarin Optimal Duration Italian Trial Investigators. *New England Journal of Medicine*. 2001;**345**(3):165–169.

Alexander JH, et al. Initial experience with a novel direct factor Xa inhibitor in percutaneous coronary intervention. *Journal of the American College of Cardiology*. 2002;**39**(suppl A):74A.

Alexander JH, et al. Effect of the direct factor Xa inhibitor, DX-9065a, on thrombin generation in patients with stable coronary artery disease. *Journal of Thrombosis and Hemostasis*. 2003;**1**(suppl 1). Abstract P2017.

Altman R, et al. Efficacy of unfractionated heparin, low-molecular-weight heparin, and both combined for releasing total and free tissue factor pathway inhibitor. *Haemostasis*. 1998;**28**:229–235.

American Thoracic Society. The diagnostic approach to acute venous thromboembolism. *American Journal of Respiratory Critical Care Medicine*. 1999;**160**:1043–1066.

Amiral J, et al. Absence of cross-reactivity of SR90107A/ORG31540 pentasaccharide with antibodies to heparin-PF4 complexes developed in heparin-induced thrombocytopenia. *Blood, Coagulation and Fibrinolysis*. 1997;**8**:114–117.

Anand SS, et al. The relation between the activated partial thromboplastin time response and recurrence in patients with venous thrombosis treated with continuous intravenous heparin. *Archives of Internal Medicine*. 1996;**156**:1677–1681.

Anand SS, et al. Does this patient have deep vein thrombosis? *Journal of the American Medical Association*. 1998;**279**(14):1094–1099.

Anderson DR. Symptomatic end points for venous thromboembolism treatment. *Hemostasis*. 1998;**28**(suppl 3):120–126.

Anderson FA Jr., et al. A population-based perspective of the hospital incidence and case-fatality rates of deep vein thrombosis and pulmonary embolism. The Worcester DVT study. *Archives of Internal Medicine*. 1991;**151**(5):933–938.

Anderson FA, Wheeler HB. Venous thromboembolism: risk factors and prophylaxis. *Clinics in Chest Medicine*. 1995;**16**:235–251.

Anderson FA Jr., Spencer FA. Risk factors for venous thromboembolism. *Circulation*. 2003;**107**:I9–I16. [a]

Anderson FA Jr., et al. Temporal trends in prevention of venous thromboembolism following primary total hip or knee arthroplasty 1996–2001: findings from the Hip and Knee Registry. *Chest*. 2003;**124**:349S–356S. [b]

Arcasoy SM, et al. Thrombolytic therapy of pulmonary embolism: a comprehensive review of current evidence. *Chest*. 1999;**115**(6):1695–1707.

Arcelus JI, et al. The management and outcome of acute venous thromboembolism: a prospective registry including 4,011 patients. *Journal of Vascular Surgery*. 2003;**38**(5):916–922.

Arnesen H, et al. A prospective study of streptokinase and heparin in the treatment of venous thrombosis. *Acta Medica Scandinavia*. 1978;**203**:457–463.

Arnold DM, et al. Missed opportunities for prevention of venous thromboembolism: an evaluation of the use of thromboprophylaxis guidelines. *Chest*. 2001;**120**(6):1964–1971.

Ascari E, et al. The epidemiology of deep vein thrombosis and pulmonary embolism. *Haematologica*. 1995;**80**:36–41.

Aschwanden M, et al. Acute deep vein thrombosis: early mobilization does not increase the frequency of pulmonary embolism. *Thrombosis and Haemostasis*. 2001;**85**(1):42–46.

Attia J, et al. Deep vein thrombosis and its prevention in critically ill adults. *Archives of Internal Medicine*. 2001;**161**:1268–1279.

Baglin T, et al. Incidence of recurrent venous thromboembolism in relation to clinical and thrombophilic risk factors: prospective cohort study. *Lancet*. 2003;**362**(9383):523–526.

Barritt DW, Jordon SC. Anticoagulant drugs in the treatment of pulmonary embolism: a controlled trial. *Lancet*. 1960;**1**:1309–1312.

Bauer K, et al. Efficacy of the first synthetic factor Xa inhibitor, pentasaccharide Org 31540/SR90107A, versus low-molecular-weight heparin (LMWH) in the prevention of venous thromboembolism (VTE) following elective major knee surgery: the Pentamaks study. *Supplement to the Journal of Thrombosis and Haemostasis*. July 2002: Abstract OC46.

Baughman RA, et al. Oral delivery of anticoagulant doses of heparin: a randomized, double-blind, controlled study in humans. *Circulation*. 1998;**16**:1610–1615.

Belcaro G, et al. Comparison of low-molecular-weight heparin, administered primarily at home, with unfractionated heparin, administered in hospital, and subcutaneous heparin, administered at home for deep vein thrombosis. *Angiology*. 1999;**50**(10):781–787.

Bergmann JF, Mouly S. Thromboprophylaxis in medical patients: focus on France. *Seminars in Thrombosis and Hemostasis*. 2002;**28**(suppl 3):51–55.

Bergqvist D, et al. Duration of prophylaxis against venous thromboembolism with enoxaparin after surgery for cancer. *New England Journal Medicine*. 2002;**346**(13):975–980.

Berube C, et al. The relationship of antiphospholipid antibodies to thromboembolic events in pediatric patients with systemic lupus erythematosus: a cross-sectional study. *Pediatric Research*. 1998;**44**(3):351–356.

Bick RL. The antiphospholipid-thrombosis syndromes: fact, fiction, confusion, and controversy. *American Journal of Clinical Pathology*. 1993;**100**(5):477–480.

Bick RL. Low-molecular-weight heparins in the outpatient management of venous thromboembolism. *Seminars in Thrombosis and Hemostasis*. 1999;**25**(3):97–99.

Bick RL, Haas S. Thromboprophylaxis and thrombosis in medical, surgical, trauma, and obstetric/gynecologic patients. *Hematology/Oncology Clinics of North America*. 2003;**17**:217–258.

Bijsterveld NR, et al. Recombinant factor VIIa reverses the anticoagulant effect of the long-acting pentasaccharide idraparinux in healthy volunteers. *British Journal of Haematology*. 2004;**124**(5):653–658.

Boneu B. Low-molecular-weight heparins: are they superior to unfractionated heparins to prevent and treat deep vein thrombosis? *Thrombosis Research*. 2000;**100**:V113–V120.

Bossuyt PMM, et al. Out-of-hospital treatment with venous thrombosis: socioeconomic aspects and patients' quality of life. *Haemostasis*. 1998;**28**(suppl 3):100–107.

Brandjes DPM, et al. Randomized trial of effect of compression stockings in patients with symptomatic proximal-vein thrombosis. *Lancet*. 1997;**349**:759–762.

Bratt G, et al. A comparison between low-molecular-weight heparin (KABI-2165) and standard heparin in the intravenous treatment of deep venous thrombosis. *Thrombosis Haemostasis*. 1985;**54**(4):813–817.

Bratzler DW, et al. Underuse of venous thromboembolism prophylaxis for general surgery patients: physician practices in the community hospital setting. *Archives of Internal Medicine*. 1998;**158**(17):1909–1912.

Bredberg E, et al. Ximelagatran, an oral direct thrombin inhibitor, has a low potential for cytochrome P450-mediated drug-drug interactions. *Clinical Pharmacokinetics*. 2003;**42**(8):765–777.

Bredberg U, et al. Effects of melagatran, a novel direct thrombin inhibitor, in healthy volunteers following intravenous, subcutaneous, and oral administration. *Blood*. 1999;**94**(suppl 1). Abstract 110.

Breddin HK. Effects of a low-molecular-weight heparin on thrombus regression and recurrent thromboembolism in patients with deep vein thrombosis. *New England Journal of Medicine*. 2001;**344**:626–631.

Bruns J, et al. The epidemiology of traumatic brain injury: a review. *Epilepsia*. 2003;**44**:2–10.

Büller HR. Arixtra (fondaparinux sodium) once daily demonstrates benefit in treating life-threatening pulmonary embolism and deep vein thrombosis in the MATISSE studies. *44th Annual Meeting of the American Society of Hematology*. 2002. Presentation.

Büller HR, et al. Subcutaneous fondaparinux versus intravenous unfractionated heparin in the initial treatment of pulmonary embolism. *New England Journal of Medicine*. 2003;**349**(18):1695–1702.

Busson JL, et al. Deep vein thrombosis in elderly patients hospitalized in subacute care facilities. *Archives of Internal Medicine*. 2003;**163**:2613–2618.

Cackett KS, et al. Thrombolytic activity of thrombin-activatable plasminogen in the anaesthetized rabbit. *British Journal of Pharmacology*. 1995;**116**(proc. suppl). Abstract 10P.

Cardosi RJ, Fiorica JV. The relationship of antiphospholipid antibodies to thromboembolic events in pediatric patients with systemic lupus erythematosus: a cross-sectional study. *Pediatric Research*. 1998;**44**(3):351–356.

Casazza F, et al. The cardiologist facing pulmonary embolism: the experience of 160 cases of acute cor pulmonale. *Italian Heart Journal*. 2000;**1**(suppl 4):520–526.

Cattaneo M, et al. Low plasma levels of vitamin B(6) are independently associated with a heightened risk of deep vein thrombosis. *Circulation*. 2001;**104**(20):2442–2446.

Charbonnier BA, et al. Comparison of a once-daily with a twice-daily subcutaneous low-molecular-weight heparin regimen in the treatment of deep vein thrombosis. FRAXODI Group. *Thrombosis and Haemostasis*. 1998;**79**(5):897–901.

Chemaly RF, et al. Venous thrombosis associated with peripherally inserted central catheters: a retrospective analysis of the Cleveland clinic experience. *Clinical Infectious Diseases*. 2002;**34**(9):1179–1183.

Cina G, et al. Epidemiology, pathophysiology, and natural history of venous thromboembolism. *Rays*. 1996;**21**:315–327.

Circlincione AS, et al. Low-molecular-weight heparin for deep vein thrombosis prophylaxis in foot and ankle surgery: a review. *Journal of Foot and Ankle Surgery*. 2000;**40**(2):96–100.

Clagett GP, et al. Prevention of venous thromboembolism. *Chest*. 1998;**114**(suppl): 531S–560S.

Clinica staff. Spanish health agency evaluates hip implant program. *Clinica*. 1999;**854**:5.

Cohen AT, et al. Fondaparinux vs. placebo for the prevention of venous thromboembolism in acutely ill medical patients (ARTEMIS). XIX Congress of the International Society on Thrombosis and Haemostasis; Birmingham, UK; July 12–18, 2003. Abstract P2406.

Colwell CW, et al. Efficacy and safety of enoxaparin versus unfractionated heparin for prevention of deep venous thrombosis after elective knee arthroplasty. Enoxaparin Clinical Trial Group. *Clinical Orthopedics*. 1995;**321**:19–27.

Colwell CW. Low-molecular-weight heparin prophylaxis in total knee arthroplasty. *Clinical Orthopedics and Related Research*. 2001;**392**:245–248.

Colwell CW, et al. Comparison of ximelagatran, an oral direct thrombin inhibitor, with enoxaparin for the prevention of venous thromboembolism following total hip replacement. A randomized, double-blind study. *Journal of Thrombosis and Haemostasis*. 2003;**1**(10):2119–2130. [a]

Colwell CW, et al. Randomized, double-blind comparison of ximelagatran, an oral direct thrombin inhibitor, and warfarin to prevent venous thromboembolism (VTE) after total knee replacement (TKR): EXULT B. *Blood*. 2003;**102**(11). Abstract 39. [b]

Comp PC, et al. A comparison of danaparoid, a subcutaneous nonheparin antithrombotic agent, with warfarin for prophylaxis against deep vein thrombosis after hip joint replacement surgery. *Orthopedics*. 1998;**21**(10):1123–1128.

Comp PC, et al. Prolonged enoxaparin therapy to prevent venous thromboembolism after primary hip or knee replacement. *Journal of Bone and Joint Surgery*. 2001;**83**:336–345.

Constans J, et al. Clinical prediction of lower-limb deep vein thrombosis in symptomatic hospitalized patients. *Thrombosis Haemostasis*. 2001;**86**:985–990.

Curtis LD, et al. Safety, pharmacokinetics, and pharmacodynamics of the novel thrombolytic BB-10153 demonstrated in healthy volunteers. *Circulation*. 2002;**106**. Abstract 3110.

Cushman M, et al. Incidence rates, case fatality, and recurrence rates of deep vein thrombosis and pulmonary embolus: the Longitudinal Investigation of Thromboembolism Etiology (LITE). *Thrombosis and Haemostasis*. 2001;**86**(suppl 1). Abstract OC2349.

Dalen JE. Pulmonary embolism: what have we learned since Virchow? Natural history, pathophysiology, and diagnosis. *Chest*. 2002;**122**:1440–1456.

Daud AN, et al. Synthetic heparin pentasaccharide depolymerization by heparinase I: molecular and biological implications. *Clinical Applied Thrombosis and Hemostasis*. 2001;**7**:58–64.

Davidson BL. DVT treatment in 2000: state of the art. *Orthopedics*. 2000;**23**:651–654.

Davis JD. Prevention, diagnosis, and treatment of venous thromboembolic complications of gynecologic surgery. *American Journal of Obstetrics and Gynecology*. 2001;**184**:759–775.

Davis R, et al. A review of its pharmacology and clinical use in the prevention and treatment of thromboembolic disorders. *Drugs Aging*. 1997;**10**(4):299–322.

Decousus H, et al. A clinical trial of vena cava filters in the prevention of pulmonary embolism in patients with proximal deep vein thrombosis. Prevention du Risque d'Embolie Pulmonaire par Interruption Cave Study Group. *New England Journal of Medicine*. 1998;**338**:409–415.

Deitcher SR. Overview of enoxaparin in the treatment of deep vein thrombosis. *American Journal of Managed Care*. 2000;**6**(suppl 20):S1026.

Department of Health (DOH). Hospital Episode Statistics. England. 2002–2003. www.statistics.gov.uk/default.asp. Accessed February 2004.

Depasse F, et al. Pharmacodynamics and pharmacokinetics of DX-9065a in renal impairment. The 45th Meeting of the American Society of Hematology; December 2003; San Diego, CA. Abstract 4193.

Devlin JW, et al. Cost-effectiveness of enoxaparin versus low-dose heparin for prophylaxis against venous thrombosis after major trauma. *Pharmacotherapy*. 1998;**18**(6):1335–1342.

Di Minno G, et al. Antithrombotic drugs for older subjects: guidelines formulated jointly by the Italian societies of hemostasis and thrombosis (SISET) and of gerontology and geriatrics (SIGG). *Nutrition Metabolism and Cardiovascular Disease*. 2001;**11**:41–62.

Douketis JD, et al. Does the location of thrombosis determine the risk of disease recurrence in patients with proximal deep vein thrombosis? *American Journal of Medicine*. 2001;**110**:515–519.

Dunn CJ, Jarvis B. Dalteparin: an update of its pharmacological properties and clinical efficacy in the prophylaxis and treatment of thromboembolic disease. *Drugs*. 2000;**60**(1):203–237.

Duplaga BA, et al. Dosing and monitoring of low-molecular-weight heparins in special populations. *Pharmacotherapy*. 2001;**21**(2):218–234.

Dyke CK, et al. First experience with direct factor Xa inhibition in patients with stable coronary disease: a pharmacokinetic and pharmacodynamic evaluation. *Circulation*. 2002;**105**(20):2385–2391.

East Anglia Cancer Registry (EACR). Data received August 30, 2003.

Editorial Committee on Japanese Guideline for Prevention of Venous Thromboembolism (digest version). *Japanese Guidelines for Prevention of Venous Thromboembolism*; Tokyo: Medical Front International Limited, 2004.

Egger B, et al. Efficacy and safety of weight-adapted nadroparin calcium vs. heparin sodium in prevention of clinically evident thromboembolic complications in 1,190 general surgical patients. *Digestive Surgery*. 2000;**17**(6):602–609.

Eichinger S, et al. Symptomatic pulmonary embolism and the risk of recurrent venous thromboembolism. *Archives of Internal Medicine*. 2004;**164**:92–96.

Eikelboom JW, et al. Extended-duration prophylaxis against venous thromboembolism after total hip or knee replacement: a meta-analysis of the randomized trials. *Lancet*. 2001;**358**(9275):9–15.

Elg M, et al. Effect of activated prothrombin complex concentrate or recombinant factor VIIa on the bleeding time and thrombus formation during anticoagulation with a direct thrombin inhibitor. *Thrombosis Research*. 2001;**101**:145–157.

Elliott CG. Pulmonary physiology during pulmonary embolism. *Chest*. 1992;**101**(suppl 4):163S–171S.

Ennis RS. Postoperative deep vein thrombosis prophylaxis: a retrospective analysis in 1,000 consecutive hip fracture patients treated in a community hospital setting. *Journal of the Southern Orthopedic Association*. 2003;**12**(1):10–17.

Eriksson BI, et al. METHRO I: dose-ranging study of H376/95, a novel, oral, direct thrombin inhibitor, and its subcutaneous formulation, melagatran, for prophylaxis of venous thromboembolism after total hip and total knee replacement. *Haemostasis*. 2000;**30**(suppl 1):1–212. [a]

Eriksson BI. New therapeutic options in deep vein thrombosis prophylaxis. *Seminars in Hematology*. 2000;**37**(suppl 5):7–9. [b]

Eriksson BI, et al. Fondaparinux compared with enoxaparin for the prevention of venous thromboembolism after hip-fracture surgery. *New England Journal of Medicine*. 2001;**345**:1298–1304.

Eriksson BI, et al. Efficacy of the first synthetic factor Xa inhibitor, pentasaccharide Org31540/SR90107A, versus low-molecular-weight heparin (LMWH) in the prevention of venous thromboembolism (VTE) following hip fracture surgery: the Penthifra study. Taken from: *Thrombosis and Haemostasis*. July 2002. Abstract OC47.

Eriksson BI, et al. Duration of prophylaxis against venous thromboembolism with fondaparinux after hip fracture surgery: a multicenter, randomized, placebo-controlled, double-blind study. *Archives of Internal Medicine*. 2003;**163**:1337–42. [a]

Eriksson BI, et al. The direct thrombin inhibitor melagatran followed by oral ximelagatran compared with enoxaparin for the prevention of venous thromboembolism after total hip or knee replacement: the EXPRESS study. *Journal of Thrombosis and Haemostasis*. 2003;**1**(12):2490–2496. [b]

Eriksson BI, et al. Direct thrombin inhibitor melagatran followed by oral ximelagatran in comparison with enoxaparin for prevention of venous thromboembolism after total hip or knee replacement. *Thrombosis and Haemostasis*. 2003;**89**(2):288–296. [c]

Eriksson H, et al. Pharmacokinetics and pharmacodynamics of melagatran, a novel synthetic LMW thrombin inhibitor, in patients with acute DVT. *Thrombosis and Haemostasis*. 1999;**81**:358–363.

Eriksson H, et al. Extended secondary prevention with the oral direct thrombin inhibitor ximelagatran for 18 months after 6 months of anticoagulation in patients with venous thromboembolism: a randomized, placebo-controlled trial. The THRIVE III Investigators. *Blood*. 2002;**100**:81a. Abstract.

Eriksson H, et al. A randomized, controlled, dose-guiding study of the oral direct thrombin inhibitor ximelagatran compared with standard therapy for the treatment of acute deep vein thrombosis: THRIVE I. *Journal of Thrombosis and Haemostasis*. 2003;**1**(1):41–47.

Eriksson UG, et al. The pharmacokinetics of ximelagatran following single and repeated dosing to healthy male subjects. Poster presented at the annual meeting for the British Society for Haemostasis and Thrombosis; October 8–11, 2001; Bath, United Kingdom.

Eriksson UG, et al. Pharmacokinetics and pharmacodynamics of ximelagatran, a novel oral direct thrombin inhibitor, in young healthy male subjects. *European Journal of Clinical Pharmacology*. 2003;**59**(1):35–43. [a]

Eriksson UG, et al. Absorption, distribution, metabolism, and excretion of ximelagatran, an oral direct thrombin inhibitor, in rats, dogs, and humans. *Drug Metabolism and Disposition*. 2003;**31**(3):294–305. [b]

Eriksson UG, et al. Influence of severe renal impairment on the pharmacokinetics and pharmacodynamics of oral ximelagatran and subcutaneous melagatran. *Clinical Pharmacokinetics*. 2003;**42**(8):743–53. [c]

Eriksson-Lepkowska M, et al. The effect of the oral direct thrombin inhibitor ximelagatran (pINN, formerly H376/95) on the pharmacokinetics of diazepam in healthy male volunteers. Taken from: *Thrombosis and Haemostasis*. July 2001. Abstract P785.

Faaij RA, et al. The oral bioavailability of pentosan polysulphate sodium in healthy volunteers. *European Journal of Clinical Pharmacology*. 1999;**54**(12):929–935.

Faioni EM, et al. Resistance to activated protein C in unselected patients with arterial and venous thrombosis. *American Journal of Hematology*. 1997;**55**(2):59–64.

Fareed J, et al. An update on heparins at the beginning of the new millennium. *Seminars in Thrombosis and Hemostasis*. 2000;**26**:5–21.

Farner B, et al. A comparison of danaparoid and lepirudin in heparin-induced thrombocytopenia. *Thrombosis Haemostasis*. 2001;**85**(6):950–957.

Feret B. Fondaparinux. A novel synthetic antithrombotic for prevention of venous thromboembolism. *Formulary*. 2001;**36**:831–837

Ferlay J, et al. *Globocan 2000. Cancer Incidence, Mortality, and Prevalence Worldwide*. Lyon, France, International Agency for Research on Cancer. World Health Organization. IARC Press; 2001.

Fiessinger JN, et al. Once-daily subcutaneous dalteparin, a low-molecular-weight heparin, for the initial treatment of acute deep vein thrombosis. *Thrombosis Haemostasis*. 1996;**76**(2):195–199.

Forbes CD. A protocol for deep vein thrombosis. *The Practitioner*. 2000;**244**:365–369.

Forster A, Wells P. Tissue plasminogen activator for the treatment of deep vein thrombosis of the lower extremity: a systematic review. *Chest*. 2001;**119**(2):572–579.

Foundation for the Promotion of Cancer Research. Cancer Statistics in Japan. 1996. www.ncc.go.jp/en/statistics/2001/tables/t07.html. Accessed June 15, 2003.

Fowkes FJI, et al. Incidence of diagnosed deep vein thrombosis in the general population: systematic review. *European Journal of Endovascular Surgery*. 2003;**25**:1–5.

Francis CW, et al. Two-step warfarin therapy. Prevention of postoperative venous thrombosis without excessive bleeding. *Journal of the American Medical Association*. 1983;**249**(3):374–378.

Francis CW, et al. Randomized, double-blind, comparative study of ximelagatran (pINN, formerly H 376/95), an oral direct thrombin inhibitor, and warfarin to prevent venous thromboembolism (VTE) after total knee arthroplasty (TKA). Taken from: *Thrombosis and Haemostasis*. July 2001. Abstract OC44.

Francis RM, Brenkel IJ. Survey of use of thromboprophylaxis for routine total hip replacement by British orthopedic surgeons. *British Journal of Hospital Medicine*. 1997;**57**(9):427–431.

Frankel S, et al. Population requirement for primary hip-replacement surgery: a cross-sectional study. *Lancet*. 1999;**353**:1304–1309.

Funfsinn N, et al. Rapid D-dimer testing and pretest clinical probability in the exclusion of deep venous thrombosis in symptomatic outpatients. *Blood Coagulation and Fibrinolysis*. 2001;**12**(3):165–170.

Gearhart MM, et al. The risk assessment profile score identifies trauma patients at risk for deep vein thrombosis. *Surgery*. 2000;**128**(4):631–640.

Geerts WH, et al. A prospective study of venous thromboembolism after major trauma. *New England Journal of Medicine*. 1994;**331**:1601–1606.

Geerts WH, et al. Prevention of venous thromboembolism. *Chest*. 2001;**119**(suppl 1):132S–175S.

Gerlach R. Postoperative nadroparin administration for prophylaxis of thromboembolic events is not associated with an increased risk of hemorrhage after spinal surgery. *European Spine Journal*. 2004;**13**(1):9–13.

German Hip Arthroplasty Trial (GHAT) Group. Prevention of deep vein thrombosis with low-molecular-weight heparin in patients undergoing total hip replacement. A randomized trial. *Archives of Orthopedic and Trauma Surgery*. 1992;**111**(2):110–120.

Giannadakis K, et al. Is a general pharmacologic thromboembolism prophylaxis necessary in ambulatory treatment by plaster cast immobilization in lower limb injuries? *Unfallchirurg*. 2000;**103**(6):475–478.

Gilbert KB, Rodgers GM. Utilization and outcomes of enoxaparin treatment for deep-vein thrombosis in a tertiary care hospital. *American Journal of Hematology*. 2000;**65**:285–288.

Ginsberg JS. Management of venous thromboembolism. *New England Journal of Medicine*. 1996;**335**:1816–1828.

Giovanni B et al. Prevention of flight-related thrombosis with elastic stockings: the JPA-Study, Final Analysis. *Journal of the American College of Cardiology*. 2004;**43**(5). Abstract 858-2.

Giuntini C, et al. Pulmonary embolism: epidemiology. *Chest*. 1995;**107**:3S–9S.

Goldhaber SZ, et al. Randomised controlled trial of recombinant tissue plasminogen activator versus urokinase in the treatment of acute pulmonary embolism. *Lancet*. 1988;**2**:293–298.

Goldhaber SZ, et al. Recombinant tissue-type plasminogen activator versus a novel dosing regimen of urokinase in acute pulmonary embolism: a randomized controlled multicenter trial. *Journal of the American College of Cardiology*. 1992;**20**(1):24–30.

Goldhaber SZ. Pulmonary embolism. *New England Journal of Medicine*. 1998;**339**:93–104.

Goldhaber SZ, et al. Acute pulmonary embolism: clinical outcomes in the International Cooperative Pulmonary Embolism Registry (ICOPER). *Lancet*. 1999;**353**(9162): 1386–1389.

Goldhaber SZ. Thrombolysis for pulmonary embolism. *New England Journal of Medicine*. 2002;**347**(15):1131–1132.

Goldhaber SZ, et al. A prospective registry of 5,451 patients with ultrasound-confirmed deep vein thrombosis. *American Journal of Cardiology*. 2004;**93**(2):259–262.

Goldman L. Urokinase in pulmonary embolism. *Lancet*. 1973;**1**(7817):1427–1428.

Gonzalez-Fajardo JA, et al. Venographic comparison of subcutaneous low-molecular weight heparin (LMWH) with oral anticoagulant therapy in the long-term treatment of deep venous thrombosis. *Journal of Vascular Surgery*. 1999;**30**:283–292.

Gori AM, et al. Tissue factor reduction and tissue factor pathway inhibitor release after heparin administration. *Thrombosis and Haemostasis*. 1999;**81**:589–593.

Greco F, et al. Results of a survey on knowledge and habits among hospital doctors concerning primary prevention of venous thromboembolism. *Minerva Medicine*. 1999;**90**(1–2):7–13.

Greinacher A, et al. Recombinant Hirudin (HBW 023) in the treatment of patients with heparin- associated thrombocytopenia (HAT): a prospective study. *Thrombosis and Haemostasis*. 1995;**73**:1452–1456.

Greinacher A. Heparin-induced thrombocytopenia. *Wiener klinische Wochenschrift*. 1997;**109**(10):343–345.

Greinacher A, et al. Recombinant hirudin (lepirudin) provides safe and effective anticoagulation in patients with heparin-induced thrombocytopenia: a prospective study. *Circulation*. 1999;**99**(1):73–80.

Gurwitz JH, et al. Risk for intracranial hemorrhage after tissue plasminogen activator treatment for acute myocardial infarction. Participants in the National Registry of MI 2. *Annals of Internal Medicine*. 1998;**129**:597–604.

Gustafsson D, et al. Pharmacodynamic properties of H 376/95. *Blood*. 1999;**94**(suppl 1):26a.

Gustafsson D, et al. The direct thrombin inhibitor melagatran and its oral pro-drug H 376/95: intestinal absorption properties, biochemical and pharmacodynamic effects. *Thrombosis Research*. 2001;**101**(3):171–181.

Gustafsson D. Oral direct thrombin inhibitors in clinical development. *Journal of Internal Medicine*. 2003;**254**(4):322–334. [a]

Gustafsson D, Elg M. The pharmacodynamics and pharmacokinetics of the oral direct thrombin inhibitor ximelagatran and its active metabolite melagatran: a mini-review. *Thrombosis Research*. 2003;**109**(suppl):S9–S15. [b]

Haas S. Deep vein thrombosis: beyond the operating table. *Orthopedics*. 2000;**23**: 629–632.

Halkin H, et al. Reduction of mortality in general medical inpatients by low-dose heparin prophylaxis. *Annals of Internal Medicine*. 1982;**96**(5):561–565.

Hall MJ, Lawrence L. Ambulatory surgery in the United States, 1996. National Center for Health Statistics. *Advance Data from Vital and Health Statistics*. 1998. No. 300:1–16.

Handoll HH, et al. Heparin, low-molecular-weight heparin and physical methods for preventing deep vein thrombosis and pulmonary embolism following surgery for hip fractures. *Cochrane Database Systems Review*. 2000;(2):CD000305.

Hansson PO, et al. Deep vein thrombosis and pulmonary embolism in the general population. The study of Men Born in 1913. *Archives of Internal Medicine*. 1997;**157**:1665–1670.

Harder S, et al. Effects of BAY 59-7939, an oral, direct factor xa inhibitor, on thrombin generation in healthy volunteers. The 4th meeting of the American Society of Hematology; December 2003; San Diego, CA. Abstract 3003.

Harenberg J, et al. Fixed-dose, body weight-independent subcutaneous LMW heparin versus adjusted-dose unfractionated intravenous heparin in the initial treatment of proximal venous thrombosis. EASTERN Investigators. *Thrombosis Haemostasis*. 2000;**83**(5):652–656.

Harrison J, et al. Economics of thromboprophylaxis in total hip replacement surgery. *Pharmacoeconomics*. 1997;**12**:30–41.

HCUPnet, Healthcare Cost and Utilization Project. December 2003. Agency for Healthcare Research and Quality, Rockville, MD. www.ahrq.gov/data/hcup/hcupnet.htm. Accessed February 2004.

Heit JA, et al. Risk factors for deep vein thrombosis and pulmonary embolism: a population-based case-control study. *Archives of Internal Medicine*. 2000;**160**(6):809–815.

Heit JA, et al. Incidence of venous thromboembolism in hospitalized patients vs. community residents. *Mayo Clinic Proceedings*. 2001;**76**:1102–1110. [a]

Heit JA, et al. The epidemiology of venous thromboembolism in the community. *Thrombosis Haemostasis*. 2001;**86**:452–63. [b]

Heit JA, et al. Comparison of the oral direct thrombin inhibitor ximelagatran with enoxaparin as prophylaxis against venous thromboembolism after total knee replacement. *Archives of Internal Medicine*. 2001;**161**:2215–2221. [c]

Heit JA, et al. Risk factors for deep vein thrombosis and pulmonary embolism: a population-based case-control study. *Archives of Internal Medicine*. 2002;**160**(6):809–815.

Heras M, et al. Guidelines of the Spanish Society of Cardiology: recommendations for the use of antithrombotic therapy in cardiology. *Revista Española de Cardiologia*. 1999;**52**:801–820.

Hirsh J. Heparin therapy in venous thromboembolism. *Annals of the New York Academy of Science*. 1989;**556**:378–385.

Hirsh J. Heparin. *New England Journal of Medicine*. 1991;**324**:1565–1574.

Hirsh J, Hoak J. Management of Deep Vein Thrombosis and Pulmonary Embolism; Dallas, TX: American Heart Association; 1996.

Hirsh J, et al. The 6th (2000) ACCP guidelines for antithrombotic therapy for prevention and treatment of thrombosis. *Chest*. 2001;**119**:3S–7S.

Horlocker TT, Heit JA. Low-molecular-weight heparin: biochemistry, pharmacology, perioperative prophylaxis regimens, and guidelines for regional anesthetic management. *Anesthesia and Analgesia*. 1997;**85**(4):874–885.

Hrebickova L, et al. Ximelagatran: a new oral anticoagulant. *Heart Disease*. 2003;**5**(6):397–408.

Huisman MV, et al. Efficacy and safety of the oral direct thrombin inhibitor ximelagatran for acute deep vein thrombosis with or without pulmonary embolism. *Program and abstracts of the XIX Congress of the International Society on Thrombosis and Haemostasis*. 2003. Abstract OC003.

Hull RD, et al. Continuous intravenous heparin compared with intermittent subcutaneous heparin in the initial treatment of proximal-vein thrombosis. *New England Journal of Medicine*. 1986;**315**(18):1109–1114.

Hull RD, et al. A comparison of subcutaneous low-molecular-weight heparin with warfarin sodium for prophylaxis against deep-vein thrombosis after hip or knee implantation. *New England Journal Medicine*. 1993;**329**:1370–1376.

Hull RD, et al. Low-molecular-weight heparin prophylaxis using dalteparin extended out-of-hospital vs. in-hospital warfarin/out-of-hospital placebo in hip arthroplasty patients: a double-blind, randomized comparison. North American Fragmin Trial Investigators. *Archives of Internal Medicine*. 2000;**160**(14):2208–2215.

Hull RD, et al. Low-molecular-weight heparin prophylaxis: preoperative versus postoperative initiation in patients undergoing elective hip surgery. *Thrombosis Research*. 2001;**101**(1):V155–162. [a]

Hull RD, et al. Timing of initial administration of low-molecular-weight heparin prophylaxis against deep vein thrombosis in patients following elective hip arthroplasty: a systematic review. *Archives of Internal Medicine*. 2001;**161**(16):1952–1960. [b]

Hyers TM. Antithrombotic therapy for venous thromboembolic disease. *Chest*. 2001;**119**(1 suppl):176S–193S.

Imamura K, Black NA. Total hip replacement: the preoperative health status of patients in Japan compared with England and the United States. *International Journal of Technological Assessment of Health Care*. 1997;**13**:1–10.

Imamura K, Black NA. Outcome of total hip replacement in Japan and England. Comparison of two retrospective cohorts. *International Journal of Technological Assessment of Health Care*. 1998;**14**:762–773.

Isawa T, et al. Incidence of pulmonary embolism in a chest hospital in Japan and importance of preoperative perfusion lung imaging in the diagnosis of postoperative pulmonary embolism. *Annals of Nuclear Medicine*. 1991;**5**:89–95.

Ito M. Pathology of pulmonary embolism. *Kokyu To Junkan*. 1991;**39**(6):567–572.

Janni W, et al. Prospective randomized study comparing the effectiveness and tolerance of various low-molecular-weight heparins in high-risk patients. *Zentralblatt fur Chirurgie*. 2001;**126**(1):32–38. Abstract.

Jerjes-Sanchez C, et al. Streptokinase and heparin versus heparin alone in massive pulmonary embolism: a randomized controlled trial. *Journal of Thrombosis and Thrombolysis*. 1995;**2**:227–229.

Jerjes-Sanchez C, et al. High dose and short-term streptokinase infusion in patients with pulmonary embolism: prospective with seven-year follow-up trial. *Journal of Thrombosis and Thrombolysis*. 2001;**12**(3):237–247.

Johansson LC, et al. A comparison of the pharmacokinetics of ximelagatran (pINN, formerly H376/95) in young and elderly healthy subjects. Taken from: *Thrombosis and Haemostasis*. July 2002. Abstract P782.

Kaboli P, et al. DVT prophylaxis and anticoagulation in the surgical patient. *Medical Clinics of North America*. 2003;**87**:77–110.

Kahn SR, et al. Long-term outcomes after deep vein thrombosis:postphlebetic syndrome and quality of life. *Journal of General Internal Medicine*. 2000;**15**:425–429.

Kakizoe T, et al., eds. Cancer Statistics in Japan 2001. Tokyo, Japan: Foundation for Promotion of Cancer Research; 2001:47. www.ncc.go.jp/en/statistics/2001/index.html. Accessed May 7, 2002.

Kakkar AK, et al. Venous thrombosis in cancer patients: insights from the FRONTLINE survey. *Oncologist*. 2003;**8**(4):381–388.

Kakkar VV. Prevention and management of venous thrombosis. *British Medical Bulletin*. 1994;**50**:871–903.

Kearon C, et al. A comparison of three months of anticoagulants with extended anticoagulation for a first episode of idiopathic venous thromboembolism. *New England Journal of Medicine*. 1999;**340**:901–907.

Kearon C, et al. A dose response study of a recombinant human soluble thrombomodulin (ART-123) for prevention of venous thromboembolism after unilateral total hip replacement *Journal of Thrombosis and Hemostasis*. 2003;**1**(suppl 1). Abstract OC330.

Kniffin WD, et al. The epidemiology of diagnosed pulmonary embolism and deep venous thrombosis in the elderly. *Archives of Internal Medicine*. 1994;**154**:861–866.

Konstantinides S, et al. Heparin plus alteplase compared with heparin alone in patients with submassive pulmonary embolism. *New England Journal of Medicine*. 2002, **347**(15):1143–1150.

Koopman MM, et al. Treatment of venous thrombosis with intravenous unfractionated heparin administered in the hospital as compared with subcutaneous low-molecular-weight heparin administered at home. The Tasman Study Group. *New England Journal of Medicine*. 1996;**334**(11):682–687.

Kroegel C, Reissig A. Principle mechanisms underlying venous thromboembolism: epidemiology, risk factors, pathophysiology and pathogenesis. *Respiration*. 2003;**70**:7–30.

Kubitza D, et al. Multiple dose escalation study investigating the pharmacodynamics, safety, and pharmacokinetics of BAY 59-7939 an oral, direct factor Xa inhibitor in healthy male subjects. *Blood*. 2003;**102**(11):811–812. [a]

Kubitza D, et al. Single-dose escalation study investigating the pharmacodynamics, safety, and pharmacokinetics of BAY 59-7939 an oral, direct factor Xa inhibitor in healthy male subjects. *Blood*. 2003;**102**(11):813–815. [b]

Kumasaka N, et al. Incidence of pulmonary thromboembolism in Japan. *Japanese Circulation Journal*. 1999;**63**:439–441.

Kyrle PA, et al. High plasma levels of factor VIII and the risk of recurrent venous thromboembolism. *New England Journal of Medicine*. 2004;**343**:457–462.

Labas P, et al. The home treatment of deep vein thrombosis with low-molecular-weight heparin, forced mobilisation and compression. *International Angiology*. 2000;**19**:303–307.

Lassen MR. Comparative efficacy of low-molecular-weight heparins in orthopedic surgery. *Seminars in Thrombosis and Hemostasis*. 2000;**26**(suppl 1):53–56.

Lassen MR, et al. Efficacy of the first synthetic factor Xa inhibitor, pentasaccharide Org31540/SR90107A, versus low-molecular-weight heparin (LMWH) in the prevention of venous thromboembolism (VTE) following elective hip replacement surgery: the Ephesus study. Taken from: *Thrombosis and Haemostasis*. July 2002. Abstract OC45.

Lassen MR, et al. A Phase II randomized, double-blind, five-arm, parallel-group, dose-response study of a new oral directly-acting factor Xa inhibitor, Razaxaban, for the prevention of deep vein thrombosis in knee replacement surgery—on behalf of the Razaxaban investigators. *Blood*. 2003;**102**(11): Abstract 41.

Lee AY. Epidemiology and management of venous thromboembolism in patients with cancer. *Thrombosis Research*. 2003;**110**:167–172.

Lee H, et al. Deep vein thrombosis is not rare in Asia—The Singapore General Hospital. *Annals of the Academy of Medicine Singapore*. 2002;**31**:761–764.

Leizorovicz A. Long-term consequences of deep vein thrombosis. *Hemostasis*. 1998;**28**(suppl 3):1–7.

Lenka H. Ximelagatran, a new oral anticoagulant. *Heart Disease*. 2003;**5**(6):397–408.

Lensing AWA, et al. Deep vein thrombosis. *Lancet*. 1999;**353**:479–485.

Leone Bay A, et al. Acylated non-alpha-amino acids as novel agents for the oral delivery of heparin sodium, USP. *Journal of Controlled Release Drugs*. 1998;**50**:1–3.

Levine M, et al. A comparison of low-molecular-weight heparin administered primarily at home with unfractionated heparin administered in the hospital for deep vein thrombosis. *New England Journal of Medicine*. 1996;**334**:677–681.

Levitan N, et al. Rates of initial and recurrent thromboembolic disease among patients with malignancy versus those without malignancy. Risk analysis using Medicare claims data. *Medicine (Baltimore)*. 1999;**78**:285–291.

Lewis BE, et al. Argatroban anticoagulant therapy in patients with heparin-induced thrombocytopenia. *Circulation*. 2001;**103**:1838–1843.

Leyvraz PF, et al. Adjusted versus fixed-dose subcutaneous heparin in the prevention of deep-vein thrombosis after total hip replacement. *New England Journal Medicine*. 1983;**309**:954–958.

Liebowitz RS. Deep vein thrombosis: thinking inside out. *Archives of Internal Medicine*. 1998;**158**(18):1964.

Lindmarker P, et al. Comparison of once-daily subcutaneous Fragmin with continuous intravenous unfractionated heparin in the treatment of deep vein thrombosis. *Thrombosis and Haemostasis*. 1994;**72**(2):186–190.

Lopez LM. Low-molecular-weight heparins are essentially the same for treatment and prevention of venous thromboembolism. *Pharmacotherapy*. 2001;**21**(6 Pt 2):56S–61S.

Lubenow N, et al. Hirudin in heparin-induced thrombocytopenia. *Seminars in thrombosis and hemostasis*. 2002;**28**(5):431–438. [a]

Lubenow N, et al. Results of a large drug-monitoring program confirm the safety and efficacy of lepirudin in patients with immune-mediated heparin-induced thrombocytopenia. *Blood*. 2002;**100**(1):502a. [b]

Lupu C, et al. Cellular effects of heparin on the production and release of tissue factor pathway inhibitor in human endothelial cells. *Arteriosclerosis, Thrombosis and Vascular Biology*. 1999;**19**:2251–2262.

Mandala M, et al. Venous thromboembolism and cancer: new issues for an old topic. *Critical Reviews in Oncology/Hematology*. 2003;**48**:65–80.

Margaglione M, et al. Increased risk for venous thrombosis in carriers of the prothrombin G— >A20210 gene variant. *Annals of Internal Medicine*. 1998;**129**(2):89–93.

Martins F, et al. Spinal cord injuries—epidemiology in Portugal's central region. *Spinal Cord*. 1998;**36**:574–578.

Meignan M, et al. Systematic lung scans reveal a high frequency of silent pulmonary embolism in patients with proximal deep vein thrombosis. *Archives of Internal Medicine*. 2000;**160**(2):145–146.

Meneveau N, et al. In-hospital and long-term outcome after sub-massive and massive pulmonary embolism submitted to thrombolytic therapy. *European Heart Journal*. 2003;**24**(15):1447–1454.

Merli GJ. Low-molecular-weight heparins versus unfractionated heparin in the treatment of deep vein thrombosis and pulmonary embolism. *American Journal of Physiology and Medical Rehabilitation*. 2000;**79**(suppl):S9–S16.

Merli GJ, et al. Subcutaneous enoxaparin once or twice daily compared with intravenous unfractionated heparin for treatment of venous thromboembolic disease. *Annals of Internal Medicine*. 2001;**134**(3):191–202. [a]

Merli GJ. Treatment of deep venous thrombosis and pulmonary embolism with low-molecular-weight heparin in the geriatric patient population. *Clinics in Geriatric Medicine*. 2001;**17**:93–106. [b]

Meyer G, et al. Subcutaneous low-molecular-weight heparin fragmin versus intravenous unfractionated heparin in the treatment of acute non massive pulmonary embolism: an open randomized pilot study. *Thrombosis and Haemostasis*. 1995;**74**(6):1432–1435.

Mismetti P, et al. Evaluation of the risk of venous thromboembolism in the medical patients. *Therapie*. 1998;**53**:565–570.

Mismetti P, et al. Meta-analysis of low-molecular-weight heparin in the prevention of venous thromboembolism in general surgery. *British Journal of Surgery*. 2001;**88**:913–930

Mizel MS, et al. Thromboembolism after foot and ankle surgery. A multicenter study. *Clinical Orthopedics*. 1998;(348):180–185.

Moll S, et al. Phase I study of a novel recombinant human soluble thrombomodulin, ART-123. *Journal of Thrombosis and Hemostasis*. 2003;**1**(suppl 1). Abstract OC329.

Monreal M, et al. Deep venous thrombosis and the risk of pulmonary embolism: a systematic study. *Chest*. 1992;**102**:677–681.

Morris RJ, Woodcock JP. Evidence-based compression: prevention of stasis and deep vein thrombosis. *Annals of Surgery*. 2004;**239**(2):162–171.

Morris TA, et al. Antithrombotic efficacies of enoxaparin, dalteparin, and unfractionated heparin in venous thromboembolism. *Thrombosis Research*. 2000;**100**(3):185–194.

Mullges W, et al. Customary use of compression stockings for prevention of thrombosis in medical intensive care units in Germany. *Dtsch Med Wochenschr*. 2001;**126**(31–32):867–871.

Murayama N, et al. Tolerability, pharmacokinetics and pharmacodynamics of DX-9065a, a new synthetic potent anticoagulant and specific factor Xa inhibitor, in healthy male volunteers. *Clinical Pharmacology and Therapeutics*. 1999;**66**(3):258–264.

Murayama N, et al. Pharmacokinetics of the anticoagulant 14C-DX-9065a, in the healthy male volunteer after a single intravenous dose. *Xenobiotica*. 2000;**30**:515–521.

Nakamura M, et al. Clinical characteristics of acute pulmonary thromboembolism in Japan: results of a multicenter registry in the Japanese Society of Pulmonary Embolism Research. *Clinical Cardiology*. 2001;**24**(2):132–138.

Nakano T, et al. Current situation for the treatment and evaluation of acute pulmonary thromboembolism in Japan. *Japanese Journal of Phlebology*. 2002;**13**(5):11–17.

Nicolaides AN, et al. Prevention of venous thromboembolism. International Consensus Statement. Guidelines compiled in accordance with the scientific evidence. *International Journal of Angiology*. 2001;**20**:1–37.

Nikparvar Fard M, et al. Utility of lower-extremity duplex sonography in patients with venous thromboembolism. *Journal of Clinical Ultrasound*. 2001;**29**:92–98.

Noble S. Enoxaparin. A reappraisal of its pharmacology and clinical applications in the prevention and treatment of thromboembolic disease. *Drugs*. 1995;**49**:388–410.

Nördstrom M, et al. A prospective study of the incidence of deep-vein thrombosis within a defined urban population. *Journal of Internal Medicine*. 1992;**232**:155–160.

O'Brien B, et al. Economic evaluation of outpatient treatment with low-molecular-weight heparin for proximal vein thrombosis. *Archives of Internal Medicine*. 1999;**159**: 2298–2304.

Office of National Statistics (ONS), 1997. Office of National Statistics: Cancer Registrations in England 1995–1997. www.statistics.uk.gov/statbase. Accessed June 18, 2002.

Ofosu FA, et al. The importance of thrombin inhibition for the expression of the anticoagulant activities of heparin, dermatan sulphate, low-molecular-weight heparin and pentosan polysulphate. *British Journal of Haematology*. 1985;**60**(4):695–704.

Oger E. Incidence of venous thromboembolism: a community-based study in Western France. EPI-GETBO Study Group. Groupe d'Étude de la Thrombose de Bretagne Occidentale. *Thrombosis and Haemostasis*. 2000;**83**:657–660.

Olsson SB, et al. Stroke prevention with the oral direct thrombin inhibitor ximelagatran compared with warfarin in patients with non-valvular atrial fibrillation (SPORTIF III): randomised controlled trial. *Lancet*. 2003;**362**(9397):1691–1698.

Otero R. Use of venous thromboembolism prophylaxis for surgical patients: a multicentre analysis of practice in Spain. *European Journal of Surgery*. 2001;**167**(3):163–167.

Ouriel K, et al. The anatomy of deep venous thrombosis of the lower extremity. *Journal of Vascular Surgery*. 2000;**31**:895–900.

Owings MF, et al. Ambulatory and in-patient procedures in the United States, 1996. National Center for Health Statistics. *Vital and Health Statistics*. 1998;**13**(139):1–119.

Page RB, et al. Head injury and pulmonary embolism: a retrospective report based on the Pennsylvania Trauma Outcomes study. *Neurosurgery*. 2004;**54**(1):143–148.

Parkin DM, et al., eds. *Cancer Incidence in Five Continents*. Volume **VIII**. Lyon, France: International Agency for Research on Cancer; 2002.

Parkin L, et al. Oral contraceptives and fatal pulmonary embolism. *Lancet*. 2000;**355** (9221):2133–2134.

Partsch H. Therapy of deep vein thrombosis with low-molecular-weight heparin, leg compression and immediate ambulation. *Vasa*. 2001;**30**(3):195–204.

PDR: Physicians' Desk Reference. 58th ed.; Montvale, NJ: Thomson, 2004.

Perrier A. Diagnostic strategies for pulmonary embolism and decision analysis. *Revue des Maladies Respiratoires*. 1999;**16**(5 pt 2):927–938.

Persist Investigators. A novel long-acting synthetic factor Xa inhibitor (idraparinux sodium) to replace warfarin for secondary prevention in deep vein thrombosis. A phase II evaluation. *Blood*. 2002;**100**(suppl). Abstract 301.

Pezzuoli G. Prophylaxis of fatal pulmonary embolism in general surgery using low-molecular-weight heparin Cy 216: a multicenter, double-blind, randomized, controlled, clinical trial versus placebo (STEP). STEP-Study Group. *Internal Surgery*. 1989;**74**(4):205–210.

Pilger E, et al. Multicenter studies of ultra-high-dose, short-duration streptokinase treatment of deep vein thrombosis. *Current Therapeutic Research*. 1996;**57**(4):251–267.

Pineda LA, et al. Clinical suspicion of fatal pulmonary embolism. *Chest*. 2001;**120**(3):791–795.

Pinide L, et al. Comparison of long versus short duration of anticoagulant therapy after a first episode of venous thromboembolism: a meta-analysis of randomized, controlled trials. *Journal of Internal Medicine*. 2000;**104**:332–338.

Pinide L, et al. Comparison of 3 and 6 months of oral anticoagulation therapy after a first episode of proximal deep vein thrombosis or pulmonary embolism and comparison of 6 and 12 weeks of therapy after isolated calf deep vein thrombosis. *Circulation*. 2001;**103**:2453–2460.

PIOPED Investigators. Value of the ventilation/perfusion scan in acute pulmonary embolism: results of the prospective investigation of pulmonary embolism diagnosis (PIOPED). *Journal of the American Medical Association*. 1990;**263**(20):2753–2759.

Planes A. An equivalence study of two low-molecular-weight heparins in the prevention and treatment of deep vein thrombosis after total hip replacement. *Seminars in Thrombosis and Hemostasis*. 2000;**26**(suppl 1):57–60.

Plasencia A, Borrell C. Population-based study of emergency department admissions and deaths from injuries in Barcelona, Spain: incidence, causes and severity. *European Journal of Epidemiology*. 1996;**12**:601–610.

Popovic JR. 1999 National Hospital Discharge Survey: annual summary with detailed diagnosis and procedure data. National Center for Health Statistics. *Vital and Health Statistics*. 2001;**13**(151):106–187.

Population Division of the Department of Economic and Social Affairs of the United Nations Secretariat. *World Population Prospects: The 2002 Revision*, vol. II, *The Sex and Age Distribution of Populations* (United Nations publication, Sales No. E.03.XIII.7), 2003.

Poulsen SH, et al. Clinical outcome of patients with suspected pulmonary embolism. A follow-up study of 588 consecutive patients. *Journal of Internal Medicine*. 2001;**250**(2):137–143.

Prandoni P, et al. Comparison of subcutaneous low-molecular-weight heparin with intravenous standard heparin in proximal deep-vein thrombosis. *Lancet*. 1992;**339**(8791):441–445.

Prandoni P, et al. The long term clinical course of acute deep venous thrombosis. *Annals of Internal Medicine*. 1996;**125**:1–7.

Prandoni P. Long-term clinical course of proximal deep venous thrombosis and detection of recurrent thrombosis. *Seminars in Thrombosis and Hemostasis*. 2001;**27**(1):9–13.

Prandoni P, et al. Recurrent Thromboembolism in cancer patients: Incidence and risk factors. *Seminars in Thrombosis and Hemostasis*. 2003;**29**(suppl 1):3–8.

Quere I, et al. Red blood cell methylfolate and plasma homocysteine as risk factors for venous thromboembolism: a matched case-control study. *Lancet*. 2002;**359**(9308):747–752.

Reiter M, et al. Idraparinux and liver enzymes: observations from the PERSIST trial. *Blood Coagulation and Fibrinolysis*. 2003;**14**(1):61–65.

Rembrandt Investigators. Treatment of proximal deep vein thrombosis with a novel synthetic compound (SR90107A/ORG31540) with pure anti-factor Xa activity. *Circulation*. 2000;**102**:2726–2731.

Remy-Jardin M. Is the spiral CT today the benchmark for diagnosing pulmonary embolism? *Revue de Medecine Interne*. 2001;**22**(6):519–521.

Research Group on Urokinase and PE. Multicenter study of 2 urokinase protocols in severe pulmonary embolism. *Archives Maladie Couer Vaiss*. 1984;**77**(7):773–781. Abstract.

Ribeiro A, et al. Pulmonary embolism: one-year follow-up with echocardiography doppler and five-year survival analysis. *Circulation*. 1999;**99**:1325–1330.

Rickles FR, Levine MN. Epidemiology of thrombosis in cancer. *Acta Haematologica*. 2001;**106**(1–2):6–12.

Ridker PM, et al. Ethnic distribution of factor V Leiden in 4,047 men and women. Implications for venous thromboembolism screening. *Journal of the American Medical Association*. 1997;**277**:1305–1307.

Ridker PM, et al. Long-term, low-intensity warfarin therapy for the prevention of recurrent venous thromboembolism. *New England Journal of Medicine*. 2003;**348**(15):1425–1434.

Ries LAG. *SEER Cancer Statistics Review, 1973–2000*. Bethesda, MD: National Cancer Institute; 2003.

Roncon L, et al. The diagnostic and therapeutic procedures in pulmonary embolism: a survey in the Veneto Region. *Cardiologia*. 1999;**44**(8):735–741.

Rosendaal FR, et al. High risk of thrombosis in patients homozygous for factor V Leiden (activated protein C resistance). *Blood*. 1995;**85**(6):1504–1508.

Rosendaal FR. Venous thrombosis: a multicausal disease. *Lancet*. 1999;**353**:1167–73.

Rubinstein I, et al. Fatal pulmonary emboli in hospitalized patients. An autopsy study. *Archives of Internal Medicine*. 1988;**148**:1425.

Rüdiger G, et al. Postoperative nadroparin administration for prophylaxis of thromboembolic events is not associated with an increased risk of hemorrhage after spinal surgery. *European Spine Journal*. 2004;**13**(1):9–13.

Saeger W, Genzkow M. Venous thrombosis and pulmonary embolisms in postmortem series: probable causes by correlations of clinical data and basic diseases. *Pathology Research and Practice*. 1994;**190**:394–399.

Sakuma M, et al. Increasing mortality from pulmonary embolism in Japan, 1951–2000. *Circulation Journal*. 2002;**66**:1144–1149.

Sakuma M, et al. Recent developments in diagnostic imaging techniques and management for acute pulmonary embolism: multicenter registry by the Japanese society of pulmonary embolism research. *Internal Medicine*. 2003;**42**(6):470–476.

Salartash K, et al. Treatment of experimentally induced caval thrombosis with oral low-molecular-weight heparin and delivery agent in a porcine model of deep vein thrombosis. *Annals of Surgery*. 2000;**231**(6):789–794.

Sallah S, et al. Pathogenesis of thrombotic disorders in patients with cancer. *In Vivo*. 2000;**14**(1):251–253.

Samama MM, et al. A comparison of enoxaparin with placebo for the prevention of venous thromboembolism in acutely ill medical patients. Prophylaxis in Medical Patients with Enoxaparin Study Group. *New England Journal of Medicine*. 1999;**341**(11):793–800.

Samama MM, et al. An epidemiologic study of risk factors for deep vein thrombosis in medical outpatients. *Archives of Internal Medicine*. 2000;**160**:3415–3420.

Sandset PM, et al. Physiologic function of tissue factor pathway inhibitor and interaction with heparins. *Haemostasis*. 2000;**30**:48–56.

Sarich TC, et al. The pharmacokinetics and pharmacodynamics of ximelagatran, an oral direct thrombin inhibitor, are unaffected by a single dose of alcohol. *Journal of Clinical Pharmacology*. 2004;**44**(4):388–393.

Sasahara AA, et al. The Urokinase Pulmonary Embolism Trial. *Circulation*. 1973;**47**(supp 2):1–108.

Sasahara AA, et al. The Phase II Urokinase-Streptokinase Pulmonary Embolism Trial. *Thrombosis et Diathesis Haemorrhagica*. 1975;**33**:464–476.

Schiele F, et al. Subcutaneous recombinant hirudin (HBW 023) versus intravenous sodium heparin in treatment of established acute deep vein thrombosis of the legs: a multicentre prospective dose-ranging randomized trial. International Multicentre Hirudin Study Group. *Thrombosis and Haemostasis*. 1997;**77**(5):834–838.

Schulman S, et al. A comparison of six weeks with six months of oral anticoagulant therapy after a first episode of venous thromboembolism. *New England Journal of Medicine*. 1995;**332**:1661–1665.

Schulman S, et al. The duration of oral anticoagulant therapy after a second episode of venous thromboembolism. The Duration of Anticoagulation Trial Study Group. *New England Journal of Medicine*. 1997;**336**(6):393–398.

Schulman S, et al. Secondary prevention of venous thromboembolism with the oral direct thrombin inhibitor ximelagatran. *New England Journal of Medicine*. 2003;**349**(18):1713–1721.

Schweizer J, et al. Comparative results of thrombolysis treatment with rt-PA and urokinase: a pilot study. *Vasa*. 1998;**27**:167–171.

Scottish Intercollegiate Guidelines Network. Antithrombotic therapy: SIGN publication number 36. Edinburgh, Scotland: SIGN, Royal College of Physicians; 1999.

Scurr JH, et al. Frequency and prevention of symptomless deep venous thrombosis in long-haul flights: a randomised trial. *Lancet*. 2001;**357**:1485–1489.

Seagroatt V, et al. Elective total hip replacement: incidence, emergency readmission rate, and postoperative mortality. *British Medical Journal*. 1991;**303**:1431–1435.

Seligsohn U, Lubetsky A. Genetic susceptibility to venous thrombosis. *New England Journal of Medicine*. 2001;**344**(16):1222–1231.

Sharma G, et al. Effect of thrombolytic therapy on pulmonary-capillary blood volume in patients with pulmonary embolism. *New England Journal of Medicine*. 1980;**303**:842–845.

Shimbo D, et al. Antithrombotic effects of DX-9065a, a direct factor Xa inhibitor: a comparative study in humans versus low-molecular-weight heparin. *Thrombosis and Haemostasis*. 2002;**88**(5):733–738.

Shingu H, et al. Spinal cord injuries in Japan: a nationwide epidemiological survey in 1990. *Paraplegia*. 1994;**32**:3–8.

Shorr AF, Ramage AS. Enoxaparin for thromboprophylaxis after major trauma: potential cost implications. *Critical Care Medicine*. 2001;**29**(9):1659–1665.

Silverstein MD, et al. Trends in the incidence of deep vein thrombosis and pulmonary embolism: a 25-year population-based study. *Archives of Internal Medicine*. 1998;**158**:585–593.

Simon P, et al. Efficacy and tolerance of low-molecular-weight heparin in the prevention of deep venous thrombosis during nonemergent total hip arthroplasty. A prospective, multicenter trial. *Journal de Chirurgie*. 1990;**127**(5):252–257.

Siragusa S, et al. Low-molecular-weight heparins and unfractionated heparin in the treatment of patients with acute venous thromboembolism: results of a meta-analysis. *American Journal of Medicine*. 1996;**100**:269–276.

Smith BJ, et al. Cost comparison of at-home treatment of deep venous thrombosis with low-molecular-weight heparin to inpatient treatment with unfractionated heparin. *Internal Medicine Journal*. 2002;**32**(1–2):29–34.

So L. Oral direct thrombin inhibition. International Society of Thrombosis and Haemostasis—XVII Congress report; July 6–12, 2001; Paris, France.

Spiro T. Enoxaparin versus heparin in the treatment of DVT/PE: the RPR-529 study. *Thrombosis and Haemostasis*. 1997;**78**(suppl):373.

Stangier J, et al. Pharmacokinetics of BIBR 953 ZW, the active form of the oral direct thrombin inhibitor BIBR-1048, in patients undergoing hip replacement. *Journal of Thrombosis and Hemostasis*. 2003;**1**(suppl 1). Abstract P1916. [a]

Stangier J, et al. The effect of BIBR 953 ZW, the active form of the oral direct thrombin inhibitor BIBR-1048, on the prolongation of aPTT and ECT in orthopedic patients: a population pharmacodynamic study. *Journal of Thrombosis and Hemostasis*. 2003;**1**(suppl 1). Abstract P1917. [b]

Stassen JM, et al. Identification and in vitro characterization of BIBR 953 ZW, a novel synthetic low-molecular-weight direct thrombin inhibitor. *Thrombosis Hemostasis*. 2001;**6–12**. Abstract 755P. [a]

Stassen JM, et al. Pharmacodynamics of the synthetic direct thrombin inhibitor BIBR 953 ZW in healthy subjects. *Thrombosis Hemostasis*. 2001; 6–12. Abstract OC160. [b]

Stein PD, Henry JW. Prevalence of acute pulmonary embolism among patients in general hospital and at autopsy. *Chest*. 1995;**108**:978–981.

Stein PD, et al. Incidence of acute pulmonary embolism in a general hospital: relation to age, sex, and race. *Chest*. 1999;**116**(4):909–913.

Stern SH. Evaluation of the safety and efficacy of enoxaparin and warfarin for prevention of deep vein thrombosis after total knee arthroplasty. *Journal of Arthroplasty*. 2000;**15**(2):153–158.

Stratton MA, et al. Prevention of venous thromboembolism: adherence to the 1995 American College of Chest Physicians consensus guidelines for surgical patients. *Archives of Internal Medicine*. 2000;**160**:334–340.

Streptase package insert. Aventis Behring LLC; 2002.

Sudo A, et al. The incidence of deep vein thrombosis after hip and knee arthroplasties in Japanese patients: a prospective study. *Journal of Orthopaedic Surgery*. 2003;**11**:174–177.

Surkin J, et al. Spinal cord injury in Mississippi. Findings and evaluation, 1992–1994. *Spine*. 2000;**25**:716–721.

Sutton GC, et al. Clinical course and late prognosis of treated subacute massive, acute minor, and chronic pulmonary thromboembolism. *British Heart Journal*. 1977;**39**:1135–1142.

Tai NR, et al. Modern management of pulmonary embolism. *British Journal of Surgery*. 1999;**86**:853–868.

Thery C, et al. Randomized trial of subcutaneous low-molecular-weight heparin CY 216 (Fraxiparine) compared with intravenous unfractionated heparin in the curative treatment of submassive pulmonary embolism. A dose-ranging study. *Circulation*. 1992;**85**(4):1380–1389.

Thodiyil PA, et al. Thromboprophylaxis in the cancer patient. *Acta Haematologica*. 2001;**106**:73–80.

Thomas DA, et al. Venous thromboembolism. A contemporary diagnostic and therapeutic approach. *Postgraduate Medical Journal*. 1997;**102**:179–194.

Thomas RH. Hypercoagulability syndromes. *Archives of Internal Medicine*. 2001;**161**(20):2433–2439.

THRIFT (Thromboembolic Risk Factors) Consensus Group. Risk of and prophylaxis for venous thromboembolism in hospital patients. *British Medical Journal*. 1992;**305**:567–571.

THRIFT II Consensus Group. Risk of and prophylaxis for venous thromboembolism in hospital patients. *Phlebology*. 1998;**13**:87–97.

TIFDED Study Group. Thromboprophylaxis in hip fracture surgery: a pilot study comparing danaparoid, enoxaparin and dalteparin. The TIFDED Study Group. *Haemostasis*. 1999;**29**(6):310–317.

Tiret L, et al. The epidemiology of head trauma in Aquitaine (France), 1986: a community based study of hospital admissions and deaths. *International Journal of Epidemiology*. 1990;**19**:133–140.

Todd CJ, et al. Differences in mortality after fracture of hip: the East Anglian audit. *British Medical Journal*. 1995;**310**:904–908.

Torbicki A, et al. Guidelines on diagnosis and management of acute pulmonary embolism (Task Force on Pulmonary Embolism, European Society of Cardiology). *European Heart Journal*. 2000;**21**:1301–1336.

Tsai AW, et al. Cardiovascular risk factors and venous thromboembolism incidence. *Archives of Internal Medicine*. 2002;**162**:1182–1189.

Turpie AGG, et al. A randomized controlled trial of a low-molecular-weight heparin (enoxaparin) to prevent deep vein thrombosis in patients undergoing elective hip surgery. *New England Journal of Medicine*. 1986;**315**(15):925–929.

Turpie AGG. Pentasaccharide Org31540/SR90107A clinical trials update: lessons for practice. *American Heart Journal*. 2001;**142**:S9–S15. [a]

Turpie AGG, et al. A synthetic pentasaccharide for the prevention of deep vein thrombosis after total hip replacement. *New England Journal of Medicine*. 2001;**344**: 619–625. [b]

Turpie AGG, et al. Fondaparinux vs enoxaparin for the prevention of venous thromboembolism in major orthopedic surgery: a meta-analysis of 4 randomized double-blind studies. *Archives of Internal Medicine*. 2002;**162**(16):1833–1840.

Turton EPL, et al. A survey of deep venous thrombosis management by consultant vascular surgeons in the United Kingdom and Ireland. *European Journal of Vascular and Endovascular Surgery*. 2001;**21**:558–563.

United Nations. *Sex and Age Quinquennial: 1950–2050* (1998 revision). 1999.

Urokinase PE Trial Coordinators. The urokinase pulmonary embolism trial. A national cooperative study. *Circulation*. 1973;**47**(2):II1–108.

U.S. Department of Health and Human Services. *Vital and Health Statistics*. 1997:41–43.

Van Aken H, et al. Anticoagulation: the present and future. *Clinical Applied Thrombosis and Hemostasis*. 2001;**7**:195–204.

Van den Belt AGM, et al. Fixed-dose subcutaneous LMWHs versus adjusted-dose UH for VTE (Cochrane Review) In: *The Cochrane Library*, Issue 2 Oxford: Update; 1998.

Van der Meer FJM, et al. Leiden Thrombophilia Study (LETS). *Thrombosis Haemostasis*. 1997;**78**(1):631–635.

Vandenbroucke JP. Increased risk of venous thrombosis in oral contraceptive users who are carriers of factor V Leiden mutation. *Lancet*. 1994;**344**(8935):1453–1457.

Varas-Lorenzo C, et al. Hormone replacement therapy and the risk of hospitalization for venous thromboembolism: a population-based study in southern Europe. *American Journal of Epidemiology*. 1998;**147**(4):387–390.

Venet C, et al. Prevention of venous thromboembolism in polytraumatized patients. Epidemiology and importance. *La Presse medicale*. 2000;**29**(2):68–75.

Villemur B, et al. Deep venous thrombosis (DVT) after hip or knee prosthesis. Evaluation of practices for prevention and prevalence of DVT on doppler ultrasonography. *Journal des Maladies Vasculaires*. 1998;**23**(4):257–262.

Wahlander K, et al. Pharmacokinetics, pharmacodynamics and clinical effects of the oral direct thrombin inhibitor ximelagatran in acute treatment of patients with pulmonary embolism and deep vein thrombosis. *Thrombosis Research*. 2002;**107**(3–4):93–99.

Wahlander K, et al. No influence of mild-to-moderate hepatic impairment on the pharmacokinetics and pharmacodynamics of ximelagatran, an oral direct thrombin inhibitor. *Clinical Pharmacokinetics*. 2003;**42**(8):755–764.

Walenga JM, et al. Fondaparinux: a synthetic heparin pentasaccharide as a new antithrombotic agent. *Expert Opinion on Investigational Drugs*. 2002;**11**(3):397–407.

Wallentin L et al. Oral ximelagatran for secondary prophylaxis after myocardial infarction: the ESTEEM randomised controlled trial. *Lancet*. 2003;**362**(9386):789–797.

Ware JE, et al. SF-36 Health survey: manual and interpretation guide; Boston, MA: Health Institute, New England Medical Center, Nimrod Press, 1993.

Weitz JI. Low-molecular-weight heparins. *New England Journal of Medicine*. 1997;**337**:688–698.

Wells PS, et al. Graduated compression stockings in the prevention of postoperative venous thromboembolism. A meta-analysis. *Archives of Internal Medicine*. 1994;**154**(1):67–72.

Wells PS, et al. Assessment of deep vein thrombosis or pulmonary embolism by the combined use of clinical model and noninvasive diagnostic tests. *Seminars in Thrombosis and Hemostasis*. 2000;**26**(6):643–656.

Wells PS, et al. Thrombolysis in deep vein thrombosis: is there still an indication? *Thrombosis and Haemostasis*. 2001;**86**:499–508.

Wessler S, Gitel SN. Warfarin. From bedside to bench. *New England Journal of Medicine*. 1984;**311**:645–652.

Westrich GH, et al. The incidence of venous thromboembolism after total hip arthroplasty: a specific hypotensive epidural anesthesia protocol. *Journal of Arthroplasty*. 1999;**14**(4):456–463.

White RH, et al. Incidence of idiopathic deep venous thrombosis and secondary thromboembolism among ethnic groups in California. *Annals of Internal Medicine*. 1998;**128**:737–740.

White RH, et al. Incidence of symptomatic venous thromboembolism after different elective or urgent surgical procedures. *Thrombosis Haemostasis*. 2003;**90**:446–55. [a]

White RH. The epidemiology of venous thromboembolism. *Circulation*. 2003;**107**: I4–I8. [b]

Wicki J, et al. Assessing clinical probability of pulmonary embolism in the emergency ward: a simple score. *Archives of Internal Medicine*. 2001;**161**(1):92–97.

Wienen W, et al. Effects of the direct thrombin inhibitor BIBR-953ZW and its orally active pro-drug BIBR-1048MS on experimentally induced clot formation and template bleeding time in rats. *Thrombosis Hemostasis*. 2001; 6–12. Abstract 761P.

Williams EV, et al. Prevention of venous thromboembolism in Wales: results of a survey among general surgeons. *Postgraduate Medical Journal*. 2002;**78**(916):88–91.

Williams HR, MacDonald DA. Audit of thromboembolic prophylaxis in hip and knee surgery. *Annals of the Royal College of Surgeons England*. 1997;**79**(1):55–57.

Wirth T, et al. Prevention of venous thromboembolism after knee arthroscopy with low-molecular-weight heparin (reviparin): results of a randomized controlled trial. *Arthroscopy*. 2001;**17**(4):393–399.

Wong JE. Are patients with cancer receiving adequate treatment for thrombosis? Results from FRONTLINE. *Cancer Treatment Reviews*. 2003;**29**(suppl 2):11–13.

Wong PC, et al. Antithrombotic effects of razaxaban, an orally-active factor Xa inhibitor, in rabbit models of thrombosis. *Blood*. 2003;**102**:11. Abstract 3011.

Wood KA, et al. Risk of thromboembolism in chronic atrial flutter. *American Journal of Cardiology*. 1997;**79**(8):1043–1047.

Yamada N. Diagnostic procedure for acute pulmonary thromboembolism. *Heart View*. 2002;**6**(13):8–14.

GENITOURINARY

Benign Prostatic Hyperplasia

ETIOLOGY AND PATHOPHYSIOLOGY

Introduction

Benign prostatic hyperplasia (BPH) is best described as a noncancerous enlargement of the prostrate gland. Clinically, BPH manifests through lower urinary tract symptoms (LUTS), which include filling symptoms such as urinary frequency, urgency, and nocturia (night-time urination), and voiding symptoms such as decreased and intermittent force of stream and the sensation of incomplete bladder emptying. The majority of men older than age 50 have histological evidence of BPH. By age 70, 70% of men report clinical symptoms of BPH (Lam JS, 2004).

Anatomy

The prostate is approximately the size and shape of a walnut and is nestled under the bladder, anterior to the rectum. The primary function of the prostate is to secrete fluids that protect and sustain sperm while in the vagina after intercourse. Prostatic fluid is produced in the 30 to 50 secretory glands distributed throughout the prostate and is emptied directly into the urethra. The secretory glands are composed of prostatic ducts, which are lined with epithelial cells that may be secretory, basal, or neuroendocrine. Structural support for the prostrate is provided by

Wiley Handbook of Current and Emerging Drug Therapies, Volumes 5–8
Copyright © 2007 Decision Resources, Inc. Published by John Wiley & Sons, Inc.

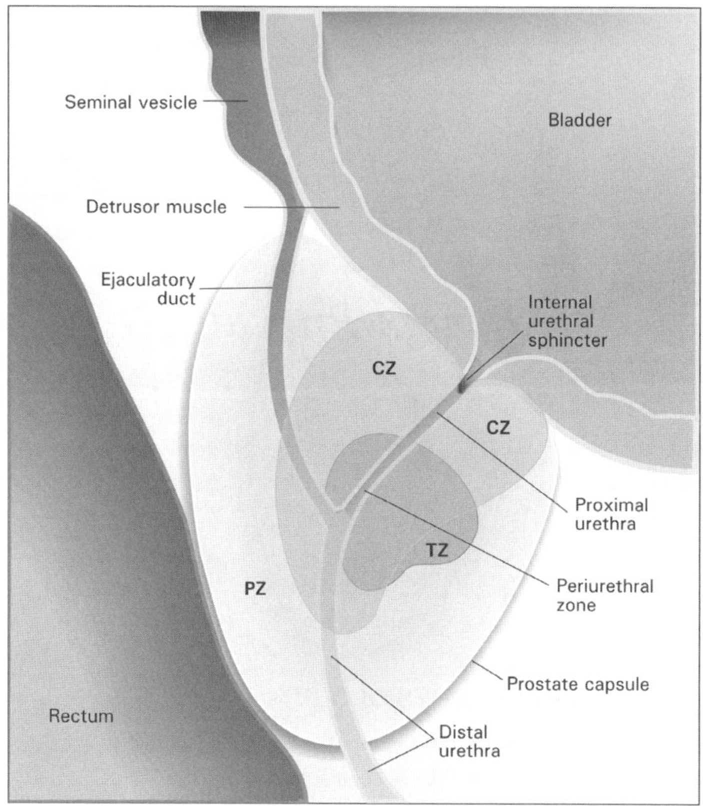

CZ = Central zone; PZ = Peripheral zone; TZ = Transitional zone.

FIGURE 1. *Anatomic location of the prostate gland.*

the stroma, which consists of smooth-muscle cells, fibroblasts, and endothelial cells and is distributed throughout the prostate around secretory glands.

As shown in Figure 1, anatomic subsections of the prostate gland that contain the epithelial and stromal cell types include the transitional zone (TZ), the central zone (CZ), and the peripheral zone (PZ). The TZ surrounds the prostatic urethra; the proximal area is called the periurethral zone. Localized enlargement of the TZ is the primary cause of bladder outlet obstruction and LUTS in men with BPH. The TZ is partially embedded in the larger, postero-inferior CZ, and both zones are encompassed by the PZ. All these zones are surrounded by the fibromuscular prostate capsule.

Components of BPH

Two pathological activities—static BPH and dynamic BPH—occur in the prostate and contribute individually or collectively to urinary symptoms (Figure 2). Histological investigation can determine which activity is taking

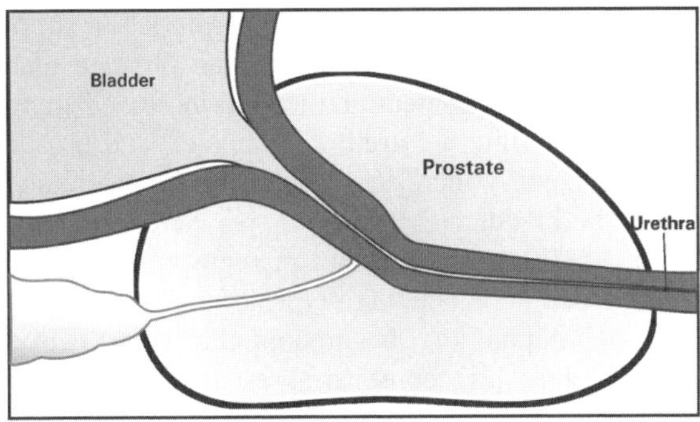

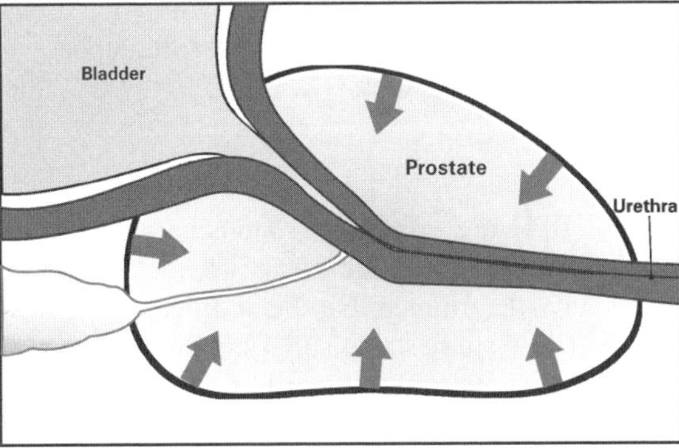

FIGURE 2. *Mechanisms of static and dynamic benign prostatic hyperplasia.*

place, but physicians usually assume, without histological testing, that both are happening.

Static BPH. Histologically, in static BPH, noncancerous hyperplasia (an increase in the number of cells) in the epithelial and stromal components of the prostate gland cause the organ to enlarge and, in most cases, impede the urethra. Static obstruction, resulting from the hyperplasia of prostatic epithelial tissue, is stimulated by androgen receptor activation in the prostate. The subsequent enlargement of the gland causes mechanical obstruction by impeding urinary flow from the bladder. This subtype of BPH, also known as androgen-dependent BPH, can involve significant enlargement of the prostate.

The primary active androgen in the prostate is dihydrotestosterone (DHT), which the enzyme 5-alpha-reductase converts from testosterone. Two 5-alpha-reductase isoenzymes exist: type 1 is found in most tissues; type 2 is found predominantly in the prostate and other genital tissues. The relevance of each isoenzyme to the pathophysiology of BPH remains to be determined—but selective inhibition of 5-alpha-reductase type 2 by finasteride (Merck's [Whitehouse Station, New Jersey] Proscar) reduces prostate size, which suggests that this isoenzyme has an important role in BPH.

Dynamic BPH. Dynamic obstruction, caused by the hyperplasia of stromal prostate tissue, may not lead to significant enlargement of the prostate gland, but it can increase prostatic smooth-muscle content and lead to increased smooth muscle contraction in the bladder neck (internal urethral sphincter) and prostatic capsule. Dynamic BPH is characterized by increased tension in the prostate and obstruction of urinary flow from the bladder.

Smooth-muscle contraction in the bladder neck and prostate is mediated by $alpha_1$-adrenergic receptors (adrenoceptors). The three types of $alpha_1$-adrenergic receptors are $alpha_{1A}$, $-_{1B}$, and $-_{1D}$. $Alpha_{1A}$ is the predominant subtype in the prostate; $alpha_{1D}$ and, in particular, $alpha_{1B}$ receptors are present in smaller quantities (Kirby R, 2000). In addition, there is a putative $alpha_{1L}$-adrenoceptor with activity similar to that of $alpha_{1A}$. Evidence exists that blocking only the $alpha_{1A}$ receptor may not relieve BPH symptoms and that inhibition of the $alpha_{1L}$ and $alpha_{1D}$ receptors may be important (Chess-Williams R, 2002; Kirby R, 2000).

Etiology

The exact mechanisms that cause BPH are unknown. Extensive research indicates that hormonal changes and increasing age are clear risk factors for BPH development. Cell culture studies have determined that the androgen DHT has an important role in prostatic growth. These studies also suggest other effects of this hormone on BPH etiology, such as disruption of the equilibrium between serum testosterone and estrogen levels and changes in cell proliferation and/or apoptosis rates. The activity of growth factors is also suspected of contributing to prostate hyperplasia; deficiency or overexpression of certain growth factors significantly changes the rate of cell multiplication and cell death. Cellular senescence also affects apoptosis; as a result of this process, prostate cells do not respond to signals that initiate apoptosis.

Dihydrotestosterone. The presence of androgens evidently influences the development of BPH. Men who are incapable of androgen activity (because of genetic mutations) or are castrated before puberty do not experience prostatic hyperplasia (endotext.org, 2004). From the embryonic stage through adulthood, prostate growth is mediated by androgens. Furthermore, pharmacological inhibition of androgen produces a clinical response in BPH patients. These findings support the hypothesis that the androgen DHT is a key player in the development of BPH.

Conversion of the steroid hormone testosterone to its active form, DHT, is catalyzed by the enzyme 5-alpha-reductase. 5-Alpha-reductase activity is seven times greater in BPH tissue than in normal tissue (Lee KL, 2004). DHT binds to soluble androgen receptors in the prostate, stimulating protein synthesis and epithelial cell multiplication. Because DHT has a higher affinity than testosterone for androgen receptors, prostate concentrations of DHT are sustained despite the major decline in the plasma level of testosterone that occurs as men age. Drug therapies, such as 5-alpha-reductase inhibitors (5-ARIs), have been designed to counteract the increased activity of 5-alpha-reductase in BPH.

Estrogen/Androgen Ratio. As a man ages, a growing imbalance develops between levels of estrogen and androgen. Approximately 75–90% of estradiol, the most active form of estrogen, is derived in men through the conversion of testicular and adrenal testosterone by an aromatase enzyme. The remaining estrogen is synthesized directly in the testes. Even as the level of free testosterone drops in aging men, estrogen levels remain relatively stable. As a result, the ratio of free estradiol to testosterone is 40% greater in older men than in younger men. Researchers hypothesize that the shift in the estrogen/androgen ratio causes the adverse effects of estrogen on the prostate.

Animal studies have demonstrated that estrogens are associated with abnormal cell proliferation and/or prostate cancer. In dogs, estrogen increases the sensitivity of the prostate gland to androgens (endotext.org, 2004). Testosterone/estradiol binding globulin (TeBG) functions as a transporter for androgens and estradiol. Researchers have proposed that with less androgen present in the aging male, there is an increase in the amount of TeBG bound to androgen receptors on the prostatic stroma. With less competition from androgens, estradiol binds the TeBG-receptor complex, activating the androgen receptor even in the absence of DHT. Estradiol also activates estrogen receptors in stromal and epithelial cells of the PZ and TZ. This alternative pathway may account for the continued growth of the prostate gland in the aging male.

Hormone therapy for BPH continues to be an area of interest for drug developers. Currently, chlormadinone acetate (Teikoku Pharma's [San Jose, California] Prostal/Prostal L), which is available only in Japan, is the only agent that directly affects the level of testosterone. Greater control of the ratio of estrogen to androgen may be important in the treatment of BPH.

Gonadotropic Hormones. Gonadotropic hormones—follicle-stimulating hormone (FSH), luteinizing hormone (LH), and chorionic gonadotropin (CG)—released from the pituitary gland induce prostatic tissue growth and function. Experimental evidence supports a potential role for their involvement in BPH development. The action of these hormones on the prostatic tissue is stimulated by the hypothalamic production of gonadotropic-releasing hormones (e.g., luteinizing hormone-releasing hormone [LHRH]). An increase of gonadotropic hormones in the blood stimulates the synthesis of testosterone in the prostate; testosterone signaling results in transcription of growth factors and cell cycle genes, both of which control the growth of prostatic tissue (Bartsch G, 2000).

Other Hormones. Other hormone-stimulated pathways may offer potential targets for BPH therapy. For example, vitamin D3 (1,25-dihydroxyvitamin-D3 [1,25(OH)2D3]) is a key regulator of cellular proliferation and differentiation. Modification of vitamin D3 activity with specific analogues prevents the occurrence of hypercalcemia while inhibiting growth of prostate cells (Crescioli C, 2003).

Growth Factors. BPH is defined by prostate enlargement as a result of prostatic tissue proliferation. Cell culture studies suggest that the rate of prostatic tissue proliferation is mediated by various growth factors, and different growth factors have been observed acting on a range of cell types. Fibroblast growth factors 2 and 7 (FGF-2 and FGF-7) are overexpressed in BPH stromal and epithelial cells (Lee KL, 2004). FGF-7 has been shown to correlate strongly with epithelial proliferation. Investigation of insulin-like growth factors (IGFs) indicates that messenger RNA (mRNA) expression of IGF-I receptor and IGF-II is higher in BPH tissue samples than in normal samples (Lee KL, 2004). Researchers hypothesize that changes in the IGF equilibrium may have a significant impact on BPH etiology, but no direct relationship has been established. Angiogenic activity (the formation of new blood vessels) in the prostate, which supports stromal and epithelial cell proliferation, is influenced by a decrease in anti-angiogenic factors and an increase in vascular endothelial growth factor (VEGF; an angiogenic factor).

Cellular Senescence. Recent studies have explored the role of cellular senescence in BPH. An examination of BPH tissues with beta-galactosidase, a biomarker associated with senescence, revealed positive staining for these cells (Lee KL, 2004). Senescent epithelial cells retain normal metabolic activity; however, they exhibit dysfunctional apoptosis as a result of their inability to respond to cell death signals (Lee KL, 2004). These cells were found to induce the secretion of FGF-7, which is responsible for enhancing epithelial proliferation. More senescent cells were observed in enlarged prostates (total mass greater than 55 g) than in smaller prostates. Greater understanding of the role of cellular senescence in BPH would create opportunities for drugs with new mechanisms of action.

Pathophysiology

Symptoms and Assessment. Clinical BPH is characterized by lower urinary tract symptoms (LUTS). As the prostate enlarges, the surrounding fibromuscular capsule stops it from expanding, causing the gland to press against the urethra and prompting obstruction and/or irritation of normal urinary flow. Failure of the lower urinary tract to empty the bladder—caused by both static and dynamic BPH—results in LUTS, which can be irritative and/or obstructive in nature. Irritative symptoms, also known as storage or filling symptoms, include urinary urgency, frequency, nocturia, dysuria, and burning. Obstructive symptoms, also known as voiding symptoms, include hesitancy, weak stream, straining, dribbling, and incomplete emptying. Although BPH is not the only cause of LUTS, it is the most common cause.

Symptom severity is measured by International Prostate Symptom Scores (IPSS), assessed by responses to a 35-point questionnaire. Scores ranging from 0 to 7, 8 to 19, and 20 to 35 indicate mild, moderate, and severe disease, respectively. Physicians use the scores to measure baseline disease severity, choose medical therapy, and gauge improvement. In general, the severity of BPH symptoms and the degree of urethral obstruction do not necessarily correlate with the size of the prostate.

Complications of BPH. BPH is associated with a variety of complications. Research has shown that patients with severe BPH and high prostate volume are at risk of experiencing acute urinary retention (AUR), which is considered the most severe stage of the disease. AUR is painful, and surgery may be required to reduce the obstruction and restore urine flow. Chronic urinary retention is not as painful as AUR; however, it can damage bladder muscles (detrusors), creating dysfunctional muscle contraction and an inability to void adequately. Also, chronic retention can cause further complications, such as recurrent urinary tract infections (UTIs), bladder stones, renal failure, and incontinence. Hematuria (blood in the urine) is another complication of BPH, owing to the increased angiogenic activity and the high probability of rupturing delicate prostatic blood vessels (endotext.org, 2004). Although most men with prostate cancer also have BPH, there is no evidence to suggest that men with BPH are more likely to develop cancer.

CURRENT THERAPIES

Treatment of benign prostatic hyperplasia (BPH) is directed primarily toward managing symptoms and improving patients' quality of life (QoL). The two dominating classes of pharmacological agents used to treat BPH are alpha blockers and 5-alpha-reductase inhibitors (5-ARIs). Both drug classes are effective in alleviating lower urinary tract symptoms (LUTS) associated with BPH, thereby improving patients' comfort level. Alpha blockers are most useful in alleviating symptoms related to dynamic BPH; 5-ARIs are used for the treatment of static BPH. The dynamic and static forms of BPH are discussed in the "Etiology and Pathophysiology" section.

Alpha blockers work by relaxing prostatic muscle involved in dynamic BPH; they cannot stop further growth of the prostate. 5-ARIs and gonadotropin modulators (used only in Japan) reduce the cellular growth seen in static BPH. LUTS are caused by bladder outlet obstruction due to prostate hyperplasia. If patients exhibit symptoms and have enlarged prostates (observed through digital rectal exam), physicians assume that they are afflicted with both static and dynamic BPH. Clinical trials have been conducted to investigate the effects of combination therapy with alpha blockers and 5-ARIs to relieve symptoms and reduce prostate volume. Also available for BPH treatment are phytopharmaceutical agents and herbal remedies; little is known of their true efficacy and long-term side effects, but available research suggests that they mimic the action of 5-ARIs. Phytopharmaceuticals are used, sometimes in combination with alpha-blocker therapy, in patients with milder disease who require a more benign side-effect profile. Table 1 summarizes the leading therapies available to treat BPH; and Figure 3 identifies symptomatic BPH targets for drug intervention.

The three primary end points used in most clinical trials of agents that target BPH are the post-treatment urinary symptom scores, post-treatment average peak urinary flow rate (Qmax), and the percentage of patients who experience a clinically meaningful improvement in these two measures. These patients (also identified as "clinical responders") achieve at least a 25% reduction in either the International Prostate Symptom Scores (IPSS) or the American Urological Association's Symptom Index (AUASI) and at least a 30% increase in Qmax. Clinical trials investigating the effects of 5-ARIs, gonadotropin modulators, and

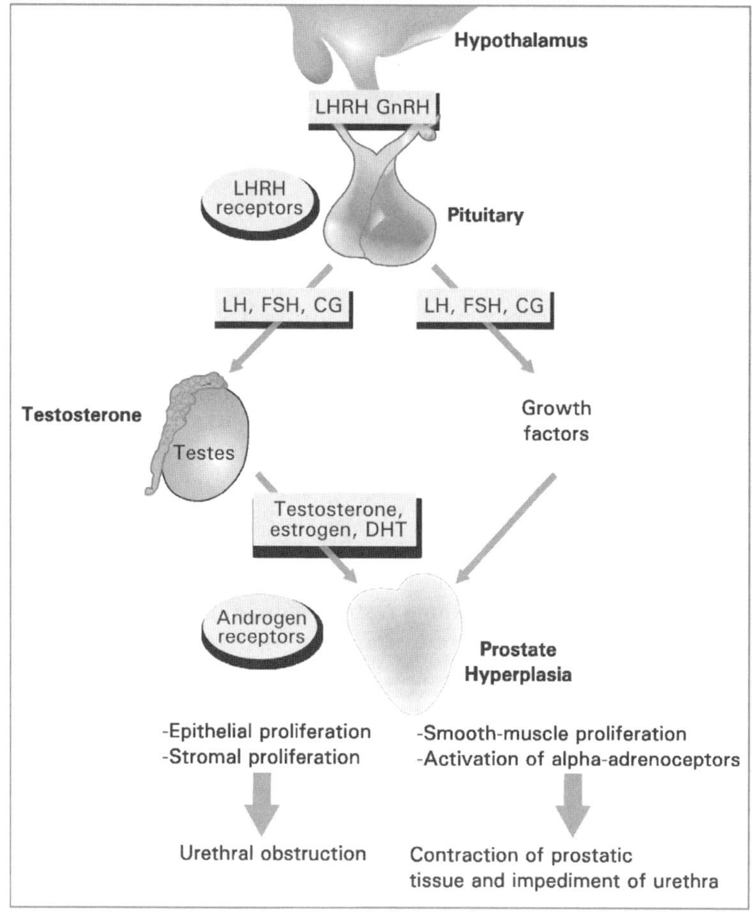

LH = Luteinizing hormone.
LHRH = Luteinizing hormone-releasing hormone.
GnRH = Gonadotropin-releasing hormone.
FSH = Folicle-stimulating hormone.
CG = Chorionic gonadotropin.
DHT = Dihydrotestosterone.

FIGURE 3. *Targets for drug intervention in symptomatic benign prostatic hyperplasia.*

TABLE 1. Select Marketed Agents Used to Treat Benign Prostatic Hyperplasia

Agent	Company/Brand	Daily Dose	Availability
Alpha blockers			
Tamsulosin	Astellas/Boehringer Ingelheim/ Abbott's Harnal/Flomax/Omnic	400 µg qd, 200 µg qd in Japan	US, F, G, I, S, UK, J
Alfuzosin	Sanofi-Aventis's Xatral/Uroxatral, others	2.5 mg tid, 5 mg bid, 10 mg qd	US, F, G, I, S, UK
Terazosin	Abbott's Hytrin, generics	1–10 mg qd or bid	US, F, G, I, S, UK, J
Doxazosin	Pfizer's Cardura/Cardura XL, generics	1–8 mg qd	US, F, G, I, S, UK, J
Naftopidil	Asahi Kasei's Flivas, Kanebo's Avishot	25–50 mg qd	J
Prazosin	Pfizer's Minipress, generics	1 mg qd or bid	US, F, G, I, S, UK, J
Indoramin	GlaxoSmithKline's Doralese	20 mg bid	UK
5-alpha-reductase inhibitors			
Finasteride	Merck's Proscar	5 mg qd	US, F, G, I, S, UK
Dutasteride	GlaxoSmithKline/Astellas' Avodart	0.5 mg qd	US, F, G, I, S, UK
Gonadotropin modulators			
Chlormidinone acetate	Teikoku's Prostal/Prostal L	50 mg qd	J

bid = Twice daily; mg = Milligrams; qd = Once daily; tid = Three times daily; µg = Micrograms. US = United States; F = France; G = Germany; I – Italy; S = Spain; UK = United Kingdom; J = Japan.

phytopharmaceuticals have the additional end point of reduced prostate volume because these drugs act by reducing hyperplasia.

Using questionnaires such as the AUASI or the IPSS is the most common method of assessing symptom severity. Patients and physicians rate symptoms on a scale of 1 to 5 for a maximum score of 35. The questionnaires differ in that the IPSS has one additional question that evaluates patient QoL. Patients rate their quality of life on a scale of 1 to 6, but the result is not added to the total symptom score. The two symptom scoring systems are considered equally adequate in evaluating LUTS. Another tool that was sometimes used in earlier clinical trials is the Boyarsky symptom score, which allows 0 to 3 points for each of nine questions for a maximum of 27 points.

Alpha Blockers

Overview. Numerous alpha blockers have been approved for the treatment of BPH in the major pharmaceutical markets (United States, France, Germany, Italy, Spain, United Kingdom, and Japan), largely replacing the need for surgical treatment in the past ten years. Alpha blockers, with tamsulosin as the leading agent, currently constitute the largest segment of the BPH drug market. Alpha-blocker drugs may differ in terms of their relative inhibitory potency and specificity for alpha$_1$-adrenergic receptors, but most seem to exhibit the same degree of efficacy in BPH patients (Clifford GM, 2000). However, the propensity for inducing side effects, such as orthostatic hypotension and retrograde ejaculation, often distinguishes one alpha blocker from another. Nevertheless, alpha-blocker activity is sustained over several years of therapy, thereby eliminating the need for dose increases that could increase side effects.

Mechanism of Action. Alpha blockers inhibit the activity of adrenergic receptors (also known as adrenoceptors), which cause smooth-muscle contraction when bound to the neurotransmitter norepinephrine. Adrenoceptors are categorized into alpha$_1$, alpha$_2$, and beta subtypes. Overstimulation of certain subtypes of alpha$_1$-adrenergic receptors (alpha$_{1A}$, alpha$_{1D}$, and alpha$_{1L}$) is largely responsible for the obstructive symptoms associated with the dynamic component of BPH.

Alpha$_{1A}$-adrenergic receptors are found in the prostate, where they are the dominant adrenoceptor subtype, and in the smooth muscle of the vascular system. The prostate also has alpha$_{1D}$-adrenergic receptors, but fewer than the number of its receptors for subtype alpha$_{1A}$. Alpha$_{1D}$-adrenergic receptors are also found in bladder muscles. Alpha$_{1B}$-adrenergic receptors are located throughout the central nervous system. When these adrenoceptors are triggered, they cause the prostatic smooth muscle and the bladder to contract, which can lead to clinical manifestations of LUTS.

Adrenoceptors are also present in other tissues; alpha$_{1B}$-adrenoceptors occur in the heart, spleen, kidney, blood vessel, and lung tissue. Inhibition of adrenoceptors in these tissues leads to the significant adverse effects associated with alpha blockers—most notably, orthostatic hypotension. As a result of vasodilation, patients may experience dizziness, postural hypotension (which may cause loss of balance and injury from falling), and/or syncope (blackout).

The development of subtype-selective alpha blockers (e.g., tamsulosin [Astellas Pharma (Tokyo, Japan)/Boehringer Ingelheim (Ingelheim, Germany)/Abbott Laboratories's (Abbott Park, llinois)] and alfuzosin [Sanofi-Aventis's (Tokyo, Japan)]) has reduced the risk of orthostatic hypotension that researchers believe results primarily from activation of the alpha$_{1B}$-adrenergic receptors. Table 2 lists alpha-blocker agents, the alpha-adrenergic receptor subtypes they bind, and the tissues where they are found.

Tamsulosin. Tamsulosin (Astellas/Boehringer Ingelheim/Abbott's Harnal/Flomax/Omnic), the leading alpha blocker, is a long-acting alpha blocker that is selective for alpha$_{1A}$- and alpha$_{1D}$-adrenoceptors found predominantly in the prostate. Astellas (formerly Yamanouchi) initially marketed tamsulosin in an immediate-release formulation (Harnal) in Japan and Europe. Boehringer Ingelheim also markets tamsulosin in the United States as a delayed-release formulation (Flomax) to provide more consistent drug levels after each dose (Lee M, 2000). In 1999, Abbott entered an agreement with Boehringer Ingelheim to comarket Flomax in the United States.

Tamsulosin selectively binds to alpha$_{1A}$- and alpha$_{1D}$-adrenergic receptors, thereby blocking activation by norepinephrine. This highly selective drug reduces

TABLE 2. Alpha Blocker Agents and Their Alpha-Adrenergic Receptor Subtype Binding and Localization

Agent	Alpha-Adrenergic Receptor Subtype/Localization
Tamsulosin	$Alpha_{1A}$: prostatic stroma, detrusor muscle, vascular smooth muscle, spinal cord $Alpha_{1D}$: prostatic stroma, detrusor muscle, spinal cord
Alfuzosin	$Alpha_{1A}$: prostatic stroma, detrusor muscle, vascular smooth muscle, spinal cord $Alpha_{1B}$: central nervous system, spleen, kidneys, lungs, heart, vascular smooth muscle, spinal cord, nonhyperplastic prostatic epithelial cells $Alpha_{1D}$: prostatic stroma, detrusor muscle, spinal cord
Terazosin	$Alpha_{1A}$: prostatic stroma, detrusor muscle, vascular smooth muscle, spinal cord $Alpha_{1B}$: central nervous system, spleen, kidneys, lungs, heart, vascular smooth muscle, spinal cord, nonhyperplastic prostatic epithelial cells $Alpha_{1D}$: prostatic stroma, detrusor muscle, spinal cord
Doxazosin	$Alpha_{1A}$: prostatic stroma, detrusor muscle, vascular smooth muscle, spinal cord $Alpha_{1B}$: central nervous system, spleen, kidneys, lungs, heart, vascular smooth muscle, spinal cord, nonhyperplastic prostatic epithelial cells $Alpha_{1D}$: prostatic stroma, detrusor muscle, spinal cord
Naftopidil	$Alpha_{1A}$: prostatic stroma, detrusor muscle, vascular smooth muscle, spinal cord $Alpha_{1D}$: prostatic stroma, detrusor muscle, spinal cord
Prazosin	$Alpha_{1A}$: prostatic stroma, detrusor muscle, vascular smooth muscle, spinal cord $Alpha_{1B}$: central nervous system, spleen, kidneys, lungs, heart, vascular smooth muscle, spinal cord, nonhyperplastic prostatic epithelial cells $Alpha_{1F}$: to be determined
Indoramin	$Alpha_{1A}$: prostatic stroma, detrusor muscle, vascular smooth muscle, spinal cord $Alpha_{1B}$: central nervous system, spleen, kidneys, lungs, heart, vascular smooth muscle, spinal cord, nonhyperplastic prostatic epithelial cells $Alpha_{1D}$: prostatic stroma, detrusor muscle, spinal cord

the incidence of adverse events because it does not affect $alpha_{1B}$-adrenoceptors located in blood vessels, spleen, or lungs to a significant extent. Tamsulosin's efficacy is only marginally better than that of other alpha blockers, but it offers a superior side-effect profile.

In a 13-week, parallel-design, double-blind trial, 756 patients with moderate to severe BPH symptoms (AUASI >13 and Qmax between 4 and 15 mL/s) were randomized to receive a daily dose of 0.4 mg of tamsulosin, 0.8 mg of tamsulosin, or placebo (Lepor H, 1998[a]). At the end of the treatment period, results showed that tamsulosin significantly alleviated symptoms as measured by the AUASI. Trial results were as follows:

- AUASI and Qmax in the tamsulosin groups were significantly better than in the placebo group ($p < 0.012$).
- Seventy percent of patients taking 0.4 mg of tamsulosin daily and 74% of patients taking 0.8 mg of tamsulosin daily had a clinically meaningful reduction in AUASI; only 51% of patients taking placebo achieved the same result.
- Thirty-one percent of patients taking 0.4 mg of tamsulosin and 36% of patients taking 0.8 mg of tamsulosin were considered responders in terms of Qmax; these patients experienced at least a 30% increase in peak urinary flow rate. Only 21% of patients taking placebo were clinical responders in terms of Qmax.

The number of patients who experienced adverse events was almost negligible:

- One out of 254 patients treated with 0.4 mg of tamsulosin and 2 out of 248 patients treated with 0.8 mg of tamsulosin experienced orthostatic hypotension (a decrease in blood pressure while standing) during the 13-week period.
- Four, six, and two patients from the 0.4 mg tamsulosin group, the 0.8 mg tamsulosin group, and the placebo group, respectively, had serious adverse effects such as overdose, cancerous development, effects involving hospitalization or fatality, or life-threatening or permanently disabling events.

Upon completion of the 13-week, double-blind phase of this study, 418 patients continued their treatment for an additional 40-week, double-blind, extension phase (Lepor H, 1998[b]). Researchers found that, by 13 weeks, the effect of tamsulosin on AUASI and Qmax achieved maximum response rates. Beyond that, the level of efficacy was maintained. Findings of this extension study were as follows:

- Treatment with 0.4 mg of tamsulosin resulted in an average decrease of 9.4 points in AUASI, and treatment with 0.8 mg of tamsulosin resulted in an average decrease of 9.7 points in AUASI, compared with an average decrease of 6.5 for patients receiving placebo ($p < 0.001$).
- Eighty-one percent of patients treated with a daily dose of 0.4 mg of tamsulosin and 78% of patients treated with a daily dose of 0.8 mg of tamsulosin were considered responders in terms of AUASI. Only 59% of patients receiving placebo had clinically meaningful AUASI improvement.
- Within the active treatment groups, the percentage of nonresponders who developed a clinical response was greater than the percentage of responders who became nonresponders (43% and 6%, respectively). In the placebo

group, similar percentages of responders and nonresponders switched status: 21% of responders became nonresponders; 23% of nonresponders became responders.

- Forty percent of patients treated with a daily dose of 0.4 mg of tamsulosin and 39% of patients treated with a daily dose of 0.8 mg of tamsulosin achieved at least a 30% increase in Qmax. Only 22% of patients receiving placebo had clinically meaningful Qmax improvement.

At the end of the 40-week extension study, researchers concluded that continued exposure to tamsulosin was not related to a significantly increased risk of adverse events. They reported the following data on side effects:

- The most commonly reported side effect was infection, which occurred in 36% of patients taking tamsulosin and 27% of patients taking placebo.
- No patients in the placebo group reported abnormal ejaculation; however, 10% of patients in the 0.4 mg tamsulosin group and 26% in the 0.8 mg tamsulosin group had at least one episode of abnormal ejaculation.
- No new occurrences of orthostatic hypotension were observed.

Comparator studies with tamsulosin have shown that it has a more favorable side-effect profile than other selective alpha blockers (Buzelin JM, 1997). A 14-week, multicenter, double-blind, parallel-group Phase III trial compared the safety and efficacy of tamsulosin and alfuzosin. Two hundred and eighty patients were randomized to receive 0.4 mg of tamsulosin once daily or 2.5 mg of alfuzosin two to three times daily. Boyarsky symptom scores and Qmax were examined after 2, 6, and 12 weeks of treatment. The Boyarsky tool allows 0 to 3 points for each of 9 questions for a maximum of 27 points. Results indicated that both treatment groups exhibited a significant improvement in symptom scores, compared with baseline values, at each visit ($p < 0.001$), but alfuzosin—not tamsulosin—demonstrated negative effects on blood pressure. Study results were as follows:

- Approximately 70% of patients in each group had at least 25% reduction in their baseline symptom score after 14 weeks. The average reduction in total Boyarsky symptom score was 4.1 for patients treated with tamsulosin and 3.8 for patients treated with alfuzosin.
- A significant increase in Qmax relative to baseline was seen in both tamsulosin-treated and alfuzosin-treated patients ($p < 0.001$): approximately 1.6 mL/s for both groups. Patients treated with tamsulosin reached maximal Qmax within two weeks; patients treated with alfuzosin reached maximal Qmax between two and six weeks. Approximately 35% of patients in each group had at least 30% improvement in their baseline Qmax after 14 weeks.

- Tamsulosin did not change patients' average blood pressure, and alfuzosin treatment produced significant blood pressure changes in older men and normotensive men. Patients 65 and older experienced an average change in standing systolic and diastolic blood pressure of $-9.7/-6.2$ mm Hg; men younger than 65 years had an average change of $-1.1/-3.0$. Hypotensive men with a supine diastolic blood pressure less than 95 mm Hg experienced an average change in standing blood pressure of $-3.2/-2.3$ mm Hg after taking alfuzosin, and men taking tamsulosin had an average blood pressure change of $-0.2/-0.2$ mm Hg.

The long-term (up to six years) safety and efficacy of tamsulosin—important because tamsulosin is often used chronically—were assessed in a multicenter, open-label, four-year extension trial (Narayan P, 2003). Patients had previously completed a one-year, open-label trial followed by either a 17-week or a 40-week double-blind study. Efficacy results were similar to those of other studies with tamsulosin. Twenty-nine patients (4.8%) experienced what were considered serious adverse events, such as skin or prostate cancer, syncope, myocardial infarction, or chest pain. Five patients (0.8%) discontinued treatment because of abnormal ejaculation. Another clinical study reported that 10% of patients taking 0.4 mg of tamsulosin and 26% of patients taking 0.8 mg had at least one episode of abnormal ejaculation (Lepor H, 1998[b]).

The risk of retrograde ejaculation increases with tamsulosin therapy because of the agent's relaxation of the bladder neck. Retrograde ejaculation does not necessarily reduce quality of life, however, and some patients see it as a sign that drug therapy is working.

Alfuzosin. The original formulation of alfuzosin, marketed in Europe since 1997, is a uroselective agent that is taken three times daily. In 2000, Sanofi-Synthélabo (now Sanofi-Aventis) launched a twice-daily, sustained-release formulation of alfuzosin, Xatral SR, in the United Kingdom, Spain, and Germany. A once-daily, controlled-release formulation of alfuzosin—called Xatral OD in the United States and Xatral XL in Europe—was developed using SkyePharma, Inc's (San Diego, California) Geomatrix technology. Xatral XL has been launched in the United Kingdom, France, Italy, and Germany. The initial European approvals triggered a milestone payment to SkyePharma from Sanofi-Aventis; SkyePharma will also receive royalty payments from product sales. In the United States, the FDA approved a new drug application (NDA) for Xatral OD in June 2003, and the agent launched in November 2003. Alfuzosin has been licensed to Astellas Pharma in Japan and is currently undergoing clinical investigation.

Alfuzosin's uroselectivity appears to be achieved through preferential distribution in prostate tissue, which allows it to have efficacy and safety comparable to that of tamsulosin. Although uroselective, alfuzosin binds $alpha_{1B}$ receptors in addition to 1A and 1D; therefore, more patients taking alfuzosin experience orthostatic hypertension than patients taking tamsulosin, which is selective for receptor 1A and 1D subtypes.

In a study published in 2000, researchers examined the safety and efficacy of the sustained-release (SR) formulation of alfuzosin in 3,095 Spanish patients with LUTS who had symptomatic BPH (Sanchez-Chapado M, 2000). The multicenter, observational Phase IV study had an active treatment period of 60 days (5 mg, three times daily). The study used the Spanish IPSS to evaluate symptoms and assessed health-related QoL using a QoL index. At the end of the study, there was a significant decrease in IPSS scores, but the absence of a placebo control should be considered when interpreting these trial results. The placebo effect in published BPH trials tends to be high. Results of this study were as follows:

- Significant decreases in IPSS scores were observed in 60% of the patients, in accord with notable improvements in the QoL index.
- Adverse events were reported in 82 patients (2.6%). Postural events— including vertigo, postural hypotension, headache, and dizziness—were reported in 55 of the patients (1.8%). Effects on sexual function were not significant, and only one patient experienced impotence. During the study, 49 (1.6%) patients dropped out because of adverse events. This large study confirms the safety and efficacy of treating BPH patients with alfuzosin SR.

A three-month, placebo-controlled study of 447 patients with symptomatic BPH demonstrated the comparable efficacy and safety of once-daily alfuzosin (10 mg) and the original three-times-daily alfuzosin (2.5 mg) (van Kerrebroeck P, 2000). Once-daily alfuzosin and the original formulation significantly lowered the IPSS (−6.9 and −6.4, respectively; placebo, −4.9) and raised Qmax (+2.3 and + 3.2 mL/s, respectively; placebo, + 1.4 mL/s); however, a lower incidence of vasodilatory side effects was observed in patients receiving alfuzosin once daily (6.3% versus 9.4%).

This study was extended for nine months in an open-label trial involving 311 patients. All patients received 10 mg of extended-release alfuzosin. IPSS decreased significantly from a baseline mean of 17.1 at the start of the placebo-controlled trial to a mean of 9.3 at the end of the nine-month extension. Mean Qmax increased 2.2 mL/s from the beginning of the placebo-controlled study. In light of these results, it is not surprising that the QoL index also improved significantly. Alfuzosin once daily was well tolerated, with orthostatic hypotension observed in only 2.8% of patients and 4.4% of patients experiencing adverse events, possibly related to drug treatment (mostly dizziness).

In a three-month trial that examined the safety and efficacy of alfuzosin once daily, 536 patients were randomized to receive alfuzosin (10 mg or 15 mg once-daily) or placebo (Roehrborn CG, 2001). At the end of the study, the mean reduction in IPSS for 10 mg alfuzosin, 15 mg alfuzosin, and placebo was −3.6, −3.4, and −1.6, respectively. A significant increase in Qmax was also observed with alfuzosin 10 mg and 15 mg, compared with placebo: + 1.1 mL/s, + 1.0 mL/s, and 0.0 mL/s, respectively. Importantly, alfuzosin was well tolerated; the incidence of orthostatic hypotension was similar among the three groups, and no abnormal ejaculation was observed.

The relative risk of orthostatic hypotension for each BPH patient is taken into consideration when selecting the most suitable alpha blocker agent. Loss of blood pressure that causes dizziness, loss of balance, and blackout puts the patient at risk of physical injury. Because alfuzosin acts locally in the prostate, it is often prescribed to normotensive patients.

Terazosin. Terazosin (Abbott's Hytrin, generics) (Figure 4) is a long-acting, alpha$_1$-adrenergic-receptor blocker with a prolonged half-life that permits once-daily dosing. Abbott markets terazosin in the United States and several European countries; Mitsubishi-Tokyo Pharmaceuticals (Tokyo, Japan) is the licensee in Japan. In March 2000, the FDA granted Mylan approval to market its generic version of terazosin; since then, several other generics have launched.

The Hytrin Community Assessment Trial (HYCAT), a 12-month, multicenter study, was conducted in the United States to investigate the clinical effectiveness of terazosin therapy (Roehrborn CG, 1996). Two thousand and eighty-four patients with AUASI scores greater than 12 (moderate to severe symptoms of BPH) were randomized to terazosin, titrated to 10 mg, or to placebo. For patients unable to tolerate high-dose terazosin, 5 mg tablets were administered instead of 10 mg. Periodic assessments during the 12-month treatment period showed a significant difference in AUASI scores between the active treatment group and the placebo group at every follow-up visit. The researchers reported the following results:

- At the end of the trial, terazosin treatment had reduced AUASI scores by 7.6 points; placebo treatment had reduced scores by 3.7 points. Of the patients taking terazosin, 55% achieved a 35% improvement in AUASI; only 28% of patients taking placebo achieved the same clinical response.

- Qmax was also measured, and terazosin was shown to increase peak urinary flow by 2.2 mL/s, while placebo increased flow by 0.8 mL/s. Forty percent of patients treated with terazosin and 26.4% of patients treated with placebo experienced an increased Qmax of at least 3 mL/s.

- A small proportion of patients did not complete the study because of lack of efficacy or intolerable side effects. The most frequently reported drug-related adverse events were dizziness and asthenia (weakness of the body).

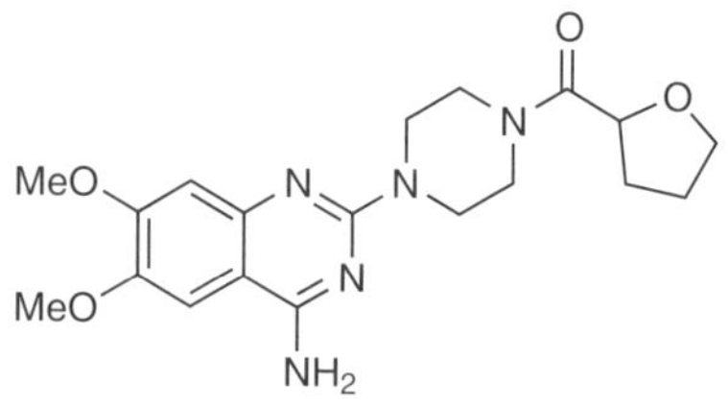

FIGURE 4. *Structure of terazosin.*

Incidence of urinary tract infections (UTIs) caused by bladder outlet obstruction increased twofold in the placebo group, compared with the terazosin group ($p = 0.03$). Ten men taking placebo and one taking terazosin experienced myocardial infarction ($p = 0.01$). Although systolic and diastolic blood pressure decreased slightly from baseline in patients treated with terazosin, this change was statistically significant ($p < 0.001$).

Data from more than 1600 patients treated with terazosin (1–20 mg/day) for a total of 1282 years of patient exposure suggest that terazosin is relatively safe compared with other alpha blockers; the main side effects of dizziness, loss of strength, and peripheral edema occurred in 10.7%, 7.5%, and 4.0% of patients, respectively (McKiernan JM, 1997). These conditions are related to the reduction in blood pressure induced by terazosin therapy. Lower occurrence rates of side effects related to hypotension are observed with tamsulosin and alfuzosin treatment. Patients receiving terazosin also experience a significantly lower risk of sexual dysfunction than is associated with other alpha blockers (Clifford GM, 2000). A particular advantage noted with terazosin therapy is a notably reduced risk of UTI and myocardial infarction (McKiernan JM, 1997). In the same analysis, patient withdrawal because of side effects (14.5%) was slightly higher than for placebo (11.4%). Because clinical data show that terazosin's safety profile is not as favorable as that of other alpha blockers (i.e., more cases of orthostatic hypotension as compared with tamsulosin), terazosin will face stiff competition from the current leader, tamsulosin.

Because terazosin is an effective hypotensive agent, it is the preferred treatment for patients with both BPH and hypertension. However, the need to slowly increase the dose of terazosin in normotensive BPH patients may reduce patient compliance, a disadvantage compared with other alpha blockers (e.g., alfuzosin), whose maximum dose can be administered immediately without amplified side effects (van Kerrebroeck P, 2000).

Doxazosin. Doxazosin (Pfizer's [New York, New York]/Cardura XL, generics) (Figure 5) is a long-acting alpha blocker selective for $alpha_1$-adrenergic receptors; this agent has been used to treat hypertension since 1991. At the end of 2001, a once-daily formulation, Cardura XL (doxazosin GITS [gastrointestinal therapeutic system]), had been launched for BPH and hypertension in 13 countries, including France, Germany, Spain, and the United Kingdom. Pfizer filed for approval of Cardura XL in April 2001 in the United States and was approved in 2005.

Although doxazosin is not as selective as some of the newer alpha blockers, it has comparable efficacy and is a good alternative for patients who may have difficulty covering the cost of tamsulosin or alfuzosin. Since publication of Medical Therapy of Prostatic Symptoms (MTOPS), a study of the effects of combination therapy on BPH progression, doxazosin is now implicated as an inhibitor of prostatic development when used in combination with finasteride. The study is described later in this section in conjunction with the 5-ARI finasteride.

The effect of doxazosin on the severity of BPH symptoms was examined in a multicenter study involving 609 normotensive and hypertensive patients (Mobley

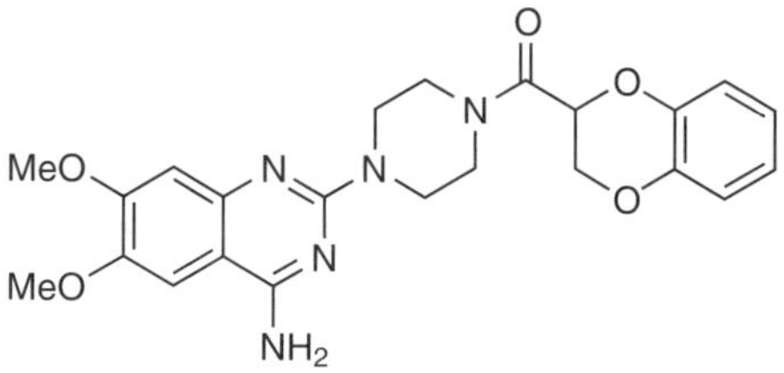

FIGURE 5. Structure of doxazosin.

DF, 1997). The placebo-controlled study was initiated at a daily dose of either 0.5 or 1.0 mg, with a final dose of up to 12.0 mg per day, during a treatment period of 12–14 weeks. In both the 0.5 mg and 1.0 mg patient populations, doxazosin was associated with significant reductions in IPSS, reflecting improvement in symptom severity and comfort levels, compared with placebo. Symptoms improved within the first two weeks of the study, and efficacy was sustained throughout the treatment period.

This study was expanded to an open-label study with continual enrollment of new patients. Four hundred and fifty men were titrated to their optimal dose of doxazosin (up to 12 mg per day) (Fawzy A, 1999). Patients' medication was increased until they achieved four consecutive weeks of stable dosing, after which they entered the stable-dose efficacy phase of the study. Treatment continued for four years or until the last day of the study, whichever came first. Primary efficacy measures included total Boyarsky symptom score (modified to accommodate a score ranging from 7 to 39 points for severity and 9 to 45 points for bother), Qmax, and residual urinary volume (the volume of urine left in the bladder after micturition). Results show that long-term treatment with doxazosin is tolerated by both normotensive and hypertensive patients and that it is effective in alleviating LUTS:

- Patients who did not complete four years of experimentation (various durations of doxazosin treatment) lowered their symptom scores by an average of 13.7%, increased Qmax by 14%, and decreased residual urine volume by 16.1 mL.

- Long-term doxazosin therapy demonstrated minimal improvement compared with shorter treatment durations. Patients who completed the four-year treatment period (28 men) attained an average symptom score of 29.8, which was a 12% reduction from baseline; an average Qmax of 12.6 mL/s, which was a 27% increase from baseline; and an average reduction in residual volume of 35.3 mL.

- Patients who experienced side effects (66%) were most likely to have dizziness or fatigue. Patients with normal blood pressure experienced fewer adverse events than hypertensive patients because their optimal doses of doxazosin were lower. Hypertensive patients benefited from the vasodilatory effects of more potent doses, but they also had a greater probability of experiencing side effects, such as dizziness and fatigue.

In a 20-week, randomized, double-blind, crossover study, doxazosin demonstrated better symptom score improvement than tamsulosin (Kirby RS, 2004). Fifty-two patients were randomized to receive 4 mg of doxazosin GITS, titrated to 8 mg, or 0.4 mg of tamsulosin, titrated to 0.8 mg, for eight weeks. After a two-week washout period, patients were switched and titrated to the other treatment arm for eight weeks. IPSS was significantly reduced from baseline for both treatment groups ($p < 0.001$). However, doxazosin GITS was significantly better than tamsulosin ($p = 0.019$) in relieving obstructive symptoms:

- After four weeks (before titration to high-dose medication), both doxazosin and tamsulosin produced a significant reduction in IPSS from baseline, which was established with the two-week washout period.
- The reduction in obstructive symptoms subscore (measured by IPSS questions 1, 3, 5, and 6) was significantly greater for 4 mg doxazosin than for 0.4 mg tamsulosin.
- The decrease in total IPSS from washout baseline was greater for 4 mg doxazosin than for 0.4 mg tamsulosin, but the difference was not significant. After four weeks of doses titrated to 8 mg of doxazosin GITS and 0.8 mg of tamsulosin, IPSS scores were further decreased.

Naftopidil. Naftopidil (Asahi Kasei Pharma's [Tokyo, Japan] Flivas, Kanebo's [Tokyo, Japan] Avishot) is an alpha$_1$-adrenergic receptor antagonist that was originally in development by Boehringer Mannheim (Gaithersburg, Maryland) for antihypertension. Roche (Basel, Switzerland) acquired Boehringer Mannheim and integrated naftopidil into its development pipeline. Roche subsequently discontinued development for the treatment of hypertension in Germany and Japan because research indicated that the drug was no more effective than already marketed therapies. Asahi Kasei and its development partner, Kanebo (now merged with Nippon Organon [Osaka, Japan]), licensed naftopidil, and it was launched in Japan in 1999 for BPH-related dysuria.

Using cloned human alpha$_1$-adrenergic-receptor subtypes, naftopidil has been shown to have a 3-fold and 17-fold higher affinity for the alpha$_{1D}$ subtype than for the alpha$_{1A}$ and alpha$_{1B}$ subtypes, respectively (Ikegaki I, 2000). Furthermore, in addition to blocking the alpha$_1$-adrenergic receptor, naftopidil inhibits platelet aggregation (Kirsten R, 1994) and antagonizes the effect of calcium on smooth muscle (Sponer G, 1992).

Researchers conducted a study in China to test the clinical efficacy and safety of naftopidil in treating BPH (Ju XB, 2002). The 42-day, randomized, double-blind study consisted of two groups of 40 patients receiving either naftopidil (25 mg/day) or tamsulosin (0.2 mg/day). At the end of the study, statistical analysis was conducted for 77 patients. The changes in IPSS, Qmax, and QoL measures differed significantly between the two groups before and after treatment ($p < 0.05$). No significant differences were noted in residual urine and prostate volumes ($p < 0.05$), and adverse reactions in both groups were mild. In conclusion, naftopidil was found to be safe and effective in treating BPH.

Another comparative study, in Japan, assessed the clinical effects of naftopidil and tamsulosin on symptomatic BPH (Hayashi T, 2002). In this crossover study, patients whose QoL scores did not improve after four weeks of treatment with naftopidil or tamsulosin were switched to the alternative drug: patients who failed naftopidil treatment (85) were dosed with 0.1–0.2 mg/day of tamsulosin for eight weeks; patients who failed treatment with tamsulosin (89) were dosed with 50–75 mg/day of naftopidil. Patients who switched from naftopidil to tamsulosin experienced significant improvement in symptoms of urgency, weak stream, and straining; patients who switched from tamsulosin to naftopidil demonstrated significant improvement in incomplete emptying, intermittency, and nocturia.

Prazosin. Prazosin (Pfizer's Minipress, generics) (Figure 6), a short-acting, selective alpha$_1$ blocker that Pfizer and Invicta originally developed for treating hypertension, can be used for its beneficial effects in reducing the symptoms of BPH. Prazosin, one of the earlier alpha blockers, is rarely the first choice of primary care physicians (PCPs) and urologists because it has a lower level of efficacy and higher rates of adverse events than other agents in its class.

A randomized, double-blind, placebo-controlled study was conducted in 93 normotensive patients to determine the effects of prazosin versus placebo on obstructive voiding in BPH patients (Chapple CR, 1992). During the 12-week study, prazosin was administered orally in doses of 0.5 mg and then 1.0 mg twice daily for four days and 2 mg twice daily for the remainder of the trial. Patients taking prazosin exhibited a significantly increased maximum urinary flow rate compared with patients on placebo (3.2 mL/s versus 0.6 mL/s) and a significant drop in maximum voiding detrusor pressure (-17.1 cm H_2O versus -1.9 cm H_2O). However, the changes in flow rate and detrusor pressure did not translate into subjective improvements in urinary symptoms. Although a similar number of patients in the prazosin and placebo groups experienced side effects (30 and 28, respectively), more patients withdrew from the active treatment arm than the control group (7 versus 3, respectively) because of adverse events. Dizziness (16.7% prazosin versus 10.0% placebo) and headache (12.6% versus 5.0%)

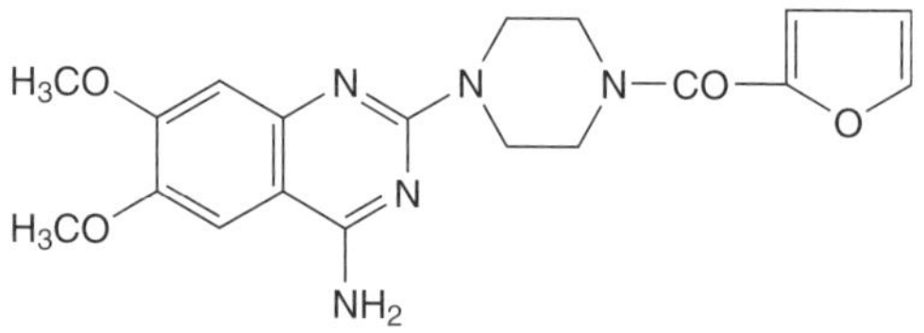

FIGURE 6. *Structure of prazosin.*

occurred more often in the prazosin group than in the placebo groups. The study demonstrates that prazosin is relatively ineffective in relieving BPH symptoms and is associated with significant hypotensive side effects.

Indoramin. Indoramin (GlaxoSmithKline's [GSK's] [Brentford, Middlesex, United Kindom]/Astella's Doralese) (Figure 7), a short-acting alpha blocker, is approved in the United Kingdom.

Of the few BPH clinical studies performed with indoramin, only two show a significant increase in Qmax. The largest study consisted of 121 patients; in this parallel group, multicenter study, patients received one of two doses of indoramin (20 mg twice daily or 20 mg once daily) or placebo (Chow W, 1990). After eight weeks, the Qmax value was 1.8 mL/s in the placebo group, 2.8 mL/s in the indoramin low-dose group, and 4.9 mL/s in the indoramin high-dose group. The effects on voiding time and volume were small in all three treatment groups, with no significant difference between them. A greater number of patients in the high-dose indoramin group reported symptomatic improvement (78%) than in the low-dose indoramin group (64%) or the placebo group (53%). Nine patients withdrew because of adverse events; five of these patients were in the placebo group, and two each were in the treatment groups. In this study, the high-dose indoramin group experienced improved BPH symptoms, and the drug was well tolerated.

5-Alpha-Reductase Inhibitors

Overview. Because inhibition of the enzyme 5-alpha-reductase is known to reduce prostate size, patients with an enlarged prostate (greater than 40 g) are often prescribed a 5-alpha-reductase inhibitor (5-ARI). Along with alpha blockers, 5-ARIs dominate the BPH drug market. The agents currently available are finasteride (Merck's Proscar) and dutasteride (GlaxoSmithKline/Astellas's Avodart). These drugs are effective in preventing further prostatic growth and in reducing prostate size, but they have a slow onset of action and cause sexual side effects. Despite these disadvantages, new data on combination therapy with alpha blockers and 5-ARIs have increased 5-ARI use.

Mechanism of Action. Research has substantiated the role of 5-alpha-reductase in the pathophysiology of BPH. The fact that men who have undergone castration before puberty or have genetic androgen deficiency are not afflicted by the disease is evidence of the vital role that androgens play in normal male development and in the progression of static BPH. 5-ARIs have proved their

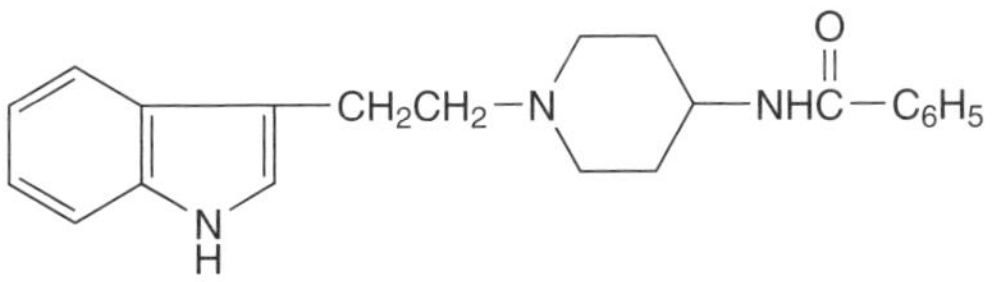

FIGURE 7. *Structure of indoramin.*

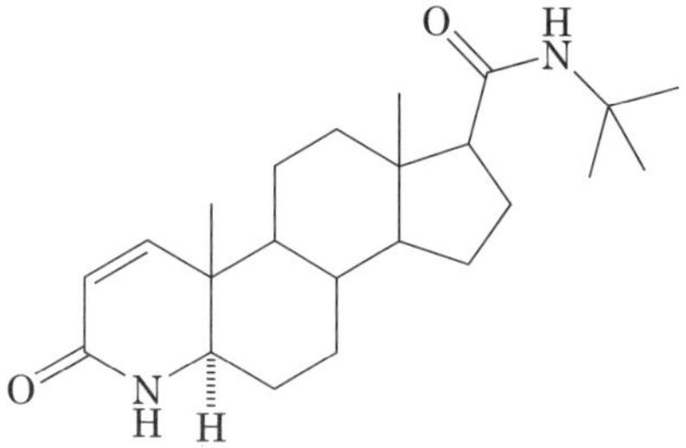

FIGURE 8. *Structure of finasteride.*

ability not only to relieve symptoms but also to change the progression of the disease, which makes them valuable in the management and treatment of BPH.

5-ARIs block the action of the 5-alpha-reductase enzyme, which converts testosterone to dihydrotestosterone (DHT). When complexed with the androgen receptor, DHT binds to nuclear DNA, thereby inciting the expression of regulatory proteins that control growth and cellular function. By preventing the formation of DHT, 5-ARIs reduce prostatic hyperplasia.

The 5-alpha-reductase enzyme has two isoenzymes: type 1 is found in various tissues of the body, such as the skin, liver, and prostate; type 2 is found predominantly in the prostate. Drugs have been developed to target only type 2 isoenzyme (Merck's finasteride [Proscar]) and to target both type 1 and type 2 isoenzymes (GSK's dutasteride [Avodart]). Both agents have proved effective in reducing symptoms and shrinking enlarged prostates. However, they are associated with sexual side effects and have a much longer onset of action than alpha blockers: patients may not experience symptom improvement for up to six months. Furthermore, use of 5-ARIs reduces prostate-specific antigen (PSA) levels, which compromises the ability to screen for prostate cancer.

Finasteride. The search for specific inhibitors of 5-alpha-reductase led to the discovery of finasteride (Merck's Proscar) (Figure 8), which has been marketed in the United States and Europe since 1992 and is now the leading agent of this class. Merck licensed finasteride to Yamanouchi and Banyu, a Merck subsidiary, in Japan, but no development has been reported since 1994.

Finasteride inhibits DHT synthesis and thereby prevents enlargement of the prostate. It acts predominantly via suppression of the type 2 isoenzyme of 5-alpha-reductase, preventing conversion of testosterone to DHT and reducing serum and prostatic tissue DHT levels by 70% and 85%, respectively (Bartsch G, 2000). Because 5-ARIs reduce prostate size, the subset of patients with static BPH is most likely to benefit from this type of therapy.

The clinical benefits and risks of finasteride treatment are best described by the Proscar Long-Term Efficacy and Safety Study (PLESS) (McConnell JD, 2003).

In this four-year, double-blind, placebo-controlled trial, 3,040 men with moderate to severe symptoms of BPH were randomized to receive 5 mg of finasteride or placebo daily. Every four months, patients were assessed for AUASI, Qmax, and prostate volume. Results indicated that finasteride improves BPH symptoms and may halt disease progression:

- At the end of four years of treatment, AUASI was reduced by an average of 3.3 points in the finasteride group and 1.3 points in the placebo group, a difference that was statistically significant ($p < 0.001$).

- Qmax improved by 1.9 mL/s for patients taking finasteride and by 0.2 mL/s for patients taking placebo; finasteride was significantly more effective in increasing peak urinary flow rate ($p < 0.001$).

- After one year of treatment, prostate volumes had been reduced to their minimal size, which was maintained during the rest of the study period. Patients receiving finasteride had an average 18% reduction in prostate size; patients receiving placebo had an average 14% reduction.

- Finasteride appeared to lower the risk of acute urinary retention (AUR) by 57% ($p < 0.001$); catheterizations and surgeries to treat AUR were reduced. Only 100 patients taking finasteride (7%) needed a procedure to treat an event of AUR, whereas twice as many patients taking placebo required emergency catheterization or surgery. Because AUR is an indicator of disease progression, finasteride shows promise as a drug that can halt further development of BPH.

Men who completed PLESS were recruited to participate in a two-year extension trial (Roehrborn CG, 2004). Nine hundred and eight patients who had taken finasteride for all four years and 785 patients who had taken placebo were given 5 mg finasteride. This division created two populations, one with six years of finasteride treatment and one with two years. The most frequently reported side effects were impotence and decreased libido, experienced by 2% and 1%, respectively, of patients receiving finasteride for six years. The overall incidence of prostate cancer was 3% in both treatment arms.

Because finasteride is known to reduce prostate size and alpha blockers have a more rapid onset of action, researchers set out to determine the safety and efficacy of the two drugs combined for the treatment of BPH and its associated symptoms. The Medical Therapy of Prostatic Symptoms (MTOPS) study was designed to last six years and measure the time to BPH progression (Bautista OM, 2003). Patients were randomized to treatment with finasteride (5 mg per day), doxazosin (4 or 8 mg per day), finasteride plus doxazosin, or placebo. The event of BPH progression was defined as an increase in AUASI of at least 4 points and one of the following: (1) a rise in creatinine because of BPH, (2) AUR, (3) two UTIs within a year, (4) urosepsis due to bladder outlet obstruction, or (5) an incontinence event. Investigators also measured the following secondary outcomes: AUASI, Qmax, prostate volume, sexual function, and QoL. Biopsies were performed before and after the start of therapy.

An interim analysis of a 4.5-year follow-up study involving 3,047 patients with AUASI scores between 8 and 30 points showed a reduction in risk of disease progression (McConnell JD, 2003). Results were as follows:

- The placebo group's overall rate of progression of BPH was 4.5 per 100 person-years.

- The risk of progression was reduced by 39%, 34%, and 66% with doxazosin, finasteride, and combination treatment, respectively ($p < 0.001$, $p = 0.002$, and $p < 0.001$, respectively). The percentage reduction was not significantly different for finasteride and doxazosin; however, both reductions were significantly lower than the reduction produced by combination therapy.

- After four years of treatment, the average improvement in AUASI was 4.9, 6.6, 5.6, and 7.4 for placebo, doxazosin, finasteride, and combination therapy, respectively. All improvement rates were significantly better than the placebo rate, and the improvement rate achieved by the combination therapy was significantly greater than that induced by either monotherapy.

- The average improvement in Qmax was 4.0 mL/s with doxazosin, 3.2 mL/s with finasteride, and 5.1 mL/s with finasteride plus doxazosin. Prostate size increased 29% in patients taking placebo or doxazosin and decreased 12% in patients taking finasteride alone or in combination.

- The most common adverse events in the doxazosin group were dizziness, postural hypotension, and asthenia (loss of strength). The most common adverse events in the finasteride group were erectile dysfunction, decreased libido, and abnormal ejaculation.

Dutasteride.   Dutasteride (GSK/Astellas's Avodart) was the first marketed dual 5-ARI. In 1999, Glaxo Wellcome (now GSK) entered an agreement with Yamanouchi Pharmaceutical (Tokyo, Japan) for this drug's copromotion for BPH in the United Kingdom. Approval in the United States was granted for the treatment of symptomatic BPH in November 2001. In October 2002, the FDA approved a supplemental NDA for dutasteride for the treatment of symptomatic BPH in men with an enlarged prostate. Subsequently, it was launched in the United States in January 2003 and in the United Kingdom in February 2003. In March 2003, GSK announced the launch of dutasteride in all major European markets.

As an inhibitor of both types 1 and 2 isoenzymes of 5-alpha-reductase, dutasteride is unique; finasteride inhibits only type 2. However, the type 2 isoenzyme is the dominant form; type 1 accounts for only 15% of the prostatic enzyme. The dual inhibition of the enzyme reduces DHT serum levels to less than 10% of normal (Clark R, 1999), but there is no evidence that inhibition of both forms of the enzyme has any therapeutic benefit.

The foremost clinical study evaluating the efficacy and safety of dutasteride was published in 2002 (Roehrborn CG, 2002). The placebo-controlled study was conducted over the course of two years in three pooled Phase III trials. Dutasteride was evaluated in 4,325 BPH patients with moderate to severe symptoms (AUASI score of 12 points or more) and an enlarged prostate of 30 grams or more. In all three trials, patients were randomized to 0.5 mg of dutasteride daily or placebo; 2,951 (68%) of the patients completed the study. Researchers reported the following results:

- At two years, the serum DHT level in dutasteride-treated patients was reduced from baseline by a mean of 90.2% (placebo increased 9.6% from baseline), the total prostate volume by a mean of 25.7% (placebo increased 1.7%), and the symptom score on average by 4.5 points (placebo by 2.3 points).
- The risk of AUR with dutasteride fell by 57%, and the risk associated with BPH surgical intervention declined 48%, compared with placebo.
- The number of discontinuations (717 placebo, 657 drug-treated) and reasons for not completing the study (e.g., adverse events, lack of efficacy) were not statistically different.
- Drug-related adverse events were observed in 5% more of the patients treated with dutasteride than with placebo (19% versus 14%). They included impotence, decreased libido, ejaculation disorders, and gynecomastia (enlarged breasts), but most effects were transient, and new events declined significantly in the second year.

Patients who completed the Phase III trials with dutasteride were eligible for enrollment in a two-year, open-label extension (Roehrborn CG, 2004). The trial consisted of two study groups: patients who continued dutasteride treatment and patients who switched to dutasteride from placebo. In this trial, as in the double-blind placebo phase, both AUASI and Qmax improved from baseline. Results were as follows:

- Patients who continued dutasteride treatment for an additional two years had an overall reduction in AUASI of 6.1 points. Qmax increased 2.8 mL/s. Patients who switched from placebo had a reduction in AUASI of 5.3 points, and Qmax increased 1.8 mL/s.
- After 24 months, researchers found that hormone levels were significantly affected by dutasteride. Both treatment arms had reduced serum DHT levels by more than 90% and serum testosterone levels by 25% from baseline.
- The most commonly reported drug-related side effects were impotence, decreased libido, and abnormal ejaculation. Results from patients taking dutasteride for four years showed that sexual adverse events decreased over the course of long-term treatment.

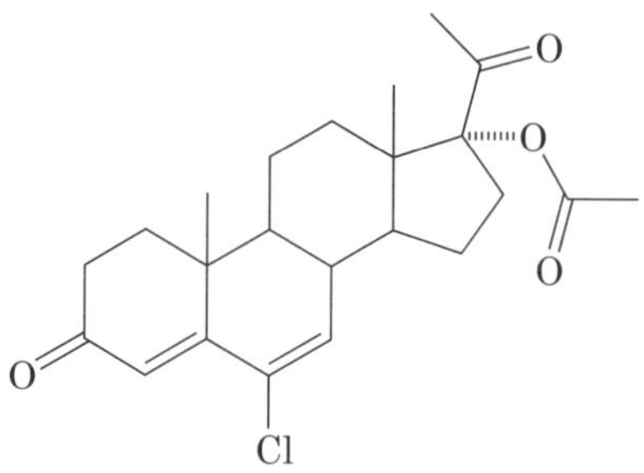

FIGURE 9. Structure of chlormadinone acetate.

Gonadotropin Modulators

Overview. Gonadotropin modulators, also known as steroid androgen antagonists (e.g., chlormadinone acetate [Teikoku's Prostal/Prostal L]), are specifically labeled for treating BPH, and their use is especially high in Japan, where finasteride and dutasteride are not approved (Akakura K, 1998). Potentially serious side effects (e.g., diarrhea, sexual dysfunction, liver toxicity) make agents in this class less desirable than less-toxic therapies such as the 5-ARIs. Because these agents are marketed primarily for prostate cancer, they are not discussed in detail here, with the exception of chlormadinone, which is often prescribed in Japan.

Mechanism of Action. The control of androgen production in the testes is directly mediated by hypothalamic/pituitary hormones (Griffin JE, 1985). Gonadotropin-releasing hormone (GnRH), also known as luteinizing hormone-releasing hormone (LHRH), is secreted by neurons in the hypothalamus, and it subsequently stimulates the release of both luteinizing hormone (LH) and follicle-stimulating hormone (FSH) in the anterior pituitary. In the testes, LH interacts with specific cell-surface receptors in the plasma membrane of Leydig cells, activating the biochemical steps that lead to the synthesis of testosterone.

Chlormadinone Acetate. Teikoku's chlormadinone acetate (Prostal) (Figure 9) was launched in Japan in 1981. In 1990, a sustained-release formulation (Prostal L) was launched there. Chlormadinone is indicated for the treatment of both BPH and prostate cancer.

Chlormadinone is a progestational hormone that reduces GnRH secretion, thereby inhibiting the production of androgens and their subsequent action in the prostate.

A double-blind study of Japanese men with BPH compared the sustained-release form of chlormadinone with finasteride (McConnell JD, 2003). After six months of chlormadinone treatment (50 mg/day), the researchers found the drug to be as effective as finasteride in reducing prostate size (29% versus 22.2%), improving symptom score (8.2 versus 7.6), and improving Qmax (3.4 mL/s versus 2.2 mL/s). Impotence, however, developed in 12.4% of chlormadinone patients, versus 4.1% of finasteride patients.

Chlormadinone has also been investigated in combination with the alpha blocker tamsulosin (Okada H, 1996). For 16 weeks, 80 patients were randomized to receive tamsulosin 0.2 mg per day, chlormadinone 50 mg per day, or a daily combination of the two drugs at doses identical to those of monotherapy. Subjective symptom improvement was greatest in patients who received tamsulosin alone and in patients who received combination therapy. Patients who received combination therapy also demonstrated the greatest improvements in urinary flow. Larger clinical studies are needed to evaluate the therapeutic efficacy and tolerability of this combination.

Phytopharmaceutical Agents

Overview. Phytotherapy is the use of naturally occurring herbal remedies to treat diseases. The use of these drugs for BPH is attractive because they are known to have a benign side-effect profile; phytopharmaceutical agents have virtually no incidence of sexual side effects. A wide range of phytopharmaceutical agents are used for the relief of BPH symptoms; the most popular is serenoa repens (saw palmetto berry). Other herbal agents used to treat symptoms of BPH include pygeum africanum, beta-sitosterol, and pollen extract, also known as cernilton. Use of specific products varies by region. Table 3 lists phytopharmaceutical agents commonly used in BPH treatment.

Mechanism of Action. Active ingredients in serenoa repens are free fatty acids, phytosterols, and other elements extracted from the plant. Researchers suspect that serenoa repens has a mechanism of action similar to that of the 5-ARIs. In vitro studies have shown that, when serenoa repens is administered, DHT

TABLE 3. Phytopharmaceutical Agents Commonly Used in Treatment of Benign Prostatic Hyperplasia

Botanical Name	Common Name	Supposed Mechanism of Action
Serenoa repens	Saw palmetto	• 5-alpha-reductase inhibitor • Anti-androgenic • Anti-edema • Anti-estrogenic • Anti-inflammatory • Inhibitor of prolactin and growth factors
Pygeum Africanum	African plum tree	• Bladder desensitizer • Anti-inflammatory • Fibroblast inhibitor
Urtica dioica	Nettle root	• 5-alpha-reductase inhibitor
Secale cereale	Rye grass pollen	• Detrusor regulator • Reduces urethra resistance • 5-alpha-reductase inhibitor
Hypoxis rooperi	South African star grass	• Anti-inflammatory

and growth factor levels decrease and testosterone levels increase (Gong EM, 2004). Cell tissue cultures show that saw palmetto extract activity is localized to the prostatic nuclear membrane, which is suspected of disrupting bound 5-alpha-reductase. Further clinical study is required to fully understand the mechanism of action of serenoa repens.

Saw Palmetto. Saw palmetto is one of many extracts of serenoa repens. It contains a heterogeneous mixture of several components. This formulation is most popular in the United States. Patients in the European Union are more likely to take Permixon (manufactured by Pierre Fabre), which is a highly purified form of saw palmetto.

Few well-designed clinical trials of saw palmetto have been conducted. A recently conducted study clearly demonstrated an improvement in BPH symptoms (Gerber GS, 1998). Eighty-five men were enrolled in a six-month, double-blind, placebo-controlled study and randomized to treatment with saw palmetto or placebo. Follow-up evaluations were conducted after months 2, 4, and 6. Results showed that IPSS was reduced by 4.4 points in patients receiving saw palmetto and by 2.2 points in patients receiving placebo ($p = 0.038$). Qmax decreased in both treatment groups; there was no significant difference between the two groups. There were no sexual side effects related to saw palmetto treatment. The most common adverse events were diarrhea and gastric distress.

Nonpharmacological Approaches

Watchful Waiting. Watchful waiting is a management strategy of close patient monitoring, without pharmacological intervention, for symptoms of BPH. This method is ideal for men with uncomplicated BPH that has not progressed to affect the upper urinary tract. Such men may have mild to moderate symptom scores and QoL. Urologists and PCPs practice watchful waiting in hope that the disease will improve on its own and postpone the need for chronic medical therapy. Patients may improve the results of watchful waiting by taking some practical measures, such as reducing fluid intake at bed time, reducing the amount of diuretics in their diets, and avoiding decongestant medication, which may exacerbate obstructive symptoms.

Minimally Invasive Therapy. When pharmacological therapy is insufficient in the treatment of LUTS associated with BPH, urologists recommend either minimally invasive therapy or surgery. Minimally invasive therapy is appropriate for patients who are unfit for operation and/or anesthesia.

In a minimally invasive procedure, a controlled amount of heat is delivered to the prostate, destroying the tissue that is causing obstructive symptoms. Minimally invasive therapies may be conducted in an office rather than a hospital, and they do not require general anesthesia. Some examples of common procedures are transurethral microwave therapy (TUMT), transurethral needle ablation (TUNA), high-intensity focused ultrasound, and water-induced thermotherapy. Table 4 describes each of the minimally invasive therapies in detail.

TABLE 4. Surgical and Minimally Invasive Treatment Options for Benign Prostatic Hyperplasia

Surgical Method	Mechanism	Comments
Open prostatectomy	Removal of prostate tissue via conventional surgery	*Advantages:* Most-effective treatment for alleviating symptoms and improving uroflow; low retreatment rate (2%); lower perioperative mortality compared with TURP; more cost-effective than TURP in the long term (i.e., >5 years). *Disadvantages:* Invasive therapy, associated with high morbidity; requires general/spinal anesthesia; increases impotence.
TURP (transurethral resection of the prostate)	Removal of prostate tissue via a low current transurethral electro-cauterizing loop	*Advantages:* Gold standard for BPH; less invasive than open prostatectomy; more effective at improving uroflow than other methods. *Disadvantages:* Normally requires general/spinal anesthesia; irrigation procedure results in TURP syndrome[a]; increases sexual dysfunction; high peri- and postoperative treatment morbidity and retreatment rates increase the cost compared with open prostatectomy
TVP (transurethral electrovapor-ization of the prostate)	Modified TURP using high-current elec-trovaporization electrodes to remove excess prostate tissue	*Advantages:* Improved TURP method using electrovaporization electrodes; enables larger volume of prostate to be removed; reduces post-TURP syndrome[a], need for catheterization, and hospitalization time; improved control of hemostasis; easy to perform and less expensive than TURP. *Disadvantages:* More time-consuming than TURP; unable to obtain tissue for histological evaluation using rollerball electrodes; long-term outcome/retreatment rate needs to be assessed (i.e., five to ten years).
TUMT (transurethral microwave therapy)	Removal of prostate tissue using low- and high-energy microwaves	*Advantages:* Minimally invasive; affords convenient 0.5–1.0 hour outpatient therapy; minimal anesthesia; safe, with low morbidity and complication rates; proven sustained efficacy (five years); may result in alpha-receptor blockade (by damaging prostatic nerve endings); high energy (HE) option improves uroflow by 65%. *Disadvantages:* Less effective than TURP at improving uroflow; HE option associated with retrograde ejaculation, AUR, and increased morbidity.

(*continued overleaf*)

TABLE 4. (*continued*)

Surgical Method	Mechanism	Comments
TUNA (transurethral needle ablation)	Removal of prostate tissue using transurethral heated needles (90–100° C)	*Advantages:* Minimally invasive, convenient outpatient therapy; no need for anesthesia; selective ablation of inner prostate spares urothelium; may result in long-term alpha-receptor blockade; fewer complications (less bleeding) compared with TURP. *Disadvantages:* Impractical for prostates >75 g; no tissue available for pathology; long-term outcome/retreatment rate and cost need to be assessed (i.e., five to ten years).
Laser techniques: TULIP (transurethral ultrasound-guided laser-induced prostatec-tomy), VLAP (visual laser ablation of the prostate), ILC (interstitial laser coagulation)	Removal of prostate tissue via pulsed laser energy	*Advantages:* Minimally invasive, convenient outpatient therapy; fewer complications (less bleeding) compared with TURP. *Disadvantages:* Less effective than TURP; higher incidence of postoperative AUR retention than TURP; long-term outcome/retreatment rate needs to be assessed (i.e., five to ten years); more costly than TURP.
HIFU (high-intensity focused ultrasound)	Removal of prostate tissue using transrectal ultrasound	*Advantages:* Minimally invasive, convenient outpatient therapy; ablates prostate without affecting surrounding tissue; no need for intra-urethral manipulation; permits imaging during treatment. *Disadvantages:* Long-term outcome/retreatment rate needs to be assessed (i.e., five to ten years).
TUIP (transurethral incision of the prostate)	Transurethral incisions in prostatic tissue to relieve urethral pressure	*Advantages:* Minimally invasive, convenient outpatient therapy; long-term efficacy comparable to TURP; lower morbidity rate than TURP; safe and less expensive than other methods. *Disadvantages:* Restricted to men with smaller prostates (<50–60 g).

TABLE 4. (*continued*)

Surgical Method	Mechanism	Comments
Stents	Insertion of a tube in the obstructed urethra to increase urine flow	*Advantages:* Improves uroflow; widely studied; new biodegradable stents eliminate need for surgical removal.
		Disadvantages: Carcinogenicity and biocompatibility concerns (increased hyperplasia and encrustation).

[a]TURP syndrome is hyponatremia resulting from excessive systemic absorption of hyponatremic irrigation fluid.
AUR = Acute urinary retention.

Surgery. Until the advent of pharmacotherapy, removal of excess prostatic tissue—by conventional surgical excision (open prostatectomy), transurethral vaporization, or transurethral incision procedures—was the main treatment for reducing the signs and symptoms of obstruction in BPH patients. Although pharmacotherapy can adequately manage the symptoms of BPH with fewer side effects than surgical techniques, surgery remains the best option for patients who have the following conditions:

- AUR.
- Recurrent UTIs.
- Recurrent severe prostatic hematuria.
- Bladder stones.
- Decreased kidney function.

Patients who are unresponsive to or intolerant of pharmacotherapy and are unable to tolerate the symptoms of BPH are also candidates for surgery, regardless of disease severity.

EMERGING THERAPIES

The ultimate goal of treatment of benign prostatic hyperplasia (BPH) and its associated comorbidities is to alleviate clinical symptoms that affect quality of life, eliminate the need for surgery, and prevent chronic and acute urinary retention. The challenge to drug developers is to create agents that have an acceptable onset of action, show a measurable level of efficacy, and induce no significant adverse events.

The pipeline of agents in development for treatment of BPH is relatively sparse. Most of the drugs currently under investigation are in early-stage development. Because BPH is not a life-threatening disease, safety is a primary area of product improvement for new therapies. Physicians are not willing to accept drugs with frequent or significant side effects because BPH is not life-threatening. Table 5 lists emerging therapies in development for BPH.

Currently, the majority of pharmaceutical research for BPH is focused on hormone therapy, as opposed to the established alpha-blocker and 5-alpha-reductase inhibitor (5-ARI) classes. The new gonadotropin modulators claim to have fewer

TABLE 5. Emerging Therapies in Development for Benign Prostatic Hyperplasia

Compound	Development Phase	Marketing Company
Alpha blockers		
Silodosin		
United States	III	Watson Pharmaceuticals
Europe	II	Recordati
Japan	PR	Kissei Pharmaceuticals/Daiichi
5-alpha-reductase inhibitors		
TF-505		
United States	—	—
Europe	—	—
Japan	I	Taiho
Gonadotropin modulators		
Cetrorelix		
United States	II	AEterna Zentaris
Europe	II	AEterna Zentaris
Japan	II	AEterna Zentaris/Shionogi/Nippon Kayaku
ML-04		
United States	II	Milkhaus Laboratory
Europe	—	—
Japan	—	—
Vitamin D3 analogues		
BXL-628		
United States	—	—
Europe	II	BioXell
Japan	—	—
Hexokinase inhibitors		
Lonidamine		
United States	II	Threshold Pharmaceuticals
Europe	III	Angelini
Japan	—	
Phosphodiesterase 5 inhibitors		
Tadalafil		
United States	II	Eli Lilly/Icos
Europe	—	—
Japan	—	—
Prostate-reducing agents		
NX-1207		
United States	II	Nymox Pharmaceuticals
Europe	—	—
Japan	—	—

adverse effects. If this claim is upheld, then the originator companies will most likely partner with overseas companies to comarket their new drugs in other regions. Because Japan is the only country where physicians and patients accept the use of gonadotropin modulators, uptake of some emerging therapies is expected to be higher in this region.

In most clinical trials of agents that target BPH, the primary end points are urinary symptom scores, average peak urinary flow rate (Qmax), and the percentage of patients who experience a clinically meaningful improvement in these two measures. These patients are also identified as "clinical responders"; they are able to achieve at least a 25% reduction in International Prostate Symptom Score (IPSS) or the American Urological Association's Symptom Index (AUASI) and at least a 30% increase in Qmax. Some drug classes, such as the 5-ARIs and the gonadotropin modulators, because they act by reducing prostate hyperplasia, have the additional end point of reducing prostate volume.

Tadalafil, a phosphodiesterase 5 inhibitor, reduces LUTS by relaxing smooth muscle in the prostate. It does so by a different mechanism of action than alpha blockers and therefore does not involve side effects such as orthostatic hypotension and retrograde ejaculation. Tadalafil will fulfill a role as supplemental therapy for symptoms of dynamic BPH, a niche not occupied by any other agent. Without competing drugs, tadalafil is expected to achieve strong commercial success.

The vitamin D3 analogue BXL-628 has shown efficacy similar to that of finasteride and dutasteride, and it has demonstrated an improved side-effect profile. If BXL-628 continues to show favorable, robust clinical trial results, it could replace 5-ARIs.

Alpha Blockers

Overview. Hyperplasia of the stromal tissue may or may not lead to significant enlargement of the prostate, but it usually leads to dynamic BPH by increasing prostatic smooth muscle, which triggers increased smooth-muscle tension and resistance to urine flow. (The dynamic and static components of BPH are discussed in the "Etiology and Pathophysiology" section.) Alpha$_1$-adrenergic receptors in the bladder neck and prostatic capsule mediate tension in these muscles. Although the alpha$_1$-adrenergic antagonists, or alpha blockers, currently used to block these receptors (e.g., doxazosin [Pfizer/AstraZeneca's Cardura/Cardura XL, generics] and terazosin [Abbott's Hytrin, generics]) reduce BPH symptoms and resistance to urine flow, some of them also cause cardiovascular side effects. The latest entrants in this field (e.g., tamsulosin [Astellas/Boehringer Ingelheim/Abbott's Harnal/Flomax/Omnic, others] and alfuzosin [Sanofi-Aventis's Xatral/Xatral SR/Uroxatral, others]) are prostate-specific or uroselective alpha blockers that reduce these side effects.

Several other reportedly selective alpha blockers that target specific receptor subtypes are under development to improve specificity and confer a better side-effect profile than current agents; the most advanced of these agents is covered in the following section. S-doxazosin, developed by Sepracor, Inc. (Marlborough,

Massachusetts) was intended to have a reduced incidence of orthostatic hypotension and offer increased efficacy, compared with its predecessor, doxazosin. In 2003, this agent was in Phase II development in the United States; however, there is no indication that the drug is still in active development. Early in 2004, Ranbaxy initiated early development of a highly selective alpha$_{1A}$-adrenoceptor antagonist, RBx-9001. Because results on the safety and efficacy of RBx-9001 have yet to be released, a full analysis of this agent is not included here.

Mechanism of Action. Enhanced sensitivity of alpha$_1$-adrenergic receptors is largely responsible for the obstructive symptoms associated with the dynamic component of BPH. By blocking these receptors in the prostate and bladder neck smooth muscle, alpha blockers relieve lower urinary tract symptoms (LUTS) associated with BPH. However, because alpha$_1$-adrenergic receptors are also present in the vascular system, broad-spectrum alpha blockers (e.g., prazosin, doxazosin, terazosin), which nonspecifically inhibit alpha$_1$-adrenergic receptor subtypes, are associated with hypotensive side effects. The development of subtype-selective alpha blockers (e.g., tamsulosin), with preferential specificity for certain subtypes (alpha$_{1A}$, alpha$_{1D}$, and alpha$_{1L}$), and the uroselective alpha blocker alfuzosin has reduced the systemic side effects that researchers believe result primarily from the activation of the alpha$_{1B}$-adrenergic receptors

Silodosin. Among the drugs in the pipeline for BPH, silodosin (Figure 10), also known as KMD-3213, is in the most advanced stage of development. The agent is being codeveloped by Kissei Pharmaceutical (Nagano Prefecture, Japan) and Daiichi Pharmaceutical (Tokyo, Japan). In June 2004, a new drug application (NDA) was submitted to the Pharmaceuticals and Medical Devices Agency (PMDA), and in 2004, Daiichi announced an expected launch date of 2006 in Japan. In April 2004, Kissei entered a licensing agreement with Watson Pharmaceuticals, which will develop and market silodosin in Mexico, Canada, and the United States, where Phase III clinical trials were in progress in 2005. In December 2004, Kissei granted Recordati (Milan, Italy) exclusive rights to the development of silodosin in 45 countries in Europe.

Silodosin is a highly selective, twice-daily oral alpha blocker that preferentially inhibits the activity of alpha$_{1A}$-adrenergic receptors, which are predominantly located in the prostate (Murata S, 2000). Other alpha blockers that are considered

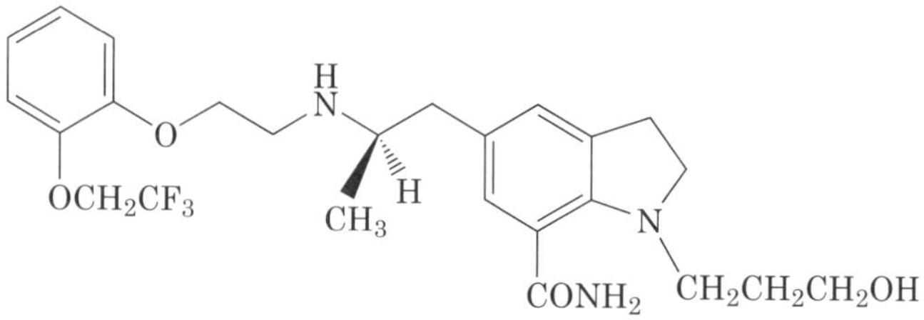

FIGURE 10. *Structure of silodosin.*

uroselective, such as tamsulosin, block not only alpha$_{1A}$-adrenoceptors but also other adrenergic receptor subtypes found in the prostate, cardiovascular system, spleen, kidney, and lungs. Although silodosin is a late-to-market agent, if it demonstrates greater efficacy in relieving BPH symptoms than currently available alpha blockers and has fewer side effects related to orthostatic hypotension and retroactive ejaculation, physicians may be willing to use the drug in BPH.

A study published in 2001 compared the uroselectivity of silodosin with that of prazosin and tamsulosin in a dog model (Akiyama K, 2001). When the drugs were administered intravenously, silodosin was 12-fold more uroselective than prazosin and 7.5-fold more than tamsulosin. When administered intraduodenally (a surrogate to oral administration), silodosin demonstrated at least 3.8-fold higher uroselectivity than tamsulosin. These results indicate that silodosin has the potential to be an effective orally administered, uroselective compound for treating the symptoms of BPH.

Phase III clinical data on silodosin were presented for the first time at the American Urological Association's (AUA's) 2005 annual meeting (Yoshida M, 2005). In a randomized, placebo-controlled, double-blind study, 457 BPH patients from 88 participating centers in Japan received treatment: 4 mg of silodosin twice daily, 0.2 mg of tamsulosin once daily, or placebo. After 12 weeks of therapy, reductions in IPSS from baseline were 8.3, 6.8, and 5.3, respectively. Of the patients taking silodosin, 76.4% achieved at least a 25% reduction in symptom score; only 65.6% of patients taking tamsulosin and 50.6% taking placebo achieved the same improvement. Silodosin induced hypotension-related adverse effects similar to those seen with tamsulosin treatment; these events affected 5.1% of the silodosin treatment group and 7.3% of the tamsulosin treatment group. Furthermore, abnormal ejaculation was more frequent in the silodosin group (22.3%) than in the tamsulosin group (1.6%).

5-Alpha-Reductase Inhibitors

Overview. The basis for using 5-alpha-reductase inhibitors (5-ARIs) to treat BPH stems from the observation that men with congenital 5-alpha-reductase deficiency have abnormally small prostates. Because 5-ARIs reduce prostate size, they are useful in treating patients with enlarged prostates—the subset of patients with static BPH. The goal in the development of new alpha-reductase inhibitors is to generate compounds that are more potent inhibitors of the enzyme but more tolerable to patients.

Mechanism of Action. 5-Alpha-reductase converts testosterone within the prostate to the androgen dihydrotestosterone (DHT). Researchers believe that DHT stimulates cell growth via paracrine and autocrine stimulation of prostatic stromal and epithelial tissue.

As discussed in the "Etiology and Pathophysiology" section, 5-alpha-reductase isoenzymes can be type 1 or type 2. The role that either type plays in the pathophysiology of androgen-dependent BPH is unclear. However, the currently marketed type 2 5-ARI, finasteride (Merck's Proscar), reduces prostate size, suggesting that this particular isoenzyme has an important role in BPH.

TF-505. Fujisawa Pharmaceutical's (Osaka, Japan) 5-ARI TF-505 entered Phase II clinical trials in Japan in 2002. In January 2004, Fujisawa's codeveloper, Taiho, confirmed that these trials were ongoing, but no new clinical data have been announced or published. TF-505 is a potential alternative to finasteride and dutasteride (GlaxoSmithKline/Astellas' Avodart).

Compared with finasteride, TF-505 exhibits a more potent inhibitory effect on testosterone-induced prostamegaly in castrated rats and is associated with a lower degree of suppression of sexual behavior (Fujita T, 2002). In a Phase I study of 12 healthy male volunteers, TF-505 induced dose-dependent inhibition of circulating 5-alpha-reductase; this inhibition peaked at 8–12 hours after dosing (Fujita T, 2000).

Gonadotropin Modulators

Overview. Chlormadinone acetate (Teikoku's Prostal/Prostal L) is the only gonadotropin modulator available for treating BPH. It is used only in Japan, where finasteride and dutasteride are not approved (Akakura K, 1998). Potentially serious side effects (e.g., diarrhea, sexual dysfunction, liver toxicity) make agents in this class less desirable than less-toxic therapies, such as the 5-ARIs. However, new agents in development may offer effective therapeutic relief and an improved side-effect profile. Because of their mechanism of action, these agents could have a greater effect on disease symptoms and progression.

Mechanism of Action. Current understanding of the etiology of BPH has established hormonal changes as a major contributor to the enlargement of prostate tissue around the urethra. The control of androgen production in the testes is directly mediated by hypothalamic/pituitary hormones (Griffin JE, 1985). Gonadotropin-releasing hormone (GnRH), also known as luteinizing hormone-releasing hormone (LHRH), is secreted by neurons in the hypothalamus; it subsequently stimulates the release of both luteinizing hormone (LH) and follicle-stimulating hormones (FSH) in the anterior pituitary. In the testes, LH interacts with specific cell-surface receptors in the plasma membrane of Leydig cells, activating the biochemical steps that lead to the synthesis of testosterone.

Cetrorelix. AEterna Zentaris (Quebec City, Quebec, Canada) recently announced a decision to continue development of cetrorelix, an LHRH antagonist, in Japan after making advances in Phase II studies in Germany and completing a broad Phase II program in endometriosis, BPH, and uterine myoma in the United States. This agent is currently the most advanced of the gonadotropin modulators in development for treatment of BPH. AEterna Zentaris's Japanese partners, Shionogi and Nippon Kayaku, planned to begin a Phase IIa clinical trial in 2005. This multicenter, placebo-controlled, randomized study will attempt to extrapolate the results from European studies to the Japanese BPH population.

Cetrorelix blocks LHRH receptors on the pituitary gland to prevent the release of luteinizing hormone (LH), thereby reducing the production of testosterone. Cetrorelix is different from other agents in the gonadotropin modulator class because of its unique, incomplete suppression of testosterone synthesis and sustained action. Without full hormone suppression, patients do not experience the side effects typically associated with gonadotropin modulators, such as depression, muscle weakness, and loss of libido. Furthermore, because cetrorelix has a longer half-life than other drugs in its class, fewer days of administration are required.

In May 2004, AEterna Zentaris presented data from Phase II trials of cetrorelix in European BPH patients (conducted by its partner, Solvay [Brussels, Belgium]) at the 18th World Congress of the International Federation of Fertility Societies (IFFS) (Aeterna Laboratories, press release [electronic], May 17, 2004). Two hundred and fifty patients were randomized into five treatment groups: placebo, one single intramuscular injection of cetrorelix via depot (30 mg or 60 mg), and four weekly subcutaneous (SC) injections of cetrorelix (5 mg or 10 mg). Following the last treatment day, patients were observed for four months. All active treatment groups showed a dose-dependent improvement in IPSS and Qmax, compared with placebo ($p < 0.001$); the therapeutic responses were maintained for three months beyond the last day of therapy. Serum testosterone decreased but did not reach castration level. Patients did not experience sexual dysfunction related to cetrorelix treatment. After clearance of the drug, patients recovered normal serum testosterone levels.

Researchers conducted an open Phase I/II study to test whether short-term administration of cetrorelix improves the treatment of BPH (Comaru-Schally AM, 1998). Thirteen patients with moderate to severe BPH were treated twice daily with 5 mg cetrorelix SC for two days followed by 1 mg/day SC for two months. They were evaluated at baseline, during treatment, and up to 18 months after therapy. Cetrorelix treatment resulted in a 52.9% decline ($p < 0.0001$) in the IPSS, a 46% improvement in QoL based on a QoL index ($p < 0.001$), a reduction of 27% ($p < 0.006$) in prostatic volume, and an increase in peak urinary flow (Qmax) rate of 2.86 mL/s at the end of therapy. Most patients continued to show a progressive improvement in urinary symptoms during long-term follow-up, with a decline in IPSS of 67% and 72% at weeks 20 and 85, respectively. This study demonstrates that short-term administration of cetrorelix produces long-term improvement. However, randomized, double-blind, placebo-controlled studies are needed to confirm these preliminary findings.

ML-04. Milkhaus Laboratory, Inc. (Boxford, Massachusetts) has ML-04 (HP-4), a patented oral form of human chorionic gonadotropin (hCG), in U.S. Phase II trials as a potential therapeutic for BPH. ML-04 is also in Phase II trials for chronic prostatitis and myelodysplastic syndrome (MDS).

In BPH, prostate cells have lost their capacity to be normally regulated, which results in hyperplasia and failure of programmed cell death (apoptosis). Prostatic cells express hCG receptors, and researchers hypothesize that hCG used therapeutically might restore normal cell regulatory controls in BPH tissue, thus blocking or reversing the disease process.

The results of a multicenter, double-blind, placebo-controlled Phase IIa trial of ML-04 in patients with moderate to severe BPH were reported in 1998 (Milkhaus Laboratory, press release, October 1998). In the 100-patient trial, the difference in symptom relief between ML-04 and placebo as measured by the AUASI score was statistically significant: over a 16-week period, the average change from baseline was -3.29 for the placebo group and -6.79 for the ML-04 group. ML-04 reportedly improved sexual function and was safe.

The company is continuing to evaluate ML-04 in a Phase IIb trial with more patients, longer treatment duration, and a broader dose range. In April 2003, enrollment was complete, with a total of 546 patients in 11 centers worldwide. The effectiveness of the drug will be measured by symptom relief as assessed by changes in the AUASI score. Final results have yet to be announced.

Vitamin D3 Analogues

Overview. The active form of vitamin D3 is calcitriol. Initially, this steroid was shown to control bone metabolism and calcium equilibrium; it has the ability to induce hypercalcemia and hyperphosphatemia. Further research proved that calcitriol also moderates cell proliferation, differentiation, and apoptosis. Vitamin D3 analogues have been developed for BPH treatment with the intention of preserving regulatory activity without causing hypercalcemic side effects. The class of vitamin D3 analogues is novel in the treatment of BPH, so elucidating its mechanism of action to practicing physicians will be necessary for this class to achieve commercial success.

Mechanism of Action. Vitamin D3 binds to vitamin D receptors, which are expressed in the human prostate gland. Vitamin D receptors are responsible for hyperproliferation of cells and are implicated in diseases such as psoriasis, cancer, and BPH. In addition to reacting directly with vitamin D receptors, vitamin-D-receptor ligands have been shown to antagonize growth factor (GF) receptors. In combination, these actions have influential regulatory effects on tissue expansion and cell death.

Synthetic analogues of vitamin-D-receptor ligands have been modified in their side chains so as to improve their therapeutic effects. Side effects related to hypercalcemia can be reduced by use of vitamin D3 analogues instead of natural vitamin D3 agents.

BXL-628. Roche has granted exclusive worldwide development and marketing rights to the novel vitamin D3 analogue BXL-628 to BioXell (Milan, Italy), an Italian company spun off from Roche Milano Richerche. BXL-628 is the company's most advanced developmental drug. BioXell's U.S. subsidiary is currently conducting clinical trials for BXL-628 in patients with BPH. A Phase IIb, dose-ranging study was initiated in July 2005.

BioXell's new agent offers a novel approach to the treatment of BPH. BXL-628 is significantly less hypercalcemic than cacitriol and other analogues in the vitamin D3 analogue class. It works by inhibiting the activity of growth factors involved in prostate proliferation. This action occurs downstream from the adrenergic receptors, which BXL-628 does not bind. Furthermore, BXL-628 does not interact with 5-alpha-reductase type 1 or type 2. Therefore, BXL-628 does not affect sex hormone secretion and potentially avoids sexual dysfunction and other side effects associated with 5-ARIs.

In September 2004, BioXell announced the results of a three-month, double-blind, randomized, placebo-controlled Phase IIa study that involved 120 men with BPH. Patients taking BXL-628 exhibited an average 7.2% reduction in prostate volume, compared with no reduction in patients taking placebo ($p < 0.0001$). Furthermore, 92% of patients treated with BXL-628 had no prostatic growth at all, compared with only 48% of patients treated with placebo who experienced no prostate enlargement ($p < 0.0001$).

Hexokinase Inhibitors

Overview. In BPH, hyperplasia of the prostate gland increases the number of smooth-muscle cells, and smooth-muscle tension causes bladder outlet obstruction leading to LUTS. Drugs that reduce total prostate volume, either by slowing cell multiplication or inducing cell apoptosis, reduce symptoms of BPH. Emerging therapies, such as hexokinase inhibitors, that can take advantage of this strategy offer a different approach to treatment than drugs that are currently available, and they may avoid associated side effects such as orthostatic hypotention, reverse ejaculation, decreased libido, and impotence.

Mechanism of Action. Recent research has shown that hexokinase inhibitors have the ability to disrupt glycolysis. Because prostate cells depend more on glycolysis than the citric acid cycle for energy to maintain and regenerate tissue, hexokinase inhibitors can cause prostate cell death, which relieves bladder outlet obstruction (Brawer M, 2005). Reducing prostate size through metabolic targeting is a novel method of treating BPH. So far, there is only one drug in this class in active development for BPH, and it has shown promise.

Lonidamine. Lonidamine, also known as TH-070, originated from the company Angelini, which licensed development outside of Europe to Threshold Pharmaceuticals (Redwood City, California). Lonidamine is currently marketed by Pfizer in Italy under the brand name Doridamina for the treatment of various cancers. For BPH, lonidamine has entered Phase III clinical trials in Europe and Phase II trials in the United States as part of a registrational program approved by the FDA. The Phase II and Phase III multicenter, double-blind, randomized trials will involve approximately 200 and 480 men and will last 4 weeks and 4.5 months, respectively. The goal of these trials is to investigate patients' dose-response in terms of safety and efficiency.

Results from a Phase II clinical trial conducted in Italy were published in August 2005. Thirty BPH patients were treated with 150 mg of oral lonidamine for 28 days, and follow-up observation was continued for six months after the end of therapy. Researchers found that lonidamine is well tolerated and correlates with a significant decrease in prostate volume and IPSS. On day 28, the average decrease in prostate size was 11.2% ($p < 0.001$). Fifteen patients (50%) had a reduction of at least 10%. Interestingly, there was no significant change in the sizes of the transitional zone of the prostate. The average decrease in IPSS was 7.3 points ($p < 0.001$); 47% of patients had an improvement of more than 7 points. Patients with higher baseline IPSS were more likely to have greater improvements in symptom scores. By day 200 (the last day of follow-up), IPSS had decreased further to a change of almost -10 points.

In addition to reductions in prostate size and symptom score, lonidamine treatment correlated with an improvement in measures of voiding symptoms, Qmax, and post-void residual volume. After 28 days of active treatment and 6 months without treatment, Qmax increased by 4.3 mL/s. Average residual volume reduced from 82 cc at baseline to 32 cc after 28 days of treatment. Lonidamine also decreased PSA levels by 17.8% at day 28 and by 14.8% at day 200.

Phosphodiesterase 5 Inhibitors

Overview. PDE 5 inhibitors have traditionally been used to treat patients with ED; several compounds are already approved and marketed for that indication. Tadalafil (Eli Lilly and Company [Indianapolis, Indiana]/ICOS Corporation's [Bothell, Washington] Cialis) is the first PDE 5 inhibitor under investigation for the treatment of BPH. Tadalafil has great potential as a supplemental treatment for dynamic BPH, a role that is not filled by any other drug.

Mechanism of Action. Researchers propose that PDE 5 inhibitors have an effect on the contractibility of prostate smooth muscle. An examination of their effect on rapid ejaculation shows that these agents can improve the symptoms of BPH by reducing the contractile response of prostatic and urethral tissues (Abdel-Hamid I, 2004). A bovine model has demonstrated that decreased blood flow to the prostate causes localized muscle contraction; treatment with a PDE 5 inhibitor relaxed muscles in the ischemic tissues (Azadzoi K, 2003). Further research is required to fully understand the mechanism of action of PDE 5 inhibitors on the prostate gland.

Tadalafil. ICOS tadalafil is currently in Phase II development for the treatment of BPH. The company initiated studies in May 2004, and by November 2004, clinical trials were under way. Icos stated that its research suggests that tadalafil can relax prostatic smooth muscle, thereby reducing obstructive symptoms associated with BPH (ICOS Corporation, press release [electronic], November 4, 2004).

Prostate-Reducing Agents

Overview. One approach to reducing LUTS resulting from BPH is to reduce prostate hyperplasia, which limits the amount of smooth-muscle development and activity associated with dynamic BPH as well as bladder outlet obstruction as a result of static BPH. Development of this type of drug treatment is needed because it would relieve not only urinary symptoms but also the progression of BPH. Nymox Pharmaceuticals (Maywood, New Jersey) is currently researching NX-1207, which has shown ability to reduce prostate size. The company has yet to release details about the exact mechanism of action, but clinical trials have focused on prostate size reduction and symptom relief.

Mechanism of Action. Drug development databases suggest that NX-1207 has cytotoxic qualities that contribute to apoptosis within the prostate. However, the specific targets involved in the mechanism of action are unclear.

NX-1207. Nymox Pharmaceuticals is currently conducting Phase II clinical trials of its new oral drug, NX-1207, for the treatment of BPH. So far, results from two major Phase I and I/II studies have been published. The Phase I study involved 20 men with BPH who did not respond to alpha blockers and 5-ARIs. They were treated with NX-1207 for 30 days and exhibited a significant reduction in prostate size ($p = 0.035$) and an average reduction in AUASI of 6.87 points ($p = 0.0352$) (Nymox Pharmaceuticals, press release [electronic], July 28, 2004).

In a follow-up Phase II study, patients continued their treatment for one year, by the end of which patients taking NX-1207 had an 8.8 point improvement in AUASI compared with the control group. A large-scale Phase II study is currently under way in the United States (Nymox Pharmaceuticals, press release [electronic], March 22, 2005).

REFERENCES

Abdel-Hamid IA. Phosphodiesterase 5 inhibitors in rapid ejaculation: potential use and possible mechanisms of action. *Drugs*. 2004;**64**(1):13–26.

Akakura K, et al. Steroidal and nonsteroidal antiandrogens: chemical structures, mechanisms of action and clinical applications. *Nippon Rinsho*. 1998;**56**(8):2124–2128.

Akiyama K, et al. Effect of KMD-3213, an α1a – adrenoceptor antagonist, on the prostatic urethral pressure and blood pressure in male decerebrate dogs. *International Journal of Urology*. 2001;**8**:177–183.

Apolone G, et al. Knowledge and opinion on prostate and prevalence of self-reported BPH and prostate-related events. A cross-sectional survey in Italy. *European Journal of Cancer Prevention*. 2002;**11**:473–479.

Azadkoi KM, et al. Chronic ischemia increases prostatic smooth muscle contraction in the rabbit. *The Journal of Urology*. 2003;**170**:659–663.

Barry MJ, Roehrborn C. Management of benign prostatic hyperplasia. *Annual Review of Medicine*. 1997;**48**:177–189.

Barry MJ. Editorial comment to Kojima M, et al. The American Urological Association symptom index for benign prostatic hyperplasia as a function of age, volume, and ultrasonic appearance of the prostate. *The Journal of Urology*. 1997;**157**:2160–2165.

Bartsch G, et al. Dihydrotestosterone and the concept of 5α-reductase in human benign prostatic hyperplasia. *European Urology*. 2000;**37**:367–380.

Bautista OM, et al. Study design of the Medical Therapy of Prostatic Symptoms (MTOPS) trial. *Control Clinical Trials*. 2003;**24**(2):224–243.

Berges RR, Pientka L. Management of the BPH syndrome in Germany: Who is treated and how? *European Urology*. 1999;(suppl 3):21–27.

Blanker MH, et al. Strong effects of definition and nonresponse bias on prevalence rates of clinical benign prostatic hyperplasia: the Krimpen study of male urogenital tract problems and general health status. *British Journal of Urology*. 2000;**85**:665–671.

Boyle P. New insights into the epidemiology and natural history of benign prostatic hyperplasia. *Progress in Clinical and Biological Research*. 1994;**386**:3–18.

Buzelin JM, et al. comparison of tamsulosin with alfuzosin in the treatment of patients with lower urinary tract symptoms suggestive of bladder outlet obstruction (symptomatic benign prostatic hyperplasia). *British Journal of Urology*. 1997;**80**(4):597–605.

Chapple CR, et al. A 12-week placebo-controlled double-blind study of prazosin in the treatment of benign prostatic hyperplasia. *British Journal of Urology*. 1992;**70**:285–294.

Chess-Williams R, et al. The role of alpha1D-adrenoceptors in prostatic contraction examine using protection studies. *Autonomic & Autacoid Pharmacology*. 2002;**22**(5–6):291–296.

Chicharro-Molero JA, et al. Prevalence of benign prostatic hyperplasia in Spanish men 40 years old or older. *The Journal of Urology*. 1998;**159**:878–882.

Chow W, et al. Multicentre controlled trial of indoramin in the symptomatic relief of benign prostatic hypertrophy. *British Journal of Urology*. 1990;**65**:36–38.

Chute CG, et al. The prevalence of prostatism: a population-based survey of urinary symptoms. *The Journal of Urology*. 1993;**150**:85–89.

Clark R, et al. Effective suppression of dihydrotestosterone (DHT) by GI98745, a novel dual 5 alpha reductase inhibitor (abstract). *The Journal of Urology*. 1999;**161**:268

Clifford GM, Farmer RDT. Medical therapy for benign prostatic hyperplasia: a review of the literature. *European Urology*. 2000;**38**:2–19.

Collins MF, et al. Underdetection of clinical benign prostatic hyperplasia in a general medical practice. *Journal of General Internal Medicine*. 1996;**11**(9):513–518.

Comaru-Schally AM, et al. Efficacy and safety of lutenizing hormone-releasing hormone antagonist cetrorelix in the treatment of symptomatic benign prostatic hyperplasia. *Journal of Clinical Endrocrinology and Metabolism*. 1998;**83**:3826–3831.

Costa P, et al. Hyperplasie Bénigne de la Prostate (HBP): prévalence en medicine générale et attitude pratique des médecins generalists français. Résultats d'une etude réalisée auprés de 17.953 patients. *Progrés en Urologie*. 2004;**14**:33–39.

Crescioli C, et al. Inhibition of Spontaneous and Androgen-Induced Prostate Growth by a Nonhypercalcemic Calcitriol Analog. *Endocrinology*. 2003;**144**:3046–3057.

Fawzy A, et al. Long-term (4 year) efficacy and tolerability of doxazosin for the treatment of concurrent benign prostatic hyperplasia and hypertension. *International Journal of Urology*. 1996;**6**:346–354.

Fawzy A, et al. Practice patterns among primary care physicians in benign prostatic hyperplasia and prostate cancer. *Family Medicine*. 1997;**29**(5):321–325.

Flam T, et al. [Screening of clinical benign prostatic hypertrophy in general practice: survey of 18,540 men.] *Progrés en Urologie*. 2003;**13**:416–424.

Fujita T. Clinical pharmacology of the urogenital system: TF-505. Seventh Conference on Clinical Pharmacology and Therapeutics and Fourth Congress of the European Association for Clinical Pharmacology and Therapeutics, Florence, Italy; 2000:July 15–20.

Fujita T, et al. Pharmacokinetics and pharmacodynamics of TF-505, a novel nonsteroidal 5-alpha-reductase inhibitor, in normal subjects treated with single or multiple doses. *British Journal of Clinical Pharmacology*. 2002;**54**:283–294.

Garraway WM, et al. High prevalence of benign prostatic hypertrophy in the community. *Lancet*. 1991;**338**:469–471.

Garraway WM, et al. Impact of previously unrecognized benign prostatic hyperplasia on the daily activities of middle-aged and elderly men. *British Journal of General Practice*. 1993;**43**:318–321.

Gee WF, et al. 1997 American Urological Association Gallup survey: Changes in diagnosis and management of prostate cancer and benign prostatic hyperplasia, and other practice trends from 1994 to 1997. *The Journal of Urology*. 1998;**160**(5):1804–1807.

Gerber GS, et al. Saw Palmetto (Sernoa repends) in men with lower urinary tract symptoms: effects on urodynamis parameters and voiding symptoms. *Urology*. 1998;**51**:1003–1007.

Girman CJ. Population-based studies of the epidemiology of benign prostatic hyperplasia. *British Journal of Urology*. 1998;**82**(suppl 1):34–43.

Gomez A, et al. Quality of life and symptomatology in benign prostate hyperplasia in active Spanish population. *Medicina Clinica*. 2000;**114**(suppl 3):81–89.

Gong EM, Gerber GS. Saw Palmetto and benign prostatic hyperplasia. *The American Journal of Chinese Medicine*. 2004;**32**:331–338.

Griffin JE, Wilson JD. Disorders of the testes and male reproductive tract. In: Wilson JD, Foster DW (eds) Williams textbook of endrocrinology. Philadelphia: Saunders; 1985:259.

Guess HA. Benign prostatic hyperplasia: antecedents and natural history. *Epidemiologic Review*. 1992;**14**:131–153.

Guthrie R. Benign prostatic hyperplasia in elderly men. What are the special issues in treatment? *Postgraduate Medicine*. 1997 May;**101**(5):141–143, 148, 141–154.

Hayashi T, et al. A comparative study assessing clinical effects of naftopidil and tamsulosin hydrochloride on benign prostatic hyperplasia. *Hinyokika Kiyo*. 2002;**48**:7–11.

Hunter DJ, et al. Health care sought and received by men with urinary symptoms, and their views on prostatectomy. *British Journal of General Practice*. 1995;**45**(390):27–30.

Ikegaki I. Pharmacological properties of naftopidil, a drug for treatment of the bladder outlet obstruction for patients with benign prostatic hyperplasia. *Nippon Yakurigaku Zasshi*. 2000;**116**:63–69.

Jacobsen SJ, et al. A population-based study of health care-seeking behavior for treatment of urinary symptoms. The Olmsted County Study of Urinary Symptoms and Health Status Among Men. *Archives of Family Medicine*. 1993;**2**:729–735.

Jacobsen SJ, et al. New diagnostic and treatment guidelines for benign prostatic hyperplasia. Potential impact in the United States. *Archives of Internal Medicine*. 1995;**155**: 477–481.

Jacobsen SJ, et al. Natural history of prostatism: risk factors for acute urinary retention. *Journalof Urology*. 1997;**158**:481–487.

Ju XB, et al. The clinical efficacy of naftopidil tablet in the treatment of benign prostatic hyperplasia. *Zhonghua Nan Ke Xue*. 2002;**8**:286–288.

Kirby R, et al. alpha(1)-Adrenoceptor selectivity and the treatment of benign prostatic hyperplasia and lower urinary tract symptoms. *Prostate Cancer & Prostatic Disease*. 2000;**3**(2):76–83.

Kirby RS, et al. Doxazosin controlled release vs tamsulosin in the management of benign prostatic hyperplasia: an efficacy analysis. *Clinical Practice*. 2004;**58**:6–10.

Kojima M, et al. The American Urological Association symptom index for benign prostatic hyperplasia as a function of age, volume and ultrasonic appearance of the prostate. *The Journal of Urology*. 1997;**157**:2160–2165.

Lam JS, et al. Changing aspects in the evaluation and treatment of patients with benign prostatic hyperplasia. *The Medical Clinics of North America*. 2004;**88**:281–308.

Lee KL, Peehl DM. Molecular and cellular pathogenesis of benign prostatic hyperplasia. *The Journal of Urology*. 2004;**172**:1784–1791.

Lee M. Tamsulosin for the treatment of benign prostatic hypertrophy. *Annals of Pharmacotherapy*. 2000;**34**:188–199.

Lepor H. Phase III multicenter placebo-controlled study of tamsulosin in benign prostatic hyperplasia. *Urology*. 1998;**51**:892–900. [a]

Lepor H. Long-term evaluation of tamsulosin in benign prostatic hyperplasia: placebo-controlled double-blind extension of Phase III trial. *Urology*. 1998;**51**:901–906. [b]

Litwin MS, et al. The National Institutes of Health chronic prostatitis symptom index: development and validation of a new outcome measure. *The Journal of Urology*. 1999;**162**:369–375.

Lukacs B. Management of symptomatic BPH in France: Who is treated and how? *European Urology*. 1999;**36**(suppl 3):14–20.

McConnell JD, et al. Benign prostatic hyperplasia: diagnosis and treatment. Clinical Practice Guideline, Number 8. AHCPR Publication No. 94–0582. Rockville, MD: Agency for Health Care Policy and Research, Public Health Service, U.S. Department of Health and Human Services. February 1994.

McConnell JD, et al. The effect of finasteride on the risk of acute urinary retention and the need for surgical treatment among men with benign prostatic hyperplasia. Finasteride Long-Term Efficacy and Safety Group. *New England Journal of Medicine*. 1998;**338**:557–562.

McConnell JD. Benign prostatic hyperplasia: other hormonal treatments. www.UroHealth.org 2003. [a]

McConnell JD. Medical therapy Post-MTOPS. Presented at the 98th Annual Meeting of the American Urological Association, April 26–May 1, 2003; Chicago, IL. [b]

McKiernan JM, Lowe FC. Side effects of terazosin in the treatment of symptomatic benign prostatic hyperplasia. *Southern Medical Journal*. 1997;**90**:509–513.

McNicholas TA. Management of symptomatic BPH in the UK: who is treated and how? *European Urology*. 1999;**36**(suppl 3):33–39.

Medina JJ, et al. Benign prostatic hyperplasia (the aging prostate). *Medical Clinics of North America*. 1999;**83**:1213–1229.

Meigs JB, et al. Risk factors for clinical benign prostatic hyperplasia in a community-based population of healthy aging men. *Journal of Clinical Epidemiology*. 2001;**54**:935–944.

Mobley DF, et al. Effect of doxazosin on the symptoms of benign prostatic hyperplasia: results from three double-blind placebo-controlled studies. *International Journal of Clinical Practice*. 1997;**51**(5):282–288.

Murata S, et al. Tissue selectivity of KMD-3213, an alpha(1)-adrenoreceptor antagonist, in human prostate and vasculature. *The Journal of Urology*. 2000;**164**(2):578–583.

Napalkov P, et al. Worldwide patterns of prevalence and mortality from benign prostatic hyperplasia. *Urology*. 1995;**46**:41–46.

Narayan P, et al. A second phase III multicenter placebo controlled study of 2 dosages of modified release tamsulosin in patients with symptoms of benign prostatic hyperplasia. *The Journal of Urology*. 1998;**160**:1701–1706.

Narayan P, et al. Long-term safety and efficacy of tamsulosin for the treatment of lower urinary tract symptoms associated with benign prostatic hyperplasia. *The Journal of Urology*. 2003;**170**:498–502.

Okada H, et al. Tamsulosin and chlormadinone for the treatment of benign prostatic hyperplasia. The Kobe University YM617 Study Group. *Scandinavian Journal of Urology and Nephrology*. 1996;**30**(5):379–285.

Population Division of the Department of Economic and Social Affairs of the United Nations Secretariat. World Population Prospects: The 2002 Revision, vol. II, The Sex and Age Distribution of Populations (United Nations publication, Sales No. E.03.XIII.7), 2003.

Roehrborn CG, et al. The Hytrin Community Assessment Trial Study: a one-year study of terazosin versus placebo in the treatment of men with symptomatic benign prostatic hyperplasia. HYCAT Investigator Group. *Urology*. 1996;**47**(2):159–168.

Roehrborn CG. Efficacy and safety of once-daily alfuzosin in the treatment of lower urinary tract symptoms and clinical benign prostatic hyperplasia: a randomized, placebo-controlled trial. *Urology*. 2001;**58**(6):953–959.

Roehrborn CG, et al. Efficacy and safety of a dual inhibitor of 5-alpha-reductase types 1 and 2 (dutasteride) in men with benign prostatic hyperplasia. *Urology*. 2002;**60**:434–441.

Roehrborn CG, et al. Sustained decrease in incidence of acute urinary retention and surgery with finasteride for 6 years in men with benign prostatic hyperplasia. *The Journal of Urology*. 2004;**171**:1194–1198.

Roehrborn CG, et al. Efficacy and safety of dutasteride in the four-year treatment of men with benign prostatic hyperplasia. *The Journal of Urology*. 2004;**63**:709–715.

Sanchez-Chapado M, et al. Safety and efficacy of sustained-release alfuzosin on lower urinary tract symptoms suggestive of benign prostatic hyperplasia in 3,095 Spanish patients evaluated during general practice. *European Urology*. 2000;**37**(4):421–427.

Sagnier P, et al. Results of an epidemiological survey using a modified American Urological Association symptom index for benign prostatic hyperplasia in France. *The Journal of Urology*. 1994;**151**:1266–1270.

Simpson RJ, et al. Consultation patterns in a community survey of men with benign prostatic hyperplasia. *British Journal of General Practice*. 1994;**44**(388):499–502.

Sponer G, et al. Naftopidil, a new adrenoceptor blocking agent with Ca(2 +)-antagonistic properties: interaction with adrenoceptors. *Journal of Cardiovascular Pharmacology*. 1992;**20**:1006–1013.

Thorpe A, et al. Benign prostatic hyperplasia. *The Lancet*. 2003;**361**:1359–1367.

Trueman P, et al. Prevalence of lower urinary tract symptoms and self-reported diagnosed 'benign prostatic hyperplasia', and their effect on quality of life in a community-based survey of men in the UK. *British Journal of Urology*. 1999;**83**:410–415.

Tsukamoto T, et al. Prevalence of prostatism in Japanese men in a community-based study with comparison to a similar American study. *The Journal of Urology*. 1995;**154**: 391–395.

Tsukamoto T, Masumori N. Epidemiology and natural history of benign prostatic hyperplasia. *International Journal of Urology*. 1997;**4**:233–246.

Tubaro A, Montanari E. Management of symptomatic BPH in Italy: who is treated and how? *European Urology*. 1999;**36**(suppl 3):28–32.

Ukimura O, et al. A statistical study of the American Urological Association symptom index for benign prostatic hyperplasia in participants of mass screening program for prostatic diseases using transrectal sonography. *The Journal of Urology*. 1996;**156**:1673–1678.

Ukimura O, et al. [A statistical study of benign prostatic hyperplasia in Japan.] *Nippon Rinsho*. 2002;**60**:577–584.

Vallancien G. How are lower urinary tract symptoms managed in real life practice? The French experience. *European Urology*. 2000;**38**(suppl 1):54–59.

van Kerrebroeck P, et al. Efficacy and safety of a new prolonged release formulation of alfuzosin 10mg once daily versus alfuzosin 2.5mg thrice daily and placebo in patients with symptomatic benign prostatic hyperplasia. ALFORTI study group. *European Urology*. 2000;**37**:306–313.

Walsh P.C. Campbell's Urology. 8th edition. 2002 W.B. Saunders Co. Epidemiology and Natural History. http://home.mdconsult.com/das /book/body/0/1049/391.html. Accessed 4/10/2003.

Yoshida M, et al. Silodosin, a new effective $\alpha 1a$ – adrenoceptor selective antagonist for the treatment of benign prostatic hyperplasia: Results of a phase 3 randomized, placebo-controlled, double-blind study. Presented at the 100th Annual Meeting of the American Urological Association, May 21–26, 2005; San Antonio, TX.

Ziada A, et al. Benign prostatic hyperplasia: an overview. *Urology*. 1999;**53**:1–6.

Stress Urinary Incontinence

ETIOLOGY AND PATHOPHYSIOLOGY

Introduction

Stress urinary incontinence (SUI) involves the involuntary leakage of small amounts of urine as a result of increased abdominal pressure (stress). This pressure occurs because of a lack of detrusor muscle contraction or overdistention of the bladder. Patients often experience SUI during physical exertion, coughing, sneezing, and laughing.

Anatomy

The Bladder. The bladder is a hollow, muscular organ found in the anterior section of the pelvic cavity (Figure 1). The organ and its outlet, the urethra, serve two functions: to store urine without leakage and to expel urine periodically through a relaxed outlet (the urethra). In males, the bladder lies in front of the rectum. In females, the organ is situated in front of the vagina, which lies in front of the rectum.

The bladder wall comprises three layers:

- The lumenal layer (mucosa) consists of a thin plane of cells, the transitional epithelium. These cells produce a protective mucosal membrane barrier and are supported by a basement membrane that provides a supportive structure

Male

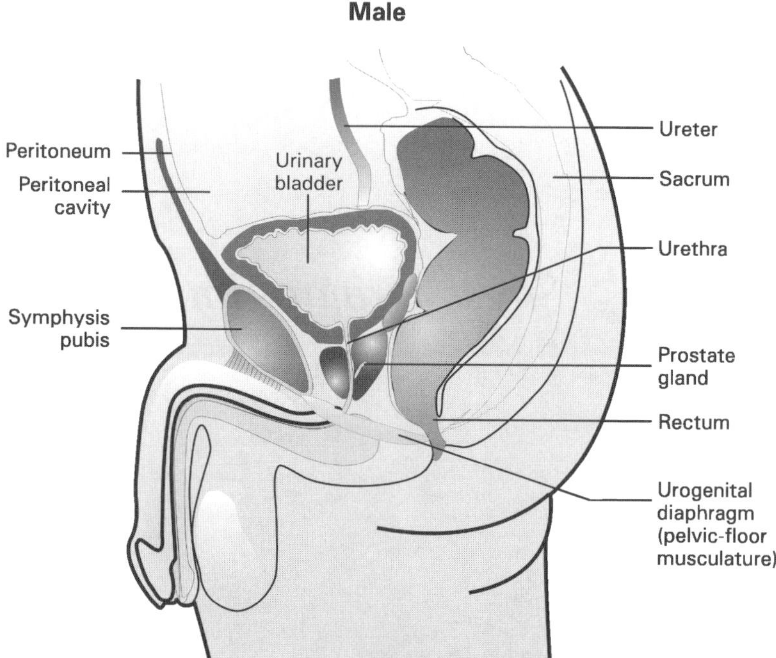

Female

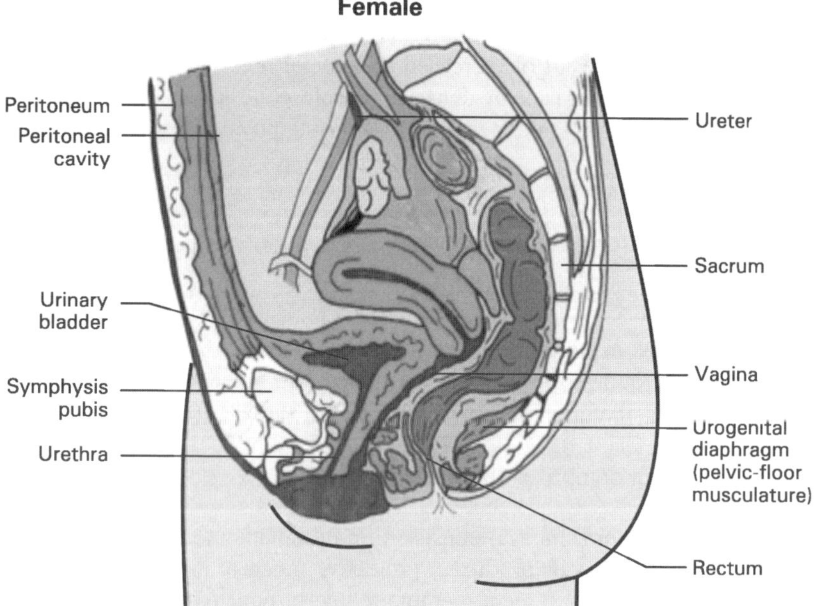

FIGURE 1. *Anatomical location of the bladder and pelvic organs.*

and filtration barrier between the submucosa (the lamina propria, which is enervated and contains blood and lymphatic vessels) and the transitional epithelium.

- The second layer is the submucosa, which consists of connective tissue that attaches the mucosal layer to the third layer, the detrusor muscle.
- The detrusor muscle consists of both longitudinal and circular muscle fibers that form an interconnecting mesh. Contractions of the detrusor muscle raise pressure within the bladder, allowing micturition (urination) to take place.

The final layer, known as the serosa, is not strictly part of the bladder. It composes the peritoneum (the sac encasing the abdominal organs) and covers only the upper surface of the bladder.

Control of the lower urinary tract is maintained by the parasympathetic and sympathetic nervous systems in an antagonistic relationship. Signal transduction through the parasympathetic nervous system induces contraction of the detrusor muscle (by activating muscarinic receptors located in the detrusor muscle) while it inhibits smooth muscle contractions in the urethra. These simultaneous actions increase the pressure in the bladder and reduce the resistance of the urethra; subsequently, urine is voided. Conversely, the sympathetic nervous system relaxes the detrusor muscle by activating β_2-adrenergic receptors in the tissue and contracts the bladder neck by stimulating α_1-adrenergic receptors located there. These actions relax the bladder, allowing it to fill with urine while keeping the urethra contracted and watertight—thus maintaining continence. Hence, voiding is typically mediated via the parasympathetic nervous system and bladder filling via the sympathetic nervous system.

A combination of peristaltic-like movements (waves of muscular contractions) within the ureters (tubes that connect the bladder to the kidneys) and gravity assist in moving urine from the hilum of the kidney toward the bladder. As the bladder fills, it is forced upward within the pelvic cavity, becoming first more spherical and then pear-shaped. Throughout this process, the pressure in the bladder remains relatively constant. This pressure control is important in maintaining continence. If the bladder were to increase in pressure as it filled, continence would be maintained until the bladder pressure exceeded the urethral resistance. At this point, urine would leak and continence would be lost. An increase in bladder urine volume from 10 mL (virtually empty) to 400 mL (virtually full) produces a pressure increase of only about 5–10 mL H_2O. This slight increase in intravesical pressure—despite a dramatic increase in the volume of liquid within the bladder—shows the bladder's effectiveness at maintaining a relatively stable pressure.

Role of the Ureters: Creation of a Control Valve. The ureters enter the bladder at a triangular area known as the trigone, then run at an oblique angle through the organ. The angle at which the ureters enter the bladder is important because the ureter, when positioned at the correct angle, forms a valve that inhibits reflux of urine. This valve mechanism works in two ways: by compressing the

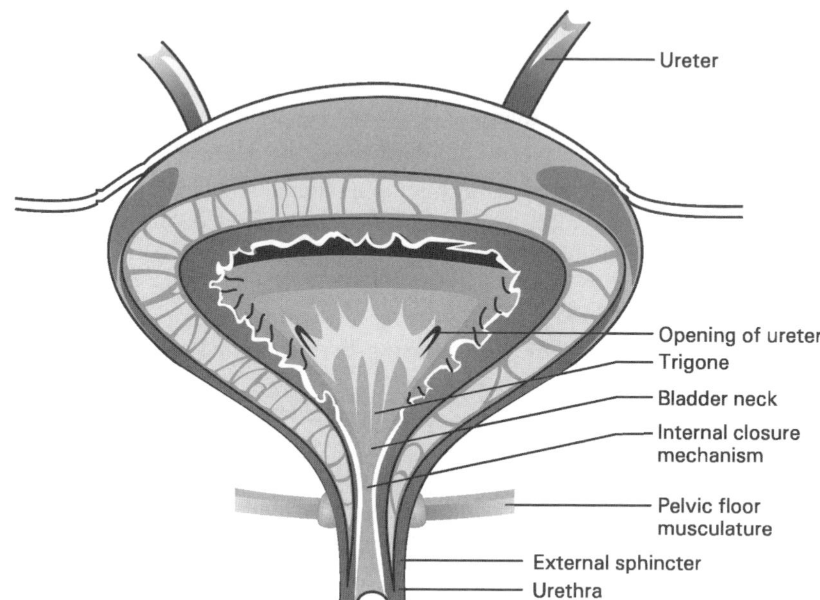

FIGURE 2. *Cross-section of the female urinary bladder.*

ureters during filling as the pressure increases and by contracting muscles within the bladder during micturition.

Figure 2 shows a cross section of the female bladder. At the base of this organ lies a closure mechanism that leads into the urethra. This mechanism is not a true sphincter; rather than being a muscle designed specifically for the purpose of urethral constriction, it relies on the pelvic-floor muscle to compress the urethra when the pressure inside the bladder increases. This compression creates a valve that controls urinary flow.

Males have a different control valve than females. In males, a circular layer of muscle extends down the prostate capsule. The contraction of this muscle group and nearby longitudinal fibers prevents semen from being ejaculated into the bladder during orgasm. Women lack this circular muscle. Instead, the female longitudinal muscle runs into the urethra and is stimulated by cholinergic, parasympathetic nerves.

Role of the Bladder Neck: Controlling the Bladder/Abdominal Pressure Balance. In both sexes, ligaments from the pelvis and fascia support the bladder neck; contraction of muscles in the pelvic floor influences the position of the bladder neck. In females, the bladder neck is partially supported by the vaginal wall as well. In a continent person, the increases in abdominal pressure during bladder filling are transferred evenly to the bladder and the bladder neck. Hence, an increase in pressure on the bladder is matched by an increase in resistance placed on the bladder neck.

The Urethra. The urethra is the tube through which urine is expelled from the bladder during micturition. Between the eighth and twelfth weeks of embryogenesis of a female fetus, the urogenital membrane develops into the upper part of the bladder, the vagina, and the distal part of the urethra. Because these three tissues evolved from the same embryogenic material, they are all equally hormone-dependent. Mucosal folds within the urethra are sensitive to the hormone estrogen; they help to provide a seal that is essential for maintaining continence.

Not surprisingly, the structure of the urethra varies significantly between males and females. The female urethra is straight and approximately 3–5 cm in length. In contrast, the male urethra has an S shape and can reach 22 cm in length. The urethra in both sexes contains layers of muscle that together constitute the urethral sphincter. The layer of smooth circular muscle is known as the internal sphincter. In women, the internal sphincter forms the entire urethra, while in men, the internal sphincter makes up only the posterior portion of the urethra. An outer circular, striated muscle, located near the pelvic floor, serves as the external sphincter in women. Males, too, have an external sphincter, which is located below the pyramid-shaped structure called the verumontanum, which in turn is close to the prostate gland.

The internal sphincter contains alpha-adrenergic receptors that respond to stimulation by causing contraction and maintaining urethral closure. This process is involuntary and arises in response to bladder filling. In contrast, the external sphincter muscle is controlled by acetylcholine receptors that are under voluntary central control. People can override the normal micturition response by using voluntary control to squeeze the external sphincter shut, thus maintaining urethral closure until a socially appropriate time for bladder voiding (Fraser MO, 2003; Ostergard DR, 2004).

Involuntary and Voluntary Control of Micturition. Micturition—the process by which the bladder's function switches from urine storage to urine voiding—involves a significant neuromuscular component. The combination of a primitive spinal reflex and higher, voluntary processes controls micturition.

When 200–300 mL of urine has accumulated in the bladder, stretch receptors become activated, sending impulses to the spinal micturition center. The spinal micturition center lies in the S2-S4 sacral area at the bottom of the spinal cord (Figure 3). This part of the spine relays information to and from the bladder. In addition, the external urethral sphincter (rhabdosphincter) and the pelvic-floor muscles are innervated by the pudendal nerve, which also originates from the S2-S4 region of the spinal cord (from an area known as Onuf's nucleus). The parasympathetic motor nucleus lies in the S3-S4 part of the spinal cord.

Micturition centers are also present in the pons and cerebral cortex of the brain. Both centers allow voluntary control over the micturition reflex via the spinothalamic nerves. Micturition is initiated by a back-and-forth reflex—the spinal-pontine-spinal reflex ("pontine" refers to the pons of the brain). This reflex coordinates the simultaneous relaxing of the external sphincter, the pelvic-floor

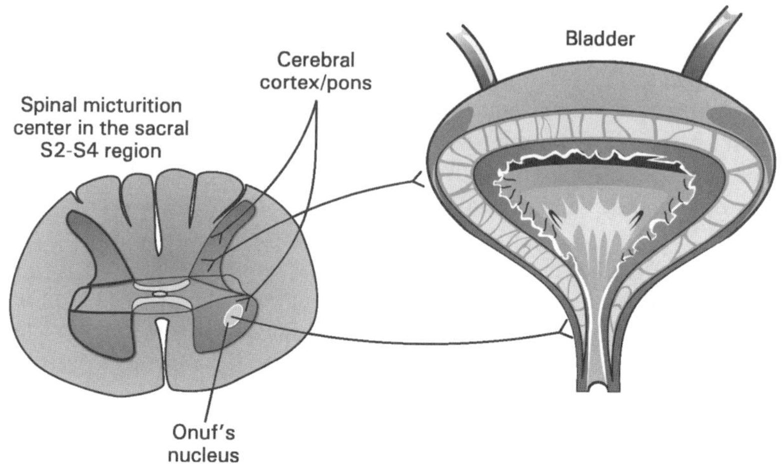

FIGURE 3. *Spinal control of micturition.*

muscles, and the bladder neck—along with contraction of the detrusor muscle. The intravesical pressure (pressure within the bladder) rises by approximately 100 cm H_2O, and urine is then expelled under pressure. Once micturition is voluntarily completed, the proximal urethra contracts, forcing any urine above the external sphincter back into the bladder. The bladder is then ready to reenter the filling phase.

Voluntary control over the bladder and external sphincter is learned as the nervous system matures. Typically, children achieve control by age three or four.

Pathophysiology

The two anatomical abnormalities that characterize SUI are weakening of the pelvic-floor musculature and deficiency of the urethral sphincter. Either of these abnormalities can compromise the body's natural ability to prevent urine loss during sudden increases in abdominal pressure.

Urethral Support Failure. In females, the urethra is supported by the levator and pelvic muscles, which surround the pelvic viscera and attach the bladder and urethra to a part of the vaginal wall known as the endopelvic fascia. The pubocervical fascia (a specific component of the endopelvic fascia that extends from the pubis to the cervix of the uterus) acts as a hammock for the vesical neck of the bladder and provides a compression surface—in essence, the pubocervical fascia pushes back against abdominal pressure forces and helps close off the bladder neck (Cundiff GW, 2004; DeLancey JO, 1996). The urethra normally has limited mobility (straining angle of less than 30 degrees from horizontal) when pelvic-floor muscles supply adequate support.

If the muscles supporting the bladder weaken, the bladder becomes able to move and descend into a lower position during periods of increased abdominal pressure. In this new position, the bladder neck is no longer within the abdominal cavity (or resting on the "hammock" of the pelvic musculature). This state is referred to as *urethral hypermobility* because the proximal urethra shifts and achieves a straining angle greater than 30 degrees from horizontal during cotton-swab testing (Ostergard DR, 2004). As the abdominal pressure increases, the bladder becomes squeezed, but a counterforce is no longer applied to the bladder neck to keep the structure closed. The result is the involuntary loss of urine that characterizes SUI.

Urethral Sphincter Deficiency. During bladder filling, parasympathetic innervation relaxes the detrusor muscle, but contraction of the bladder neck and the external sphincter prevents urine leakage. The external sphincter plays only a minor role in maintaining continence because it tires easily and, therefore, can contract for only a short period of time. For example, it normally contracts in response to increases in abdominal pressure, such as occur with coughing, sneezing, and laughing.

However, if the urethral sphincter is weakened, it is often unable to maintain urethral closure during stress (increased abdominal pressure) or while at rest. This condition is known as *intrinsic sphincter deficiency* (ISD), and it may be present alone or in conjunction with urethral hypermobility in patients with SUI. Although ISD may arise from physical damage to the sphincter muscles themselves, it may also be associated with neurological damage or impairment that interferes with normal sympathetic and/or parasympathetic control of the urethral sphincter. Pudendal nerve damage, for example, may impair or completely block voluntary contraction of the external sphincter. Because prostate surgery may damage urogenital innervation, ISD is a common feature of SUI in post-prostatectomy patients.

Classification. As the roles of urethral hypermobility and ISD in the pathogenesis of SUI have become well defined, researchers have developed a system for classifying SUI subtypes based on the nature of bladder neck descent and the degree of urethral sphincter function in SUI patients (Cundiff GW, 2004). The original classification system (Green TH, 1968) has been modified to include further subdivision of clinically relevant features of SUI (Blaivas JG, 1988; McGuire EJ, 1976). Blaivas and Olsson's version of SUI classification comprises the following types of SUI:

- *Type 0*. During increased abdominal pressure, the bladder neck and urethra are hypermobile and descend, but no urine leakage occurs.
- *Type 1*. During abdominal stress, the bladder neck and urethra are open and slightly hypermobile, with the urethra descending less than 2 cm during stress. The angle of the urethra has changed less than 45 degrees. Type I patients show little or no sign of cystocele (a condition where the bladder herniates, often into the vagina).

- *Type IIA*. The bladder neck and urethra are closed and very hypermobile, with the urethra descending more than 2 cm (greater than 45 degrees) during increased abdominal stress. Cystocele is more common.
- *Type IIB*. Similar to type IIA SUI in that the bladder neck and urethra are closed and very hypermobile, with the urethra descending more than 2 cm (greater than 45 degrees) during increased abdominal stress. At rest, the base of the bladder rests below the pubis so that, during stress, the bladder neck and urethra descend significantly more than with type IIA SUI.
- *Type III*. Synonymous with ISD, type III incontinence refers to serious SUI in which the angle of the urethra and the support of the vagina are not the cause of the urinary leakage; rather, the urethral sphincter is too weak to maintain continence during increased abdominal stress (Blaivas JG, 1988; Cundiff GW, 2004).

SUI subtypes in this classification generally correlate with severity of incontinence, with Type 0 being the mildest and Type III being the most severe. However, patient assessments of SUI severity do not consistently correlate to the frequency or severity of incontinent episodes: patients with very frequent incontinent episodes may rate their condition as mild, while SUI patients with only a handful of incontinent episodes per month may rate their condition as intolerable.

Etiology

The causes of SUI are primarily related to stress or trauma that damages the pelvic-floor musculature or other supporting tissues that normally prevent urethral hypermobility. Biochemical mediators may also play a role in disease etiology, particularly those that may amplify existing physical deficiencies or leave pelvic tissues more susceptible to damage. This section outlines some of the major risk factors for the development of SUI.

Child-Bearing History. A woman's history of vaginal deliveries is significantly associated with an increased risk of SUI. An Italian observational study found the odds ratios for SUI were 5.4 and 5.1 for women reporting one to two vaginal deliveries and three or more vaginal deliveries, respectively (Parazzini F, 2003). Vaginal deliveries exact profound pressure on the pelvic-floor musculature and contribute to the relaxation and weakening of those muscles over time. The result is the loss of the "hammock" that normally prevents urethral hypermobility. Additionally, the physical strain of child-bearing can damage urethral innervation that normally allows voluntary constriction of the urethral sphincter to prevent urine loss during increased abdominal pressure. The incidence of SUI may be particularly high immediately postpartum, but researchers have found that nearly one third of women will have some degree of SUI at least four years postdelivery (Fritel X, 2004; Schytt E, 2004).

Interestingly, caesarean delivery also confers an excess risk of developing SUI. In the previously mentioned Italian study, women with a history of any number of caesarean deliveries had an increased risk of SUI when compared with nulliparous women (Parazzini F, 2003). Estrogen deficiency and/or excess progesterone during pregnancy may play a role in this phenomenon. As described previously, bladder and urethral tissues share the same embryogenic source as many parts of the female reproductive tract and thus are equally hormone-dependent. Low estrogen levels cause the urethral lining to lose its previously abundant mucus layer and muscle tone and lead to thinning of vaginal tissues that normally provide structural support to the bladder neck and proximal urethra. Indeed, many women develop SUI while pregnant or while breast-feeding an infant, presumably because of estrogen deficiency during these periods; the risk of SUI 15 years postchildbirth is approximately doubled in women who developed antenatal SUI (Dolan LM, 2003).

Urogenital Surgery. Along with erectile dysfunction, urinary incontinence (including SUI) is one of the most common complications in post-prostatectomy patients. Studies have demonstrated that incontinence (SUI, urge UI, or mixed UI) occurs in up to 70% of post-prostatectomy patients, with prevalence falling as time postoperative increases (Alivizatos G, 2003; Bate TS, 1998; Sebesta M, 2002; van Kampen M, 1997). Researchers suggest that the specific surgical procedure (nerve-sparing versus non-nerve-sparing, or transvesical versus transurethral versus radical) and the expertise of the practicing surgeon are significant determinants of the rate of incontinence following prostatectomy (Alivizatos G, 2003; van Kampen M, 1997).

Data on the risk of developing SUI posthysterectomy are conflicting. Anecdotal evidence suggests that hysterectomized women are at increased risk of developing SUI either immediately posthysterectomy or later in life; some observational studies have confirmed this link (Benedetti-Panici P, 2004; Parazzini F, 2003). However, a prospective Swedish study found that neither abdominal nor vaginal hysterectomy was associated with a significant change in the prevalence of SUI or urge UI (UUI) 12 months postoperatively (Altman D, 2003).

Comorbid Conditions. An increased risk of SUI is associated with a number of comorbid conditions. Obesity has been shown to predispose both men and women to SUI (Jackson RA, 2004; Maher C, 2002; Parazzini F, 2003; Rasmussen KL, 1997; Van Oyen H, 2002). A history of chronic obstructive pulmonary disease (COPD) (Jackson RA, 2004) or constipation (Maher C, 2002) has also been linked to SUI. All three conditions are linked to SUI presumably because they inflict chronic and/or intense increased pressure on the pelvic-floor musculature, leaving it prone to relaxation. Neurological conditions such as Parkinson's disease are also associated with many types of incontinence—including SUI—because of central nervous system dysfunction that disrupts voluntary and/or involuntary control of bladder function.

Reduction in Endogenous Estrogen. In peri- and postmenopausal women, reductions in endogenous estrogen production can result in the development or exacerbation of SUI symptoms. Low estrogen levels cause the urethral lining to lose its previously abundant mucus layer and muscle tone and lead to thinning of the vaginal tissues that normally provide structural support to the bladder neck and proximal urethra. As a result, either urethral hypermobility or ISD can develop in women during or immediately after menopause and in women who suffer estrogen deficiency secondary to disease.

Heredity. Some researchers believe that a familial factor may be involved in the development of SUI, and several published studies have shown that SUI prevalence is up to three times higher in first-degree relatives of female patients with SUI than in people without first-degree relatives afflicted by the condition. A Turkish study of 254 women, for example, found that the prevalence of SUI was 1.8–2.1 times higher among the first-degree female relative of SUI patients compared with the relatives of non-SUI patients (Ertunc D, 2004). This increased prevalence rate may reflect the presence of a genetic defect in connective tissue that could predispose people to SUI.

CURRENT THERAPIES

The three major approaches to stress urinary incontinence (SUI) treatment are rehabilitation, pharmacotherapy, and surgery. The Agency for Health Care Research and Quality (AHRQ; formerly the Agency for Health Care Policy and Research [AHCPR]) recommends behavioral modification or rehabilitation as the first-line therapy for SUI (AHCPR, 1996). Most behavioral modifications involve reducing fluid consumption and using absorbent pads and sponges, urethral plugs, and continence guards to reduce or absorb the result of an incontinence episode. Rehabilitation techniques are commonly encouraged, including bladder retraining and pelvic-floor exercises. Rehabilitation requires long-term commitment, and compliance to a physical therapy regimen is typically low. Although these techniques do not correct SUI, they may adequately reduce or manage incontinence symptoms while avoiding the worrisome side effects often seen with pharmacotherapy and surgery.

As discussed in the "Etiology and Pathophysiology" section, SUI is caused by malfunctions or defects in the mechanics of the pelvic-floor muscles or the urethral sphincter. In contrast to urge urinary incontinence (UUI), for which approved pharmacological treatments are available, the only pharmacological agents employed for SUI are off-label agents with only marginal efficacy. Phenyl-propanolamine (PPA, a constituent of numerous over-the-counter cold remedies and diet preparations) is an alpha-adrenergic agonist that was used until recently to treat SUI. In late 2000, regulatory authorities in both the United States and Europe asked manufacturers to voluntarily withdraw products containing PPA from the market following results of a five-year study that indicated an increased risk of hemorrhagic stroke in young women taking the compound (Kernan WN, 2000). PPA was subsequently withdrawn from sale in the United States and

TABLE 1. Current Therapies Used for Stress Urinary Incontinence

Agent	Company/Brand	Dose	Availability
Serotonin and norepinephrine reuptake inhibitors (SNRIs)			
Duloxetine	Eli Lilly/Boehringer Ingelheim's Yentreve/ Ariclaim	40 mg bid	G, UK
Hormone replacement therapies			
Estradiol vaginal cream	Galen's Estrace, others	100–200 µg qd or three times per week	G, S, UK, US
Estriol vaginal cream	Organon's Ovestin, others	500 µg qd or three times per week	F, G, I, J, S, UK, US
Conjugated estrogens vaginal cream	Wyeth's Premarin	0.3–1.25 mg qd or three times per week	US, I, UK
Estradiol vaginal ring	Pfizer's Estring	2 mg (approximately 7.5 µg/24 hours); replace ring every three months	G, UK, US
Estradiol vaginal tablet	Novo Nordisk's Vagifem	25 µg twice per week	G, I, UK, US
Beta-adrenergic agonists			
Clenbuterol	Teijin's Spiropent	20 µg bid	J

US = United States; F = France; G = Germany; I = Italy; S = Spain; UK = United Kingdom; J = Japan.

bid = Twice daily; qd = Once daily.

Europe, and its distribution was restricted to a small set of cold remedies in Japan. Surgery remains the most successful method for treating the mechanical malfunctions that characterize SUI.

Duloxetine (Eli Lilly and Company [Indianapolis, Indiana]/Boehringer Ingelheim's [Ingellheim, Germany] Yentreve/Ariclaim), a serotonin and norepinephrine reuptake inhibitor (SNRI), is the first agent formally indicated for treatment of SUI in Europe; it was approved there for SUI in 2004. Based on the mechanism of action, the use of alpha-adrenergic agonists and tricyclic antidepressants (TCAs) is theoretically appropriate, but clinical trial data supporting their use for SUI are scarce, and these agents are seldom used off-label to treat the condition. Table 1 summarizes the leading pharmacological therapies available to treat SUI.

Serotonin and Norepinephrine Reuptake Inhibitors

Overview. Originally developed as antidepressants, serotonin and norepinephrine reuptake inhibitors (SNRIs) have also been found to have benefits in SUI patients. Three SNRIs are currently marketed: duloxetine, venlafaxine (Wyeth's Effexor), and milnacipran (Sanofi-Aventis's [Tokyo, Japan] Ixel/Dalcipran in Europe; Asahi Kasei [Tokyo, Japan] and Janssen Pharmaceutical's [Antwerpen, Belgium] Toledomin in Japan). Although other drug classes, such as the TCAs, also function as serotonin and norepinephrine reuptake inhibitors, SNRIs were developed in the hope that a more balanced inhibition of the two neurotransmitters would result in greater efficacy—with fewer side effects—in treating both the emotional and physical symptoms of depression. The discovery of the role of serotonin and norepinephrine in the relaxation and contraction of urinary tract musculature prompted the development of SNRIs for SUI. Duloxetine's European approval for SUI in 2004 made it the only SNRI approved for this indication.

Mechanism of Action. Neurotransmitters such as serotonin and norepinephrine help regulate the sympathetic nervous system; they relax the detrusor muscle by stimulating beta-adrenergic receptors and induce contraction of the bladder neck by stimulating alpha-adrenergic receptors. By blocking the reabsorption of these neurotransmitters, SNRIs prolong their activity, effectively reducing pressure in the bladder while the bladder neck is contracted, thus inhibiting urine loss in SUI patients.

Duloxetine. In August 2004, duloxetine (Eli Lilly/Boehringer Ingelheim's Yentreve/Ariclaim) (Figure 4) was approved in Europe for treatment of moderate-to-severe SUI in women; it was launched the following month in the United Kingdom, Germany, and a few other European nations. In November 2002, Lilly and Boehringer Ingelheim submitted a new drug application (NDA) for duloxetine to the FDA for the treatment of SUI in the United States. In August 2003, the FDA issued an approvable letter—approval, according to Lilly, that was contingent on resolution of manufacturing issues, product labeling, and additional pharmacology studies specific to the drug's use in treating SUI. In mid 2004, a complete response to the approvable letter was submitted to the FDA's Division of Reproductive and Urologic Drug Products, but in January 2005, Lilly and Boehringer Ingelheim announced that they had withdrawn duloxetine's NDA for the treatment of SUI. According to the manufacturers, the FDA was unwilling to approve duloxetine for SUI based on the data contained in the existing NDA (Lilly press release, January 28, 2005).

In most markets, duloxetine is approved for more than one indication. In the United States, for example, it is approved under the trade name Cymbalta to treat major depression, and it is the first drug approved to treat diabetic peripheral

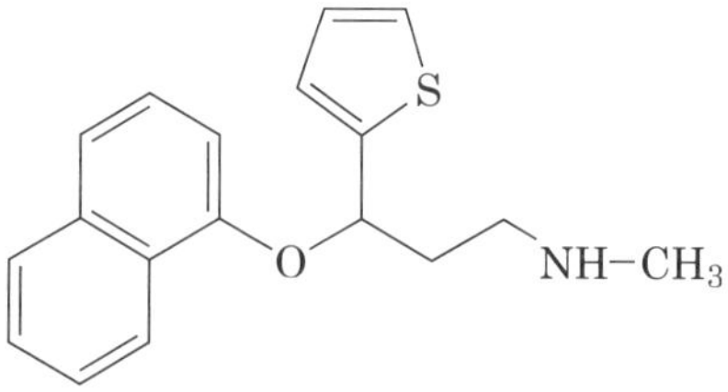

FIGURE 4. *Structure of duloxetine.*

neuropathy (DPN). In Europe, duloxetine was approved to treat major depression under the trade names Cymbalta and Xeristar in January 2005. Eli Lilly and Boehringer Ingelheim have agreed to develop and market duloxetine for all indications worldwide and for SUI only in the United States. Lilly and Quintiles Transnationals Corp. (Durham, North Carolina) are in a five-year commitment to copromote duloxetine for depression in the United States. Elan Pharmaceuticals (South San Francisco, California) has entered into a manufacturing and supply agreement with Lilly to supplement the latter's production of duloxetine worldwide beginning in mid 2005.

Duloxetine inhibits the activity of serotonin, adrenaline, and norepinephrine transporters, reducing the cellular reuptake of these neurotransmitters. In the case of SUI, the resulting prolonged serotonin and norepinephrine activity increases the stimulation and contraction of the urethral sphincter, which acts like a valve controlling the flow of fluids out of the bladder.

Several Phase III trials have demonstrated duloxetine's efficacy in female SUI patients. The first published Phase III trial of duloxetine in SUI enrolled 683 North American women with a weekly incontinence episode frequency (IEF) of seven or more (Dmochowski R, 2003). After a two-week washout period with placebo, the double-blind, placebo-controlled trial randomized patients to either placebo or 40 mg duloxetine twice daily for 12 weeks. Trial end points were change in IEF and change in Urinary Incontinence-Specific Quality-of-Life Instrument (I-QoL) score. The I-QoL instrument is a 22-item, incontinence-specific measure of the effects of incontinence on behavior, social functioning, and psychosocial domains. After 12 weeks, average IEF fell 50% in duloxetine-treated patients and 27% in patients receiving placebo. Average I-QoL scores increased 11 points in the duloxetine group compared with 7 points in the placebo group.

Another double-blind, placebo-controlled Phase III study enrolled 458 women in Australia, Brazil, Finland, Poland, South Africa, and Spain (Millard RJ, 2004). Eligible participants had SUI for at least the previous three months and IEF of seven or more episodes per week. The treatment protocol was similar to that of the North American study: after a two-week placebo lead-in period, patients were randomized to either placebo or 40 mg duloxetine twice daily for 12 weeks. Change in IEF and change in I-QoL score were the primary efficacy end points. The median drop in IEF was significantly greater with duloxetine (54%) than with placebo (40%), while the median increase in I-QoL score was significantly greater with duloxetine (10.3 points) than with placebo (6.4 points). Although slightly more duloxetine-treated patients (7.1%) than placebo-treated patients (6.1%) reported having no incontinent episodes after 12 weeks of treatment, the difference was not statistically significant.

A double-blind, randomized, placebo-controlled study of women with SUI in Australia, Canada, the Netherlands, and the United Kingdom examined the impact of duloxetine therapy on patients' interest in undergoing scheduled SUI surgery (Cardozo L, 2004). The researchers randomized 109 SUI sufferers with pure urodynamic SUI (no urge UI component) who were scheduled for SUI surgery to either placebo or duloxetine daily for eight weeks. Duloxetine dosing was 80 mg/day for the first four weeks and 120 mg/day for the remaining four weeks. At the end of the eight weeks, the median number of incontinent episodes (IEF) fell 60% in patients receiving duloxetine and 27% in the placebo group. In the duloxetine-treated group, the use of continence pads dropped 35%, compared with 5% in the placebo group, and I-QoL scores increased 10.6 points, compared with 2.4 points in the placebo group. Approximately 20% of duloxetine-treated patients were somewhat not interested or strongly not interested in SUI surgery (measured by a Willingness to Consider Surgery rating), compared with none of the placebo-treated patients.

The body of clinical data on duloxetine's efficacy demonstrates that it effectively reduces IEF in female SUI patients while improving a number of QoL parameters. A meta-analysis of four double-blind, placebo-controlled studies of similar design summarized the data supporting duloxetine's efficacy in a total of 1,913 women with SUI. Trial end points were significant reductions in IEF and significant increases in incontinence QoL scores (determined from the I-QoL). The meta-analysis of these four studies demonstrates that duloxetine treatment reduces the median IEF by 52% in comparison to a 33% reduction in IEF within the placebo-treated group (Eli Lilly, press release, June 2004). After one year of treatment, 82% of women on duloxetine reported improvements in their condition.

The most common adverse effects associated with duloxetine therapy include nausea, fatigue and drowsiness, dry mouth, insomnia, constipation, and dizziness. In clinical trials, these effects tend to occur with less frequency after four weeks of treatment.

Hormone Replacement Therapies

Overview. Estrogen (generics) is frequently given to postmenopausal women as part of hormone replacement therapy (HRT). Some researchers have suggested that this hormone may be efficacious in the treatment of SUI, but this assumption has not been supported by the available clinical trial data (detailed further on). Estrogen treatment can be given orally, transdermally (via a patch), or intravaginally (via topical cream or tablets); patients often must take the therapy for six weeks before the full benefits become evident.

Mechanism of Action. As a woman ages, reductions in the level of circulating estrogen can cause atrophy of the muscles, ligaments, and fascia involved in controlling and supporting the bladder; this atrophy can predispose the patient to SUI. Estrogen treatment—both local and systemic—increases urethral closure pressure, restores perivaginal tissue integrity, and increases urine storage capacity within the bladder. All these actions are believed to help reduce SUI symptoms.

Vaginal Estrogen. Available in intravaginal ring or tablet or in topical cream or gel, vaginal estrogens are primarily used to relieve the atrophic symptoms of menopause, such as dryness, and other climacteric complaints, including burning and overall discomfort. Like systemic estrogen, unopposed topical estrogen (e.g., estrogen replacement therapy without a concomitant progestin product) stimulates the endometrium and can put patients at increased risk of uterine cancer. In women with intact uteri, a progestin is therefore added if a topical product is used for more than six weeks; alternatively, the topical product dose is tapered or the product is discontinued. Estradiol cream (such as Galen's [County Armagh, Ireland] Estrace) and vaginal tablets (such as Novo Nordisk's [Bagsvaerd, Denmark] Vagifem) dominate the U.S. market for vaginal estrogens, but these products have little presence outside the United States, where estriol creams (Organon's [Roseland, New Jersey] Ovestin, others) are more popular. Conjugated estrogen cream (Wyeth's [Madison, New Jersey] Premarin) is another commonly used vaginal estrogen product; its popularity is confined largely to the U.S. market. These agents are administered either daily or three times per week. This relatively frequent dosing schedule (along with the cream's potential for leakage) makes these agents somewhat inconvenient. Relatively new estrogen vaginal rings (Pfizer's [New York, New York] Estring), which remain in place for three months, offer more suitable options for patients who do not mind their presence in the vagina.

A study of 83 hypoestrogenic women reporting an IEF of at least once per week showed that systemic HRT did not provide a significant benefit with regard to incontinence (Fantl JA, 1996). In addition, a meta-analysis of the available studies on estrogen therapy for the treatment of SUI noted that only those with nonrandomized study populations demonstrated clinical or symptomatic improvements; the randomized trials showed no benefit in reducing episodes of incontinence, regardless of the method of estrogen administration or the presence or absence of pharmacological cotherapies (Al-Badr A, 2003).

Beta-Adrenergic Agonists

Overview. Beta-adrenergic receptors are located on the dome of the bladder, and adrenoreceptor-2 agonists are reportedly effective in reducing the symptoms of SUI.

Mechanism of Action. While often prescribed for use as bronchodilators, beta-adrenoreceptor agonists may be used to treat symptoms of SUI. The activation of beta-adrenergic receptors leads to both relaxation of the smooth muscles lining the bladder, reducing voiding pressure, and contraction of the skeletal muscles that make up the external urethral sphincter, thus reducing the possibility of leakage.

Clenbuterol. Clenbuterol (Teijin Pharma's [Tokyo, Japan] Spiropent) (Figure 5), a beta-adrenoreceptor-2 agonist, was approved for treatment of SUI in Japan in 1995; it was first marketed in 1986 as a bronchodilator for treatment of asthma and other respiratory ailments. The drug is typically administered in oral tablet form (10 µg per tablet); the usual dose is 20 µg twice per day.

A few small clinical studies have demonstrated clenbuterol's efficacy in reducing the symptoms of urinary incontinence in SUI sufferers. A randomized study conducted in 61 women compared the efficacy of clenbuterol (20 µg, twice per

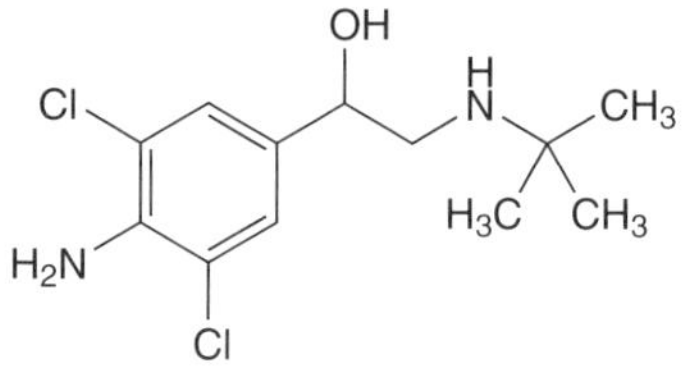

FIGURE 5. *Structure of clenbuterol.*

day for 12 weeks) with that of physical therapy (pelvic-floor muscle exercises) or a combination of physical therapy and clenbuterol (Ishiko O, 2000). Determination of efficacy relied on the patient's own impression of improvement. After 12 weeks, 77% of clenbuterol-treated patients observed improvement, compared with 53% of patients taking physical therapy alone and 90% of patients taking clenbuterol and physical therapy. Another study, conducted in a population of 89 postmenopausal women, found that after eight weeks of clenbuterol treatment, 41% of treated patients experienced a reduction in the frequency of incontinence and improvements in their quality of life (Ushiroyama T, 2000).

However, subsequent reviews of adrenergic agents have cast doubt on their efficacy for SUI. For example, a meta-analysis of clinical trials of adrenergic drugs in the treatment of urinary incontinence concluded that agents like clenbuterol are only marginally more effective than placebo (Alhasso A, 2003).

Side effects of oral clenbuterol treatment include tremor (3.6% of patients), abdominal pain (1%), and hypertension (0.2%). Clenbuterol has also been associated with palpitations, skin rash, reductions in serum potassium levels, muscle spasms, headache, nausea, and hepatic ailments (Spiropent package insert, Teijin Pharma).

Nonpharmacological Approaches

Noninvasive Management. Because SUI is most commonly caused by either the weakening of the pelvic-floor muscles or the weakening of the urethral sphincter, many nonpharmacological, noninvasive methods focus on strengthening these muscles. Collectively, these methods are often referred to as conservative management. Patients can strengthen their pubococcygeal muscles through a number of methods, including Kegel exercises, electromyographic biofeedback, electrostimulation, and the use of vaginal cones. Because these methods require regular repetition (for example, to be effective, Kegel exercises must be performed at least twice a day for five minutes per workout), they are reasonably effective only when compliance is high. The use of pessaries to support and constrict the bladder neck can be mildly effective, but this method is not often used because, unlike muscle training or surgery, it does not correct or improve the pathophysiological problems that cause SUI, and it typically interferes with the patient's lifestyle. Table 2 describes conservative management therapies for patients with SUI.

TABLE 2. Nonpharmacological Therapies for Stress Urinary Incontinence

Nonpharmacological Therapy	Description
Bladder retraining	• Patients systematically increase the time between visits to the toilet, which teaches them to inhibit the sensation of urgency, to delay voiding, and to use the toilet on a schedule rather than in response to the urge to void.
Pelvic-floor exercises	• Pelvic-floor exercises (PFEs) may be conducted by both men and women to strengthen muscles and ligaments on the pelvic floor that help support the bladder. PFEs involve repeated contractions of the muscles located in the pelvic floor, particularly the pubococcygeus muscle. They are designed to increase both muscle bulk and maximum urethral closure pressure, which then gives stronger reflex contractions to sudden increases in abdominal pressure, such as during sneezing.
Weighted vaginal cones	• Weighted vaginal cones may be used for strengthening the pelvic-floor muscles in female patients. After insertion of the cone, the patient is instructed to contract the pelvic-floor muscles to hold the weight in place. The cones come in many different weights, which can be increased as patients become more proficient in manipulating the muscles.
Biofeedback	• Biofeedback involves reeducating and retraining patients' bladder control mechanisms. This technique relies on muscle pressure sensor readings, taken from electrodes placed in the vagina and/or the anus, that provide information about neuromuscular and bladder activity, particularly during pelvic-muscle exercises.
Modification of fluid consumption	• Physicians use voiding diaries and frequency and volume charts to assess patients' fluid intake. Frequency and volume charts might reveal that a patient is drinking abnormally large amounts of water. In such cases, symptoms can be reduced by simply advising the patient to reduce his or her intake to a normal level. Older patients with lower-extremity edema produce more urine at night and, therefore, can benefit from fluid restriction after dinner.
UI management products	• Absorbent undergarments and pads. • Intravaginal sponges: help support the bladder neck during exercise and physical exertion. • Urethral plugs: a fluid-filled or inflated plug is inserted into the urethra to prevent urine passage. • Continence guards: inserted into the vagina to support the bladder neck and aid continence. • FemAssist: a silicone, nipple-shaped device that the patient applies over the urethral opening. • Reliance: a urethral insert made of the plastic elastomer dynaflex that contains a valve and releasing string that can be pulled to allow for micturition. • In-dwelling permanent catheter.

Surgical Procedures. The number of surgical procedures performed to treat SUI is immense, and the choice of procedure often depends on whether the surgeon is a gynecologist, urologist, or urogynecologist. The most widely used (and successful) surgical procedures for female SUI patients are tension-free vaginal tape (TVT), transobturator tape (TOT), and colposuspension. The most common surgical procedure for male SUI patients is the installation of an artificial urethral sphincter. Table 3 summarizes the main surgical procedures used for SUI.

TVT and TOT are minimally invasive techniques that use a polypropylene mesh tape to create a sling that increases support, normally provided by the vaginal wall, to the middle of the urethra. The main difference between the two procedures is the location of the incisions and how the mesh tape tracks across the bladder. In TVT, the incisions are made in the abdomen and the tape comes across the bladder at an acute angle, risking contact with blood vessels supplying the bladder and retropubic area. This procedure leads to an approximate 3% risk of bladder perforation and 3–10% risk of bleeding and bruising. In TOT, the incisions are made through the obturator muscle of the inner thigh, allowing the tape to be threaded across the bladder at a more obtuse angle, thus avoiding most of the blood vessels lining the bladder and retropubic area and reducing the risk of bladder perforation, bleeding, and bruising to less than 1%. Both techniques are extremely successful: 63–90% of SUI sufferers remain "dry" one to two years after the surgery (Delorme E, 2004; Tsivian A, 2004; Ward KL, 2004).

Colposuspension, sometimes called Burch's colposuspension or laparoscopic colposuspension, involves the placement of sutures through the vaginal wall (at the position proximal to the bladder neck, the point where the urethra meets the bladder) to Cooper's ligament, a stretch of connective tissue that spans the top of the pelvis. The attachment to this ligament increases tension on the bladder neck, thus increasing regulatory control of urine leakage. Laparoscopic colposuspension simply involves the use of a laparoscope to minimize the invasive components of this procedure. Colposuspension is extremely successful: about 90% of patients remain "dry" after surgery (McCrery RJ, 2004; Ward KL, 2004).

In men, the most common surgical procedure for SUI involves the placement of an artificial sphincter around the urethra. This device consists of three fluid (saline)-filled parts: a cuff, a pump, and a balloon-like reservoir. The cuff is placed around the urethra and is connected to a pump that has been surgically implanted in the scrotum. Upon activation of the pump—by pressing a button or squeezing—the saline in the cuff empties into the reservoir, releasing the tension on the urethra and allowing the flow of urine out of the bladder. The cuff then refills to clamp the urethra shut.

EMERGING THERAPIES

Although the clinical features of stress urinary incontinence (SUI) are well understood, researchers have had a difficult time developing therapies targeted to this indication. Development has been largely hampered by the essentially mechanical

TABLE 3. Surgical Interventions for Stress Urinary Incontinence

Procedure	Mechanism	Advantages and Disadvantages
Sling procedures	Autologous (or, rarely, cadaveric) tissue from the fascia lata of lateral thigh or rectus sheath used as a sling around the bladder neck. Artificial tension-free vaginal tape (TVT) or transobturator tape (TOT) and bone anchors are common modifications.	*Advantages:* 90% success rate. *Disadvantages:* Urethral obstruction can result from excess of tissue tension. Depending on the technique used, complication rate can be moderate (3–10%), including frequency and urgency.
Anterior repair	Lifting of the bladder off vaginal wall and repositioning of bladder neck through the vagina.	*Advantages:* Easiest procedure to perform. Most rapid recovery time. Allows simultaneous repair of other vaginal defects. *Disadvantages:* Wide variation of success rates reported (from 36% to 92%). Highest failure rate of the listed procedures.
Retropubic cystourethropexy	Surgical fixation of the bladder neck and urethra.	*Advantages:* Estimated 50–68% of patients have no incontinent episodes 5–20 years after surgery. *Disadvantages:* Higher morbidity compared with transvaginal and laparoscopic bladder neck suspensions, which offer similar results.
Burch/laparoscopic colposuspension	Elevation of the bladder via an incision in the suprapubic region. Two to four long-term sutures lift the bladder and bladder neck off underlying fascia.	*Advantages:* Used for both primary and recurrent stress urinary incontinence. Has an 80–90% success rate. *Disadvantages:* The higher the bladder neck is raised, the greater the chances of postoperative voiding problems and obstruction.
Needle suspension	Suture passed through anterior abdominal wall to vaginal vault on both sides of the bladder neck and tied to the anterior rectus, elevating the vagina.	*Advantages:* Success rates range from 40% to 72%. *Disadvantages:* Risks include infection, nerve entrapment, urethral obstruction, urinary retention, and de novo urge urinary incontinence.

(*continued overleaf*)

TABLE 3. (*continued*)

Procedure	Mechanism	Advantages and Disadvantages
Ingelmann-Sunberg denervation	Disruption of motor supply to the bladder by diversion of nerves at the bladder base via a small vaginal incision.	*Advantages:* Used for patients who are resistant to medication and for whom major surgery is contraindicated. *Disadvantages:* Overall efficacy is unreliable.
Injectable bulking agents	A bulking agent injected into periurethral tissues at the bladder neck, closing the lumen over the urethral opening to reduce urine leakage.	*Advantages:* Performed in outpatient setting with minimal postoperative morbidity. Cost-effective. *Disadvantages:* Risks include de novo urge urinary incontinence, hematuria, and urinary retention. Less successful in males.
Artificial sphincters	Pump placed in scrotum or labia majora controls reservoir balloon that fills and drains a cuff placed around the urethra.	*Advantages:* Used for patients of both sexes. Very effective for men with stress urinary incontinence following prostate surgery. *Disadvantages:* The benefit over surgical slings in women is debatable, as the two approaches have not been directly compared.

nature of SUI: urethral hypermobility during increased abdominal stress is due to faulty pelvic-floor support and not primarily to any biochemical defect. Therefore, the pipeline of emerging pharmacological therapies for SUI is sparsely populated. Additionally, although the recent success of duloxetine (Eli Lilly/Boehringer Ingelheim/Shionogi's [Osaka, Japan] Yentreve/Ariclaim) in Europe has created hope for new pharmaceutical opportunities, the subsequent withdrawal of the drug's U.S. new drug application highlights the difficulties involved in drug development for this indication.

Nevertheless, the potential to develop pharmaceuticals that alleviate SUI symptoms via other mechanisms—such as increasing urethral close pressure or reducing overall urine production—has encouraged a handful of companies to explore novel SUI drug targets. Table 4 lists agents under investigation. Dr. Esteve Laboratories (Barcelona, Spain) announced in February 2005 that the substance P/CGRP inhibitor cizolirtine will be studied in Phase II European clinical trials for SUI, but this section does not describe this agent or mechanism in detail because data on its utility in SUI are scanty.

TABLE 4. Emerging Therapies in Development for Stress Urinary Incontinence

Compound	Development Phase	Marketing Company
AA-10025		
United States	—	—
Europe	PC	Arachnova
Japan	—	—
Venlafaxine[a]		
United States	—	Wyeth
Europe	—	Wyeth
Japan	—	—
Desmopressin[b]		
United States	—	Ferring
Europe	—	Ferring
Japan	—	Ferring
FE-106483		
United States	—	—
Europe	I	Ferring
Japan	—	—

[a]Venlafaxine is marketed for depression, generalized anxiety disorder, and social anxiety disorder in the United States and Europe. It is in Phase II development for depression in Japan.

[b]Desmopressin is marketed in the major pharmaceutical markets for the treatment of nocturnal enuresis and diabetes insipidus; it is also approved for the treatment of nocturia in multiple sclerosis patients in the United Kingdom.

PC = Preclinical (including discovery).

Serotonin and Norepinephrine Reuptake Inhibitors

Overview. Serotonin and norepinephrine reuptake inhibitors (SNRIs) are a new class of drugs that were designed to be effective antidepressants, based on the success of the serotonin reuptake inhibitor fluoxetine (Eli Lilly's Prozac, generics) and the norepinephrine reuptake inhibitor atomoxetine (Eli Lilly's Strattera). Like tricyclic antidepressants (TCAs), SNRIs inhibit the presynaptic reuptake of serotonin and norepinephrine, but unlike TCAs, they have little effect on histaminergic, cholinergic, dopaminergic, and alpha-adrenergic receptors and so are associated with fewer side effects (Mattia C, 2002).

Three SNRIs are currently available in the major pharmaceutical markets: duloxetine (Eli Lilly/Boehringer Ingelheim's Cymbalta/Yentreve/Ariclaim), venlafaxine (Wyeth's Effexor), and milnacipran (Sanofi-Aventis's Ixel/Dalcipran in the European Union; Asahi Kasei and Janssen Pharmaceutical's Toledomin in Japan). Following duloxetine's European approval for SUI (making it the first pharmacological therapy indicated for SUI), manufacturers are hoping to capitalize on this newly defined market by developing additional SNRIs for SUI.

Mechanism of Action. Serotonin and norepinephrine help regulate the sympathetic nervous system; they relax the detrusor muscle by stimulating beta-adrenergic receptors and induce contraction of the bladder neck by stimulating alpha-adrenergic receptors. By blocking the reabsorption of these neurotransmitters, SNRIs prolong the neurotransmitters' activity, effectively reducing pressure in the bladder while the bladder neck is contracted and thereby inhibiting urine loss in SUI patients.

AA-10025. AA-10025 is an SNRI in preclinical development in the United Kingdom for the treatment of SUI as well as several neuropathic pain indications. The agent had previously been in development with Mitsubishi-Tokyo Pharmaceuticals, Inc. (Tokyo, Japan) for Alzheimer's disease and depression (as MCI-225) and had reached Phase II trials for the latter indication before its development for these indications was discontinued. In early 2004, Arachnova Therapeutics (Cambridge, United Kingdom) licensed the development rights to the compound for a number of newly identified target indications, including SUI. Dynogen Pharmaceuticals (Waltham, Massachusetts) entered a similar agreement with Mitsubishi in 2004 under which Dynogen will develop the compound (as DDP-225) for irritable bowel syndrome.

Venlafaxine. Venlafaxine (Wyeth's Effexor/Effexor XR) (Figure 6) has been approved for depression, generalized anxiety disorder, and social anxiety disorder and is available in the United States and Europe in immediate- and extended-release (XR or once-daily) formulations. In Japan, venlafaxine is in Phase II trials for depression. It is not in formal development for SUI in any market.

Venlafaxine blocks the uptake of serotonin and norepinephrine almost equally and has little effect on muscarinic, cholinergic, histaminergic, and noradrenergic receptors. It also has some dopaminergic activity, but the extent to which this activity translates into clinical benefit is unclear. Its mechanism of action in norepinephrine reuptake inhibition is like that of the TCAs, but because of its serotonergic component, it has a relatively benign side-effect profile, more like that of the selective serotonin reuptake inhibitors (SSRIs).

No clinical trials have tested venlafaxine's efficacy in SUI patients, but pre-clinical data from animal models suggest it can increase urethral sphincter activity and urethral close pressure. In in vitro studies, venlafaxine significantly increased the contraction of urethral muscle while reducing bladder contractility; in vivo data from rats demonstrated that venlafaxine increased urethral perfusion pressure (Bae JH, 2001). Using a cat model of incontinence, researchers also demonstrated that 0.1–10 mg/kg venlafaxine increases electromyographic (EMG) activity in the urethral sphincter and bladder capacity (Katofiasc MA, 2002).

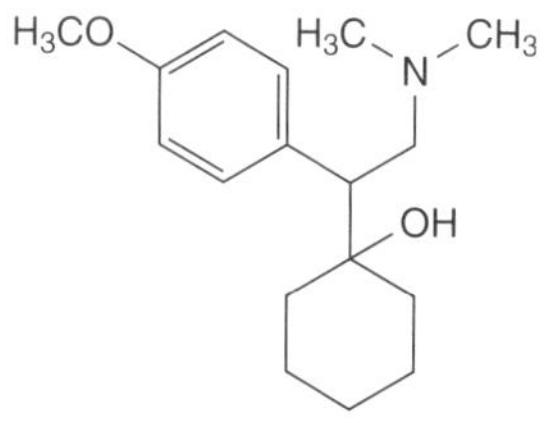

FIGURE 6. *Structure of venlafaxine.*

Although venlafaxine is generally better tolerated than the TCAs, it can trigger sustained blood pressure increases in some patients at doses higher than 200 mg/day. It also requires gradual titration at the start of therapy to minimize its gastrointestinal side effects, and like the SSRIs, it can disrupt sleeping patterns and cause sexual dysfunction (Effexor XL prescribing information). Comparative preclinical data appear to show that venlafaxine is not as potent as duloxetine in increasing urethral close pressure (Katofiasc MA, 2002).

Vasopressin Agonists

Overview. Vasopressin agonists mimic the actions of the endogenous antidiuretic hormone vasopressin and have been employed in the treatment of nocturnal enuresis (childhood bed-wetting) for several years. By reducing urine production, vasopressin agonists delay bladder filling and help reduce the number of nocturnal voids. Most vasopressin agonists have relatively rapid onset of action and short-to-medium duration of action. Vasopressin agonists appear particularly appealing as "on demand" therapies for patients who are unwilling to take pharmacotherapy that requires chronic, consistent dosing.

Mechanism of Action. Arginine vasopressin is an antidiuretic hormone secreted by the pituitary gland. Vasopressin acts on V_2 receptors in the kidney to promote water and sodium reabsorption; in higher concentrations, vasopressin may stimulate contraction of vascular smooth muscle via V_1 receptor agonism. As renal water reabsorption increases in response to increased vasopressin concentrations, urine becomes more concentrated and the total volume of urine produced drops. In healthy adults, vasopressin levels are markedly higher during sleep to reduce the number of voids and allow continuous sleep. Analogues of vasopressin are used therapeutically for patients with nocturnal voiding frequency to reduce nightly voids and enable longer sleep periods in between voids.

Desmopressin. Desmopressin is marketed extensively in nasal and oral formulations as Ferring's Minirin for the treatment of nocturnal enuresis (bed-wetting) in children and diabetes insipidus; in the United Kingdom, desmopressin is also approved for nocturia caused by multiple sclerosis. Desmopressin is a synthetic vasopressin analogue that directly agonizes V_2 receptors in the kidney.

Although desmopressin is not in formal development for SUI, a small trial involving female incontinents suggests it may be an effective option for some patients (Robinson D, 2004). The multicenter, randomized, placebo-controlled, double-blind, crossover study enrolled 64 women with severe daytime incontinence. Approximately 25% of the enrollees had SUI, and 53% had mixed UI; therefore, approximately 78% of the study group had some degree of SUI symptoms. All patients received seven single 40 µg of intranasal desmopressin and three single doses of placebo. Patients were randomized to receive active and placebo treatment in one of four patterns: seven desmopressin treatments followed by three placebo; three placebo followed by seven desmopressin; two desmopressin, then three placebo, then five desmopressin; or five desmopressin, then three placebo, then two desmopressin.

The study investigators found that desmopressin increased the mean incidence of leak-free periods in the first four hours after administration (62% in patients taking desmopressin, compared with 48% of patients taking placebo). During the four- to eight-hour period after dosing, the difference between desmopressin and placebo was smaller and statistically insignificant. The time to first incontinent episode postadministration was longer in desmopressin-treated patients (6.3 hours) than in placebo-treated patients (5.2 hours), and the total volume voided was lower in desmopressin-treated patients than in the placebo group.

Clinical trials of desmopressin demonstrate that it is generally safe and well tolerated. The most common side effects are headache and nausea (Lose G, 2003; Robinson D, 2004). In rare cases, desmopressin may cause hyponatremia (also known as water intoxication), a drop in serum sodium concentration due to excess water volume. Severe hyponatremia may occur in up to 1% of treated patients; reducing water intake during desmopressin therapy generally reduces the risk of this adverse event (Beach PS, 1992; Ferrer J, 1990; Lose G, 2003).

FE-106483. Ferring (Noord-Holland, The Netherlands) is developing the vasopressin agonist FE-106483 for the treatment of urinary incontinence; it is in Phase I testing in the United Kingdom. To date, it is unclear whether FE-106483 is in development specifically for SUI or for indications such as those for which desmopressin was developed (nocturnal enuresis, nocturia, diabetes insipidus). According to the developer, FE-106483 is an oral nonpeptide vasopressin agonist that is highly selective for the V_2 receptor. Theoretically, the compound would have a clinical profile similar to that of other vasopressin agonists.

REFERENCES

Abrams P, et al. The standardization of terminology of lower urinary tract function: report from the standardization sub-committee of the International Continence Society. *American Journal of Obstetrics and Gynecology*. 2003;**187**(1):116–126.

Agency for Health Care Policy and Research (AHCPR). Urinary incontinence in adults: acute and chronic management. Clinical Practice Guideline Number 2 (1996 Update) AHCPR Publication No. 96-0682: March 1996.

Al-Badr A, et al. What is the available evidence for hormone replacement therapy in women with stress urinary incontinence? *Journal of Obstetrics and Gynaecology Canada*. 2003;**25**(7):567–574.

Alhasso A, et al. Adrenergic drugs for urinary incontinence in adults. *Cochrane Database of Systematic Reviews*. 2003.

Alivizatos G, et al. Recent data upon impotence, incontinence and quality of life issues concerning radical prostatectomy. *Archivos Espanoles de Urologia*. 2003;**56**(3):321–330.

Altman D, et al. The impact of hysterectomy on lower urinary tract symptoms. *International Urogynecology and Pelvic Floor Dysfunction*. 2003;**14**(6):418–423.

Andersen JT, et al. ICS 7th Report on the standardization of terminology of lower urinary tract function—lower urinary tract rehabilitation techniques. *Neurourology and Urodynamics*. 1992;**11**:593–603.

Artibani W, et al. Epidemiology of urinary incontinence. *Urodinamica*. 1992;**2**:127–150.

Bae JH, et al. The effects of a selective noradrenaline reuptake inhibitor on the urethra: an in vitro and in vivo study. *BJU International*. 2001;**88**(7):771–775.

Bate TS, et al. Prevalence and impact of incontinence and impotence following total prostatectomy assessed anonymously by the ICS-male questionnaire. *European Urology*. 1998;**33**(2):165–169.

Beach PS, et al. Hyponatremic seizures in a child treated with desmopressin to control enuresis: a rational approach to fluid intake. *Clinical Pediatrics*. 1992;**31**:566–569.

Benedetti-Panici P, et al. Long-term bladder function in patient with locally advanced cervical carcinoma treated with neoadjuvant chemotherapy and type 3–4 radical hysterectomy. *Cancer*. 2004;**100**(10):2110–2117.

Blaivas JG, Olsson CA. Stress incontinence: classification and surgical approach. *Journal of Urology*. 1988;**139**:727–731.

Bortolotti A, et al. Prevalence and risk factors for urinary incontinence in Italy. *European Urology*. 2000;**37**:30–35.

Boyle P, et al. The prevalence of male urinary incontinence in four centres: the UREPIK study. *BJU International*. 2003;**92**:943–947.

Brocklehurst J. Urinary incontinence in the community-analysis of a MORI poll. *BMJ*. 1993;**306**:832–834.

Butaud JP, et al. Enquete nationale sur l'incontinence urinaire. *Journal of Radiology*. 1992;**73**:139–142.

Cardozo L, et al. Pharmacological treatment of women awaiting surgery for stress urinary incontinence. *Obstetrics and Gynecology*. 2004;**104**:511–519.

Cheater FM, et al. Epidemiology and classification of urinary incontinence. *Bailliere's Best Practice and Research. Clinical Obstetrics and Gynaecology*. 2000;**14**:183–205.

Cundiff GW. The pathophysiology of stress urinary incontinence: a historical perspective. *Revista de Urologia*. 2004;**6**(suppl 3):S10–S18.

Damián J, et al. Prevalence of urinary incontinence among Spanish older people living at home. *European Urology*. 1998;**34**:333–338.

DeLancey JO. Stress urinary incontinence: where are we now, where should we go? *American Journal of Obstetrics and Gynecology*. 1996;**175**:311–319.

Delorme E, et al. Transobturator tape (Uratape): a new minimally-invasive procedure to treat female urinary incontinence. *European Urology*. 2004;**45**(2):203–207.

Diokno AC, et al. Prevalence of urinary incontinence and other urological symptoms in the noninstitutionalized elderly. *Journal of Urology*. 1986;**136**:1022–1025.

Diokno AC. Epidemiology of urinary incontinence. *Journals of Gerontology. Series A. Biological Sciences and Medical Sciences*. 2001;**56**:M3–M4.

Dmochowski R, et al. Duloxetine versus placebo in the treatment of North American women with stress urinary incontinence. *Journal of Urology*. 2003;**170**(4):1259–1263.

Dolan LM, et al. Stress incontinence and pelvic floor neurophysiology 15 years after the first delivery. *BJOG*. 2003;**110**(12):1107–1114.

Engström G, et al. Prevalence of three lower urinary tract symptoms in men—a population-based study. *Family Practice*. 2003;**20**(1):7–10.

Ertunc D, et al. Is stress urinary incontinence a familial condition? *Acta Obstetricia et Gynecologica Scandinavia*. 2004;**83**(10):912–916.

Fantl JA, et al. Efficacy of estrogen supplementation in the treatment of urinary incontinence. The Continence Program for Women Research Group. *Obstetrics and Gynecology*. 1996;**88**(5):745–749.

Ferrer J, et al. Acute water intoxication after intranasal desmopressin in a patient with primary polydipsia. *Journal of Endocrinological Investigation*. 1990;**13**:663–666.

Fraser MO, Chancellor MB. Neural control of the urethra and development of pharmacotherapy for stress urinary incontinence. *BJU International*. 2003;**91**(8):743–748.

Fritel X, et al. Stress urinary incontinence four years after the first delivery: a retrospective cohort study. *Acta Obstetricia et Gynecologica Scandinavia*. 2004;**83**(10):941–945.

Fultz NH, et al. Prevalence of urinary incontinence in middle-aged and older women: a survey-based methodological experiment. *Journal of Aging and Health*. 2000;**12**:459–469.

Fultz NH, et al. Burden of stress urinary incontinence for community-dwelling women. *American Journal of Obstetrics and Gynecology*. 2003;**189**(5):1275–1282.

Gavira Iglesias FJ. Prevalence and psychosocial impact of urinary incontinence in older people of a Spanish rural population. *Journals of Gerontology. Series A. Biological Sciences and Medical Sciences*. 2000;**55A**:M207–M214.

Green TH Jr. Classification of stress urinary incontinence in the female: an appraisal of its current status. *Obstetrical & Gynecological Survey*. 1968;**23**:632–634.

Hagglund D, et al. Urinary incontinence: an unexpected large problem among young females. Results from a population-based study. *Family Practice*. 1999;**16**:506–509.

Hampel C, et al. Definition of overactive bladder and epidemiology of urinary incontinence. *Urology*. 1997;**50**(suppl 6A):4–14.

Hannestad YS, et al. A community-based epidemiological survey of female urinary incontinence: the Norwegian EPICONT study. *Journal of Clinical Epidemiology*. 2000;**53**:1150–1157.

Herzog AR, et al. Two-year incidence, remission, and change patterns of urinary incontinence in noninstitutionalized older adults. *Journal of Gerontology: Medical Sciences*. 1990;**45**:M67–M74.

Hirai K, et al. Indifference and resignation of Japanese women toward urinary incontinence. *International Journal of Gynecology and Obstetrics*. 2001;**75**:89–91.

Hoshi T, et al. Prevalence estimation of urinary incontinence among non-institutionalized persons aged 60 and over in Japan. *Nippon Koshu Eisei Zasshi*. 1994;**41**:910–919.

Hunskaar S, et al. Epidemiology and natural history of urinary incontinence. *International Urogynecology Journal and Pelvic Floor Dysfunction*. 2000;**11**:301–319.

Hunskaar S, et al. The prevalence of urinary incontinence in women in four European countries. *British Journal of Urology*. 2004;**93**:324–330.

Ishiko O, et al. Beta(2)-adrenergic agonists and pelvic floor exercises for female stress incontinence. *International Journal of Gynaecology and Obstetrics*. 2000;**71**:39–44.

Jackson RA, et al. Urinary incontinence in elderly women: findings from the Health, Aging, and Body Composition Study. *Obstetrics and Gynecology*. 2004;**104**(2):301–307.

Jolleys JV, et al. Urinary symptoms in the community: how bothersome are they? *British Journal of Urology*. 1994;**74**:551–555.

Katofiasc MA, et al. Comparison of the effects of serotonin selective, norepinephrine selective, and dual serotonin and norepinephrine reuptake inhibitors on lower urinary tract function in cats. *Life Sciences*. 2002;**71**(11):1227–1236.

Kernan WN, et al. Phenylpropanolamine and the risk of hemorrhagic stroke. *New England Journal of Medicine*. 2000;**343**:1826–1832.

Koskimaki J. Prevalence of lower urinary tract symptoms in Finnish men: A population-based study. *British Journal of Urology*. 1998;**81**(3):364–369.

Koyama W, et al. Prevalence and conditions of urinary incontinence among the elderly. *Methods of Information in Medicine*. 1998;**37**:151–155.

Lagace E, et al. Prevalence and severity of urinary incontinence in ambulatory adults: an UPRNet study. *Journal of Family Practice*. 1993;**36**:610–614.

Langa KM, et al. Informal caregiving time and costs for urinary incontinence in older individuals in the United States. *Journal of the American Geriatrics Society*. 2002;**50**:733–737.

Liberman JN, et al. Health-related quality of life among adults with symptoms of overactive bladder: results from a U.S. community-based survey. *Urology*. 2001;**57**:1044–1050.

Lose G, et al. Efficacy of desmopressin (Minirin) in the treatment of nocturia: a double-blind placebo-controlled study in women. *American Journal of Obstetrics and Gynecology*. 2003;**189**(4):1106–1113.

Maher C. Female urinary stress incontinence: what causes it and how to treat it. *Medicine Today*. 2002;**3**(2):16–21.

Malmsten UGH, et al. Urinary incontinence and lower urinary tract symptoms: an epidemiological study of men aged 45 to 99 years. *Journal of Urology*. 1997;**158**:1733–1737.

Mattia C, et al. New antidepressants in the treatment of neuropathic pain. A review. *Minerva Anestesiologica*. 2002;**68**:105–114.

McCrery RJ, Thompson PK. Outcomes of urethropexy added to paravaginal defect repair: A randomized trial of Burch versus Marshall-Marchetti-Krantz. *Joint meeting of the American Urogynecologic Society and the Society of Gynecologic Surgeons;* 2004; Presentation of abstract.

McGuire EJ, et al. Stress urinary incontinence. *Obstetrics and Gynecology*. 1976;**47**:255–264.

Millard RJ, et al. Duloxetine versus placebo in the treatment of stress urinary incontinence: a four-continent randomized clinical trial. *BJU International*. 2004;**93**:311–318.

Milsom I, et al. The prevalence of overactive bladder. *American Journal of Managed Care*. 2000;**6**(suppl):S565–S573.

Milsom I, et al. How widespread are the symptoms of an overactive bladder and how are they managed? A population-based prevalence study. *British Journal of Urology International*. 2001;**87**:760–766.

Minaire P, Jacquetin B. La prevalence de l'incontinence urinaire feminine en medicine generale. *Journal de Gynecologie Obstetrique et Biologie de la Reproduction*. 1992;**21**:731–738.

Nuotio M, et al. Urgency, urge incontinence and voiding symptoms in men and women aged 70 years and over. *British Journal of Urology International*. 2002;**89**:350–355.

Nygaard IE, et al. Urinary incontinence in rural older women: prevalence, incidence and remission. *Journal of the American Geriatrics Society*. 1996;**44**:1049–1054.

O'Brien J, et al. Urinary incontinence: prevalence, need for treatment, and effectiveness of intervention by nurse. *BMJ*. 1991;**303**:1308–1312.

Ostergard DR. New target for intervention: the neurourology connection. *Advanced Studies in Medicine*. 2004;**4**(3C):S220–S224.

Parazzini F, et al. Risk factors for stress, urge or mixed urinary incontinence in Italy. *BJOG*. 2003;**110**(10):927–933.

Payne CK. Epidemiology, pathophysiology, and evaluation of urinary incontinence and overactive bladder. *Urology*. 1998;**51**(suppl 2A):3–10.

Perry S, et al. An epidemiological study to establish the prevalence of urinary symptoms and felt need in the community: the Leicestershire MRC Incontinence Study. Leicestershire MRC Incontinence Study Team. *Journal of Public Health Medicine*. 2000;**22**:427–434.

Population Division of the Department of Economic and Social Affairs of the United Nations Secretariat. *World Population Prospects: The 2002 Revision*, vol. II, *The Sex and Age Distribution of Populations* (United Nations publication, Sales No. E.03.XIII.7), 2003.

Rasmussen KL, et al. Obesity as a predictor of postpartum urinary symptoms. *Acta Obstetricia et Gynecologica Scandinavia*. 1997;**76**(4):359–362.

Ricci JA, et al. Coping strategies and health care-seeking behavior in a US national sample of adults with symptoms suggestive of overactive bladder. *Clinical Therapeutics*. 2001;**23**:1245–1259.

Roberts RO, et al. Urinary incontinence in a community-based prevalence cohort: prevalence and healthcare-seeking. *Journal of the American Geriatric Society*. 1998;**46**:467–472.

Robinson D, et al. Antidiuresis: a new concept in managing female daytime urinary incontinence. *BJU International*. 2004;**93**:996–1000.

Roe B, et al. Prevalence of urinary incontinence and its relationship with health status. *Journal of Clinical Nursing*. 2000;**9**:178–187.

Romanzi LJ. Urinary incontinence in women and men. *Journal of Gender Specific Medicine*. 2001;**4**:14–20.

Schulman C, et al. Urinary incontinence in Belgium: a population-based epidemiological survey. *European Urology*. 1997;**32**:315–320.

Schytt E, et al. Symptoms of stress urinary incontinence one year after childbirth: prevalence and predictors in a national Swedish sample. *Acta Obstetricia et Gynecologica Scandinavia*. 2004;**83**(10):928–936.

Sebesta M, et al. Questionnaire-based outcomes of urinary incontinence and satisfaction rates after radical prostatectomy in a national study population. *Urology*. 2002;**60**(6):1055–1058.

Smoger SH, et al. Urinary incontinence among male veterans receiving care in primary care clinics. *Annals of Internal Medicine*. 2000;**132**(7):547–551.

Temml C, et al. Urinary incontinence in both sexes: prevalence rates and impact on quality of life and sexual life. *Neurourology and Urodynamics*. 2000;**19**:259–271.

Thom D. Variation in estimates of urinary incontinence in general practice: effects of differences in definition, population characteristics, and study type. *Journal of the American Geriatrics Society*. 1998;**46**:473–480.

Tsivian A, et al. Tension-free vaginal tape procedure for the treatment of female stress urinary incontinence: long-term results. *Journal of Urology*. 2004;**172**(3):998–1000.

Ueda T, et al. Urinary incontinence among community-dwelling people aged 40 years or older in Japan: prevalence, risk factors, knowledge, and self-perception. *International Journal of Urology*. 2000;**7**:95–103.

Ushiroyama T, et al. Prevalence, incidence, and awareness in the treatment of menopausal urinary incontinence. *Maturitas*. 1999;**33**:127–132.

Ushiroyama T, et al. Clinical efficacy of clenbuterol and propiverine in menopausal women with urinary incontinence: improvement in quality of life. *Journal of Medicine*. 2000;**31**:311–319.

Van Kampen M, et al. Urinary incontinence following transurethral, transvesical, and radical prostatectomy: retrospective study of 489 patients. *Acta Urologica Belgica*. 1997;**65**(4):1–7.

Van Oyen H, Van Oyen P. Urinary incontinence in Belgium; prevalence, correlates, and psychosocial consequences. *Acta Clinica Belgica*. 2002;**57**(4):207–218.

Ward KL, et al. A prospective multicenter randomized trial of tension-free vaginal tape and colposuspension for primary urodynamic stress incontinence: two-year follow-up. *American Journal of Obstetrics and Gynecology*. 2004;**190**(2):324–331.

Welz-Barth A, et al. 1999 rerun of the 1996 German Urinary Incontinence Survey: will doctors ever ask? *World Journal of Urology*. 2000;**18**:436–438.

Urge Urinary Incontinence

ETIOLOGY AND PATHOPHYSIOLOGY
Introduction

Urge urinary incontinence (UUI) is an involuntary urine loss associated with a strong desire to void, even when the bladder contains a very small amount of urine. UUI is primarily associated with an overactive detrusor muscle that contracts unexpectedly, opening the bladder neck. Patients experience involuntary leakage accompanied by or immediately preceded by urgency.

Anatomy

The Bladder. The urinary bladder is a hollow, muscular organ found in the anterior section of the pelvic cavity (Figure 1). The organ—and its outlet, the urethra—serve two functions: to store urine without leakage and to expel urine periodically through a relaxed outlet (the urethra). In males, the bladder lies in front of the rectum. In females, the organ is situated in front of the vagina, which lies in front of the rectum.

The bladder wall comprises three layers:

- The lumenal layer (mucosa) consists of a thin plane of cells making up the transitional epithelium. These cells constitute a protective mucosal membrane barrier and are supported by a basement membrane that provides a

Wiley Handbook of Current and Emerging Drug Therapies, Volumes 5–8
Copyright © 2007 Decision Resources, Inc. Published by John Wiley & Sons, Inc.

Male

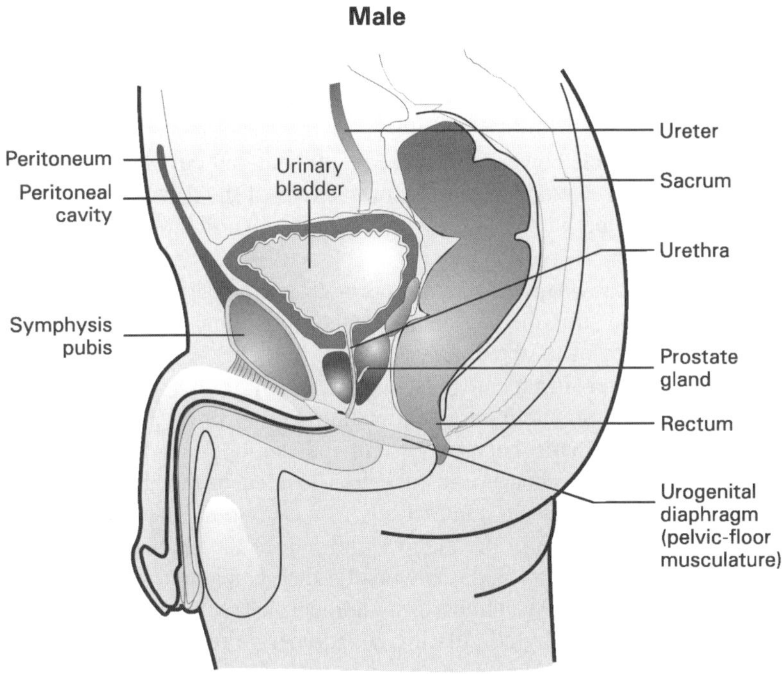

Female

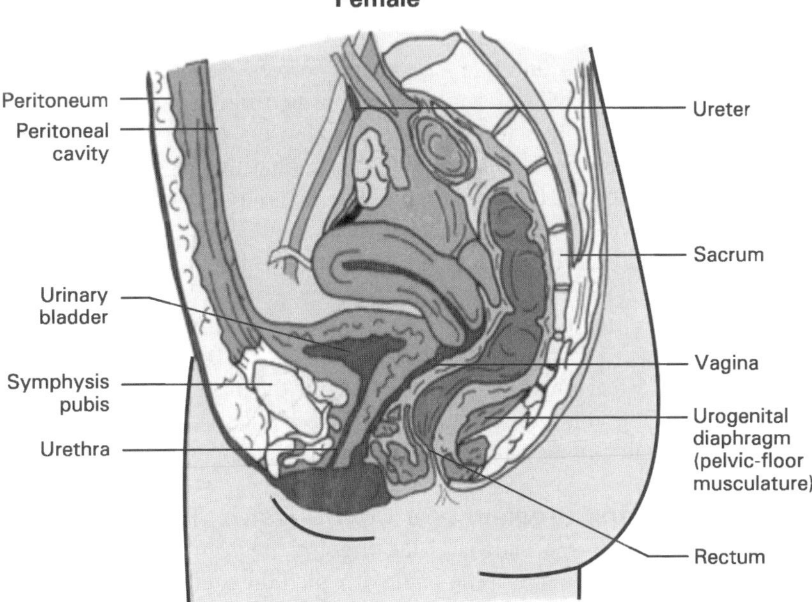

FIGURE 1. *Anatomical location of the bladder and pelvic organs.*

    supportive structure and filtration barrier between the submucosa (the lamina propria, which is innervated and contains blood and lymphatic vessels) and the transitional epithelium.

- The second layer is the submucosa, which consists of connective tissue that attaches the mucosal layer to the third layer, the detrusor muscle.
- The detrusor muscle consists of both longitudinal and circular muscle fibers that form an interconnecting mesh. Contractions of the detrusor muscle raise pressure within the bladder, allowing micturition (urination) to take place.

The final layer, known as the serosa, is not strictly part of the bladder. It comprises the peritoneum (the sac encasing the abdominal organs) and covers only the upper surface of the bladder.

Control of the lower urinary tract is maintained by the parasympathetic and sympathetic nervous systems in an antagonistic relationship. Signal transduction through the parasympathetic nervous system induces contraction of the detrusor muscle (by activating muscarinic receptors located in the detrusor muscle) while inhibiting smooth muscle contractions in the urethra. These simultaneous actions increase the pressure in the bladder and reduce the resistance of the urethra; subsequently, urine is voided. Conversely, the sympathetic nervous system relaxes the detrusor muscle by activating β_2-adrenergic receptors in the tissue and contracts the bladder neck by stimulating α_1-adrenergic receptors located there. These actions relax the bladder, allowing it to fill with urine while keeping the urethra contracted and watertight—thus maintaining continence. Hence, voiding is typically mediated via the parasympathetic nervous system and bladder filling via the sympathetic nervous system.

A combination of peristaltic-like movements (waves of muscular contractions) within the ureters and gravity assist in moving urine from the kidney to the bladder. As the bladder fills, it is forced upward within the pelvic cavity, becoming first more spherical and then pear-shaped. Throughout this process, the pressure in the bladder remains relatively constant. This pressure control is important in maintaining continence. If the bladder increases in pressure as it is filled, continence is maintained until the bladder pressure exceeds the urethral resistance. At this point, urine leaks and continence is lost. An increase in bladder urine volume from 10 mL (virtually empty) to 400 mL (virtually full) produces a pressure increase equivalent to that produced by only about 5–10 mL H_2O. This slight increase in intravesical pressure (pressure within the bladder)—despite a dramatic increase in the volume of liquid within the bladder—shows the bladder's effectiveness at maintaining a relatively stable pressure.

Role of the Ureters: Creation of a Control Valve. The ureters enter the bladder at a triangular area known as the trigone, then run at an oblique angle through the wall of the bladder. The angle at which the ureters enter the bladder is important because the ureter, when positioned at the correct angle, forms a valve that inhibits reflux of urine. This valve mechanism works in two ways to compress the ureters; as the pressure increases during filling and as the muscles

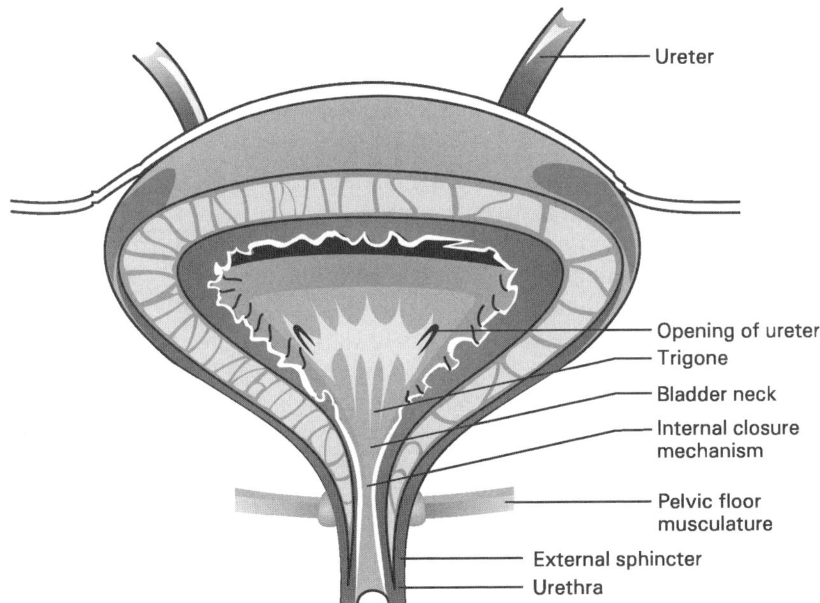

FIGURE 2. *Cross section of the female urinary bladder.*

within the bladder contract during micturition (the process by which the bladder's function switches from urine storage to urine voiding), the ureters are compressed.

Figure 2 shows a cross-section of the female bladder. At the base of this organ lies a closure mechanism that leads into the urethra. This mechanism is not a true sphincter; rather than being a muscle designed specifically for the purpose of urethral constriction, it relies on the pelvic-floor muscle to compress the urethra when the pressure inside the bladder increases. This compression creates a valve that controls urinary flow.

Males have a different control valve than that found in females. In males, a circular layer of muscle extends down the prostate capsule. The contraction of this muscle group and nearby longitudinal fibers prevents semen from being ejaculated into the bladder during orgasm. Women lack this circular muscle. Instead, in females the longitudinal muscle extends into the urethra and is stimulated by cholinergic, parasympathetic nerves.

Role of the Bladder Neck: Controlling the Bladder/Abdominal Pressure Balance.

In both sexes, ligaments from the pelvis and fascia support the bladder neck; contraction of muscles in the pelvic floor also influences the position of the bladder neck. In females, the bladder neck is partially supported by the vaginal wall as well. In a continent person, the increases in abdominal pressure during bladder filling are transferred evenly to the bladder and the bladder neck. Hence, an increase in pressure on the bladder is matched by an increase in resistance placed on the bladder neck.

The Urethra. The urethra is the tube through which urine is expelled from the bladder during micturition. Between the eighth and twelfth weeks of embryogenesis of a female fetus, the urogenital membrane develops into the upper part of the bladder, the vagina, and the distal part of the urethra. Because these three tissues evolved from the same embryogenic material, they are all equally hormone-dependent. Mucosal folds within the urethra are sensitive to the hormone estrogen; they help provide a seal that is essential for maintaining continence.

Not surprisingly, the structure of the urethra varies significantly between males and females. The female urethra is straight and approximately 3–5 cm in length. In contrast, the male urethra has an S shape and can reach 22 cm in length. The urethra in both sexes contains layers of muscle that together constitute the urethral sphincter. The layer of smooth circular muscle is known as the internal sphincter. In women, the internal sphincter forms the entire urethra, while in men, the internal sphincter makes up only the posterior portion of the urethra. An outer circular, striated muscle, located near the pelvic floor, serves as the external sphincter in women. Males, too, have an external sphincter, which is located below the pyramid-shaped structure called the verumontanum, which in turn is close to the prostate gland.

The internal sphincter contains α-adrenergic receptors that respond to stimulation by causing contraction and maintaining urethral closure. This process is involuntary and arises in response to bladder filling. In contrast, the external sphincter muscle is controlled by acetylcholine receptors that are under voluntary central control. People are able to override the normal micturition response by using voluntary control to squeeze the external sphincter shut, thus maintaining urethral closure until a socially appropriate time for bladder voiding (Fraser MO, 2003; Ostergard DR, 2004).

Involuntary and Voluntary Control of Micturition. Micturition involves a significant neuromuscular component. The combination of a primitive spinal reflex and higher, voluntary processes controls micturition.

When 200–300 mL of urine has accumulated in the bladder, stretch receptors become activated, sending impulses to the spinal micturition center. The spinal micturition center lies in the S2-S4 sacral area at the bottom of the spinal cord (Figure 3). This part of the spine relays information to and from the bladder. In addition, the external urethral sphincter (rhabdosphincter) and the pelvic-floor muscles are innervated by the pudendal nerve, which also originates from the S2-S4 region of the spinal cord (from an area known as Onuf's nucleus). The parasympathetic motor nucleus lies in the S3-S4 part of the spinal cord.

Pathophysiology

The primary dysfunction associated with UUI is aberrant detrusor muscle function. Detrusor overactivity is a urodynamic observation in which the bladder is objectively shown to contract either spontaneously or with provocation during the filling phase of a cystometrogram (the recording of neuromuscular function of

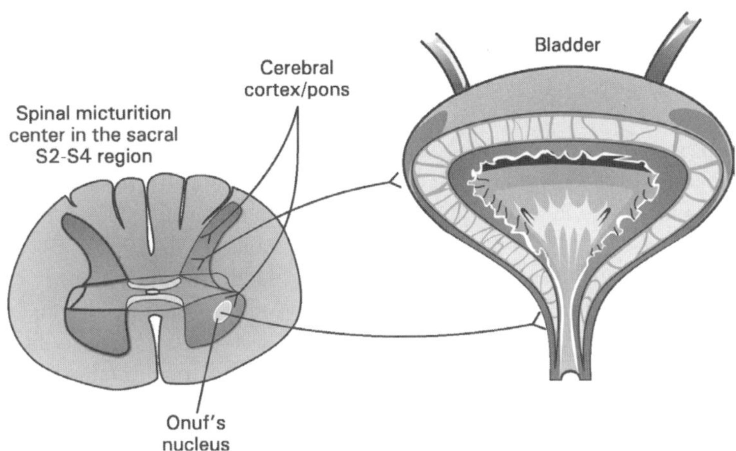

FIGURE 3. *Spinal control of micturition.*

the bladder by means of pressure and capacity) in neurologically intact patients attempting to inhibit micturition. There are two primary types of aberrant detrusor overactivity:

- *Idiopathic detrusor overactivity* (also called detrusor instability) has no known precipitating cause. This is the result of an oversensitive detrusor muscle that contracts unexpectedly, opening the bladder neck.

- *Neurogenic detrusor overactivity* (also called detrusor hyperreflexia) is caused by disturbances of the central nervous system such as multiple sclerosis. Detrusor hyperactivity with impaired contractility (DHIC) is a subgroup of detrusor overactivity. DHIC is characterized by involuntary detrusor contractions that do not completely empty the bladder following micturition, which results in elevated postvoid residual urine volume. The larger the amount of postvoid residual urine retained in the bladder, the greater the patient's chance of developing a urinary tract infection. DHIC may represent the late stage of neurogenic detrusor overactivity, characterized by further deterioration of detrusor muscle function.

Activation of muscarinic receptors via release of acetylcholine from post-ganglionic parasympathetic nerves is suspected to be the ultimate mechanism driving abnormal detrusor activity in the diseased bladder (De Groat WC, 1997). It has also been hypothesized that non-neuronal acetylcholine, acting through afferent muscarinic mechanisms, may play a role in detrusor overactivity (Anderson KE, 2003).

The muscarinic receptor population in the human detrusor is composed primarily of M_3 and M_2 subtypes, with the later predominating in number (Wang P, 1995; Hegde SS, 1999). M_3 receptors mediate direct contraction of the detrusor (Chess-Williams R, 2001; Fetscher C, 2002). This M_3 mechanism mediates physiological voiding contractions during the emptying phase of the micturition cycle (Matsui M, 2000). M_2 receptors mediate a smaller component of the direct contraction, by a mechanism that might involve closure of calcium-activated potassium channels (Bymaster FP, 2001; Nakamura T, 2002). However, M_2 receptor activation mediates detrusor contraction through an indirect mechanism that involves reversal of sympathetically mediated (β_3-adrenoreceptor-evoked) relaxation via a cyclic AMP-dependent mechanism (Braverman AS, 1998; Hegde SS, 1997; Ymamnishi T, 2000; Matsui M, 2003). Because the sympathetic nervous system is involved in the bladder-filling phase, it has been hypothesized that unstable detrusor contractions maybe also be driven by these M_2 receptor-mediated mechanisms. Although M_1 and M_4 receptors have been shown to modulate neuronal acetylcholine release, their functional roles have not been elucidated (Hegde SS, 2004).

Classification. UUI may be further subdivided into motor urge incontinence and sensory urge incontinence. Motor urge incontinence occurs when a sense of urgency is accompanied by involuntary detrusor contractions. Sensory urge incontinence involves a sense of urgency without detrusor contractions.

Other Types of Incontinence and Their Relationship to UUI

Overactive Bladder. Overactive bladder (OAB) encompasses an array of symptoms and disorders known to affect the lower urinary tract. The symptoms of OAB include urinary frequency and urgency, both of which can occur with or without incontinence. Within the category of urinary incontinence (UI), there are three distinct subtypes: UUI, stress urinary incontinence (SUI), and mixed urinary incontinence (MUI). Although the focus of interest in UI has been broadened in some epidemiological and clinical studies to include OAB, this expanded definition of UI is not yet universally accepted in clinical practice. Thus, OAB is not included in the definition of UUI used here.

Mixed Urinary Incontinence. MUI accounts for approximately one-fourth of all UI cases and is generally recognized as a combination of UUI and stress urinary incontinence (SUI). SUI involves the involuntary leakage of small amounts of urine resulting from increased abdominal pressure. Patients often experience SUI during physical exertion, coughing, sneezing, or laughing.

MUI is more prevalent in women than in men and is more frequently observed in the population aged 60 or older. MUI patients are often classified by their predominant form of incontinence (UUI or SUI) and treated for the predominant form. The same therapies employed for UUI and SUI are employed in MUI management.

Etiology

Detrusor Overactivity. The etiology of detrusor overactivity associated with UUI is not well defined—the majority of detrusor overactivity cases are idiopathic

(90%). Two factors are known to produce involuntary contractions of the bladder: outflow obstruction and neurologic dysfunction.

Detrusor overactivity secondary to outlet obstruction is most commonly associated with prostate hypertrophy in men. Outflow obstruction is rare in women. The most common causes in women are prior anti-incontinence surgery and advanced pelvic organ prolapse.

Neurological conditions associated with detrusor overactivity include multiple sclerosis, Parkinson's disease, dementia, spinal cord injury, and neoplasia. These conditions all interfere with the brain's ability to exert inhibitory neuronal control over the detrusor muscle. This interference allows the sacral reflex to predominate, such that patients lose voluntary control of micturition. In multiple sclerosis, the majority of patients with lower urinary tract dysfunction show neurogenic detrusor overactivity on cystometry (Blaivas JG, 1985). In Parkinson's disease, loss of dopamine activity results in loss of detrusor inhibition, leading to neurogenic detrusor overactivity. The loss of input is associated with the D_1 dopaminergic receptor. In dementia, bladder dysfunction is secondary to direct involvement of cerebrocortical areas, leading to neurogenic detrusor overactivity. Alzheimer's-type dementia is thought to be mediated by downregulation of M_1 muscarinic receptor inhibitory mechanisms (Yokoyama O, 2002).

Risk Factors. Several risk factors are associated with the development of detrusor overactivity:

- Increasing age.
- Diminished cognitive function.
- Decreased ambulation.
- Inflammation.
- Hypoestrogenism/genital atrophy.
- Altered immune function.
- Poor nutrition and fluid intake.
- Infections.
- Emotional disorders.
- Medications.
- Genetic factors.
- Hysterectomy.
- Prostate surgical procedures.

Many of these factors are a direct consequence of aging. The aging process itself can sometimes cause the bladder to shrink, thereby increasing urinary frequency. In addition, early detrusor contractions, even at low bladder volumes, can create a sense of urgency to empty the bladder. On the whole, elderly people are less capable of suppressing these early detrusor contractions. UUI is not an inevitable part of aging, however, and sufferers should be encouraged to seek medical assistance regardless of their age.

CURRENT THERAPIES

The three major approaches to urge urinary incontinence (UUI) treatment are behavioral treatment, pharmacology, and surgery. The Agency for Healthcare Research and Quality (AHRQ) (formerly the Agency for Health Care Policy and Research [AHCPR]) recommends behavioral treatment (lifestyle modification, physical therapy) as the first-line therapy for UUI (AHCPR, 1996). These approaches seek to reduce or manage UUI symptoms while avoiding the worrisome side effects often seen with pharmacotherapy or surgery. Many of the drugs used to treat UUI are associated with anticholinergic effects such as dry mouth, blurred vision, and constipation. The severity of these symptoms, however, is less with the newer anticholinergic agents and with newer formulations of older agents on the market. Table 1 highlights the major drugs prescribed for UUI.

The same therapies used for UUI and stress urinary incontinence (SUI) treatment are employed in mixed urinary incontinence (MUI) management. Patients with MUI generally receive pharmacological therapy first to address the UUI component of their symptoms. If the remaining SUI symptoms are significant, they will then be treated for SUI, usually with surgery.

In countries where it is available, extended-release (ER) tolterodine (Pfizer's [New York, New York] Detrol LA/Detrusitol XL) is generally considered the current standard of care for UUI treatment. Its superior side-effect profile combined with an efficacy comparable to that of oxybutynin (Johnson & Johnson's [New Brunswick, New Jersey] Ditropan XL/Lyrinel XL) (which was considered the first-line treatment for UUI prior to tolterodine's launch) is largely responsible for tolterodine's success. However, ER tolterodine's superior side-effect profile may come at the expense of efficacy, so some physicians continue to prescribe oxybutynin where efficacy is placed at a premium over side effects. Similarly, oxybutynin is used in price-sensitive markets or where tolterodine is not available. Of the newer agents, extended-release formulations are prescribed more frequently than immediate-release formulations; the exceptions are when the adjustable dosing made possible by the immediate-release formulations allows greater flexibility in dose escalation for patients who require higher efficacy or in situations where cost or availability are concerns.

Based on clinical trials of the newer anticholinergic agents, transdermal oxybutynin is expected to provide similar efficacy and an improved anticholinergic side-effect profile compared with ER tolterodine, although its nonanticholinergic adverse effects include skin irritation. Solifenacin (Astellas Pharma, Inc.'s [Tokyo, Japan] Vesicare), an M_3 muscarinic receptor-selective antagonist, has been shown to have greater efficacy and similar side-effect profile compared with ER tolterodine, though its efficacy compared with oxybutynin (considered the most effective agent for UUI) is not clear. Darifenacin (Novartis's [Basel, Switzerland] Enablex/Emselex), another M_3-selective antagonist, is as effective as oxybutynin but with better tolerability (as would be expected from an M_3-selective antagonist). However, less information comparing darifenacin with ER tolterodine or with solifenacin is available.

TABLE 1. Current Therapies Used for Urge Urinary Incontinence

Agent	Company/Brand	Daily Dose	Availability
Anticholinergics			
Tolterodine	Pfizer's Detrol/Detrusitol	2 mg bid	US, F, G, I, S, UK
Extended-release tolterodine	Pfizer's Detrol LA/Detrusitol XL	4 mg qd	US, G, S, UK
Oxybutynin	Johnson & Johnson's Ditropan, generics	5 mg bid	US, F, G, I, S, UK, J
Extended-release oxybutynin	Johnson & Johnson's Ditropan XL/Lyrinel XL	10 mg qd	US, F, G, UK
Transdermal oxybutynin	Watson Pharmaceuticals' Oxytrol	3 mg/day patch applied twice weekly	US, G
Trospium chloride	Madaus's Sanctura/Spasmolyt, others	20 mg bid	US, F, G, I, S, UK
Solifenacin succinate	Astellas Pharma's Vesicare	5 mg qd	US, F, G, S, UK
Darifenacin	Novartis's Enablex/Emselex	7.5 mg qd	US, G
Propiverine	Apogepha/Taiho Pharmaceutical/Schering-Plough's Detrunorm/BUP-4	10 mg tid	G, UK, J
Tricyclic antidepressants			
Imipramine	Mallinckrodt's Tofranil, generics	25 mg bid	US, F, G, I, S, UK, J
Doxepin	Pfizer's Sinequan, generics	50 mg qd at night	US, F, G, I, S, UK, J
Hormone replacement therapies			
Estradiol vaginal cream	Galen's Estrace, others	100–200 µg qd or three times per week	G, S, UK, US
Estriol vaginal cream	Organon's Ovestin, others	500 µg qd or three times per week	US, F, G, I, S, UK, J
Conjugated estrogen vaginal cream	Wyeth's Premarin, others	0.3–1.25 mg qd or three times per week	US, F, G, I, S, UK, J
Estradiol vaginal ring	Pfizer's Estring	2 mg (approximately 7.5 µg/24 hours); replace ring every three months	US, G, UK
Estradiol vaginal tablet	Novo Nordisk's Vagifem	25 µg twice per week	US, G, I, UK

bid = Twice per day; qd = Once per day; tid = Three times per day.

US = United States; F = France; G = Germany; I = Italy; S = Spain; UK = United Kingdom; J = Japan.

Tricyclic antidepressants (TCAs) exert anticholinergic as well as musculotropic effects, increasing bladder outlet resistance. The combination of anticholinergic effects and increased bladder outlet resistance allows better storage of urine (Cannon T, 2002). Imipramine hydrochloride (Mallinckrodt, Inc. [Hazelwood, Missouri] Tofranil, generics) and doxepin (Pfizer's Sinequan, generics) are TCAs prescribed mainly as an antidepressant agents, but they may also be used for UUI. Unfortunately, TCAs can lead to adverse events in elderly patients, a group that accounts for a significant proportion of the UUI population. In particular, TCAs have the potential to cause cardiac events, which necessitates constant monitoring for these effects in patients with cardiovascular disease. Also of concern is the potential for multiple drug interactions. When combined with multiple medications, TCAs can pose serious dangers, including hepatic failure. Because elderly patients are often treated for multiple conditions, the risks of prescribing a TCA for UUI can greatly outweigh the benefits for this specific group. Because TCAs are rarely used in UUI, they are not covered in detail here.

Anticholinergics

Overview. Anticholinergics are the most common class used to treat UUI. The most-used agents in this class are tolterodine (Pfizer's Detrol/Detrusitol, extended-release Detrol LA/Detrusitol XL) and oxybutynin (Johnson & Johnson's Ditropan and generics; extended-release Ditropan XL/Lyrinel XL), which combine anticholinergic properties with direct muscular relaxant or local anesthetic actions. Although these agents are sometimes classified as musculorelaxants, they are included under the general heading of anticholinergic agents here.

Historically, the side-effect profile of anticholinergic drugs has been very poor, causing many patients to discontinue therapy or show poor compliance if they continue taking the drugs. The most frequently reported problems with anticholinergic treatment for UUI include dry mouth and constipation, but blurred vision, delirium, and cardiac arrhythmias can occur as well. Unfortunately, when patients develop dry mouth, they have a tendency to drink more fluids—potentially exacerbating their incontinence.

Various other anticholinergic agents are available for treatment of UUI. However, some of these agents are infrequently used and therefore will not be discussed in detail here. Dicyclomine hydrochloride (Sanofi-Aventis's [Tokyo, Japan] Bentyl, generics) is a muscarinic antagonist that has some direct smooth-muscle-relaxing properties. It is occasionally (albeit rarely) prescribed for UUI. This compound is used primarily to treat gastrointestinal hypermotility disorders; no large controlled studies have investigated its use in the treatment of UUI. A small pilot study published in 1987 showed that 30 mg of dicyclomine hydrochloride given three times daily was no better than placebo in relieving UUI symptoms. Propantheline bromide (Shire Pharmaceuticals's [Wayne, Pennsylvania] Pro-Banthine, generics) has anticholinergic effects on the lower urinary tract. To date, few large controlled studies have examined the use of this agent for the treatment of UUI. Flavoxate (Johnson & Johnson's Urispas) is a weak anticholinergic agent with some direct smooth-muscle-relaxing properties. Although flavoxate is associated with fewer side effects than many of the other anticholinergic agents (including oxybutynin), it provides fewer benefits. In fact, several studies have shown the compound to be ineffective compared with placebo. The 1996 AHRQ guidelines do not recommend the use of flavoxate. Flavoxate is also a relatively expensive anticholinergic agent.

Mechanism of Action. Anticholinergic agents act by inhibiting the effects of the parasympathetic nervous system (mediated via acetylcholine) on the bladder, thereby reducing the frequency of bladder contractions, relaxing the smooth muscle, and increasing bladder capacity.

Tolterodine. First launched in Sweden at the end of 1997, Pfizer's immediate-release (IR) tolterodine (Detrol/Detrusitol) was introduced in the United States in April 1998. Tolterodine was initially developed by Pharmacia Corp. (Bridgewater, New Jersey), which was acquired by Pfizer in 2003. This agent is available in all of the major pharmaceutical markets except Japan, where it is preregistered. Tolterodine is indicated for the treatment of overactive bladder (OAB) with symptoms of urinary frequency, urgency, and urge incontinence. It is the first agent to significantly challenge oxybutynin's market dominance in the past 20 years.

Tolterodine is reportedly as potent as oxybutynin in blocking muscarinic receptors in isolated human and guinea pig tissue. In cats, however, this compound is more selective for muscarinic receptors on the bladder (primarily M_2 and M_3 receptors are present and involved in bladder control) than for muscarinic receptors on the salivary glands (primarily M_3 receptors, although M_1, M_4, and M_5 receptors may play a role). Antagonism of M_3 receptors on the salivary gland is believed to result in dry mouth. Oxybutynin has the opposite selectivity, which may partially explain tolterodine's better side-effect profile (Hegde SS, 2004; Nilvebrant L, 1997). The mechanisms underlying profiles selective for the bladder over the salivary glands are not clear. Tolterodine shows little selectivity for any one of the five muscarinic receptors over another; except for a twofold greater selectivity for M_3 receptors over M_4 receptors (Moreland RB, 2005).

Trials in patients with confirmed UUI have shown that 2 mg of tolterodine taken twice daily significantly reduces the number of micturition episodes and incontinence events in a 24-hour period. This regimen was almost as effective as 5 mg tolterodine given three times daily and was far better tolerated. In an Australian trial involving 316 patients with overactive bladder, 2 mg tolterodine twice daily reduced micturition episodes from 11.2 per 24 hours to 9 per 24 hours after 12 weeks of therapy. Importantly, the number of incontinence episodes per 24 hours decreased from 3.6 to 1.8. Severe dry mouth was not significantly worse in the tolterodine group than in the placebo group (Millard R, 1999). According to data presented at the 1999 annual meeting of the International Incontinence Society, in a trial involving 2220 patients, 75% of the participants elected to continue tolterodine therapy after the trial ended.

The side-effect profile of tolterodine comprises the classic side effects of anticholinergic drugs, although the effects are less severe than those noted with older anticholinergic drugs (e.g., oxybutynin). Therefore, tolterodine should not be given to patients with urinary retention, gastric retention, or narrow-angle glaucoma—all of which are exacerbated by anticholinergic drugs. A trial of tolterodine involving three doses between 3.2 mg and 12.8 mg found a dose-dependent reduction in paraffin-stimulated saliva production, with the high dose causing virtual cessation of salivation. Thus, this drug has the potential to block salivary function at high doses, leading to dry mouth.

Unwanted drug interactions with tolterodine may pose a challenge in prescribing this agent. Tolterodine is metabolized by the cytochrome P450 2D6 isoenzyme and could potentially interact with other drugs that are metabolized by the same isoenzyme (e.g., phenytoin, imipramine). Little information is available about the extent of these potential drug interactions. Doses must be adjusted in patients with impaired hepatic function (e.g., cirrhosis patients), in whom exposure to the unbound, active fraction can be double that noted in the normal population.

At the 1997 American Urological Association (AUA) meeting, researchers presented the results of a head-to-head trial comparing tolterodine and oxybutynin. Of the 293 UUI patients who participated in the study, 118 received tolterodine (2 mg twice daily), 118 received oxybutynin (5 mg three times daily), and 57 received placebo. Although the trial showed that oxybutynin produced a higher reduction in the number of incontinent episodes, its side-effect profile was considerably worse.

A retrospective analysis of a pharmacy claims database evaluated patients' adherence to treatment with IR oxybutynin (515 patients) and tolterodine (505 patients). In this study, 32% of patients in the tolterodine group were found to continue therapy for six months, compared with 22% of patients in the IR oxybutynin group. Patients in the IR oxybutynin group discontinued treatment significantly earlier (mean = 45 days) than patients taking tolterodine (mean = 59 days) and were switched to another therapy more often than the tolterodine-treated individuals (19% and 14%, respectively). Although the study showed statistically significant differences between study treatments in favor of tolterodine, fewer than one third of patients continued therapy with either drug for the entire six months. Also, investigators were not able to determine whether adverse effects or lack of effectiveness—or a combination of the two—prompted therapy discontinuation (Lawrence M, 2000).

Extended-Release Tolterodine. In December 2000, the FDA approved Pfizer's ER tolterodine (Detrol LA/Detrusitol XL) as a once-daily therapy for the treatment of OAB with symptoms of UUI, urgency, and frequency. ER tolterodine is also available in the United Kingdom, Germany, and Spain.

In studies comparing IR tolterodine and ER tolterodine, treatment with the latter is associated with a greater reduction in urge incontinence episodes and a lower incidence of dry mouth. In a 12-week study involving 1529 patients (81% female) with overactive bladder, patients took 4 mg of ER tolterodine (once daily), 2 mg of IR tolterodine (twice daily), or placebo. Patients in both tolterodine groups reported statistically significant reductions in urge incontinence episodes per week. Compared with baseline, a 71% reduction of incontinence episodes was seen in the ER tolterodine group, a 60% reduction in episodes was seen in the IR tolterodine group, and a 33% reduction in episodes was seen in the placebo group. Dry mouth was seen in 23% of ER tolterodine patients, 30% of IR tolterodine patients, and 8% of placebo patients (Van Kerrebroeck P, 2001).

Another study points to ER tolterodine's efficacy over a longer period. This 12-month, open-label study of ER tolterodine enrolled 1,077 patients who had completed a 12-week comparison study of IR tolterodine, ER tolterodine, and placebo. In the 12-month trial, the median decrease in micturitions per 24 hours was 21% and weekly incontinence episodes decreased by a median 83%. Dry mouth was the most common adverse event, occurring in 13% of patients (Kreder K, 2002).

Oxybutynin. The original oxybutynin (IR) formulation (Johnson & Johnson's Ditropan, generics) (Figure 4), which is given three or four times daily, received FDA approval in July 1975. Until the launch of tolterodine, IR oxybutynin was considered the first-line treatment for UUI. A second available oxybutynin formulation is an ER formulation given once daily. These two formulations are available in all major markets. A third, recently approved form of oxybutynin is transdermal oxybutynin (Watson Pharmaceuticals's [Corona, California] Oxytrol) delivered via a skin patch.

Oral oxybutynin's side-effect profile includes dry mouth, blurred vision, and bowel irregularities. These side effects have significantly hindered patient compliance with this compound.

Unlike tolterodine, oxybutynin has greater selectivity for muscarinic receptors on the salivary glands than for muscarinic receptors on the bladder. This selectivity partially explains the side effects associated with the drug (M_3 receptors are located in the bladder, salivary glands, and smooth muscles of the eye and lower bowel), such as serious dry mouth as well as the other typical anticholinergic side effects (Hegde SS, 2004; Nilvebrant L, 1997). Oxybutynin displays modest specificity for the M_1 and M_3 receptors over the other three subtypes (Yarker YE, 1995). Oxybutynin also has direct muscle relaxant and some local anesthetic actions.

The 1996 AHCPR UI guidelines state that oxybutynin is the drug of choice for treating UUI, based on a series of clinical trials demonstrating a 28–44% cure rate (this rate was reduced to approximately 30% when the placebo level was extracted) and a reduction in symptoms of as much as 56% with this agent (AHCPR, 1996). The patient dropout rate because of side effects ranged from 3% to 45%.

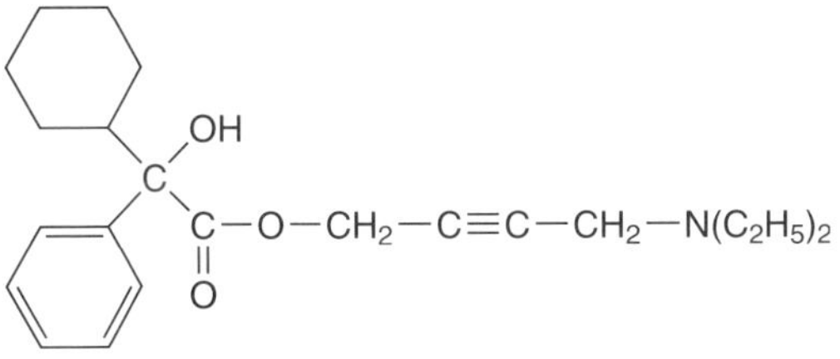

FIGURE 4. *Structure of oxybutynin.*

Extended-Release Oxybutynin. Extended-release oxybutynin (Johnson & Johnson's Ditropan XL/Lyrinel XL) was developed in an attempt to improve the side-effect profile associated with oxybutynin. In February 1999, UCB, Inc. (Smyrna, Georgia) and ALZA Corporation (Mountain View, California, acquired by Johnson & Johnson in 2001) copromoted the new formulation and launched the product in the United States. ER oxybutynin is available in several European countries, including France, Germany, and the United Kingdom. In May 2003 in the United Kingdom, Ditropan XL was renamed Lyrinel XL; Janssen-Cilag (Issy-les-Moulineaux, France), a Johnson & Johnson company, is marketing the new brand in the United Kingdom.

Previous studies have shown ER and IR versions of oxybutynin to have similar efficacy, with ER oxybutynin having a better (albeit sometimes only slightly better) side-effect profile. In a double-blind study involving 105 patients with UUI or MUI, 87% of patients taking the ER oxybutynin experienced some form of anticholinergic side effects, compared with 94% in the group taking the immediate-release drug. Dry mouth was reportedly less severe in the ER oxybutynin group, with 68% of recipients experiencing this problem, compared with 87% in the IR oxybutynin group (Anderson RU, 1999). Another small study of both formulations revealed their comparable efficacy in reducing UUI episodes, with equivalent rates of anticholinergic side effects experienced by patients (e.g., dry mouth was evident in 47.7% and 59.1% of patients taking ER and IR oxybutynin, respectively); however, patients' first reports of moderate to severe dry mouth were significantly later in the extended-release group (Versi E, 2000).

The OBJECT (Overactive Bladder: Judging Effective Control and Treatment) trial was designed to determine the relative tolerability and efficacy of ER oxybutynin and IR tolterodine. In this randomized, double-blind trial, patients received either 10 mg ER oxybutynin once daily or 2 mg tolterodine twice daily over a 12-week period. Data from the trial showed that patients using ER oxybutynin had significantly fewer episodes of UUI and urinary frequency than did those using IR tolterodine. Patients taking ER oxybutynin experienced 19.5 fewer weekly episodes of UUI, while patients taking IR tolterodine experienced 16.3 fewer such episodes. (Additionally, urinary frequency decreased by 24.7 episodes/week in patients treated with ER oxybutynin; urinary frequency decreased by 20.1 episodes/week in patients treated with IR tolterodine.) Adverse effects, including dry mouth and central nervous system (CNS) effects, occurred with similar frequency in both groups, and both drugs were equally tolerated, resulting in similar discontinuation rates for both drugs (Appell RA, 2001; Hashim H, 2004).

Another clinical trial, the Overactive Bladder Performance of Extended-Release Agents (OPERA) trial, was designed to compare the efficacy and safety of ER tolterodine and ER oxybutynin. In this randomized, double-blind trial, 790 women with severe UUI (21 to 60 UUI episodes/week and an average of 10 or more voids per 24 hours) received either 10 mg ER oxybutynin once daily or 4 mg ER tolterodine once daily. Both patient groups had similar improvements in total incontinence episodes and in weekly UUI episodes. Oxybutynin was statistically more effective in reducing mean weekly micturition frequency and in producing total dryness (no incontinence episodes). Dry mouth, though mild, was significantly more common with oxybutynin. Other adverse events, including CNS effects, had similar frequencies for both drugs. Both groups had similar discontinuation rates of treatment (Diokno AC, 2003).

Transdermal Oxybutynin. Transdermal oxybutynin (Watson Pharmaceuticals' Oxytrol) was approved by the FDA in February 2003 for treatment of OAB with symptoms of UUI. In September 2004, Watson entered into a marketing and supply agreement with UCB to market transdermal oxybutynin in Europe. Transdermal oxybutynin received approval from the European Medicines Agency (EMEA) under the brand name Kentera in November 2004 and was launched initially in Germany, with a launch in other European countries to follow.

Transdermal administration of oxybutynin achieves a higher plasma concentration of the drug with a lower daily dose and less inhibition of saliva production. Overall, this route seems to produce fewer systemic side effects than the oral route, as it bypasses the presystemic gastrointestinal and first-pass metabolism seen with oral administration; this-first pass metabolism generates high levels of the active metabolite (N-desethyloxybutynin) associated with anticholinergic adverse effects, which is avoided in transdermal delivery (Bang LM, 2003 Dmochowski RR, 2002). Skin irritation at the site of administration is an adverse effect in some patients (Dmochowski RR, 2003).

Previously published Phase II trial data showed that transdermal oxybutynin is as effective as IR oxybutynin, but with fewer anticholinergic side effects. In a 76-patient study, 38% of patients receiving transdermal oxybutynin reported having dry mouth, while 94% of patients in the IR oxybutynin (at a dose of 5 mg administered bid or tid) group reported this side effect. Less than 10% of patients given the transdermal formulation had a skin reaction or mild redness at the site of therapy application (Davila GW, 2001).

In a study of 361 adult patients with UUI or MUI, twice-weekly transdermal oxybutynin (designed to deliver a dose of 3.9 mg/day) was compared with daily ER tolterodine (4 mg) or placebo. Both transdermal oxybutynin and ER tolterodine significantly reduced the number of daily incontinence episodes (median change of −3 for transdermal oxybutynin, −3 for ER tolterodine, and −2 for placebo), increased the average void volume (median change 24 and 29 mL versus 5.5 mL), and improved the quality of life (assessed by the incontinence impact questionnaire and Urogenital Distress Inventory Irritative Symptom subscale) compared with placebo. The most common adverse event for transdermal oxybutynin was localized application site pruritis (14% versus 4% for placebo). Dry mouth was seen in 7.3% of patients who received ER tolterodine and 4.1% of patients who received transdermal oxybutynin, compared with 4% who received placebo. The two treatments appear to have comparable efficacy, with transdermal oxybutynin offering an improved anticholinergic side-effect profile (Dmochowski RR, 2003).

Trospium. Trospium (Madaus's [Koln, Germany] Sanctura/Spasmolyt, others) (Figure 5) is a quaternary ammonium derivative and anticholinergic agent available in Europe (Austria, France, Germany, Luxembourg, Spain, and the United

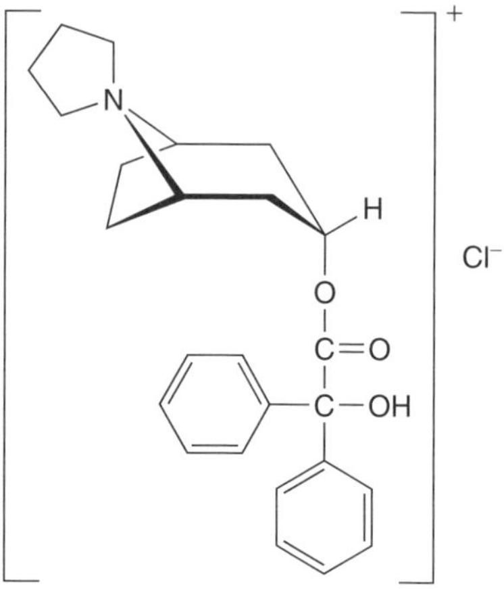

FIGURE 5. *Structure of trospium.*

Kingdom). This drug has been used for several years in Germany and Spain but was introduced to the French and U.K. markets only in late 2000. Trospium has been licensed to Indevus (formerly Interneuron) for development in the United States. In April 2004, Indevus Pharmaceuticals, Inc. (Lexington, Massachusetts) entered into an agreement with PLIVA, Inc. (East Hanover, New Jersey) to copromote trospium. Odyssey Pharmaceuticals, Inc. (East Hanover, New Jersey) a subsidiary of PLIVA, launched trospium in the United States in August 2004.

Trospium appears as effective as and better tolerated than IR oxybutynin. In a randomized, double-blind, 52-week study involving 358 patients with urge symptoms or UI, both agents improved urodynamic variables, including maximum bladder capacity, and there were no significant differences between the two agents. Similarly, micturition frequency, incontinence, and number of urgency events were similar in patients treated with trospium or IR oxybutynin. However, the incidence of adverse effects was significantly lower in the trospium groups compared with the oxybutynin group (Halaska M, 2003).

The efficacy of trospium was compared with that of IR tolterodine (2 mg administered twice daily) in 234 patients with overactive bladder. While both agents reduced urinary frequency relative to placebo, only the decrease observed with trospium was significant. The agents appear to have similar safety profiles (Jüncmann KP, 2000).

While trospium appears to offer a superior side-effect profile relative to that associated with IR oxybutynin, no head-to-head trials have been conducted to compare trospium chloride with ER oxybutynin, ER tolterodine, or to the newer agents solifenacin and darifenacin.

Solifenacin. Solifenacin succinate (Astellas Pharma's Vesicare) received regulatory approval from both the FDA and the EMEA in November 2004. Solifenacin is preregistered in Japan.

Solifenacin is a bladder-selective M_3 receptor antagonist. In an in vitro study of monkey and rat cells, solifenacin displayed tissue selectivity toward bladder smooth muscle cells over salivary gland cells. Solifenacin also showed higher bladder selectivity compared with tolterodine, oxybutynin, and darifenacin. This bladder-selective profile may allow for desired effects in UUI and minimize adverse effects such as dry mouth (Hatanaka T, 2003).

A randomized, double-blind, placebo-controlled Phase IIIa study in 1281 patients with symptoms of urge frequency and incontinence compared solifenacin with tolterodine. Participants received 5 or 10 mg solifenacin once daily, 2 mg tolterodine twice daily, or placebo. Solifenacin at both doses significantly reduced the mean number of urgency and urge incontinence episodes in 24 hours compared with tolterodine and placebo. Solifenacin and tolterodine both reduced the number of voids and increased the mean volume voided per void compared with placebo. Solifenacin was well tolerated; dry mouth, the most common side effect, was reported in 14.0% of patients receiving 5 mg solifenacin, in 21.3% receiving 10 mg solifenacin, in 18.6% receiving tolterodine, compared with 4.9% receiving placebo (Chapple C, 2004).

The recent Solifenacin Versus Tolterodine ER (STAR) study compared solifenacin with ER tolterodine for UUI associated with overactive bladder; results were presented at the 2005 European Association of Urology meeting in Istanbul, Turkey (Astellas, press release, March 2005). The study, which involved 1355 patients, was a double-blind, double-dummy, randomized trial conducted in 17 European countries. Solifenacin was administered at 5 and 10 mg doses, and ER tolterodine was administered at a 4 mg dose. The results demonstrated that solifenacin was superior to ER tolterodine on all end points: incontinence episodes, urge incontinence, urgency, and volume voided. Significantly more incontinent patients experienced no urinary leakage with solifenacin (59%) than ER tolterodine (49%). Adverse anticholinergic side effects (dry mouth, constipation, blurred vision) were similar in both the solifenacin- and the ER tolterodine-treated groups, and they were mild to moderate in both groups. In addition, discontinuation rates due to adverse events were less than 5% in both groups. Overall, the data demonstrated that solifenacin was 65% more effective than ER tolterodine in treating UUI.

Darifenacin. Darifenacin (Novartis's Enablex/Emselex) received FDA approval in the United States in December 2004. Darifenacin was being developed by Pfizer until April 2003, when Pfizer divested darifenacin as a result of its merger with Pharmacia; darifenacin was sold to Novartis at this time. In 2004, Novartis announced a collaboration with Bayer Pharmaceuticals Corporation (West Haven, Connecticut) for commercialization and distribution of darifenacin in Germany, where it is marketed under the brand name Emselex. Novartis remains the owner of marketing authorization for darifenacin, while Bayer gains exclusive commercialization rights for Emselex in Germany.

Darifenacin is an anticholinergic agent selective for the M_3 muscarinic receptor. In vitro studies using human recombinant muscarinic receptor subtypes showed that darifenacin had a 9-fold and 12-fold greater affinity for M_3 receptors than for M_1 and M_5 receptors, respectively. Darifenacin also had a 59-fold greater affinity for M_3 receptors than for either M_2 or M_4 receptors (Napier C, 2002). Data from animal models also indicate that this drug has a heightened selectivity for the M_3 receptor. In rabbits, darifenacin has been shown to have a 100-fold selectivity for the M_3 receptor in the ileum compared with M_2 receptors on the atria and a 30-fold selectivity for the M_3 receptor compared with M_1 receptors in the vas deferens. The M_3 receptor is believed to be involved in bladder overactivity; hence, darifenacin might reduce bladder contractions while having a lesser effect on other muscarinic receptor subtypes, thereby reducing side effects.

A multicenter, double-blind, placebo-controlled Phase III trial studied the effect of darifenacin on 561 patients (85% female) with symptoms of urinary urge, urinary frequency, and urinary incontinence. At both 7.5 and 15 mg once-daily doses, darifenacin induced a significant reduction in micturition frequency, median number of urgency and incontinence episodes, and increased bladder capacity compared with placebo. At 12 weeks after treatment, darifenacin administered at 7.5 and 15 mg reduced the weekly number of incontinence episodes from baseline by 67.7% and 72.8% respectively, compared with 55.9% for placebo. Darifenacin also induced a higher incidence of dry mouth and constipation compared with placebo. However, no blurred vision was reported with darifenacin treatment, and CNS and cardiac adverse events were comparable to those seen with placebo (Haab F, 2004).

A small crossover study in 76 patients (93% female) compared darifenacin and oxybutynin in patients who had a significant number of urge incontinence episodes (four or more per week) and eight or more voids per day. Darifenacin (15 mg once daily for two weeks) was as effective as oxybutynin in reducing the frequency of urinary incontinence and the frequency and severity of urgency. The mean number of weekly incontinence episodes in week 2 was similar in the darifenacin and oxybutynin groups, and both treatments were significantly more effective than placebo (10.9 and 9.4 episodes for both groups, respectively, versus for 14.6 for placebo). Oxybutynin was associated with a higher incidence of dry mouth (36%) than either darifenacin (13%) or placebo (5%). Rates of constipation were comparable between darifenacin (10%) and oxybutynin (8%), although both tended to be higher than placebo (3%). Blurred vision and dizziness were reported only during oxybutynin therapy. Darifenacin's comparable clinical efficacy and improved tolerability versus that of oxybutynin was attributed to the former drug's high selectivity for M_3 receptors, combined with M_1 receptor and M_2 receptor-sparing characteristics (Zinner N, 2004).

Propiverine. Propiverine (Schering-Plough's [Kenilworth, New Jersey] Detrunorm/BUP-4) (Figure 6) was launched in the former East Germany in 1981 as a treatment for UI. In 1993, Taiho acquired the marketing rights in Japan and launched the product jointly with Fujirebio, Inc. (Tokyo, Japan) as BUP-4. The compound has also been introduced in the United Kingdom, where Schering-Plough has the rights.

Propiverine is a tertiary amine anticholinergic with calcium channel antagonizing action in vitro. It has neurotrophic and musculotrophic effects on the urinary bladder smooth muscle (Hashim H, 2004).

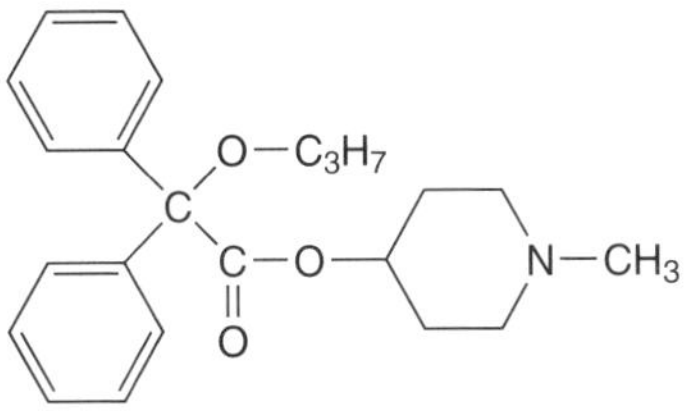

FIGURE 6. *Structure of propiverine.*

A randomized, double-blind, placebo controlled study demonstrated that propiverine has similar efficacy and a better side-effect profile compared with oxybutynin. In this study, 366 patients with symptoms of urgency and urinary incontinence were treated with propiverine (15 mg three times daily), oxybutynin (5 mg twice daily), or placebo for four weeks. Propiverine improved urodynamic measurements, including cystometric bladder capacity at first desire to void and mean maximal cystometric capacity, as effectively as oxybutynin. Dry mouth was less common and less severe with propiverine than oxybutynin (Maderbacher H, 1999).

Hormone Replacement Therapies

Overview. Some researchers have suggested that estrogen (generics) may have efficacy in the treatment of UUI. The treatment can be given orally, transdermally (via a patch), or intravaginally; patients often must take the therapy for six weeks before the full benefits become evident. Women with an intact uterus should also receive supplementary progesterone to reduce the risk of endometrial cancer. In the treatment of UUI, estrogen is typically reserved for postmenopausal UUI patients with atrophic vaginitis (inflammation of the vagina with thinning of the epithelial lining due to estrogen deficiency).

Mechanism of Action. Estrogen therapy may improve the symptoms of UI via the reversal of urogenital atrophy (Klutke JJ, 1995). As a woman ages, decreases in the level of circulating estrogen can cause atrophy of the muscles, ligaments, and fascia involved in controlling and supporting the bladder. Estrogen treatment—both local and systemic—increases urethral closure pressure, restores perivaginal tissue integrity, and increases urine storage capacity within the bladder. All these actions help reduce UI symptoms.

Vaginal Estrogen. Available in intravaginal ring or tablet or in topical cream or gel, vaginal estrogens are primarily used to relieve the atrophic symptoms of menopause, such as dryness, and other climacteric complaints, including burning and overall discomfort. Like systemic estrogen, unopposed topical estrogen (e.g., estrogen replacement therapy without a concomitant progestin product) stimulates the endometrium and can put patients at increased risk of uterine cancer. In women with an intact uterus, a progestin is therefore added if a topical product is used for more than six weeks; alternatively, the topical product dose is tapered or the product is discontinued. Estradiol cream (such as Galen's [Country Armagh, Ireland] Estrace) and vaginal tablets (such as Novo Nordisk's [Bagsvaerd, Denmark] Vagifem) dominate the U.S. market for vaginal estrogens, but these products have little presence outside the United States, where estriol creams (Organon's [Roseland, New Jersey] Ovestin, others) are more popular. Conjugated estrogen cream Wyeth's (Madison, New Jersey) is another commonly used vaginal estrogen product; its popularity is confined largely to the U.S. market. These agents are administered either daily or three times per week. This relatively frequent dosing schedule (along with the cream's potential for leakage) makes these agents somewhat inconvenient. Relatively new estrogen vaginal rings (Pfizer's Estring), which remain in place for three months, offer more suitable options for patients who do not mind their presence in the vagina.

A meta-analysis reviewed the effects of estrogen in 430 overactive bladder patients from 11 randomized trials (Cardozo L, 2004). The analysis included patients who had symptoms of overactive bladder and who were treated with systemic estrogen, local estrogen, or placebo. Overall, estrogen therapy was associated with statistically significant improvements in all outcome variables, including diurnal frequency, nocturnal frequency, urgency, first sensation to void, and number of incontinence episodes. However, when analyzed separately, local therapies had statistically significant benefits on all variables; systemic therapies were associated with significant improvements only in incontinence episodes and first sensation to void, while nocturnal frequency actually worsened. These results suggest that estrogen may be effective in relieving some UUI symptoms, and local administration may be more beneficial than systemic administration.

Nonpharmacological Therapies

The AHRQ recommends behavioral treatment as the first-line therapy for UUI (AHCPR, 1996). Behavioral treatments include lifestyle interventions such as stopping caffeine (which acts as a mild diuretic and stimulant to the detrusor muscle) and alcohol intake and voiding before going to bed if nocturia is a problem.

Bladder training aims to regain bladder control by suppressing involuntary detrusor contractions through feedback inhibition, thereby increasing the time interval between voids and the voided volumes. Bladder training is usually supplemented by pelvic floor exercises (Kegel exercises), which teaches patients to tighten the pelvic floor when they get an involuntary contraction. Biofeedback involves reeducating and retraining patients' bladder control mechanisms and can be used as adjunct to bladder training. Nonpharmacological therapies for UUI are described in Table 2.

The AHRQ guidelines recommend behavioral techniques for motivated individuals who wish to avoid more invasive procedures or dependence on protective garments, external devices, and medications. Although the precise level of effectiveness of behavioral interventions has not been accurately assessed, the AHRQ

TABLE 2. Nonpharmacological Therapies for Urge Urinary Incontinence

Nonpharmacological Therapy	Description
Bladder retraining	Patients systematically increase the time between visits to the toilet, which teaches them to inhibit the sensation of urgency, to delay voiding, and to use the toilet on a schedule rather than in response to the urge to void. According to the AHRQ guidelines, bladder retraining can achieve a 16% cure rate and a 54% improvement in UUI patients.
Pelvic-floor exercises	Pelvic-floor exercises (PFE) may be conducted by both men and women to strengthen muscles and ligaments on the pelvic floor that help support the bladder. PFE involve repeated contractions of the muscles located in the pelvic floor, particularly the pubococcygeus muscle. The exercises are designed to increase both muscle bulk and maximum urethral closure pressure, which then gives stronger reflex contractions to sudden increases in abdominal pressure or to involuntary detrusor contractions.
Biofeedback	Biofeedback involves reeducating and retraining patients' bladder control mechanisms. This technique relies on muscle pressure sensor readings, taken from electrodes placed in the vagina and/or the anus, that provide information about neuromuscular and bladder activity, particularly during pelvic muscle exercises.
Modification of fluid consumption	Physicians use voiding diaries and frequency and volume charts to assess patients' fluid intake. Frequency and volume charts might reveal that a patient is drinking abnormally large amounts of water. In such cases, symptoms can be reduced by simply advising the patient to decrease his or her intake to a normal level. Older patients with lower-extremity edema produce more urine at night and, therefore, can benefit from fluid restriction after dinner.
UUI management products	• Absorbent undergarments and pads. • Intravaginal sponges: help support the bladder neck during exercise and physical exertion. • Urethral plugs: a fluid-filled or inflated plug is inserted into the urethra to prevent urine passage. • Continence guards: inserted into the vagina to support the bladder neck and aid continence. • FemAssist: a silicone, nipple-shaped device that the patient applies over the urethral opening. • Reliance: a urethral insert made of the plastic elastomer dynaflex that contains a valve and releasing string that can be pulled to allow for micturition. • Indwelling permanent catheter: a closed sterile system inserted through the urethra to allow bladder drainage.

AHRQ = Agency for Healthcare Research and Quality.
UUI = Urge urinary incontinence.

TABLE 3. Surgical Interventions for Urge Urinary Incontinence

Procedure	Mechanism	Advantages and Disadvantages
Augmentation cystoplasty	Segment of the intestine introduced into the bladder to increase capacity and reduce end-filling pressure	*Advantages*: Effective in patients with neurogenic bladder dysfunction. *Disadvantages*: Bowel disturbances in as many as one third of patients. Risk of cancer. As many as 30% of patients have to perform intermittent self-catheterization.
Autoaugmentation	Excision of bladder muscle to produce a large cellule to expand bladder volume	*Advantages*: Increases bladder capacity without using bowel or stomach segments. *Disadvantages*: Not advised for patients unable to perform self-catheterization or who have kidney disorders, bowel disease, or urethral disease.
Neuromodulation	Electrical stimulation of sacral somatic nerve afferents to inhibit the micturition reflex	*Advantages*: Implanted nerve stimulators provide continuous and effective treatment. *Disadvantages*: Expensive. Intermittent nerve stimulators (anal and vaginal plugs) have rapid onset of effect but the effect does not persist when therapy is temporarily stopped.

guidelines note that, in general, studies suggest that behavioral interventions are effective in reducing incontinence. Behavioral interventions, alone or in combination with pharmacological treatments, are often recommended as a first-line therapy for UUI.

The use of surgical procedures in UUI is uncommon and is usually considered only in highly symptomatic patients for whom nonsurgical methods of treatment have failed repeatedly. Surgical procedures used for UUI are listed in Table 3.

EMERGING THERAPIES

Researchers are investigating several potential drug targets in the search for novel agents to treat UUI. Nevertheless, the most advanced research and late-stage clinical development efforts remain focused on modification of existing therapeutic approaches, with several new anticholinergic agents being investigated for UUI; novel agents based on noncholinergic mechanisms of action are mainly in preclinical or early-stage clinical development. With the recent launches of solifenacin and darifenacin, the availability of low-cost oxybutynin, the introduction of an extended-release (ER) formulation of oxybutynin (in the United States and several European markets), the successful launch of the better-tolerated tolterodine in most of the major pharmaceutical markets, and the launch of ER tolterodine (in the United States and several European markets), any new therapy will need to show a significant improvement in efficacy and side-effect profile if it is to be

TABLE 4. Emerging Therapies in Development for Urge Urinary Incontinence

Compound	Development Phase	Marketing Company
Anticholinergics		
Fesoterodine		
United States	III	Schwarz Pharma
Europe	III	Schwarz Pharma
Japan	—	—
Imidafenacin		
United States	—	—
Europe	I	Kyorin Pharmaceutical
Japan	PR	Kyorin Pharmaceutical
Oxybutynin vaginal ring		
United States	II	Barr Laboratories
Europe	II	Barr Laboratories
Japan	—	—
Neuromuscular blocking agents		
Botulinum toxin A		
United States	III	Allergan
Europe	II	Allergan
Japan	—	—
Potassium-channel activators		
KW-7158		
United States	II	Kyowa Hakko
Europe	II	Kyowa Hakko
Japan	I	Kyowa Hakko
NS-8		
United States	—	—
Europe	II	Nippon Shinyaku
Japan	I	Nippon Shinyaku
Beta$_3$-adrenergic receptor agonists		
KUC-7483		
United States	—	—
Europe	II	Kissei Pharmaceutical/Boehringer Ingelheim
Japan	I	Kissei Pharmaceutical/Boehringer Ingelheim
Tachykinin-release modulators		
Cizolirtine		
United States	—	—
Europe	II	Esteve Laboratories
Japan	—	—

PR = Preregistered.

widely prescribed and win market share. Table 4 summarizes the drug therapies in development for UUI.

A number of potential UUI treatments in the neurokinin antagonists class have proceeded to clinical trials, only to be discontinued later in the trial process. These include Takeda Pharmaceutical's (Osaka, Japan) TAK-637, GlaxoSmithKline's (Brentford, Middlesex, United Kingdom) talnetant, and Pfizer's UK-224671 and UK-290795. A few new agents are in development: AstraZeneca's (Wilmington, Delaware) AZ-311 and AZ-685 (neurokinin-2 receptor antagonists, in preclinical development) and Tanabe Seiyaku Company's (Osaka, Japan) TA-5538 (a neurokinin-1 receptor antagonist, in Phase I development). However, no clinical data have been released for any of these agents, so this class is not covered in detail here.

Besipirdine, a compound with multiple mechanisms of action, is currently in Phase II development by UroGene (Evry, France) in Europe for treatment of UUI associated with overactive bladder. The drug's effects on central monoaminergic systems include inhibition of norepinephrine and serotonin uptake, antagonism of the $alpha_2$ (α_2)-adrenergic receptor, stimulation of norepinephrine release, and inhibition of central neurotransmitter release (Hubbard JW, 1997; Tang L, 1996). Because very little information is available on besipirdine's utility in the treatment of UUI, it is not discussed further.

Anticholinergic Agents

Overview. Developers of emerging therapies in the anticholinergics class have focused on compounds that have better selectivity profiles for different muscarinic receptors. These agents would be expected to have better side-effect profiles than currently marketed anticholinergics.

Several anticholinergics are in early-stage development for the treatment of UUI. SALVAT's (Barcelona, Spain) SVT-40776 is in Phase II clinical trials in Spain for UUI associated with overactive bladder. SVT-40776 is an anticholinergic that is highly selective for M_3 over M_2 receptors (M_2 receptors are likely to mediate adverse cardiac effects). Unlike darifenacin, another M_3-selective anticholinergic, SVT-40776 lacks selectivity for M_3 over M_1, M_4, and M_5 receptors (Salcedo C, 2003). RO-320-2904 is in preclinical development by Roche Bioscience (a pharmaceutical research division of Roche [Basel, Switzerland]) for the treatment of UUI. In rats and dogs, this compound was more selective than tolterodine and oxybutynin, inhibiting urinary bladder contractions without inhibiting saliva production (Greene B, 2000; Shetty SG, 2002). These effects suggest that this compound may be effective against UUI without causing dry mouth. No other published information is available on these early-stage compounds; therefore, they are not covered in detail here.

Mechanism of Action. Anticholinergic agents act by inhibiting the effects of the parasympathetic nervous system (mediated via acetylcholine) on the bladder, thereby reducing the frequency of bladder contractions, relaxing the bladder smooth muscle, and increasing bladder capacity.

Fesoterodine. Schwarz Pharma (Milwaukee, Wisconsin) is developing a selective M_3 muscarinic antagonist, fesoterodine (SPM-007), for treatment of UUI. In 2005, fesoterodine completed Phase III clinical trials in the United States and Germany.

In vivo, fesoterodine is rapidly hydrolyzed by esterases to an active metabolite, SPM-7605, that is chemically identical to the 5-hyroxymethyl metabolite of tolterodine. Although release of the active metabolite occurs by different mechanisms for fesoterodine and tolterodine, this does not result in an apparent pharmacokinetic advantage for fesoterodine compared with tolterodine (Hedge SS, 2004; Brynne N, 1998). In rats, both fesoterodine and its active metabolite produce potent increases in bladder capacity (Breidenbach A, 2002).

While no peer-reviewed, published clinical trial data are available, a 2005 company press release reported the results of recent clinical trials for UUI associated with overactive bladder. A Phase III clinical study in 1900 patients in Europe and the United States studied the effect of treatment with 4 mg or 8 mg fesoterodine compared with placebo; one group in the European arm received 4 mg of ER tolterodine. Results showed significant improvements in the number of micturitions and urge incontinence episodes per day in fesoterodine-treated patients compared with placebo. Fesoterodine had a favorable profile over tolterodine, and the most common adverse event was dry mouth. In addition, more than 90% of patients chose to enter a follow-on, open-label study.

Although company-reported results suggest that fesoterodine may have an efficacy and/or safety profile at least comparable to that of tolterodine, there is insufficient information to show whether fesoterodine will have significant advantages over marketed anticholinergics—specifically, tolterodine, solifenacin, and darifenacin.

Imidafenacin. Imidafenacin (KRP-197) (Kyorin Pharmaceutical's [Tokyo, Japan] Uritos) was submitted for approval in Japan for treatment of pollakiuria (extraordinary urinary frequency) and UUI in 2004. The compound is also in Phase I development in the United Kingdom for UUI. Kyorin and Ono Pharmaceutical Company (Osaka, Japan) signed a codevelopment and comarketing agreement for KRP-197 in Japan in February 2001.

Imidafenacin is an imidazole derivative that displays selectivity for M_1 and M_3 muscarinic receptors. In rats, imidafenacin has shown tenfold greater selectivity for muscarinic receptors in the bladder than for muscarinic receptors in the salivary gland (Miyachi H, 1999; Yoshida M, 2000).

Oxybutynin Vaginal Ring. Barr Laboratories's (Pomona, New York) oxybutynin-releasing vaginal ring (Enhance UI) is currently in Phase II development for the treatment of UUI; Barr acquired the technology from Enhance Pharmaceuticals (Plainsboro, New Jersey) in 2002. In 2004, Schering AG (Berlin, Germany), which had previously entered into a development agreement with Enhance Pharmaceuticals, assigned worldwide rights to Barr.

The vaginal ring delivers oxybutynin slowly over a 28-day period, and patients will be able to remove and insert the ring themselves. While no trial data have been released, the company claims that the oxybutynin vaginal ring has fewer side effects than oral oxybutynin.

Neuromuscular Blocking Agents

Overview. Neuromuscular blocking agents are used to relax muscles or suppress overactive glands. The major agent in this class is botulinum toxin A, which has been previously approved for treatment of other medical conditions, such as strabismus (a deviation of the eye that the patient cannot overcome).

Mechanism of Action. When injected into overactive muscles, neuromuscular blocking agents inhibit acetylcholine release from nerve endings. This inhibition of acetylcholine consequently inhibits muscle overactivity and is therefore believed to inhibit detrusor muscle overactivity in UUI (Hashim H, 2004).

Botulinum Toxin A. Allergan is developing its botulinum toxin type A (Botox) for UUI associated with overactive bladder. It is in Phase II trials in Germany and in Phase III trials in the United States for UUI associated with neurogenic overactive bladder. It is also in Phase II trials in the United States for UUI associated with idiopathic overactive bladder.

Botulinum toxin A is a purified neurotoxin, administered by intravesical (within the bladder) injection into the detrusor muscle. In addition to its inhibition of acetylcholine release, botulinum toxin A has been shown to induce a state of nerve growth factor (NGF) deprivation in the bladder tissue of patients with neurogenic detrusor overactivity (Giannantoni A, 2005). This depletion of NGF decreased the hyperexcitability of C-fiber bladder afferents, which subsequently reduced detrusor overactivity.

In a small study of 21 patients with neurogenic overactive bladder with incontinence resulting from spinal cord injury, botulinum toxin A doses of 200–300 units per patient were administered by injection to the detrusor muscle at 20–30 random sites, sparing the trigone (Schurch B, 2000[a]; Schurch B, 2000[b]; Stohrer M, 2000). Of these patients, 90% were fully continent after six weeks' treatment, 28% were able to discontinue anticholinergic therapy, and 61% reduced their doses of anticholinergics to 50% or less of levels required before botulinum toxin A treatment. Reflex volume and maximal bladder capacity were significantly increased and maximal detrusor pressure was significantly decreased, relative to baseline. These improvements were maintained in the 52% of patients assessed at weeks 16 and 26 after treatment.

In a Phase II, retrospective, multicenter study of 231 patients, botulinum toxin A was injected cytoscopically into the detrusor muscle at 30 different sites, sparing the trigone (Reitz A, 2003). The injections enabled patients with neurogenic incontinence to stop or considerably reduce anticholinergic drugs without experiencing reflux incontinence. The mean bladder capacity and mean reflex volume were significantly increased at 12- and 36-week urodynamic follow-up examinations.

At the May 2005 American Urology Association (AUA) meeting in San Antonio, Texas, the effect of botulinum toxin A treatment in 100 UUI patients with overactive bladder (who were also refractory to anticholinergic therapy and physiotherapy) was reported (Schmid DM, 2005). Treatment was accomplished by injection under cystoscopic control of 100 units of botulinum toxin A into the detrusor muscle. Of these patients, 88% showed an improvement in bladder function with regard to subjective symptoms and urodynamic parameters. Urgency was abolished in 76% of patients and incontinence was abolished in 80% of patients within one to two weeks after botulinum toxin A injections. Frequency decreased from 14 to 7 micturitions/day. There were no severe side effects except temporary urine retention in three patients. The mean duration of efficacy was nine months.

Potassium-Channel Activators

Overview. In the laboratory, several agents (e.g., tachycardia) have demonstrated activity on potassium-channel targets (e.g., cromakalin, pinacidil), though few clinical trials have been conducted with members of this drug class because of concerns about negative cardiovascular effects previously seen in investigations of some agents.

A number of potential UUI treatments that boast enhanced uroselectivity have proceeded to clinical trials, only to be discontinued later in the trial process. These include AstraZeneca's ZD-0947 and ZD-6169, both of which proceeded to Phase II clinical trials before being discontinued. There are also a number of candidates in preclinical and early clinical development. These include Abbott Laboratories (Abbott Park, Illinois) A-278637 and Wyeth's WAY-13357, which are in preclinical development, and Abbott's ABT-598, which is in Phase I clinical development.

Mechanism of Action. Potassium-channel activators directly hyperpolarize (increase the amount of electrical charge separated by the membrane) the smooth-muscle membrane in the bladder, making it less excitable and less likely to contract involuntarily. It has also been proposed that activation of potassium channels on the primary afferent neurons that innervate the bladder may also inhibit UUI by directly decreasing afferent drive to the spinal cord (Burgard EC, 2005).

KW-7158. Kyowa Hakko's (New York, New York) KW-7158 is currently in Phase II trials in United States and Western Europe and in Phase I trials in Japan for UUI associated with overactive bladder. KW-7158 is an activator of the neuronal A-type potassium currents on bladder sensory neurons (Sculptoreanu A, 2004). This compound has been shown to depress bladder activity (Lu SH, 2002). Selective modulation of bladder afferent activity by KW-7158 may alleviate the problems commonly associated with using potassium-channel activators, such as adverse cardiovascular effects.

NS-8. Nippon Shinyaku's (Kyoto, Japan) NS-8 is currently in Phase II development in Western Europe and in Phase I development in Japan for pollakiuria and UUI. In 2003, Nippon Shinyaku granted exclusive European marketing and development rights to Apogepha.

NS-8 acts on a large-conductance calcium-activated potassium channel (the BK channel) in bladder smooth muscle cells. NS-8 is a potassium channel opener that preferentially inhibits pelvic nerve afferent firing without a coincident decrease in amplitude of bladder contractions (Tanaka N, 2003). Selective modulation of afferent nerve activity via BK channel activation may maintain efficient bladder contractility and therefore be effective in treatment of UUI.

Beta$_3$-Adrenergic Receptor Agonists

Overview. Several beta$_3$-adrenergic receptor agonists are in early-stage clinical development for UUI. These include Kissei Pharmaceutical's (Tokyo, Japan) KUC-7483 and Astellas Pharma's YM-178, both of which are in Phase II clinical trials for UUI in Europe and the United States and in Phase I in Japan (Astellas Pharma, R&D meeting summary, July 6, 2005). Little clinical information is available on YM-178, so it is not discussed in detail here.

Mechanism of Action. Beta$_3$-adrenergic receptor agonists augment the storage phase of the micturition cycle, which is mediated by the sympathetic nervous system, without interfering with the voiding phase. Selective stimulation of beta$_3$ receptors relaxes the bladder and increases bladder capacity. In previous preclinical studies in rats, beta$_3$ agonists were shown to increase the inter-micturition interval and bladder capacity with no increase in residual volume during continuous cystometry (Woods M, 2001; Takeda H, 2000).

KUC-7483. Kissei Pharmaceutical's KUC-7483 is in Phase II clinical development in Western Europe for UUI associated with overactive bladder. In November 2002, Kissei Pharmaceutical granted Boehringer Ingelheim (Ingelheim, Germany) exclusive worldwide rights to develop and market KUC-7483.

KUC-7483 showed potent and selective beta$_3$-adrenergic receptor agonistic activity in rat preclinical models. KUC-7483 prolonged the micturition interval and increased micturition volume as well as well as dose-dependently decreased intravesical pressure. The ability to prevent bladder overactivity in these models suggests a potential use for this compound in treatment of UUI associated with overactive bladder in humans (Yamakazi Y, 2002).

Tachykinin-Release Modulators

Overview. Compounds in development for UUI in this class have multiple mechanisms of action. For example, cizolirtine has analgesic activity and was originally developed for treatment of pain; however, its effects on substance P, calcitonin-gene related peptide (CGRP), and noradrenergic pathways, which may be involved in UUI, may have beneficial effects in the treatment of UUI.

Mechanism of Action. Tachykinins such as substance P activate neurokinin (NK1) receptors are located within the spinal cord and are associated with peripheral sensory innervation. In UUI, antagonists of NK1 receptors interrupt aberrant sensory signaling from the overactive detrusor (Burgard EC, 2005). In addition, NK1 receptors are located in the blood vessels in the bladder, where they mediate vasodilation and plasma extravasation. Therefore, agents that block NK1 receptors may also reduce inflammatory conditions that would otherwise stimulate afferent pathways involved in UUI (Cannon TW, 2002).

Cizolirtine. Cizolirtine is currently in Phase II development in Barcelona, Spain by Dr. Esteve Laboratories for treatment of UUI. This compound has multiple mechanisms of action. Cizolirtine inhibits the release of the tachykinin substance P and of the neurotransmitter calcitonin-gene related peptide (CGRP) in the spinal cord. Substance P and CGRP are believed to be involved in the pathogenesis of UUI. In addition, the main metabolite of cizolirtine is a serotonin reuptake inhibitor (Farre AJ, 2002; Ballet S, 2001).

The mechanism by which cizolirtine inhibits the release of substance P and CGRP is not clearly defined, although it is believed to involve noradrenergic pathways. Cizolirtine increases serotonin and noradrenaline release in different parts of the brain; this increase is believed to inhibit the release of substance P and CGRP in the spinal cord. Substance P activates NK1 receptors located within the spinal cord that are associated with peripheral sensory innervation; inhibition of substance P release is believed to interrupt aberrant NK1 receptor-mediated sensory signaling from the overactive detrusor in UUI (Farre AJ, 2002; Ballet S, 2001; Burgard EC, 2005).

In June 2004, Esteve announced positive results from two double-blind, Phase II trials of cizolirtine for the treatment of patients with UUI (Esteve, press release, June 26, 2004). In the first trial, 135 patients were randomized to receive cizolirtine, oxybutynin, or placebo. The trial achieved the primary efficacy end points (decrease in the number of incontinence episodes and urgencies) in a statistically significant manner versus placebo. The second trial involved 79 patients in three arms: two different doses of cizolirtine and placebo. Cizolirtine showed a dose-response relationship, with the higher dose showing significantly better efficacy versus placebo. Cizolirtine was generally well tolerated in both studies. Subsequent Phase III programs in UUI will be carried out with a modified-release formulation of cizolirtine, which is currently being developed by Esteve (Esteve, press release, March 8, 2005).

REFERENCES

Abrams P, et al. The standardization of terminology of lower urinary tract function: report from the standardization sub-committee of the International Continence Society. *Neurourology and Urodynamics*. 2002;**21**:167–178.

Agency for Health Care Policy and Research (AHCPR). Urinary incontinence in adults: acute and chronic management. Clinical Practice Guideline Number 2 (1996 Update), AHCPR Publication No. 96-0682. March 1996.

Andersen JT, et al. ICS 7th report on the standardization of terminology of lower urinary tract function—lower urinary tract rehabilitation techniques. *Neurourology and Urodynamics*. 1992;**11**:593–603.

Andersson KE, Yoshida M. Antimuscarinics and the overactive detrusor—which is the main mechanism of action? *European Urology*. 2003;**43**(1):1–5.

Anderson RU, et al. Once-daily controlled- versus immediate-release oxybutynin chloride for urge urinary incontinence. *Journal of Urology*. 1999;**161**:1809–1812.

Appell RA, et al. Prospective randomized controlled trial of extended-release oxybutynin chloride and tolterodine tartrate in the treatment of overactive bladder: results of the OBJECT study. *Mayo Clinic Proceedings*. 2001;**76**(4):358–363.

Ballet S, et al. The novel analgesic, cizolirtine, inhibits the spinal release of substance P and CGRP in rats. *Neuropharmacology*. 2001;**40**(4):578–589.

Bang LM, et al. Transdermal oxybutynin for overactive bladder. *Drugs Aging*. 2003; **20**(11):857–864.

Blaivas JG. Nontraumatic neurogenic voiding dysfunction in the adult, II: multiple sclerosis and diabetes mellitus. *AUA Update Series*. 1985;**4**.

Bortolotti A, et al. Prevalence and risk factors for urinary incontinence in Italy. *European Urology*. 2000;**37**:30–35.

Braverman AS, et al. M2 muscarinic receptor contributes to contraction of the denervated rat urinary bladder. *American Journal of Physiology*. 1998;**275**(5 Pt 2):R1654–R1660.

Breidenbach A, et al. Pharmacodynamic profiling of the novel antimuscarinic drug fesoterodine on rat bladder. Annual Meeting of the International Continence Society; August 28–30, 2002; Heidelberg, Germany. Abstract 449.

Brynne N, et al. Influence of CYP2D6 polymorphism on the pharmacokinetics and pharmacodynamic of tolterodine. *Clinical Pharmacology and Therapeutics*. 1998;**63**(5):529–539.

Burgard EC, et al. New pharmacological treatments for urinary incontinence and overactive bladder. *Current Opinion in Investigational Drugs*. 2005;**6**(1):81–89.

Bymaster FP, et al. Investigations into the physiological role of muscarinic M2 and M4 muscarinic and M4 receptor subtypes using receptor knockout mice. *Life Science*. 2001;**68**(22–23):2473–2479.

Cannon TW, Chancellor MB. Pharmacotherapy of the overactive bladder and advances in drug delivery. *Clinical Obstetrics and Gynecology*. 2002;**45**(1):205–217.

Cardozo L, et al. A systematic review of the effects of estrogens for symptoms suggestive of overactive bladder. *Acta Obstetricia et Gynecologica Scandinavica*. 2004;**83**(10):892–897.

Chapple C, et al. Randomised, double-blind placebo-and tolterodine-controlled trial of the once daily antimuscarinic agent solifenacin in patients with symptomatic overactive bladder. *BJU International*. 2004;**93**(3):303–310.

Cheater FM, et al. Epidemiology and classification of urinary incontinence. *Baillieres Best Practice and Research. Clinical Obstetrics and Gynaecology*. 2000;**14**:183–205.

Chess-Williams R, et al. The minor population of M3-receptors mediate contraction of human detrusor muscle in vitro. *Journal of Autonomic Pharmacology*. 2001;**21**(5–6):243–248.

Damián J, et al. Prevalence of urinary incontinence among Spanish older people living at home. *European Urology*. 1998;**34**:333–338.

Davila GW, et al. A short-tern, multicenter, randomized double-blind dose titration study of the efficacy and anticholinergic side effects of transdermal compared to immediate release oral oxybutynin treatment of patients with urge urinary incontinence. *Journal of Urology*. 2001;**166**(1):140–145.

De Groat WC. A neurologic basis for the overactive bladder. *Urology*. 1997;**50**(6A): 36–52.

Diokno AC, et al. Prospective, randomized, double-blind study of the efficacy and tolerability of the extended-release formulations of oxybutynin and tolterodine for overactive bladder: results of the OPERA trial. *Mayo Clinic Proceedings*. 2003;**78**(6):687–695.

Diokno AC. Epidemiology of urinary incontinence. *Journal of Gerontology*. 2001;**56A**: M3–M4.

Dmochowski RR, et al. Efficacy and safety of oxybutynin in patients with urge and mixed urinary incontinence. *Journal of Urology*. 2002;**168**:580–586.

Dmochowski RR, et al. Comparative efficacy and safety of transdermal oxybutynin and oral tolterodine in previously treated patients with urge and mixed urinary incontinence. *Urology*. 2003;**62**(2):237–242.

Dunn JS, et al. Pathophysiology of detrusor overactivity. *Journal of Pelvic Medicine and Surgery*. 2004;**10**:43–51.

Engström G, et al. Prevalence of three lower urinary tract symptoms in men—a population-based study. *Family Practice*. 2003;**20**(1):7–10.

Farre AJ, Figola J. Cizolirtine citrate. *Drugs Future*. 2002;**27**(8):721.

Fraser MO, Chancellor MB. Neural control of the urethra and development of pharmacotherapy for stress urinary incontinence. *BJU International*. 2003;**91**(8):743–748.

Fetscher C, et al. M3 muscarinic receptors mediate contraction of human urinary bladder. *British Journal of Pharmacology*. 2002;**136**(5):641–643.

Fultz NH, et al. Prevalence of urinary incontinence in middle-aged and older women: a survey-based methodological experiment. *Journal of Aging and Health*. 2000;**12**:459–469.

Gavira Iglesias FJ. Prevalence and psychosocial impact of urinary incontinence in older people of a Spanish rural population. *Journals of Gerontology. Series A. Biological Sciences and Medical Sciences*. 2000;**55A**:M207–M214.

Giannantoni A, et al. Botulinum A toxin intravesical treatment induces a reduction of nerve growth factor bladder tissue levels in patients with neurogenic detrusor overactivity. *Journal of Urology*. 2005;**173**(suppl):330.

Greene B, et al. The effect of the muscarinic antagonists, RO320-2904 (RO), tolterodine (TOL) and oxybutynin (OXY) on pilocarpine (PIL)-induced bladder contraction and salivation in conscious dogs. *Pharmacologist*. 2000;**44**(2 suppl 1):25.12.

Haab F, et al. Darifenacin, an M3 selective is an effective and well-tolerated daily treatment for overactive bladder. *European Urology*. 2004;**45**(4):420–429.

Halaska M, et al. Controlled, double-blind, multicentre clinical trial to investigate long term tolerability and efficacy of trospium chloride in patients with detrusor instability. *World Journal of Urology*. 2003;**20**(6):392–399.

Hampel C, et al. Definition of overactive bladder and epidemiology of urinary incontinence. *Urology*. 1997;**50**(suppl 6A):4–14.

Hannestad YS, et al. A community-based epidemiological survey of female urinary incontinence: the Norwegian EPICONT study. *Journal of Clinical Epidemiology*. 2000;**53**:1150–1157.

Hashim H, Abrams P. Drug treatment of overactive bladder: efficacy, cost and quality of life considerations. *Drugs*. 2004;**64**(15):1643–1656.

Hatanaka T, et al. In vitro tissue selective profile of solifenacin succinate (YM905) for urinary bladder over salivary gland in rats and monkeys. *Proceedings of the International Continence Society 33rd Annual Meeting*; October 5–9, 2003; Florence, Italy. Abstract 312.

Hegde SS, Eglen RM. Muscarinic receptor subtypes modulating smooth muscle contractility in the urinary bladder. *Life Science*. 1999;**64**(6–7):419–428.

Hedge SS, et al. Antimuscarinics for treatment of overactive bladder: current options and emerging therapies. *Current Opinion in Investigational Drugs*. 2004: **5**:40–49.

Herzog AR, et al. Two-year incidence, remission, and change patterns of urinary incontinence in noninstitutionalized older adults. *Journal of Gerontology: Medical Sciences*. 1990;**45**:M67–M74.

Hirai K, et al. Indifference and resignation of Japanese women toward urinary incontinence. *International Journal of Gynecology and Obstetrics*. 2001;**75**:89–91.

Homma Y, et al. Epidemiologic survey on lower urinary tract symptoms in Japan. *Journal of Neurogenic Bladder Society*. 2003;**14**:266–277.

Hubbard JW, et al. α-Adrenergic activity and cardiovascular effects of besipirdine HCl (HP 749) and metabolite P7480 in vitro and in the conscious rat and dog. *Journal of Pharmacology and Experimental Therapeutics*. 1997;**281**(1):337–346.

Hunskaar S, et al. Epidemiology and natural history of urinary incontinence. *International Urogynecology Journal and Pelvic Floor Dysfunction*. 2000;**11**:301–319.

Hunskaar S, et al. The prevalence of urinary incontinence in women in four European countries. *British Journal of Urology*. 2004;**93**:324–330.

Jünemann KP, Al-Shukri S. Efficacy and tolerability of trospium chloride and tolterodine in 234 patients with urge-syndrome: a double-blind, placebo-controlled, multicentre trial. *Neurourology and Urodynamics*. 2000;**19**:488–90. Abstract.

Klutke, JJ, Bergman A. Hormonal influence on the urinary tract. *Urologic Clinics of North America*. 1995;**22**(3):629–639.

Kreder K, et al. Long-term safety, tolerability and efficacy of extended-release tolterodine in the treatment of overactive bladder. *European Urology*. 2002;**41**(6):588–595.

Kuh D, et al. Urinary incontinence in middle-aged women: childhood enuresis and other lifetime risk factors in a British prospective cohort. *Journal of Epidemiology and Community Health*. 1999;**53**:453–458.

Lagace E, et al. Prevalence and severity of urinary incontinence in ambulatory adults: an UPRNet study. *Journal of Family Practice*. 1993;**36**:610–614.

Langa KM, et al. Informal caregiving time and costs for urinary incontinence in older individuals in the United States. *Journal of the American Geriatrics Society*. 2002;**50**:733–737.

Lawrence M, et al. Immediate-release oxybutynin versus tolterodine in detrusor overactivity: a population analysis. *Pharmacotherapy*. 2000;**20**(4):470–475.

Lu SH, et al. Effect of KW-7158, a putative afferent nerve inhibitor, on bladder and vesico-vascular reflexes in rats. *Brain Research*. 2002;**946**(1):72–78.

Madersbacher H, et al. A placebo-controlled, multicentre study comparing the tolerability and efficacy of propiverine and oxybutynin in patients with urgency and urge incontinence. *BJU International*. 1999;**84**(6):646–651.

Maggi S, et al. Prevalence rate of urinary incontinence in community-dwelling elderly individuals: The Veneto Study. *Journal of Gerontology*. 2001;**56A**:M14–M18.

Malmsten UGH, et al. Urinary incontinence and lower urinary tract symptoms: an epidemiological study of men aged 45 to 99 years. *Journal of Urology*. 1997;**158**:1733–1737.

Matsui M, et al. Multiple functional defects in peripheral autonomic organs in mice lacking muscarinic acetylcholine receptor gene for the M3 subtype. *Proceedings of the National Academy of Sciences U S A*. 2000;**97**(17):9579–9584.

Matsui M, et al. Increased relaxant action of forskolin and isoproterenol against muscarinic agonist-induced contractions in smooth muscle from M2 receptor knockout mice. *Journal of Pharmacology and Experimental Therapeutics*. 2003;**305**(1):106–113.

Millard R, et al. Clinical efficacy and safety of tolterodine compared to placebo in detrusor overactivity. *Journal of Urology*. 1999;**161**(5):1551–1555.

Milsom I, et al. The prevalence of overactive bladder. *American Journal of Managed Care*. 2000;**6**(suppl):S565–S573.

Minassian VA, et al. Urinary incontinence as a worldwide problem. *International Journal of Gynecology and Obstetrics*. 2003;**82**; 327–338.

Miyachi H, et al. Synthesis and antimuscarinic activity of a series of 4-(1-imidazolyl)-2,2-diphenylbutyramides: Discovery of potent and subtype-selective antimuscarinic agents. *Bioorganic & Medicinal Chemistry*. 1997;(6):1151–1161.

Moreland RB, et al. Emerging pharmacological approaches for treatment of lower urinary tract disorders. *Journal of Pharmacology and Experimental Therapeutics*. 2004;**308**:797–804.

Nakamura T, et al. Muscarinic M2 receptors inhibit Ca2+-activated K + channels in rat bladder smooth muscle. *International Journal of Urology*. 2002;**9**(12):689–696.

Napier C, Gupta P. Darifenacin is selective for the human recombinant M3 receptor subtype [electronic]. 32nd Annual Meeting of the International Continence Society; August 27–30, 2002; Heidelberg, Germany. Abstract 445. www.icsoffice.org/publications.

Nilvebrant L, et al. Tolterodine-a new bladder-selective antimuscarinic agent. *European Journal of Pharmacology*. 1997;**327**; 195–207.

Nuotio M, et al. Urgency, urge incontinence and voiding symptoms in men and women aged 70 years and over. *British Journal of Urology International*. 2002;**89**:350–355.

Nygaard I, et al. Urinary incontinence in rural older women: prevalence, incidence and remission. *Journal of the American Geriatrics Society*. 1996;**44**:1049–1054.

O'Brien J, et al. Urinary incontinence: prevalence, need for treatment, and effectiveness of intervention by nurse. *British Medical Journal*. 1991;**303**:1308–1312.

Ostergard DR. New target for intervention: the neurourology connection. *Advanced Studies in Medicine*. 2004;**4**(3C):S220–S224.

Payne K. Epidemiology, pathophysiology, and evaluation of urinary incontinence and overactive bladder. *Urology*. 1998;**51**(suppl 2A):3–10.

Peyrat L, et al. Prevalence and risk factors of urinary incontinence in young and middle-aged women. *British Journal of Urology International*. 2002;**89**:61–66.

Population Division of the Department of Economic and Social Affairs of the United Nations Secretariat. *World Population Prospects: The 2002 Revision*, vol. II, *The*

Sex and Age Distribution of Populations (United Nations publication, Sales No. E.03.XIII.7), 2003.

Reitz A, et al. European experience of 200 cases treated with botulinum-A toxin injections into the detrusor muscle for neurogenic incontinence. *Journal of Urology*. 2003; **169**(suppl):373.

Roberts RO, et al. Urinary incontinence in a community-based prevalence cohort: prevalence and healthcare-seeking. *Journal of the American Geriatric Society*. 1998;**46**:467–472.

Roe B, et al. Prevalence of urinary incontinence and its relationship with health status. *Journal of Clinical Nursing*. 2000;**9**:178–187.

Romanzi LJ. Urinary incontinence in women and men. *Journal of Gender Specific Medicine*. 2001;**4**:14–20.

Salcedo C, et al. SVT-40776, a new selective M3 muscarinic antagonist: human receptor binding profile and bladder effects in the guinea pig. *Neurourology and Urodynamics*. 2003;**22**(5):382–384.

Schmid DM, et al. Experience of 100 cases treated with botulinum toxin A injections into the detrusor muscle for overactive bladder refractory to anticholinergics. *Journal of Urology*. 2005;**173**(suppl):149.

Schurch B, et al. Botulinum A toxin for treating detrusor hyperreflexia in spinal cord injured patients: A new alternative to anticholinergic drugs? Preliminary results. *Journal of Urology*. 2000;**164**:692–697. [a]

Schurch B, et al. Treatment of neurogenic incontinence with botulinum toxin A. *New England Journal of Medicine*. 2000;**342**:665. [b]

Sculptoreanu A, et al. KW-7158 [(2S)-(+)-3,3,3-trifluoro-2-hydroxy-2-methyl-N-(5,5,10-trioxo-4,10-dihydrothieno[3,2-c]-[1]benzothiepin-9-yl)propanamide] enhances A-type K + currents in neurons of the dorsal root ganglion of the adult rat. *Journal of Pharmacology and Experimental Therapeutics*. 2004;**310**(1):159–168.

Shetty SG, et al. RO320-2904, A novel bladder selective anti-muscarinic. *Pharmacologist*. 2002;**44**(2 suppl 1):25.7.

Siracusano S, et al. Prevalence of urinary incontinence in young and middle-aged women in an Italian urban area. *European Journal of Obstetrics and Gynecology and Reproductive Biology*. 2002;**107**:201–204.

Smoger SH, et al. Urinary incontinence among male veterans receiving care in primary care clinics. *Annals of Internal Medicine*. 2000;**132**(7):547–551.

Stewart WF, et al. Prevalence and burden of overactive bladder in the United States. *World Journal of Urology*. 2003;**20**:327–336.

Stöhrer M, et al. Botulinum A-toxin detrusor injections in the treatment of detrusor hyperreflexia. *Journal of Urology*. 2000;**163**(suppl):244.

Takeda H, et al. Role of the β3-adrenoceptor in urine storage in the rat: Comparison between the selective β3-adrenoceptor agonist, CL316, 243, and various smooth muscle relaxants. *Journal of Pharmacology and Experimental Therapeutics*. 2000;**293**(3):939–945.

Tanaka M, et al. A novel pyrrole derivative, NS-8 suppresses the rat micturition reflex by inhibition afferent pelvic nerve activity. *BJU International*. 2003;**92**(9):1031–1036.

Tang L, Kongsamut S. Frequency-dependent inhibition of neurotransmitter release by besipirdine and HP 184. *European Journal of Pharmacology*. 1996;**300**(1–2):71–74.

Temml C, et al. Urinary incontinence in both sexes: prevalence rates and impact on quality of life and sexual life. *Neurourology and Urodynamics*. 2000;**19**:259–271.

Thom D. Variation in estimates of urinary incontinence in general practice: effects of differences in definition, population characteristics, and study type. *Journal of the American Geriatrics Society*. 1998;**46**:473–480.

Thom DH, et al. Urologic diseases in America project: urinary incontinence in women-national trends in hospitalization, office visits, treatment and economic impact. *Journal of Urology*. 2005;**173**:1295–1301.

Tsukamoto T, et al. Prevalence of prostatism in Japanese men in a community-based study with comparison to a similar American study. *Journal of Urology*. 1995;**154**:391–395.

Ueda T, et al. Urinary incontinence among community-dwelling people aged 40 years or older in Japan: prevalence, risk factors, knowledge, and self-perception. *International Journal of Urology*. 2000;**7**:95–103.

Ushiroyama T, et al. Prevalence, incidence, and awareness in the treatment of menopausal urinary incontinence. *Maturitas*. 1999;**33**:127–132.

Van Kerrebroeck P, et al. Tolterodine once-daily: superior efficacy and tolerability in the treatment of the overactive bladder. *Urology*. 2001;**57**:414–421.

Versi E, et al. Dry mouth with conventional and controlled-release oxybutynin in urinary incontinence. *Obstetrics and Gynecology*. 2000;**95**:718–721.

Wang P, et al. Muscarinic acetylcholine receptor subtypes mediating urinary bladder contractility and coupling to GTP binding proteins. *Journal of Pharmacology and Experimental Therapeutics*. 1995;**273**(2):959–966.

Welz-Barth A, et al. 1999 rerun of the 1996 German Urinary Incontinence Survey: will doctors ever ask? *World Journal of Urology*. 2000;**18**:436–438.

Woods M, et al. Efficacy of the β3-adrenergic receptor agonist CL-316243 on experimental bladder hyperreflexia and detrusor instability in the rat. *Journal of Urology*. 2001;**166**(3):1142–1147.

Yamanishi T, et al. The role of M2-muscarinic receptors in mediating contraction of the pig urinary bladder in vitro. *British Journal of Pharmacology*. 2000;**131**(7):1482–1488.

Yamazaki Y, et al. Characterization of KUC-7483 and its active metabolite, KUC-7322, a selective beta3-adrenoceptor agonist, on bladder function in rats. *Neurourology and Urodynamics*. 2002, **21**(4):405–406.

Yarker YE, et al. Oxybutynin: a review of its pharmacodynamic and pharmacokinetic properties, and its therapeutic use in detrusor instability. *Drugs Aging*. 1995;**6**(3):243–262.

Yokoyama O, et al. Overactive bladder—experimental aspects. *Scandinavian Journal of Urology and Nephrology*. 2002;**210**(suppl):59–64.

Yoshida M, et al. Pharmacological effects of a new muscarinic receptors antagonist: KRP-197 on human isolated urinary bladder. *Neurourology and Urodynamics*. 2000;**19**(4):435–436.

Zinner N, et al. Efficacy and tolerability of darifenacin, a muscarinic M3 selective receptor antagonist, compared with oxybutynin in the treatment of patients with overactive bladder [electronic]. Joint Meeting of the International Continence Society and the International Urogynecological Association; August 23–27, 2004; Paris. Abstract 378. www.icsoffice.org.

PAIN TREATMENT

Chronic Low Back Pain

ETIOLOGY AND PATHOPHYSIOLOGY

Introduction

In the United States, low back pain (LBP) is one of the leading reasons for visits to primary care physicians (PCPs) (Toth PP, 2004). In fact, LBP is the second most common cause for visits to physicians in ambulatory settings in the United States (Boden SD, 1998). Back pain is likely the most common worldwide cause of worker absenteeism and long-term disability for adults in middle age (Andersson GB, 1999; Ehrlich GE, 2003). Indeed, LBP occurs in most adults at some point in their life; estimates of lifetime prevalence range between 50% and 80% of the population. The economic burden of LBP is substantial. Direct medical costs for treating back pain patients approach $25 million per year in the United States (Boden SD, 1998). Total health care expenditures incurred by back pain patients in the United States reached $90.7 billion in 1998, $26.3 billion of which is directly attributable to the back pain itself (Luo X, 2004). In addition, LBP gives rise to an annual loss in labor productivity of approximately $28 billion in the United States (Rizzo JA, 1998). In the "Low Back Pain Initiative," a report released in 1999, the World Health Organization suggests that LBP has reached epidemic proportions in developed nations (World Health Organization, 2001). While the vast majority of LBP cases (approximately 85–90%) resolve within one to three months without residual loss of function, the condition persists

Wiley Handbook of Current and Emerging Drug Therapies, Volumes 5–8
Copyright © 2007 Decision Resources, Inc. Published by John Wiley & Sons, Inc.

for an extended period for the remaining patients (Bartleson JD, 2001; Coste J, 1994; Croft PR, 1998).

Chronic pain is generally defined as pain that persists beyond the usual course of an acute disease or beyond a reasonable time for an injury to heal (Andersson GB, 1999). Although this definition is accurate, pain that recurs at intervals for months or years is also included in the classification of chronic pain. In fact, recent studies reiterate that chronic low back pain (CLBP) is not a static, continuous phenomenon; it is episodic in nature, with events characterized by increased pain intensity recurring throughout the course of the condition (McGorry RW, 2000; Waxman R, 2000). For the purposes here, CLBP is defined as pain in the area between the gluteal folds and the 12th rib that persists for a period greater than three months.

In patients whose pain persists beyond 12 weeks, the chances for full recovery diminish substantially and decline even further with the passage of time (Andersson GB, 1999). The likelihood of resuming work declines with the duration of sick leave for CLBP; chances for a return to work are 20–40% after one year and drop to nearly 0% after two years of sick leave (Valat JP, 1997).

Between 2% and 20% of the total populations in the major pharmaceutical markets (United States, France, Germany, Italy, Spain, United Kingdom, and Japan) are considered disabled by CLBP. As previously noted, 85–90% of LBP resolves itself within a short time; however, one study found that only 25% of patients who had presented with LBP had completely recovered in terms of pain and function within one year (Croft PR, 2001). This finding suggests that the actual size of the CLBP population is larger than current estimates suggest and that the economic burden related to CLBP may therefore be underestimated.

Etiology

By most estimates, 80–85% of CLBP is idiopathic—i.e., no significant anatomical or structural defect is detected (Cole MH, 2003; Deyo RA, 1996). Determining the precise etiology is difficult because CLBP often results from multiple interacting dynamics, including mechanical, psychological, social, and neurophysiological factors (Carragee EJ, 2004). Because physicians are rarely able to detect clinical features indicating a serious underlying pathology, few diagnostic exams result in a precise anatomic diagnosis (Carragee EJ, 2004). Therefore, most physicians provide a symptomatic diagnosis based on the patient's description of the type of pain and the region in which it is occurring. Although the exact structure that is the source of pain is often unknown in CLBP, it is known that the pain often originates from conditions such as osteoarthritis, muscle strain, and/or disc herniation. Table 1 lists the common causes of CLBP (Atlas SJ, 2003; Deyo RA, 2001).

Most nonspecific (i.e., idiopathic) CLBP can be categorized as either mechanical (inflammatory or nociceptive) or neuropathic pain. Mechanical pain refers to pain that derives from somatic tissue such as muscle, joint, tendon, bursa, or fascia. Structural damage, injury, or wear and tear within the tissues and skeletal structures can result in the transmission of painful sensations via nerves. In

TABLE 1. Common Causes of Chronic Low Back Pain

Cause	% of CLBP Population
Idiopathic origins	85
Muscle strain, ligament/tendon strain, nonspecific sprain, intervertebral disc herniation, facet joints, sacroiliac strain	
Fracture	5
Traumatic and osteoporotic	
Spinal stenosis	4
Spondylolisthesis	2
Neoplastic diseases	1
Carcinomas, myelomas, leukemia, tumors, metastatic spine disease	
Inflammatory arthritis	1
Ankylosing spondylitis, psoriatic spondylitis, Reiter's syndrome	
Infections	0.5
Osteomyelitis, discitis, epidural abscess, herpes zoster	
Cauda equine syndrome	0.5
Vascular or hematologic origins	1
Abdominal aortic aneurysm, epidural hematoma, hemoglobinopathy	

Source: Based on: Deyo RA, Weinstein JN. Low back pain. New England Journal of Medicine. 2001;344:363–370; Atlas SJ, Nardin RA. Evaluation and treatment of low back pain: an evidence-based approach to clinical care. Muscle Nerve. 2003;27:265–284.

contrast, neuropathic pain arises directly from injured nerves. Radicular neuropathic pain associated with CLBP (i.e., sciatica) results from nerve root damage. The nerve damage most commonly results from compression by a spinal disc, which subsequently leads to pain that radiates down the leg, below the knee. Nerve roots are especially prone to compression because there is little fat and connective tissue at the root level (Atlas SJ, 2003). Peripheral or other central nervous system (CNS) nerve damage—resulting in changes to nerve pathways or transmission—can also lead to neuropathic pain.

A compressed nerve root may be caused by either a herniated or a degenerated spinal disc. Disc herniation, the outward bulge of a disc from the spinal cord structure, can produce pressure on nerve roots where they exit the spinal cord and project peripherally. Not all herniated discs, however, result in neuropathic pain; as many as 50% of the general population have spinal disc herniation that can be seen via imagery, yet these individuals are asymptomatic for LBP. It is theorized that disc herniation triggers infiltration at the site of compression by inflammatory cells, which then secrete cytokines. Indeed, studies confirm that proinflammatory molecules, including cytokines, are found in and around herniated and degenerated discs (Brisby H, 2003). The inflammatory agents have a negative effect on the nerve roots, eventually leading to CLBP. Two agents that are thought to be integral to the development of nerve root injury are tumor necrosis factor (TNF) and nitric oxide (NO) (Brisby H, 2003). Research suggests that some cytokines, including TNF, also enhance matrix metalloproteinase

(MMP) production; these proteinases subsequently act to cause further disc degradation. Indeed, the role of MMPs in the pathophysiology of back pain is widely recognized (Biyani A, 2004).

Disc degeneration, another cause of radicular neuropathic pain, is the result of spinal discs collapsing together following skeletal damage or the natural deterioration of aging. As the discs compress, nerves are pinched between them. However, some patients with considerable disc deterioration do not report painful symptoms (Biyani A, 2004). Figure 1 shows a section of the spine with structures subject to disc compression.

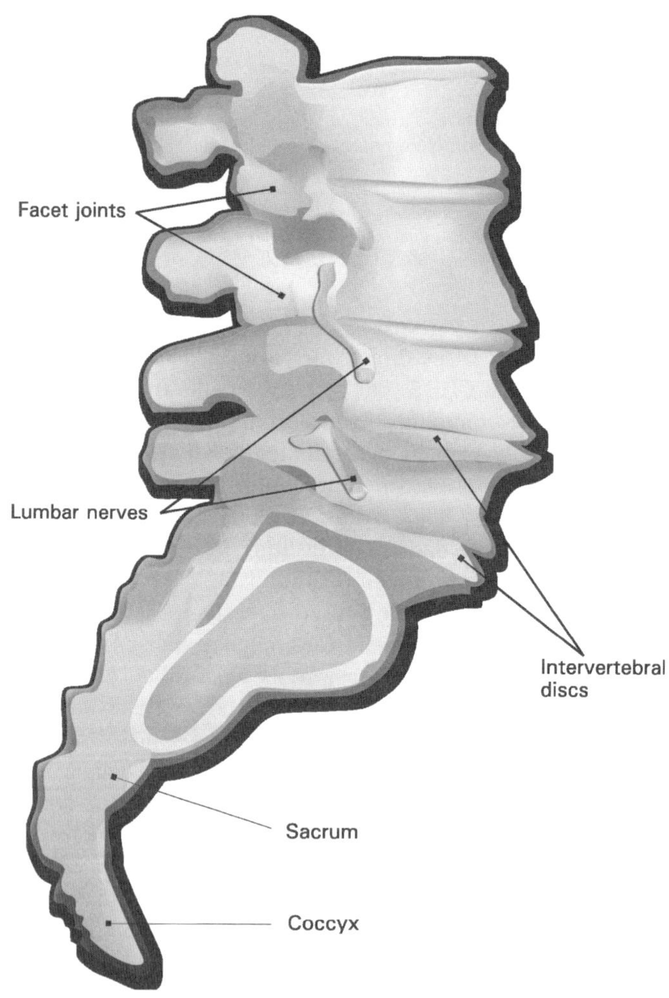

FIGURE 1. *Spinal column cross-section.*

Many CLBP patients experience pain from more than one source; they can suffer from nociceptive, inflammatory, and/or neuropathic pain mechanisms.

Determining which LBP patients will suffer from chronic symptoms remains difficult; chronicity of LBP is not directly linked to the cause of injury. Many studies have examined the risk factors associated with the chronicity and disability of CLBP; a review of these studies found that risk factors are more closely related to demographic, psychosocial, and occupational factors than to medical conditions (Valat JP, 1997). The risk factors that most strongly correlate with CLBP include advancing age, rigorous physical labor, and home- or work-related stress. One note of interest from these studies is that LBP patients involved in worker's compensation and litigation issues are at a higher risk for long-term chronicity and tend to have poorer prognosis (Vaccaro AR, 1997).

Pathophysiology

The CLBP population is highly heterogeneous, yet chronic pain involves certain common aberrations in somatosensory processing in the central and/or peripheral nervous system. This section describes the basic mechanisms of pain transmission and modulation that underlie most forms of chronic pain. Researchers generally identify three distinct categories of pain that result from diverse mechanisms: nociceptive, inflammatory, and neuropathic pain. As mentioned previously, in some CLBP patients, a single mechanism may be responsible for their pain; in others, multiple mechanisms may contribute. In addition, while continuous physical injury may be required for CLBP in some patients, in others the initial injury may eventually result in an alteration in the pain processing pathways. Consequently, pain may be independently produced within the CNS even in the absence of stimulation from the primary injury (Atlas SJ, 2003). To complicate matters further, in different patients the same painful symptom may be generated by a number of mechanisms, or one mechanism may be responsible for a variety of painful symptoms. Therein lies the difficulty in identifying the etiology of CLBP and successfully treating this condition

The Pain Pathways. Pain messages are modified at many levels in the nervous system as they pass from the periphery into the brain. As illustrated in Figure 2, the complexity of this system and the diversity of its mechanisms make it difficult to understand the intricacies of pain, yet it provides a plethora of potential sites for drug targets. Although the details are not completely known, the basic mechanisms of pain perception are known to proceed in two distinct steps. First, harmful stimuli are detected peripherally by nociceptors. Second, stimulated nociceptors transmit their pain signals to the CNS, where pain is perceived.

Pain Receptors. Peripheral nociceptors, which are found in the nerve terminals of peripheral afferent fibers, are present in abdominal organs, musculoskeletal structures, and cutaneous tissues. Once stimulated, peripheral nociceptors transmit nerve signals along any one of three major types of afferent nerve fibers: Aβ,

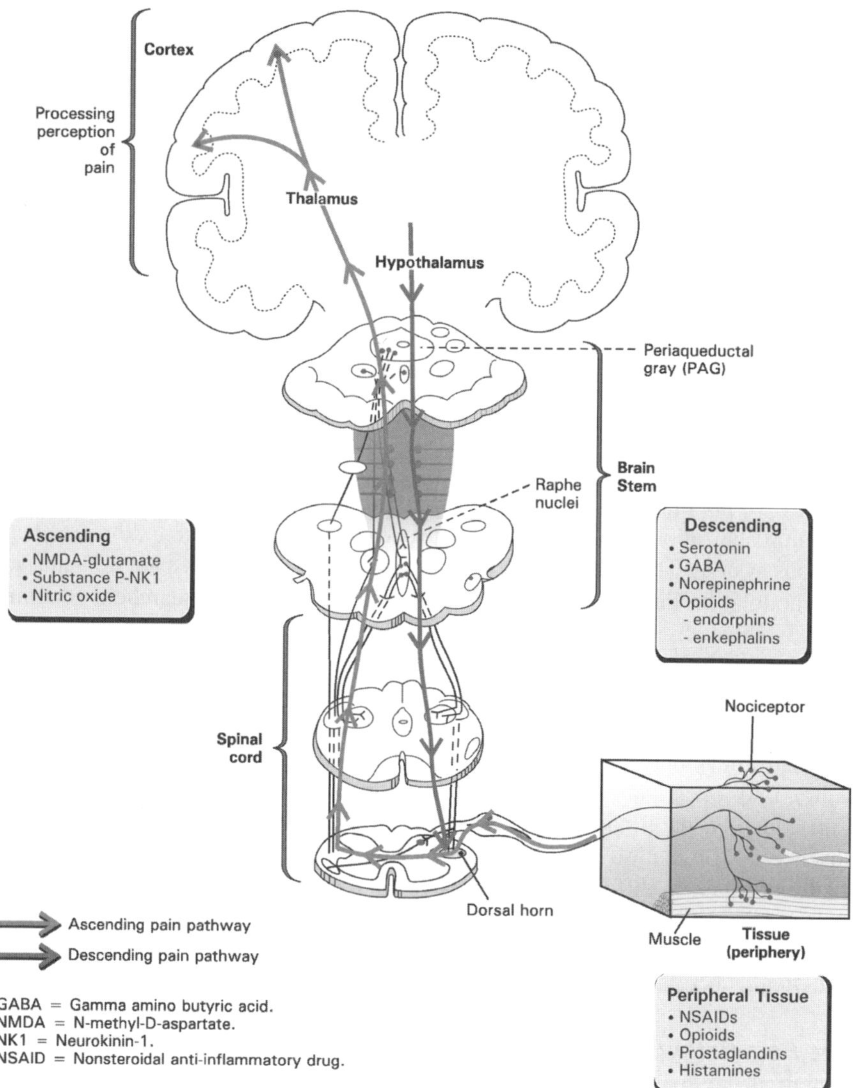

FIGURE 2. *Ascending and descending pain pathways.*

Aδ, and C fibers. These fibers are differentiated by their diameter and thickness of myelination, both of which affect the speed of conduction. For example, large-diameter, myelinated Aβ afferent fibers rapidly transmit pain signals, while small-diameter, unmyelinated C fibers convey signals more slowly.

Transmission of Pain. Neuronal signals carrying pain inputs are mediated via electrical impulses known as action potentials. The action potential is generated by ion gradients (involving sodium and potassium ions) that are established across the neuronal cell membrane. Damage to nerve axons and aggravation of nociceptors by inflammatory agents may lead to altered expression of sodium channels. This alteration can lead to abnormal neuronal excitability, whereby neurons become unusually sensitive to stimuli. Because of their critical role in pain transmission, ion channels are important drug targets in pain research. Some compounds proven effective in neuropathic pain, for example, bind sodium channels and stabilize them in their inactive state, thus impeding the flow of ions after an electrical stimulus and disrupting action potentials.

Although action potentials relay signals via the axon, additional mechanisms are required to carry electrical information from one neuron to another. Intercellular transmission among neurons occurs at the synapse, a functional contact between neurons where electrical information is both transmitted and modulated. Most synaptic contacts in the brain are chemical in nature. An action potential arriving at the presynaptic terminal triggers the release of a neurotransmitter and/or neuromodulator, a chemical substance that diffuses across the synapse to bind at the postsynaptic membrane.

Receptors for neurotransmitters and neuromodulators represent key targets for neuropathic pain drug development. Glutamate receptors, which are the principal mediators of excitatory electrical activity in the brain, have attracted particular attention. The dorsal root ganglia, believed to be critical in the modulation of CLBP, demonstrate a high concentration of these receptors. Blocking the glutamate receptors could theoretically inhibit the transmission of excitatory pain signals from one neuron to another. The N-methyl-D-aspartate (NMDA) receptor, a target for the amino acid L-glutamate, is a voltage-gated ion channel that has been especially well studied in this context. Serotonin and norepinephrine are also important neurotransmitters in pain modulation. These neurotransmitters play an important role in the release of endogenous opioids, pain-relieving substances capable of acting on opiate receptors in a way similar to that of the opioid drug morphine.

Researchers have identified three classes of endogenous opioid peptides—enkaphalins, dynorphins, and endorphins. These endogenous opioids are distributed throughout the descending pain pathway. Enkaphalins and dynorphins concentrate in several areas of the brain and in the dorsal horn of the spinal cord. Beta-endorphin, the most powerful known endogenous opioid peptide, can be found in basal hypothalamic neurons whose axons terminate in the periaqueductal gray (PAG) area of the mesencephalon portion of the brain stem. Three classes of opioid receptors (MOR, DOR, and KOR) are localized throughout the central and peripheral nervous systems, and the endogenous opioids are capable of binding to all three receptors. For many years, researchers believed that opioids exerted the bulk of their action centrally, in the spinal cord and brain stem, although recent findings suggest that peripheral mechanisms are at least as important (Stein C, 2003). Opioids function centrally by binding to opioid receptors in the brain and spinal cord, so as to impede the transmission of pain signals to the brain. They also work within the brain to modulate the sensation of pain. At the supraspinal level, opioid receptors regulate incoming pain signals by sending inhibitory signals along the descending pain modulation pathway.

According to recent research, peripheral opioid receptors may actually play a dominant role (more influential than that of the spinal and supraspinal receptors) in the analgesic mechanism of opioid agonists; study results suggest that injected opioid agonists function principally through peripheral receptors (Stein C, 2003). Opioids achieve their analgesic effect through a variety of mechanisms; these molecules may hinder signaling in sensory neurons by inhibiting the transduction of ion channel currents, moderate the excitability of peripheral nociceptor terminals, diminish action potential propagation, attenuate proinflammatory neuropeptide release from the terminals of sensory nerves, or reverse the vasodilatation caused by C-fiber stimulation (Stein C, 2003).

Researchers recently discovered opioid receptors on the dorsal root ganglion (DRG), on peripheral extensions of sensory neurons, and on C fibers and A fibers. Furthermore, expression of opioid receptors on the DRG is increased in response to inflammation of peripheral tissues, a process that is upregulated by inflammatory cytokines such as interleukin-1. This upregulation results in increased axonal transport of receptors toward peripheral nerve terminals and hence in amplified efficacy of opioid agonists at these peripheral locations. Interestingly, the opioid receptor ligands are produced in large amounts by immune cells, as well as by sensory neurons, a fact that suggests an integrative link between the immune system and the pain arm of the neurological system. Although the development of tolerance at central opioid receptors is well documented, investigations of tolerance at peripheral receptors are so far inconclusive. Furthermore, because it is theorized that the side effects commonly associated with opioid use are based on the central actions of the molecules, the development of drugs that function exclusively peripherally could prove to be a major step forward in the treatment of CLBP. At the current time, however, the development of such drugs is in early stages.

Ascending Tracts. Afferent (i.e., sensory) nerve fibers arise from cell bodies in the DRG on the spinal cord; these cell bodies relay signals to the dorsal horn of the spinal cord and synapse via neurons that carry and integrate pain signals to the brain (see Figure 3). The dorsal root ganglia are believed to be critical in the modulation of CLBP; the ganglia serve as an important integrative link, and nociceptors on the DRG are believed to produce several neuropeptides, including substance P (Biyani A, 2004).

Afferents join the CNS at the dorsal horn of the spinal cord, where neuronal signals are channeled via ascending neural pathways to the brain. The key ascending sensory neural pathway is the spinothalamic tract. Nociceptive impulses from the entire body below the head are transmitted via fibers along the spinothalamic pathway.

Descending Tracts. Descending pain pathways from brain centers pass through the PAG region to the dorsal horn in the spinal cord, where efferent fibers synapse

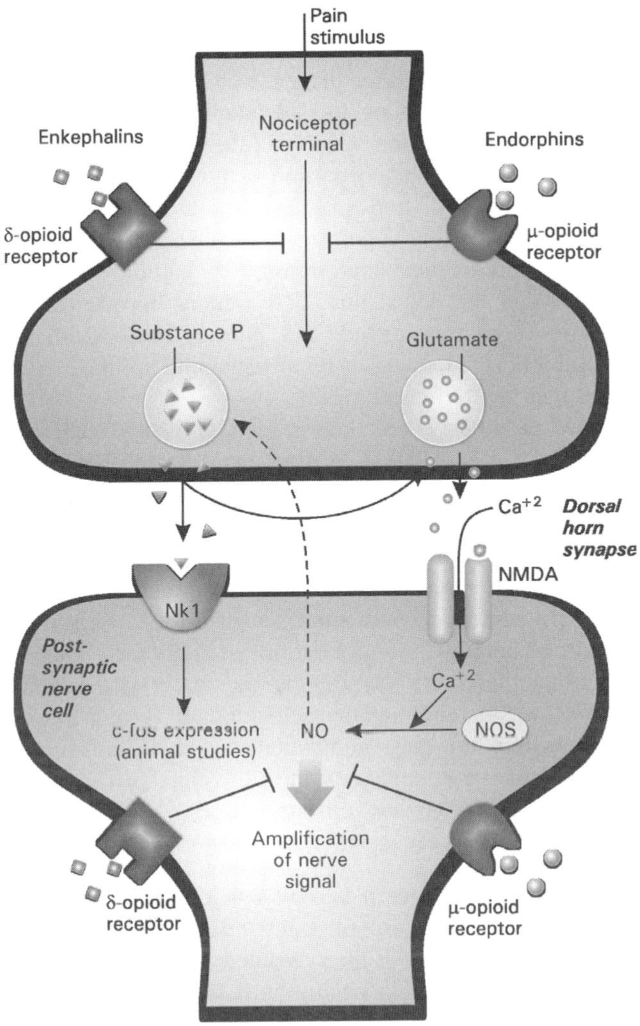

FIGURE 3. *Schematic of nociceptive and antinociceptive pathways in the dorsal horn.*

with neurons and are involved in nociceptive inhibition and facilitation (pain regulation and response). Also contained within the dorsal horn are interneurons, localized nerve fibers that synapse with ascending and descending pathways, providing inhibitory functions. In addition, interneurons facilitate reflex responses to nociceptive transmissions (i.e., quick withdrawal responses to painful stimuli).

The various neurotransmitters and neuromodulators involved in these pathways are potential therapeutic targets for CLBP.

Researchers have established the presence of a pain modulation system within the CNS, and they are beginning to understand the intricacies of endogenous pain mitigation. Pain modulation occurs via descending pathways that originate in the PAG of the mesencephalon portion of the brain stem (Fields HL, 2000; Gebhart GF, 2004). The PAG transmits signals to the raphe nuclei in the medulla, which then relay input to dorsal horn neurons of the spinal cord via descending fibers. Using serotonin as their neurotransmitter, neurons in the medulla inhibit ascending neurons in the dorsal horn and thereby impede the transmission of pain signals from these areas to the CNS. Normal sensory afferent flow is also controlled by inhibitory interneurons that use gamma-aminobutyric acid (GABA) and glycine as their neurotransmitters.

As mentioned previously, neurotransmitters and their receptors are potential drug targets for analgesia. Pathological changes to the descending pain modulation pathway, resulting from injury or damage, can cause changes in the functioning of the receptors or in the synthesis of neurotransmitters. Changing the architecture of the pathway alters the inhibitory function of the descending pain modulation system and increases pain transmission to the brain (a process discussed later in the section on central sensitization). Because of their central role in the pain modulation system, neurotransmitters have long been viewed as key targets for pain therapies. For example, the analgesic mechanism of tricyclic antidepressants (TCAs) relies on the activation of serotonergic and noradrenergic pathways within the pain-modulation system (Mattia C, 2002), as does the mechanism of the new antidepressant duloxetine (Eli Lilly and Company's [Indianapolis, Indiana] Cymbalta/Xeristar).

Basic Pain Mechanisms.
Nociceptive Pain. Nociceptive pain, or somatic pain, is the "normal" physiological response to pain. This form of pain is relayed to the CNS via nociceptors, which are primary afferent nerve fibers located in peripheral tissues and organs (see Figure 3). Nociceptive pain occurs with any form of acute pain, such as a sharp needle prick against the skin. However, nociceptive pain may also contribute to pain when nociceptors transduce chemical, mechanical, or heat stimuli—for example, when pain is caused by acute trauma (before inflammation is established). Pain drugs in development target nociceptive receptors such as ion channels that are selectively expressed in sensory neurons.

Inflammatory Pain. Inflammatory pain is triggered by nociceptive afferents that become irritated when surrounded by inflamed tissue. In most cases, pain sensitivity is proportional to the degree of inflammation, and pain generally declines when the injury heals. Inflammatory pain is common in patients experiencing inflammation following back injuries. Anti-inflammatory drugs specifically designed for selective targets in the inflammatory pathway (see Figure 4), including prostaglandins, continue to be developed and refined. Drugs targeting inflammatory mediators such as cytokines are also in development for pain.

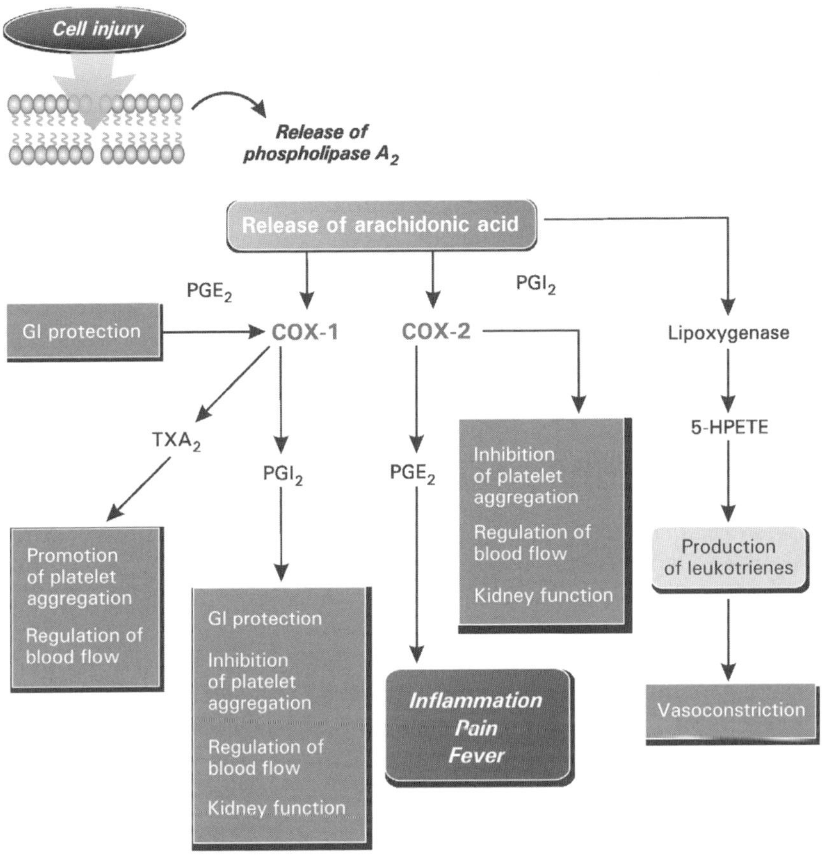

5-HPETE = 5-hydroperoxyeicosatetraenoic acid.
COX = Cyclooxygenase.
GI = Gastrointestinal.
PGE$_2$ = Prostaglandin E$_2$.
PGI$_2$ = Prostaglandin I$_2$.
TXA$_2$ = Thromboxane A$_2$.

FIGURE 4. *Effect of nonsteroidal anti-inflammatory drugs on the arachidonic acid pathway.*

Neuropathic Pain. Neuropathic pain involves an aberration in the somatosensory processing in the central or peripheral nervous system, an aberration that occurs specifically from nerve injury and that may persist even after the injured nerve is healed. Neuropathic pain exists in a significant proportion of patients with CLBP; some experts estimate this subpopulation to be 14% of the total CLBP population. Neuropathic pain is associated with numerous other conditions, including postherpetic neuralgia, trigeminal neuralgia, painful diabetic neuropathy, and nerve destruction by the human immunodeficiency virus.

Drugs that target nociceptive and inflammatory mechanisms are generally ineffective for neuropathic pain. Most of the drugs currently indicated for neuropathic pain—used off-label in CLBP patients with neuropathic pain symptoms—were approved for painful diabetic neuropathy, postherpetic neuralgia, or trigeminal neuralgia. However, some patients' pain does not respond to these drugs, suggesting that the mechanisms involved in neuropathic pain are not fully understood. Drugs targeting neuropathic pain mechanisms represent an unmet need in CLBP management.

Mechanisms of Chronic Pain. Although nociceptive pain is often considered an adaptive biological response essential for the avoidance of tissue injury, chronic pain (mechanical and neuropathic) is a maladaptive response to tissue inflammation or neurological damage, producing pain of no apparent biological value. The development of the chronic pain state in CLBP is thought to involve the following mechanisms.

Peripheral Sensitization. Peripheral sensitization of pain involves two different mechanisms: autosensitization and heterosensitization.

In peripheral autosensitization, repeated stimulation of peripheral nociceptors lowers the threshold of pain by directly altering the physiological properties of nociceptive transducers (i.e., ion channels that generate depolarizing currents in nociceptors in response to noxious stimuli). Changes in receptor sensitivity are thought to be mediated by conformational changes in the transducer protein induced by the stimuli.

The onset of chronic pain is provoked by hypersensitivity among peripheral afferent nociceptors that have been repeatedly activated. This hypersensitivity leads to the clinical expression of allodynia (perception of pain following nonpainful stimuli) and hyperalgesia (heightened sensitivity to painful stimuli). However, chronic pain caused by autosensitization occurs only with continuous transducer activation; increases in nociceptor sensitivity are readily reversible with diminished frequency of the activating stimuli.

In peripheral heterosensitization, the sensitization of primary afferent nociceptors may also be caused by the localized release of chemical mediators in an inflamed area of a damaged or diseased tissue. A variety of cytokines and metabolites of arachidonic acid (eicasonoids) and bradykinin appear to play the most important roles in the sensitization of nociceptors. Nonsteroidal anti-inflammatory drugs (NSAIDs) block pain by inhibiting the enzyme cyclooxygenase (COX), which converts arachidonic acid into inflammatory mediators; NSAIDs reduce pain by easing the inflammation that causes sensitization of nociceptors over time, and they may have a direct analgesic effect as well.

Neuropeptide release is another potentially sensitizing response to injured tissue. Substance P is a neuropeptide of particular interest to researchers of neuropathic pain because it is found in large quantities in primary afferent nerve terminals. Researchers theorize that substance P-induced vasodilation increases capillary permeability, thus allowing the extravasation of additional neuroactive and vasoactive chemicals from the blood into injured tissue or nerves. These extravasated substances render the physiological and chemical environment of nociceptors unstable, increasing nociceptive excitability and pain perception. The continued release of vasoactive and neuroactive substances from the bloodstream may provoke spontaneous impulse transduction along sensitized peripheral afferent nerves. However, some researchers question the importance of substance P in pain because the clinical effectiveness of substance P inhibitors in treating pain is still unclear.

Biochemical mediators that increase sensitivity of peripheral nociceptors (such as PGE2, bradykinin, 5-HT, epinephrine, and adenosine) act through modulation of intracellular kinases that are coupled with cell surface proteins. These kinases phosphorylate ion channels and receptors to change their physical properties. Phosphorylation of tetrodotoxin-resistant (TTX-r) sodium channels, for example, alters their activation threshold, rate of activation and inactivation, and magnitude of sodium current depolarization. More specifically, the binding of bradykinin to its B1 or B2 receptor stimulates a mechanism that ultimately results in activation of the vanilloid receptor 1 (VR1) ion channels (Premkumar LS, 2000). The VR1 channel is widely acknowledged to be a molecular integrator of noxious pain stimuli. Activation of the VR1 receptor allows for an influx of positively charged ions into the neuron and a resultant increased sensitization of peripheral nociceptors. The prostaglandin pathway functions analogously, though this pathway can result in activation of not only the VR1 but also the TTX-r sodium channels (De PL, 2001; England S, 1996). The mediators and receptors involved in these inflammatory response pathways may represent viable therapeutic targets for the development of new analgesics to attenuate pain and inflammation. Because many different sensitizing molecules acting at different receptors and ion channels effect the same result, inhibiting a single sensitizing agent is unlikely to completely eliminate peripheral sensitization.

Central Sensitization. The injured portion of the peripheral nerve may not be the only source of neuronal excitability. Cells in the dorsal root ganglion may also become a source of abnormal impulse generation in response to injury in the peripheral nerve. Indeed, in experimental studies, hyperactivity in the dorsal root ganglion persists even after peripheral injury has been treated and the hyperactivity in the peripheral nerve has ceased (Gammaitoni A, 2000). Researchers refer to the process by which peripheral afferent input sensitizes dorsal horn neurons as central sensitization, or "wind-up."

Wind-up commences when unmyelinated C fibers, in a reaction to nerve injury or inflammation, release glutamate into the dorsal horn. Glutamate exerts a potent excitatory effect on neurons through its binding to the NMDA receptor. Stimulation of the NMDA receptor prompts large amounts of calcium ions to enter neuronal cells. The calcium influx provokes enzyme cascades, including the synthesis of prostaglandins, nitric oxide (NO), and other cytotoxic reactions that likely exacerbate nerve injury. The calcium surplus also lowers the cell's firing threshold, provoking spontaneous firing.

The input of unmyelinated C fibers appears to be necessary for the induction of wind-up. Although it remains unclear why C fibers are prone to wind-up, researchers suspect that these fibers' slower transduction may be a factor. Once the dorsal horn neurons have been sensitized, C-fiber activation is no longer necessary to maintain a state of central sensitization. In experimental models, central sensitization can be maintained even after the administration of a local anesthetic has halted C-fiber activation. Central sensitization, therefore, is probably a mechanism that is dependent on, but separate from, peripheral nociceptor input from unmyelinated C fibers.

Once the CNS neurons have been sensitized, even input from uninjured primary afferent nerves may provoke a pain-like response from the dorsal horn neurons. Several drug developers are investigating agents that antagonize the NMDA receptor as potential analgesic therapies in the hope that these agents will prevent sensitization-induced hyperalgesia. Historically, side effects associated with existing NMDA receptor antagonists, such as sedation, dry mouth, and gastrointestinal distress, have prevented the widespread use of these agents in CLBP. However, drug manufacturers are developing new NMDA receptor antagonists that will likely have improved side-effect profiles.

Activity-Dependent Modification. The maintenance of chronic pain can occur with activity-dependent modification, a process during which repeated stimulation induces permanent structural changes in the anatomy of the nervous system. This process is driven by intracellular cascades (e.g., G-protein signaling, calcium influx via NMDA receptors) that ultimately lead to actual changes in gene transcription. Once gene transcription is modified, new synaptic connections may be formed following nerve damage, acting as a source of excess and abnormal neuronal transmission. These connections may form when injured axons regenerate, a process known as "sprouting." Such axon sprouts are presumed to have increased sensitivity to mechanical or chemical stimuli, tissue ischemia, and inflammation. Additionally, increased sensitivity may occur with "phenotype switching" of the primary afferent nerve fibers. Researchers claim that nerve injury results in a delayed loss of sensory neurons that is more prominent for C fibers than for A fibers. This loss is believed to be compensated for by a central reorganization of A fibers, which branch into the area of the spinal cord where C fibers normally terminate and create functional contacts.

Research has also demonstrated that both chronic neuropathic pain and musculoskeletal pain lead to the reorganization of the somatosensory and motor systems, specifically in the thalamus and cortex (Flor H, 2003). This cortical reorganization results in an altered representation of the pain-afflicted area in the brain, or "pain memory." This type of memory can cause pain perception in the absence of peripheral stimulation. However, agents that prevent or reverse cortical reorganization may be able to prevent the formation of pain memories; of these agents, the GABA agonists, NMDA receptor agonists, and anticholinergic agents are believed to hold the most promise (Flor H, 2003).

Awakening of Silent Nociceptors. Nociception may be enhanced by the activation of so-called silent nociceptors, or nociceptors that cannot be activated under normal physiological conditions. These nociceptors can be activated only under pathological conditions as sensitizing agents are released, synthesized, or attracted to the site of tissue injury. Silent nociceptors were first identified in the spinal cord and have since been found in visceral and cutaneous tissues (Schaible HG, 1993).

Complexity of Nervous System Function. Many transmitters and receptors, such as ion channels, peptides, and excitatory amino acid receptors, are widely distributed throughout the nervous system and have multiple physiological roles in addition to the transmission and/or modulation of pain. Any agent developed to target these systems could potentially produce undesirable side effects. Thus, drug development efforts have begun focusing heavily on the identification of more-specific targets (e.g., specific receptors and ion channel subtypes) that are involved in biochemical pathways active only under pathophysiological conditions. This research, still in its early stages, has already pointed to new targets.

CURRENT THERAPIES

Many pain therapies used to treat chronic low back pain (CLBP) (e.g., traditional nonsteroidal anti-inflammatory drugs [NSAIDs], selective cyclooxygenase-2 [COX-2] inhibitors) target specific inflammatory mechanisms. Although these agents are beneficial for many patients with nonradiating CLBP, they are usually not effective for patients with sciatica (neuropathic CLBP radiating down the back of the thigh to below the knee). For these patients, physicians typically prescribe therapies from drug classes not traditionally used to treat pain (e.g., antiepileptic drugs [AEDs], antidepressants). Narcotic analgesics are also used to treat patients with sciatica or nonradiating CLBP who do not respond to other treatment.

In the major pharmaceutical markets, no drugs have been approved specifically to treat CLBP, except in Japan, where multiple agents are approved for use in LBP. Most drugs used for CLBP have not been studied in the types of rigorous, double-blind, placebo-controlled clinical trials required to gain regulatory approval for this indication. Physicians must therefore rely on data from studies of drugs in other types of chronic pain.

The following sections discuss the leading therapies used to treat CLBP. Table 2 reviews these drugs, and Table 3 explains clinical end points used in CLBP trials.

TABLE 2. Current Therapies Used for Chronic Low Back Pain

Agent	Company/Brand	Daily Dose	Availability
Traditional NSAIDs			
Ibuprofen	Pfizer's Motrin, Knoll's Brufen, generics	1,200–2,400 mg	US, F, G, I, S, UK, J
Ketoprofen	Wyeth's Orudis/Oruvail, generics	150–300 mg	US, F, G, I, S, UK, J
Diclofenac	Novartis's Voltaren/Cataflam, generics	75–150 mg	US, F, G, I, S, UK, J
Preferential COX-2 inhibitors			
Meloxicam	Boehringer Ingelheim/Abbott's Mobic	7.5–15 mg	US, F, G, I, S, UK, J
Selective COX-2 inhibitors			
Celecoxib	Pfizer's Celebrex	200–400 mg	US, F, G, I, S, UK
Narcotic analgesics			
Codeine	Generics	60–120 mg	US, F, G, I, S, UK, J
Morphine SR	Purdue's MS Contin, Napp/Mundipharma's MST Continus, Elan/Ligand Pharmaceutical's Avinza, Alpharma/MGI's Kadian, generics	60–120 mg	US, F, G, I, S, UK, J
Oxycodone CR	Purdue/Napp's Oxycontin, generics	60–200 mg	US, F, G, S, UK, J
Fentanyl patch	Janssen/Alza's Duragesic/Durogesic, generics	25–300 µg/hour; patch is replaced every three days	US, F, G, I, S, UK, J
Other analgesics			
Tramadol	Johnson & Johnson's Ultram, generics	50–100 mg	US, F, G, I, S, UK, J
Antiepileptic drugs			
Gabapentin	Pfizer's Neurontin, generics	900–3,600 mg	US, F, G, I, S, UK
Antidepressants			
Amitriptyline[a]	AstraZeneca's Elavil, Roche's Laroxyl, generics	25–100 mg	US, F, G, I, S, UK, J
Local anesthetics			
Lidocaine patch	Endo's Lidoderm	1–3 patches (700 mg each) for up to 12 hours (12 hours on, 12 hours off)	US

[a]Other tricyclic antidepressants (TCAs) used as alternatives to amitriptyline include desipramine (Sanofi-Aventis's Norpramin, Novartis's Pertofran, generics), imipramine (Novartis's Tofranil, generics), and nortriptyline (Novartis's Pamelor, Eli Lilly's Aventyl, generics).

US = United States; F = France; G = Germany; I = Italy; S = Spain; UK = United Kingdom; J = Japan.

TABLE 3. Clinical End Points Used In Chronic Low Back Pain Trials

End Point	Description
Pain measures	
Brief Pain Inventory (BPI)	Measures pain based on patient's answers to series of short questions
Categorical Scale	Measures pain using a scale consisting of sentences indicating a range of pain levels
Gracely Pain Scale	Measures level of pain using a 13-point ratio scale consisting of verbal pain intensity descriptors
Likert Scale	Assesses level of pain using an 11-point scale
Neuropathic Pain Scale (NPS)	Assesses global dimensions of pain intensity and pain unpleasantness considered specific to neuropathic pain
Numerical Pain Scale	Measures pain based on association of numerical values with varying levels of pain
Pain Relief Scale (VAS-PR)	Measures degree of pain relief on line scale
Patient Global Impression of Change (PGIC), Clinical Global Impression of Change (CGIC)	Assesses change in overall pain status as determined by patient (PGIC) or investigator (CGIC)
Short Form McGill Pain Questionnaire (SF-MPQ)	Derives single pain score based on the intensity rank values of the words chosen for sensory, affective, and total descriptors
Total Pain Relief (TOTPAR)	Measures summed pain relief over a period of time
Verbal Pain Scale/Verbal Rating Scale	Assesses pain based on patient's choice of verbal descriptors
Visual Analogue Pain Intensity Scale (VAS-PI)	Measures pain intensity on line scale
Visual Analogue Scale (VAS)/Pain Visual Analogue (PVA) Scale	Measures level of pain based on straight-line scale
Function/disability measures	
Oswestry Disability Questionnaire (ODQ)	Measures permanent functional disability
Pain Disability Index (PDI)	Assesses patient perception of the impact of pain on disability
Profile of Mood States (POMS)	Assesses mood states to determine effect of pain on emotion
Roland Morris Disability Questionnaire	Evaluates disability level
Short Form-36 Quality-of-Life (SF-36 QOL) Questionnaire	Determines overall quality of life to gauge impact of pain on everyday functioning
SF-12 Health Survey	Measures everyday functioning using subset of SF-36 Questionnaire questions
Sleep Interference Diary	Determines degree to which pain interferes with patient's ability to sleep
Treatment Outcomes in Pain Survey (TOPS) Instrument	Measures health-related quality of life, using the SF-36 and a pain-specific component
Verran and Snyder-Halpern (VSH) Sleep Scale	Assesses impact of pain on sleep characteristics

Traditional Nonsteroidal Anti-Inflammatory Drugs

Overview. NSAIDs, which have a long history of use in pain, are the most frequently prescribed therapies for CLBP. NSAIDs are also popular over-the-counter (OTC) therapies for CLBP patients.

Despite NSAIDs' popularity and historically strong presence in pain treatment, data demonstrating that these drugs provide effective pain relief for CLBP are still scarce (van Tulder MW, 2000). Although neuropathic pain rarely responds to treatment with anti-inflammatory agents, patients with sciatica often self-treat with NSAIDS, and primary care physicians (PCPs) occasionally prescribe NSAIDs alone or in conjunction with other pain medications to improve a patient's response to treatment. In some cases, sciatica patients improve with NSAID treatment because of a coexisting inflammatory pain component.

Although the scarcity of efficacy data for CLBP has not curtailed the popularity of NSAIDs as first-line therapy for CLBP, increasing concerns regarding the safety of drugs in this class may affect their use in the future. In April 2005, the FDA asked manufacturers of prescription NSAIDs to revise their drug labeling to include a boxed warning regarding the potential for increased risk of cardiovascular (CV) events and gastrointestinal (GI) bleeding. The FDA also requested that package inserts for OTC NSAIDs include strengthened warnings about GI and CV risks. This action by the U.S. regulatory agency followed earlier concerns raised about naproxen in December 2004, when the National Institutes of Health (NIH) halted a five-year study investigating the efficacy of naproxen (and celecoxib) for preventing Alzheimer's disease; in the Alzheimer's Disease Anti-Inflammatory Prevention Trial (ADAPT), naproxen increased the risk of heart attack and stroke.

Numerous NSAIDs, many of which are available as inexpensive OTC preparations, are available to treat CLBP. The following sections discuss ibuprofen (Pfizer's [New York, New York] Motrin, Knoll Pharmaceutical's [Mount Olive, New Jersey] Brufen, generics), ketoprofen (Wyeth's [Madison, New Jersey] Orudis/Oruvail, generics), and diclofenac (Novartis's [Basel, Switzerland] Voltaren/Cataflam, generics)—all of which have been specifically studied in back pain.

Mechanism of Action. Although the mechanism of NSAID action is not fully understood, these drugs are known to block the arachidonic acid pathway at an early stage. (Figure 4 illustrates a condensed version of the arachidonic acid pathway and the recognized role of NSAIDs in blocking this pathway.) Arachidonic acid is the major fatty acid incorporated into cell membranes; its metabolites serve as precursors to the synthesis of inflammatory mediators known as prostaglandins. The enzyme COX—which is present in platelets, endothelial cells, the GI tract, and the kidneys—initially converts arachidonic acid into intermediary cyclic endoperoxides, which in turn are converted into prostaglandins. Prostaglandin inflammatory mediators (especially prostaglandin-E_2 [PGE_2]) cause inflammation by increasing the vascular permeability of the blood vessels. NSAIDs inhibit the activity of COX, thereby preventing the production of prostaglandins.

As mentioned previously, NSAID use is complicated by potentially serious GI side effects. The most common complications include gastritis, mucosal damage, peptic erosions, ulcers, and bleeding. Patients who use these drugs for chronic treatment are especially vulnerable to NSAIDs' GI effects because the risk increases with length of therapy; in addition, patients who take higher than recommended dosages of NSAIDs are more likely to experience additional serious side effects.

In addition to the risk of GI problems, NSAIDs are associated with impaired renal function. Epidemiological studies suggest that NSAID use among elderly patients may, for example, increase the risk of acute renal failure by as much as 58% (Griffin MR, 2000).

Studies also suggest that the use of NSAIDs—specifically ibuprofen—may reduce the cardioprotection of aspirin (Catella-Lawson F, 2001; MacDonald TM, 2003). This reduction in cardioprotection (due to a rise in both thromboxane levels and platelet aggregation) may be caused by the competitive interaction between ibuprofen and aspirin, the binding sites of which lie close together on cyclooxygenase (COX-1).

Although other studies have not detected significant CV risks associated with NSAID use (Ray WA, 2002; Kimmel SE, 2004), some physicians are cautious about prescribing these drugs to elderly patients. Many older individuals use long-term, low-dose aspirin therapy for both cardioprotection and ischemic stroke prevention, and chronic NSAID use by CLBP patients may interfere with aspirin's anticipated benefits.

Ibuprofen. Ibuprofen (Figure 5) is approved for a wide variety of indications, including the relief of mild-to-moderate pain. Throughout its long history—and despite the emergence of newer therapies used to treat pain (e.g., COX-2 inhibitors)—ibuprofen has remained a mainstay of pain therapy. Combination drugs in which ibuprofen is the NSAID component (e.g., hydrocodone/ibuprofen [Abbott Laboratories's (Abbott Park, Illinois) Vicoprofen, generics]) are also prescribed for CLBP. In addition to its broad use as a prescription therapy, ibuprofen is available OTC. CLBP patients often self-treat with OTC ibuprofen, either alone or in combination with prescription medications.

Ibuprofen is a propionic acid derivative with anti-inflammatory, antipyretic, and analgesic properties. Although it is as effective as aspirin for relieving pain, it is generally better tolerated than other NSAIDs because, unlike aspirin, it does not interfere significantly with blood platelets and is therefore less likely to exacerbate GI bleeding.

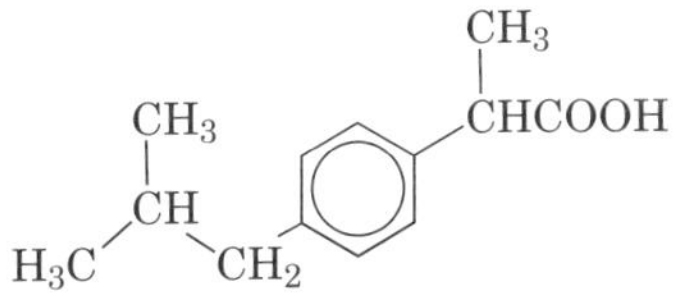

FIGURE 5. *Structure of Ibuprofen.*

Very few well-designed published studies have investigated the efficacy of ibuprofen in CLBP. Although results from one small ($n = 60$) CLBP crossover study suggest that ibuprofen is effective for treating CLBP (Pownall R, 1985), these data are inconclusive and do not confirm ibuprofen's efficacy in this indication. Furthermore, a randomized, double-blind, placebo-controlled study ($n = 372$) in acute LBP patients found that, although ibuprofen was superior to placebo on one primary outcomes measure, it was not as effective as diclofenac on other end points (Dreiser RL, 2003).

Similar to other NSAIDs, ibuprofen is associated with GI events—such as dyspepsia and ulcers—and renal failure. According to the drug's package insert, 4–16% of adults reported one or more GI complaints in clinical trials with ibuprofen.

Ketoprofen. Like ibuprofen, ketoprofen (Figure 6) is available in both OTC and prescription strengths. Wyeth also markets a controlled-release formulation (Oruvail).

Ketoprofen's pharmacology is somewhat different from that of other traditional NSAIDs. It has a short plasma half-life (less than two hours), but it can suppress prostaglandin E2 production for up to 24 hours and inhibit platelet aggregation for up to 36 hours after a 100 mg dose. Studies indicate that ketoprofen can also inhibit 5-lipoxygenase and thus block the production of leukotrienes—an activity that no other NSAID is known to have.

As is the case with ibuprofen, very few well-designed published studies have investigated the efficacy of ketoprofen for CLBP. One double-blind study ($n = 155$), conducted in 1981, found that ketoprofen was as effective as diclofenac in reducing CLBP (Matsumo S, 1981). However, because the trial did not include a placebo control, the results are not sufficient to prove ketoprofen's efficacy in CLBP.

The side effects associated with ketoprofen treatment are primarily GI-related, as is the case with other NSAIDs. According to the drug's package insert, common GI side effects include dyspepsia (11%), nausea (3–9%), constipation (3–9%), and vomiting (3–9%).

Diclofenac. Diclofenac (Figure 7), a phenylacetic acid derivative, is available both OTC and by prescription. Diclofenac sodium (Novartis's Voltaren/Voltaren XR, generics) is available in original and extended-release formulations; diclofenac potassium (Novartis's Cataflam, generics) is available in an immediate-release formulation.

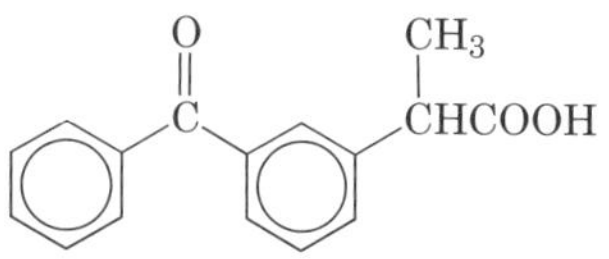

FIGURE 6. *Structure of ketoprofen.*

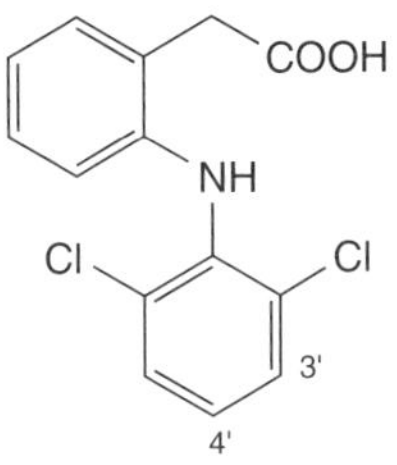

FIGURE 7. Structure of Diclofenac.

In addition to inhibiting cyclooxygenase, diclofenac reduces the availability of arachidonic acid and inhibits production of leukotrienes. It is a rapidly metabolized NSAID with a plasma half-life of less than two hours, requiring multiple doses daily (although the extended-release formulation is typically administered once daily).

Although few well-designed clinical studies have investigated diclofenac's efficacy in CLBP, one randomized, double-blind, placebo-controlled study ($n = 372$) in acute LBP patients found that diclofenac was more effective than ibuprofen or placebo (Dreiser RL, 2003). Another double-blind study found that diclofenac provides pain relief similar to that offered by its metabolite, aceclofenac (Schattenkirchner M, 2003). However, because these studies were conducted in acute LBP patients, their results are not conclusive regarding diclofenac's efficacy in CLBP.

Like other traditional NSAIDs, diclofenac's side effects are predominantly GI-related; its labeling reports an incidence of 1–10% GI adverse reactions, including abdominal pain, constipation, dyspepsia, flatulence, nausea, and vomiting. Hepatotoxicity is also a concern with diclofenac. According to 180 cases reviewed by the FDA between 1988 and 1991, diclofenac poses a risk of liver damage to all patients, particularly women (Banks AT, 1995).

Preferential Cyclooxygenase-2 Inhibitors

Overview. In 1991, researchers achieved a major breakthrough when they discovered that two distinct isoforms of COX exist. COX-1—also called constitutive cyclooxygenase—is present in cells under normal physiological conditions and stimulates the synthesis of prostaglandins (including PGE2) that help regulate renal function, blood flow, platelet activity, and protection of the mucous membrane along the GI tract. COX-2, otherwise known as inducible cyclooxygenase, occurs only under pathological conditions. Its production is induced by proinflammatory cytokines, mitogens, or endotoxins, and it stimulates the production of prostaglandins (including PGE2) that drive the inflammatory process. Researchers believe that inhibition of COX-2 by NSAIDs is responsible for their analgesic and anti-inflammatory properties, while inhibition of COX-1 causes GI side effects by reducing the production of gastroprotective prostaglandins.

Although drugs in this class were developed with the goal of reducing GI side effects, recent findings have caused many to question whether preferential COX-2 drugs are safer than traditional NSAIDs. In April 2005, the FDA asked that a boxed warning be added to drug labeling for all preferential COX-2 inhibitors, similar to that for NSAIDs (and for selective COX-2 inhibitors, discussed later). The warning would indicate a potentially increased risk of CV events and GI bleeding.

Although a number of preferential COX-2 inhibitors have been developed (including nimesulide [Roche's (Basel, Switzerland) Guaxon, Novartis's Mesulid, generics], piroxicam [Pfizer's Feldene, generics], and meloxicam [Boehringer Ingelheim (Ingelheim, Germany)/Abbott's Mobic]), none has been proven to have a significantly better GI safety profile than that of traditional NSAIDs. Researchers postulate that either these agents do not inhibit COX-2 strongly enough or their degree of COX-1 inhibition is still too great to prevent gastroenteropathies. Because meloxicam is one of the most popular preferential COX-2 inhibitors used for CLBP, it is discussed here in greater detail.

Mechanism of Action. COX-1, also called constitutive cyclooxygenase, is present in cells under normal physiological conditions; it stimulates the synthesis of prostaglandins (including PGE2) that help regulate renal function, blood flow, platelet activity, and protection of the mucous membrane along the GI tract. COX-2, otherwise known as inducible cyclooxygenase, occurs only under pathological conditions. Its production is induced by proinflammatory cytokines, mitogens, and endotoxins, and it stimulates the production of prostaglandins (including PGE2) that drive the inflammatory process. Preferential COX-2 inhibitors block both COX isoforms, yet agents in this class favor the suppression of COX-2 over COX-1, unlike traditional NSAIDs, which inhibit both COX isoforms fairly indiscriminately.

Meloxicam. Meloxicam (Figure 8) has been available in Europe since 1996 and was launched in 2000 in the United States for the treatment of osteoarthritis (OA). In Japan, where the drug launched in 2001, meloxicam is approved for the treatment of back pain and arthritis.

Meloxicam preferentially inhibits COX-2 over COX-1, so the inhibition of COX-2-stimulated proinflammatory prostaglandin production is greater than the inhibition of the production of COX-1-stimulated prostaglandins, which regulate

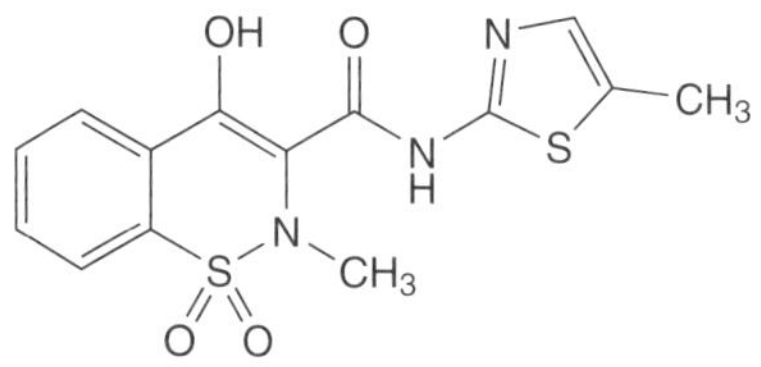

FIGURE 8. *Structure of Meloxicam.*

renal function, blood flow, platelet activity, and the protection of the mucous membrane along the GI tract.

Despite its use for CLBP and its approval for back pain in Japan, there is a dearth of published clinical trial data for meloxicam in this indication. One placebo-controlled study of patients with acute CLBP ($n = 180$) found that meloxicam was superior to the NSAID diclofenac in terms of efficacy and tolerability (Colberg K, 1996).

The most common side effects of meloxicam are GI disturbances, including dyspepsia, nausea and vomiting, abdominal pain, and diarrhea (Dequeker J, 1998; Hawkey C, 1998). Meloxicam's packaging indicates that more than 15% of patients in placebo-controlled trials experienced adverse GI events. Researchers and physicians were originally hopeful that preferential COX-2 inhibitors were safer than traditional NSAIDs, but postmarketing surveillance pointed to a different conclusion. In meloxicam's first two years on the market in the United Kingdom, the U.K. Medicines Control Agency and the Committee on Safety of Medicines received 733 reports that included 1,339 suspected adverse drug reactions (ADRs) involving meloxicam. Gastric perforation, ulcers, and bleeding accounted for 18% of the reports, and five patients died as a result of GI side effects. Because of these ADRs, U.S. packaging for meloxicam was updated to include warnings about potentially serious GI side effects. Nevertheless, current concerns regarding the selective COX-2 inhibitors (discussed in the next section) have boosted meloxicam's popularity as physicians seek alternatives to COX-2 agents. However, because meloxicam will carry the same boxed warning as selective COX-2 therapies, the recent surge in prescriptions for the drug may be short-lived.

Selective Cyclooxygenase-2 Inhibitors

Overview. Most research in the development of novel NSAIDs has concentrated on the elimination of side effects. In 1991, researchers discovered that two distinct isoforms of COX exist and that selective inhibition of just one of these isoforms could achieve the same level of pain relief as NSAIDs (which inhibit both COX isoforms) with fewer GI side effects. This finding ushered in the new class of anti-inflammatory drugs, the COX-2 inhibitors. Several clinical studies show that patients treated with selective COX-2 inhibitors have significantly lower rates of GI-related adverse events compared with traditional NSAID users (Bombardier C, 2000; Silverstein FE, 2000; Watson DJ, 2004). Based on these findings, many physicians began prescribing COX-2 inhibitors to CLBP patients at risk for GI complications.

However, recent concerns regarding the CV and cerebrovascular effects of COX-2 inhibitors have tainted many physicians' and patients' perceptions of this drug class, leaving patients and physicians wondering whether COX-2 inhibitors are safe. Doubts about the safety of the COX-2 inhibitors made headlines in September 2004 when Merck announced a worldwide withdrawal of rofecoxib (Vioxx). Rofecoxib's withdrawal was based on three-year data from the Adenomatous Polyp Prevention on Vioxx (APPROVE) trial. The data demonstrated a doubling in the risk of myocardial infarction and cerebrovascular accident (compared with placebo) at 18 months (Bresalier RS, 2005). Close on the heels of the rofecoxib news, valdecoxib (Pfizer's Bextra) was also shown to increase the risk of CV/thromboembolic events for patients treated with valdecoxib following coronary artery bypass graft (CABG) surgery (Furberg CD, 2005). Soon after, a study investigating Pfizer's other COX-2 inhibitor, celecoxib (Celebrex), in cancer patients was halted because of data suggesting that celecoxib increased patients' risk of myocardial infarction and stroke.

In February 2005, the FDA Advisory Committee recommended that COX-2 inhibitors be allowed to remain on the market. Although a majority voted in favor of all three COX-2 agents currently available in the United States, the committee ruled most strongly in favor of celecoxib, whose lower degree of selectivity is believed to result in a lower safety risk. Margins in favor of rofecoxib (to allow it to return to the market) and valdecoxib were much narrower. The committee also recommended that a black box warning be added to COX-2 package inserts and that direct-to-consumer (DTC) advertising be curtailed.

In April 2005, the FDA itself took action, asking Pfizer to withdraw valdecoxib from the market because of its unfavorable cost/benefit profile. At the same time, the European Medicines Agency (EMEA) asked Pfizer to remove the drug from all European markets. Although the FDA allowed celecoxib to remain on the market, it requested that Pfizer add a boxed warning highlighting the potential for increased risk of CV events and GI bleeding.

Based on safety concerns and on resultant actions by regulatory agencies in the United States and Europe, it is clear that future prescriptions of COX-2 drugs will be severely curtailed compared with historical use.

Mechanism of Action. As noted earlier, traditional NSAIDs combat inflammation by blocking both isoforms of COX fairly indiscriminately. Selective COX-2 inhibitors, by contrast, predominantly inhibit COX-2 and therefore have little effect on COX-1. As a result, they act specifically to reduce pathological inflammation caused by prostaglandins without disrupting their beneficial effects.

Celecoxib. Celecoxib (Pfizer's Celebrex) (Figure 9) is marketed for osteoarthritis (OA), rheumatoid arthritis (RA), familial adenomatous polyposis (FAP), and the management of acute pain and primary dysmenorrhea. Pfizer markets celecoxib

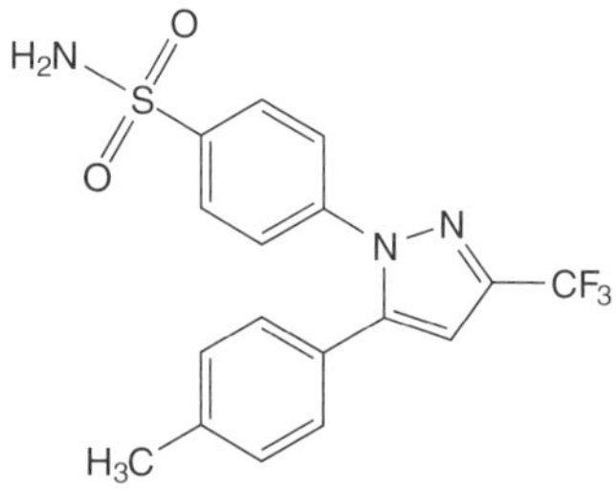

FIGURE 9. *Structure of Celecoxib.*

in all of the major markets except Japan, where Yamanouchi Pharmaceutical (Tokyo, Japan, now Astellas Pharma, Inc. [Tokyo, Japan]) is developing the drug and has submitted it for approval.

Celecoxib acts by the same mechanism as that of other selective COX-2 inhibitors, primarily inhibiting COX-2. Although few published trials have studied celecoxib's effect on CLBP, studies in other indications (e.g., OA, RA) have demonstrated that the incidence of GI toxicity with celecoxib is lower than that with traditional NSAIDs (Silverstein FE, 2000). The Celecoxib Long-Term Arthritis Safety Study (CLASS) assigned 8059 OA and RA patients to receive daily doses of 800 mg celecoxib, 2400 mg ibuprofen (a traditional NSAID), or 150 mg diclofenac for at least six months. The celecoxib dose used was four times that recommended for OA and twice the highest recommended RA dose. The incidence of upper GI ulcer complications for patients receiving 800 mg of celecoxib daily and for those receiving the other NSAIDs was 0.76% and 1.45%, respectively; the incidence rates of these complications combined with symptomatic ulcers were 2.08% and 3.54%, respectively. Upon completion of CLASS, Pfizer successfully petitioned the FDA for a revision of celecoxib's labeling. The FDA determined that the results of this study demonstrate sufficient GI safety superiority of celecoxib over diclofenac to warrant a label change.

Because other agents in its class (i.e., rofecoxib, valdecoxib) have been pulled from the market, experts are increasingly concerned about the risks associated with long term celecoxib treatment. Indeed, although celecoxib remains on the market, in April 2005 the FDA asked Pfizer to add a boxed warning to the drug's label that will indicate a potentially increased risk of CV events and GI bleeding. Data from the Adenoma Prevention with Celecoxib (APC) study provides evidence for an increased CV risk (Solomon SD, 2005). A review of potentially serious CV events among the 2035 patients enrolled in the APC trial found that treatment with celecoxib (200 or 400 mg) led to a dose-related increase in the risk of serious CV events, including death, myocardial infarction, stroke, and heart failure. This finding reflects similar conclusions from a 2001 meta-analysis, in which investigators compared the annual rates of myocardial infarctions for all patients in the CLASS and Vioxx Gastrointestinal Outcomes Research (VIGOR) studies with a placebo meta-analysis of 23,407 patients from recent aspirin prevention trials (Mukherjee D, 2001). The analysis revealed that the annualized myocardial infarction rates for rofecoxib and celecoxib were significantly higher than that of the placebo meta-analysis group (0.74% for rofecoxib, 0.8% for celecoxib, and 0.54% for placebo).

However, other studies refute both findings of the 2001 meta-analysis and the APC study. For example, evaluation of the CLASS trial showed no difference between COX-2- and traditional NSAID-treated patient groups in terms of CV event rates (Silverstein FE, 2000). In addition, a study presented at the 2003 American College of Rheumatology (ACR) Annual Scientific Meeting in Orlando, Florida, compared the adjusted relative risk of acute myocardial infarction (MI) in more than 54,000 Medicare beneficiaries treated with celecoxib, rofecoxib, or other NSAIDs (Solomon DH, 2003). Results from this study demonstrated that there was no difference in MI risk between patients treated with celecoxib and those not treated with an NSAID or selective COX-2 inhibitor (odds ratio [OR] = 0.93). However, patients treated with rofecoxib had a 14% increased risk of an acute MI compared with patients not treated with an NSAID or selective COX-2 inhibitor (OR = 1.1.4) and a 24% increased risk of an acute MI compared with patients treated with celecoxib (OR = 1.24).

Narcotic Analgesics

Overview. Because of their powerful ability to control pain, narcotic analgesics, also known as opioids, are often used to treat chronic pain conditions. However, long-term narcotic use remains controversial because of concerns about tolerance, addiction, and regulatory sanctions. Narcotic analgesics are also associated with side effects that are intolerable for many patients (e.g., sedation, nausea, constipation). Therefore, chronic narcotic analgesic treatment remains a last resort for CLBP. However, as discussed in the "Emerging Therapies" section, drug manufacturers are developing narcotic agents that they hope will deliver potent narcotic efficacy without the risk of tolerance or dependency and—much further in the future—perhaps without the problematic side-effect profile.

Long-acting or sustained-release opioid agonists (e.g., morphine SR, oxycodone CR) are often preferred over short-acting or immediate-release opioid agonists (e.g., codeine, hydromorphone) for CLBP because they deliver steady pain relief without the euphoric effect associated with immediate-release opioids, thus reducing the risk of inducing dependence or withdrawal symptoms. Short-acting or immediate-release opioids are generally reserved for controlling breakthrough or acute episodes of LBP; physicians are unlikely to treat patients chronically with these drugs. Although many different narcotic analgesics are used to treat CLBP, this section discusses four of the more commonly prescribed agents in this class—codeine (generics), morphine (Purdue's [Wilson, North Carolina] MS Contin, Napp Pharmaceutical [Cambridge, United Kingdom]/Mundipharma's [Basel, Switzerland] MST Continus, Elan Pharmaceutical [South San Francisco, California]/Ligand Pharmaceuticals Inc.'s [San Diego, California] Avinza, Alpharma, Inc. [Fort Lee, New Jersey]/MGI PHARMA, Inc.'s [Bloomington, Minnesota] Kadian, generics), oxycodone controlled-release (CR) (Purdue's Oxycontin CR, Napp's Oxycontin M/R, generics), and the fentanyl patch (Janssen [Titusville, New Jersey]/ALZA Corporation's [Mountain View, California] Duragesic/Durogesic, generics).

Mechanism of Action. Currently available narcotic analgesics relieve pain via agonist activity at opiate receptors in the central nervous system (CNS), primarily the mu and kappa opioid receptors (some evidence suggests these agents also act at the delta opioid receptors). These agents are classified as either full or partial agonists by their activity at opioid receptors. Clinically, mu opioid receptor agonists are used more often than kappa agonists because they are full rather than partial agonists (Holdcroft A, 2003) and are therefore more effective (the analgesic potency of opioids is believed to correlate directly with their affinity for the mu receptor).

Narcotic analgesics' activity at these receptors also mediates their adverse effects; the mu receptor mediates euphoria, respiratory depression, and constipation, and the kappa receptor mediates sedation. Because narcotic analgesics typically cause sedation, physicians prefer prescribing drugs in this class at bedtime. Other common side effects include constipation, nausea or vomiting, and, more seriously, possible tolerance and dependency. At high doses, respiratory depression is a potential risk. Because of the abuse potential associated with narcotic analgesics, their use is strictly monitored in most countries (i.e., narcotic analgesics are "scheduled" compounds in the United States), a practice that often limits their use in CLBP.

Codeine. An opium alkaloid, codeine (Figure 10) resembles morphine pharmacologically but has milder effects and somewhat less addictive potential. As such, it is generally prescribed for relief of mild-to-moderate pain, and in CLBP management it is used more often for acute back pain or breakthrough pain. Physicians are likely to prescribe codeine in combination with the less potent analgesics aspirin (generics) or acetaminophen (generics) to create an incremental increase in analgesic efficacy.

Because codeine is typically given in combination with an analgesic, few published studies have investigated its use as a monotherapy for CLBP. However, one small double-blind crossover study ($n = 55$) found that combination codeine/acetaminophen (Johnson & Johnson's [New Brunswick, New Jersey] Tylenol with Codeine, generics) was as effective as tramadol (Johnson & Johnson's Ultram, generics) for treating patients with refractory back pain (Muller FO, 1998). Additionally, the acetaminophen/codeine combination was better tolerated: 81% of patients tolerated the combination drug "well," compared with 69% of tramadol patients.

Morphine. Morphine (Figure 11), an opium alkaloid, has a long history of use for chronic pain and remains a cornerstone of pain therapy because of its high analgesic potency and rapid onset of action. Morphine's popularity over other opioid agonists stems primarily from physicians' extensive experience with its dosing and side effects, its availability in both short- and long-acting formulations, and its multiple routes of administration.

Short-acting morphine (generics) is rarely used in CLBP because of its euphoric effect and associated risk of dependence. Morphine sustained-release

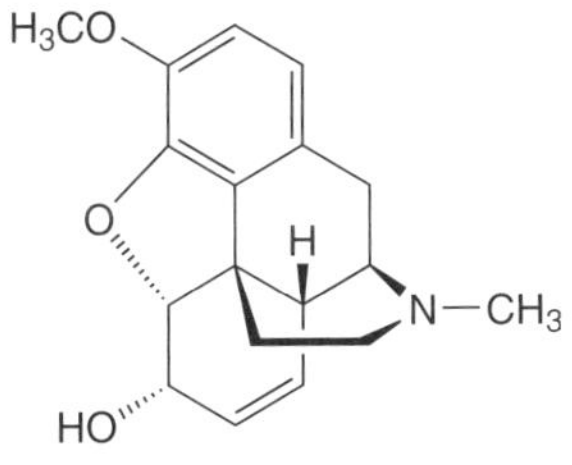

FIGURE 10. Structure of codeine.

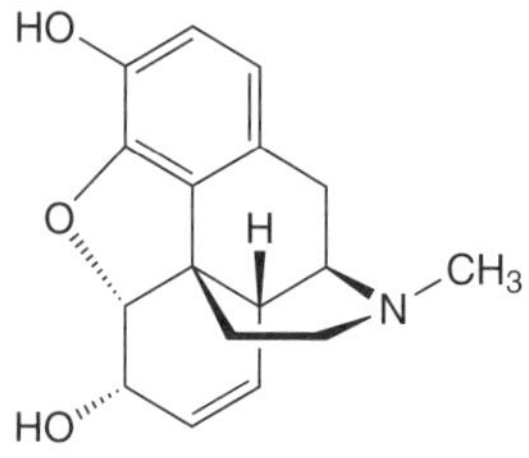

FIGURE 11. Structure of morphine.

(SR) is available in twice-daily and once-daily formulations (Purdue's MS Contin, Napp/Mundipharma's MST Continus, Elan/Ligand Pharmaceutical's Avinza, Alpharma/MGI's Kadian, generics). Elan/Ligand Pharmaceutical's once-daily oral morphine formulation Avinza, which was approved in the United States in 2002, is intended for patients with moderate-to-severe pain who require continuous opioid therapy. Ligand developed the agent using spheroidal oral drug absorption system (SODAS) technology developed by Elan. SODAS involves encapsulation of morphine in spherical beads 1–2 mm in diameter that are coated with modified-release polymers. Avinza contains both immediate-release and extended-release polymers that offer fast onset of action and sustained relief for up to 24 hours. Alpharma's sustained-release morphine product Kadian, which requires once-daily dosing, has a similar, innovative polymer-coated shell technology. Kadian will continue to be marketed by Alpharma to pain specialists in the United States.

Few published studies have investigated morphine's efficacy in CLBP. One open-label study ($n = 128$) demonstrated that once-daily morphine SR (Avinza) provided stable analgesia for one year in CLBP patients, with no dose increases or use of rescue medications (Keeton W, 2003). A small crossover study ($n = 49$) found that morphine SR was an effective treatment for patients with chronic non-tumor-associated pain syndromes (Maier C, 2002).

As with other narcotic analgesics, common side effects of morphine SR include constipation, lightheadedness, dizziness, sedation, nausea, vomiting, sweating, dysphoria, and euphoria.

Oxycodone CR. A semisynthetic opium analogue, oxycodone (Figure 12) controlled-release (CR) is marketed in the United States, France, Germany, Spain, the United Kingdom, and Japan. Oxycodone CR is a mu agonist that has twice the oral potency of oral morphine. Oxycodone is also available in an immediate-release (IR) formulation (Endo Pharmaceuticals [Chadds Ford, Pennsylvania] Endocodone, generics). In comparison with oxycodone IR, oxycodone CR is generally considered more convenient for chronic pain because of its longer duration of action and more convenient (every 12 hours) dosing (Hale ME, 1999). The availability of less expensive oxycodone CR—following the recent launch of generic formulations of the agent—will likely lead to increased use in countries with stringent cost restrictions. However, oxycodone CR's potential for and

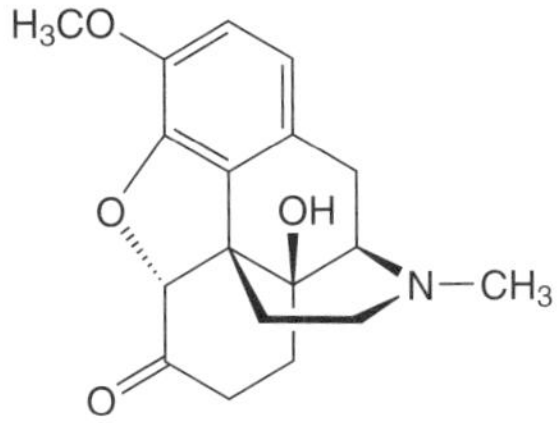

FIGURE 12. *Structure of oxycodone.*

history of abuse will continue to limit its use, particularly in the primary care setting. Oxycodone IR is also available in combination with ibuprofen (Forest Laboratories, Inc.'s [New York, New York] Combunox) or acetaminophen (Endo's Percocet, generics).

Although only limited data are available for CLBP, oxycodone CR has thus far proven to be an effective treatment for this indication. In a double-blind, placebo-controlled study ($n = 110$), CLBP patients were randomized to receive either oxycodone CR (10 mg every 12 hours) or placebo for three months (Richards P, 2002). Inclusion criteria for the study were a 3- to-12-month history of moderate-to-severe persistent low back pain and previous lack of response to NSAIDs and/or low-dose combination opioid analgesics. The primary outcome measure was pain intensity, assessed using the Brief Pain Inventory (BPI), an 11-point numeric scale ranging from 0 (no pain) to 10 (worst possible pain). Functionality and quality of life were also evaluated, based on the Roland-Morris Functionality Questionnaire and the MOS 35-Item Short-Form Health Survey (SF-36). At study completion, oxycodone CR was significantly superior to placebo with regard to BPI scores (4.6 with oxycodone CR versus 5.4 with placebo). No significant differences between oxycodone CR and placebo were found in terms of the Roland Morris or SF-36 scores.

A prospective, open-label, nonrandomized, four-week trial ($n = 33$) found that combination oxycodone/acetaminophen with a reduced dose of acetaminophen relieved pain in CLBP patients unresponsive to other medications (Gammaitoni AR, 2003). After four weeks, treatment with combination oxycodone/acetaminophen significantly reduced pain intensity.

Like other narcotic agents, oxycodone CR is associated with a number of common side effects. According to the drug's labeling, the most frequently reported side effects are constipation (23%), nausea (23%), somnolence (23%), dizziness (13%), pruritis (13%), and vomiting (12%).

Fentanyl Patch. Launched in 1991, the transdermal opioid fentanyl (Figure 13) patch has enabled what was once only an intravenous agent to become an option for the management of chronic pain. (As an IV agent, fentanyl was used almost exclusively in pre- and perioperative settings for induction and maintenance of anesthesia and postoperatively for short-term analgesia.) The fentanyl patch is available in all the markets under study. Although its high cost has been somewhat

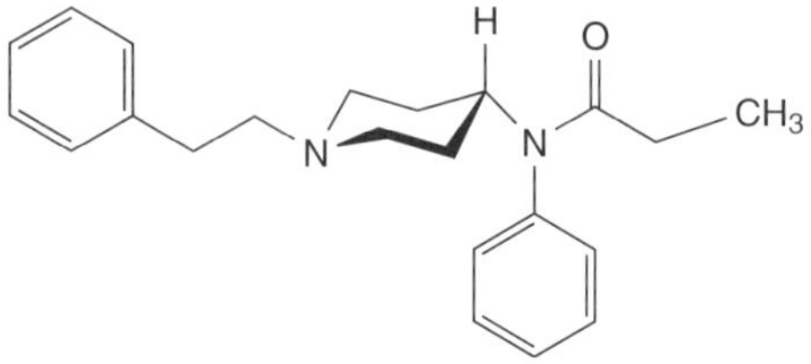

FIGURE 13. *Structure of fentanyl.*

prohibitive to its use in the past, a less expensive generic fentanyl patch (made by Mylan Laboratories, Inc. [Canonsburg, Pennsylvania]) reached the market in early 2005, following the expiration of Janssen/Alza's six-month pediatric exclusivity. Labtec is also developing a matrix formulation (i.e., a slightly altered delivery system) of the fentanyl patch, which will be marketed by an undisclosed partner.

Fentanyl is a low-molecular-weight, highly lipophilic, short-acting opiate that binds selectively to mu receptors. The transdermal (patch) system is a long-acting, controlled-release preparation of fentanyl in which the amount of drug released is proportional to the surface area of the patch (25, 50, 75, or 100 µg/hour). After the first application, the drug takes approximately four hours to reach effective levels in the bloodstream and maintains a steady release over three days.

Although controlled trials investigating the use of the fentanyl patch for CLBP are lacking, open-label studies have demonstrated that the patch provides pain relief similar to that offered by oral narcotic analgesics. One open-label study ($n = 50$) of CLBP patients who had previously had an unsatisfactory response to conventional CLBP treatment and had been receiving short-acting oral narcotic analgesics for at least six months found the fentanyl patch to be an effective alternative to oral opioid therapy (Simpson RK, Jr., 1997). A second, open-label study ($n = 680$) found that the transdermal fentanyl patch provides pain relief comparable to that of oral morphine SR (Allan L, 2004; Allan L, 2003). This trial also concluded that the fentanyl patch was more tolerable than morphine SR; only 31% of patients on the patch suffered from constipation at study completion, compared with 48% of patients on morphine SR.

The fentanyl patch has also been shown to improve quality of life (QoL) better than combination oxycodone/acetaminophen for CLBP patients. A six-month two-way crossover study ($n = 229$) compared health-related QoL outcomes (as measured with the Treatment Outcomes in Pain Survey [TOPS] instrument) in CLBP patients randomized to receive oxycodone/acetaminophen for three months followed by three months of the fentanyl patch or vice versa (Katz N, 2003). During the first three months, patients in both treatment groups showed significant improvements in physical functioning, bodily pain, vitality, and social functioning scales relative to baseline scores. Patients treated with the fentanyl patch also demonstrated significant improvements in mental health scores. Patients who crossed over to the patch showed continued improvement in their health-related QoL scales, while patients who received oxycodone/acetaminophen during the second treatment phase experienced declines in their health-related QoL scales. An additional, observational study confirmed the fentanyl patch's positive impact on QoL for CLBP patients, finding significant improvements in physical and social functioning as well as significantly improved activity limitation (Kosinski M, 2004; Schein J, 2004).

Trial results reveal a patient preference for the fentanyl patch over oral morphine SR. A randomized crossover trial ($n = 256$) with chronic noncancer pain (40% with CLBP) assessed patient preference for the patch versus oral morphine SR (Allan L, 2001). Although both therapies provided adequate pain relief, 65% of the study's participants preferred transdermal fentanyl over morphine. Patients using fentanyl had higher quality-of-life scores as measured by the SF-36 and experienced greater pain relief compared with morphine.

In general, the fentanyl patch is somewhat better tolerated than morphine because of a lower propensity for causing respiratory distress and nausea. However, the patch can cause itching and discomfort at the application site—a troublesome side effect that forces some patients to discontinue therapy with the patch in favor of long-acting oral opioids. Additionally, because peak plasma concentrations are not reached until 12–18 hours after the administration of transdermal fentanyl, some patients require rescue doses of short-acting opioids. Patients who fail on transdermal fentanyl, either because of side effects or inadequate analgesia, must wait 12–18 hours to allow serum concentrations of the drug to diminish sufficiently before switching to another opioid. This lengthy elimination often requires that fentanyl-induced side effects be treated for an extended period following fentanyl discontinuation.

Other Analgesics

Overview. The only drug in this category reviewed here is tramadol (Johnson & Johnson's Ultram, generics), a synthetic analogue of codeine. The FDA classifies tramadol as a non-narcotic analgesic because, despite binding to opioid receptors (albeit weakly, at 6000 times lower affinity than morphine), its analgesic activity is only partially inhibited by the opioid antagonist naloxone. This fact suggests that tramadol derives at least some of its pain-relieving properties from a separate, nonopioid mechanism, indicating a dual mechanism of action and earning the drug a non-narcotic classification.

Mechanism of Action. Although chemically unrelated to opioids, tramadol has some affinity for opioid receptors, likely exerting analgesia through a mechanism similar to that of opioids. Like some antidepressants with analgesic properties, tramadol inhibits norepinephrine and serotonin reuptake (Sindrup SH, 1999).

Tramadol. Tramadol (Johnson & Johnson's Ultram, generics) (Figure 14) was launched for the treatment of pain in Europe in 1992 and in the United States in 1995. In Japan, tramadol is not yet available in an oral formulation. In January

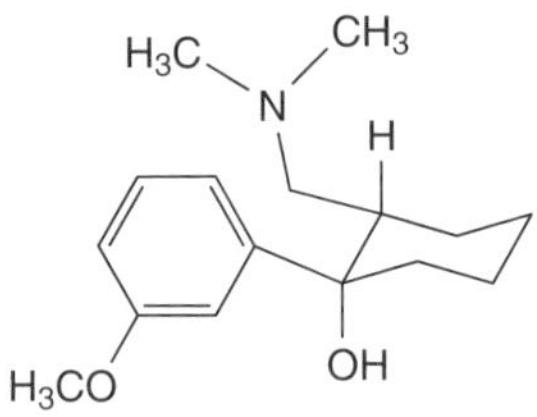

FIGURE 14. Structure of tramadol.

2005, Biovail received an FDA "approvable" letter for a once-daily formulation of tramadol (Ralivia ER); however, the FDA requested that Biovail submit additional clinical trial data. Labopharm is also developing—in Phase III in the United States and Europe—a once-daily formulation of tramadol for pain; Labopharm has signed licensing agreements with several European companies that will market the tramadol formulation in Europe once the drug is launched. Another once-daily controlled-release formulation of tramadol is under development by Purdue Pharma and is preregistered in the United States.

Tramadol is available in most markets in combination with acetaminophen (Ortho-McNeil Pharmaceutical's [Raritan, New Jersey] Ultracet). Although tramadol is prescribed on its own for CLBP, the combination tramadol/acetaminophen drug (37.5 mg tramadol/325 mg acetaminophen) is also frequently prescribed for this condition; this combination is thought to have a faster onset of action and a longer duration of pain relief than tramadol alone. Therefore, most studies have focused on the combination treatment rather than on tramadol monotherapy.

One study of tramadol/acetaminophen demonstrated that the combination drug effectively reduced CLBP. In this three-month, double-blind, placebo-controlled study ($n = 338$), CLBP patients with at least moderate pain (i.e., score ≥ 40 mm, measured on a 100 mm VAS) were randomized to receive either tramadol (37.5 mg)/acetaminophen (325 mg) or placebo (Peloso PM, 2004). Over a period of ten days, treatment was titrated from one combination tablet per day (at bedtime) to one combination tablet four times a day; following the titration phase, patients were allowed to adjust their dose as needed (to a maximum of two tablets four times a day and a minimum of three tablets per day). The primary efficacy measure was pain, measured using a 100 mm VAS. Secondary measures included the six-point pain relief scale (-1 = worse pain, 0 = no relief, 1 = slight relief, 2 = moderate relief, 3 = a lot of relief, 4 = complete relief), the SF-MPQ, RDQ, SF-26 Health Survey, and an overall assessment of how well study medication controlled pain (rated by patients and investigators on a five-point scale; -2 = very poor, 2 = very good).

At study completion, patients in the tramadol/acetaminophen group had a significantly lower mean pain VAS score than patients in the placebo group (47.4 versus 62.9). In addition, patients receiving tramadol/acetaminophen had significantly superior final pain relief scores compared with patients receiving placebo (1.8 versus 0.7). Patients in the tramadol/acetaminophen group also had better SF-36 Health Survey, SF-MPQ, RDQ, and overall medication assessments scores than their placebo counterparts.

An earlier, similarly constructed, three-month study also found tramadol/acetaminophen to be an effective treatment for CLBP. In this double-blind, placebo-controlled study ($n = 318$), patients with at least moderate pain (i.e., pain visual analogue (PVA) score $\geq 40\,$mm, measured on a $100\,$mm scale) were randomized to receive either tramadol ($37.5\,$mg)/acetaminophen ($325\,$mg) or placebo after a three-week screening and washout phase (Ruoff GE, 2003). Over a ten-day period, treatment was titrated from one combination tablet to four combination tablets per day; following the titration phase, dosage was adjusted according to individual patient requirements (up to a maximum of eight tablets/day). The primary efficacy measure was PVA score at study completion. At study completion, the tramadol/acetaminophen group had a significantly lower mean PVA score compared with the placebo group; PVA scores in the tramadol/acetaminophen group fell from a baseline 71.1 to 44.4, while scores in the placebo group dropped from a baseline 68.8 to 52.3.

One three-phase study ($n = 380$) investigated the efficacy of tramadol alone (instead of combination tramadol/acetaminophen) and found that the drug effectively relieved pain in patients with CLBP (Schnitzer TJ, 2000). The study included a washout/screening phase, an open-label run-in phase (three weeks), and a randomized, placebo-controlled phase (four weeks). At study completion, the discontinuation rate in the tramadol group was significantly lower than in the placebo group (20.7% versus 51.3%). Compared with patients who received placebo, patients taking tramadol experienced significant improvements in all secondary measures; mean pain VAS scores, pain relief, SF-MPQ, and RDQ scores were significantly lower in the tramadol group after four weeks.

With regard to side effects, tramadol is better tolerated than older NSAIDs over the long term because it does not cause GI ulcers or bleeding. However, it is associated with side effects that some patients find difficult to tolerate; according to tramadol's packaging, the drug's most common side effects are dizziness/vertigo (33%), nausea (40%), constipation (46%), headache (32%), somnolence (25%), and vomiting (17%). Compared with the narcotic analgesics, tramadol is associated with a lower risk of tolerance and/or dependence, a characteristic that earned the drug its classification as a non-narcotic analgesic. Because of this advantage, many physicians—particularly PCPs, who tend to be more cautious about prescribing narcotic agents—try tramadol rather than resorting to treatment with stronger narcotic drugs.

Antiepileptic Drugs

Overview. Although originally developed and launched for the treatment of epileptic seizures, AEDs are also effective therapies for various types of neuropathic pain, including sciatica (neuropathic CLBP radiating down the back of the thigh to below the knee), most likely because of strong similarities between the pathophysiological and biochemical mechanisms of epilepsy and neuropathic pain (Backonja MM, 2002). Because AEDs have greater utility in managing sciatica than they do in addressing nonradiating CLBP, many physicians employ these agents when a patient is suspected to have a neuropathic component to their CLBP, regardless of whether the patient has signs of inflammatory pain as well.

Because older AEDs have pronounced side effects (e.g., sedation, cerebellar symptoms, hematological changes, cardiac arrhythmia, teratogenicity), second-generation AEDs are the most commonly used to treat sciatica. In the past, physicians typically chose gabapentin (Pfizer's Neurontin, generics) as first-line therapy because of its relatively benign side-effect profile compared with that of other second-generation AEDs and because it is approved for neuropathic pain (postherpetic neuralgia in the United States, peripheral neuropathic pain in Europe). However, the recent approval of pregabalin (Pfizer's Lyrica)—the follow-on compound to gabapentin—has presented physicians with an alternative treatment option that is approved specifically for neuropathic pain (painful diabetic neuropathy and postherpetic neuralgia in the United States, peripheral neuropathic pain in Europe). Gabapentin is discussed in the following section (see "Emerging Therapies" for a discussion of pregabalin). AEDs prescribed less frequently than gabapentin include lamotrigine (GlaxoSmithKline's [Brentford, Middlesex, United Kingdom] Lamictal; discussed in "Emerging Therapies"), carbamazepine (Novartis's Tegretol/Tegretal, generics), oxcarbazepine (Novartis's Trileptal), topiramate (Ortho-McNeil's Topamax, Janssen's Epitomax), levetiracetam (UCB, Inc.'s [Smyrna, Georgia] Keppra), phenytoin (Pfizer's Dilantin, generics), and clonazepam (Roche's Klonopin, generics).

The few clinical trials that have been conducted to corroborate the analgesic effectiveness of AEDs have been targeted to niche patient populations (e.g., patients with painful diabetic neuropathy or postherpetic neuralgia). No large-scale trials to date have studied AED use specifically in CLBP. The design of such trials would be complicated due to the heterogeneity of this patient population (the pain can be of any of a variety of etiologies).

Mechanism of Action. AEDs curb or prevent the runaway neuronal excitation and subsequent depolarization in the CNS that results in sciatica. Drugs in this class tend to work through more than one pharmacological mechanism, but most often they block neuronal sodium or calcium channels or inhibit the neuronal reuptake of the major antiexcitatory neurotransmitter, gamma-aminobutyric acid (GABA).

Gabapentin. Gabapentin (Pfizer's Neurontin, generics) (Figure 15) is often the AED of choice for treating sciatica because of its relatively superior side-effect profile compared with that of other available AEDs and its generic availability. Gabapentin is also widely prescribed because it is one of the only AEDs approved specifically for treating neuropathic pain. Initially approved for the treatment of epilepsy in the United States and Europe in the early 1990s, gabapentin received expanded European approval for broad treatment of neuropathic pain in 2001 and was approved for postherpetic neuralgia in the United States in 2002. In Japan,

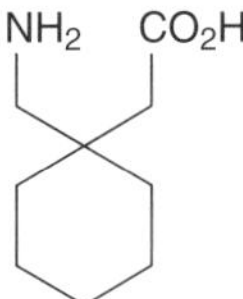

FIGURE 15. *Structure of gabapentin.*

where gabapentin is licensed to Astellas Pharma (Tokyo, Japan; the result of the merger of Fujisawa and Yamanouchi), the agent is in Phase III development for the treatment of epilepsy.

Despite much research, gabapentin's precise mechanism of action remains unknown. It is structurally related to the amino acid neurotransmitter GABA and was initially believed to mimic its inhibitory effects on synaptic neurotransmission, an action that would relieve pain by disrupting the transmission of nociceptive signals across neurons. However, it has since been shown that the drug does not interact with GABA receptors and is not converted into GABA or a GABA agonist, although its activity does result in increased GABA levels in the brain (Backonja M, 2002).

Studies suggest that gabapentin binds to the alpha-2-delta subunit of voltage-dependent calcium channels (VDCCs), a high-affinity binding site in neuronal membranes. This subunit has been implicated in the maintenance of mechanical hypersensitivity in models of neuropathic pain (Field MJ, 2000), and the drug's interaction with the site may play a role in its ability to exert analgesia. Calcium ions enable neurotransmitters to bind vesicles at the presynaptic membrane terminal; thus, it has been hypothesized that gabapentin exerts its therapeutic effect by blocking calcium influx via the alpha-2-delta receptor and reducing the release of neurotransmitters that transmit nociceptive signals between neurons. Specifically, in vitro findings suggest gabapentin may reduce the presynaptic release of excitatory neurotransmitters such as glutamate and norepinephrine (Dooley DJ, 2000).

Although data are scarce regarding the efficacy of gabapentin for sciatica, several studies have confirmed the benefit of gabapentin for various neuropathic pain conditions (Backonja M, 1998; Rice AS, 2001; Rowbotham M, 1998; Serpell MG, 2002). One double-blind, placebo-controlled study ($n = 307$) investigated gabapentin's efficacy across a range of neuropathic pain syndromes (Serpell MG, 2002). Patients enrolled in this eight-week study were required to have a definite diagnosis of neuropathic pain and at least two of the following nonspecific symptoms: allodynia (i.e., painful response to normally nonpainful stimuli), burning pain, shooting pain, or hyperalgesia (i.e., increased sensitivity to painful stimuli). Following randomization, patients were administered either gabapentin or placebo. After a one-week baseline period, patients randomized to gabapentin entered a five-week titration period with an initial dose of 900 mg/day (tid), titrated up over three days. Patients who did not demonstrate at least a 50% reduction in overall pain (evaluated every two weeks) were titrated to 1800 mg/day (tid) and further increased to 2400 mg/day (tid) if necessary. The primary efficacy measure used in the trial was change in mean weekly pain score from baseline to final study week, based on an 11-point Likert scale (0 = no pain; 10 = worst possible pain). At study completion, statistically significant differences in mean pain scores were found between the gabapentin-treated and placebo-treated groups; mean pain scores among patients in the gabapentin group had dropped by 1.5 points compared with only a 1-point decline in the placebo group.

Physicians frequently choose gabapentin because of its superior safety and tolerability profile compared with that of other AEDs. The agent is a water-soluble compound excreted in its unchanged form by the kidneys. In contrast, most AEDs are metabolized in the liver, where they may be broken down into toxic metabolites that frequently trigger side effects, idiosyncratic adverse events, and drug interactions. The most common side effects of gabapentin are somnolence, dizziness, and nausea. Among patients who participated in two neuropathic pain pivotal trials included in gabapentin's prescribing information, 16% of gabapentin-treated patients discontinued treatment because of adverse events, compared with 9% of placebo-treated patients.

Antidepressants

Overview. Antidepressants are usually reserved for patients with sciatica, although some nonradiating CLBP patients with comorbid depression may derive benefit from antidepressant treatment. Tricyclic antidepressants (e.g., amitriptyline [AstraZeneca's (Wilmington, Delaware) Elavil, Roche's Laroxyl, generics]) have historically been the most frequently used of the antidepressants for sciatica because they were considered to be the most effective. Although numerous TCAs are used to treat sciatica, the discussion here is limited to amitriptyline (AstraZeneca's Elavil, Roche's Laroxyl, generics), the most widely used agent.

Despite their superior side-effect profile (and broad use in mood disorders), newer antidepressants (e.g., selective serotonin reuptake inhibitors [SSRIs], serotonin and norepinephrine reuptake inhibitors [SNRIs]) have typically been used only for sciatica patients who cannot tolerate TCA therapy; SSRIs and SNRIs have not been studied as extensively in sciatica and were generally not believed to be very effective for neuropathic pain conditions. In particular, SSRIs are thought to be relatively ineffective because they do not affect neurotransmitters other than serotonin. However, like TCAs, SNRIs do affect both serotonin and norepinephrine and therefore hold more potential than SSRIs for sciatica (and other types of neuropathic pain).

Capitalizing on the potential for an SNRI to provide pain relief similar to that offered by the TCAs but with fewer side effects, Eli Lilly developed and launched the SNRI duloxetine (Eli Lilly's Cymbalta/Ariclaim/Xeristar); the drug—detailed in "Emerging Therapies"—was approved for peripheral diabetic neuropathy in the United States in September 2004. Duloxetine's approval marks the first time the FDA has approved an antidepressant to treat pain. Duloxetine's approval for pain, as well as its superior tolerability compared with older TCAs, will likely make it a favorite among physicians treating patients with sciatica.

In addition to being prescribed to relieve the pain itself, antidepressants are potentially beneficial for treating any comorbid depression. The 1997 Practice Guidelines for Chronic Pain Management, published by the American Society of Anesthesiologists, recommends that antidepressants be used as adjunct therapy for chronic pain conditions (Practice guidelines for chronic pain management: A report by the American Society of Anesthesiologists Task Force on Pain Management, Chronic Pain Section, 1997).

Mechanism of Action. TCAs appear to relieve pain by blocking the synaptic uptake of two neurotransmitters, serotonin (5-HT) and norepinephrine, thereby increasing local levels of these neuromediators and increasing their inhibitory effects on the nociceptive pathway (Mattia C, 2002). TCAs are also potent blockers of muscarinic, alpha-1-adrenergic, cholinergic, and histaminergic receptors. This blockade desensitizes afferent nerve fibers that transmit pain signals from the body to the brain.

Like TCAs, SNRIs inhibit the presynaptic reuptake of serotonin and norepinephrine, but they have little effect on histaminergic, cholinergic, dopaminergic, and alpha-adrenergic receptors and are therefore associated with fewer side effects than TCAs (Mattia C, 2002). SSRIs, in contrast, selectively inhibit the presynaptic reuptake of 5-HT while exerting little effect on norepinephrine reuptake (Mattia C, 2002). Like SNRIs, SSRIs as a class have little effect on histaminergic, cholinergic, dopaminergic, and alpha-adrenergic receptors and so are much more tolerable than the TCAs.

Amitriptyline. Amitriptyline (AstraZeneca's Elavil, Roche's Laroxyl, generics) (Figure 16) was first introduced in the early 1960s for the treatment of depression. Since its launch, it has become the most commonly prescribed antidepressant for the treatment of pain disorders, including sciatica, because it has accumulated a strong set of data to support its efficacy in treating patients with various forms of neuropathic pain. However, amitriptyline is associated with numerous side effects that often make the drug poorly tolerated, especially for elderly patients. Like other TCAs, amitriptyline appears to relieve pain by blocking the synaptic uptake of serotonin and norepinephrine.

Although many studies have investigated the efficacy of amitriptyline in other types of neuropathic pain, few trials have focused on sciatica. Data from existing studies (detailed here) suggest that amitriptyline is effective for treating sciatica; however, these trials involved only small patient populations.

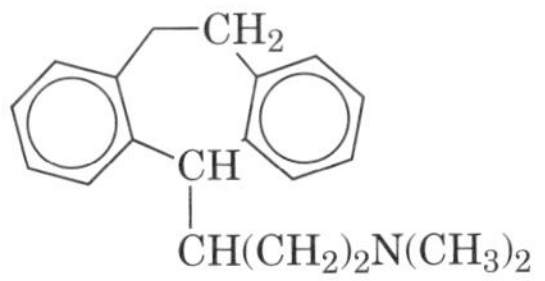

FIGURE 16. *Structure of amitriptyline.*

A six-week, double-blind, crossover study ($n = 9$) found that, although it did not improve activity levels, amitriptyline did reduce the need for analgesic medications. In this trial, patients who had suffered from CLBP for at least one year were randomized to one of two treatment sequences: patients in sequence A received amitriptyline (50–150 mg/day) for six weeks, bitter lactose washout for two weeks, placebo for six weeks, and bitter lactose washout for another two weeks; patients in sequence B received placebo, washout, amitriptyline, and another washout (Pheasant H, 1983). Outcome measures included changes in activity level (measured by a functional rating and an activity questionnaire) and average weekly usage of concomitant analgesic drugs. Amitriptyline-treated patients did not experience any significant change in activity level, but they were able to reduce concomitant use of analgesics by 46% compared with placebo-treated patients.

Another trial found that amitriptyline was as effective as acetaminophen for reducing pain in patients with acute LBP. In this five-week double-blind comparator trial ($n = 39$), patients were randomized to receive either amitriptyline (150 mg/day) or acetaminophen (2000 mg/day); dosage was titrated to the therapeutic level over the initial four days of the study (Stein D, 1996). Pain was measured by the UCLA Pain Profile (UCLA-PP), a pain scale that uses a 15-cm VAS and a 7-point rating scale (1 = no pain; 7 ="worst pain imaginable"). At study completion, both the amitriptyline and the acetaminophen groups demonstrated significant improvements in pain; 79% of amitriptyline-treated patients and 75% of acetaminophen-treated patients reported a significant reduction in pain intensity. In addition, patients receiving amitriptyline had greater reductions in pain from the second week of treatment.

With regard to tolerability, amitriptyline's side effects, such as dry mouth, sedation, weight gain, orthostatic hypotension, and urinary retention, lead to a high rate of treatment discontinuation. Additionally, unlike gabapentin, amitriptyline treatment poses numerous potential problems with regard to drug interactions and contraindications, thereby limiting its use in various subsegments of the patient population (e.g., those taking monoamine oxidase inhibitors, anticholinergic agents, or anticoagulant therapy; those with glaucoma, prostatic hypertrophy, or a recent myocardial infarction).

Local Anesthetics

Overview. Local anesthetics, either as monotherapy or in combination with other agents, are occasionally used to treat chronic pain. The lidocaine patch (Endo's Lidoderm) is the most widely used lidocaine formulation for CLBP.

Mechanism of Action. Lidocaine exerts its analgesic effect by blocking voltage-activated sodium channels, which are responsible for nerve conduction. Neuronal signals carrying pain inputs are mediated via electrical impulses known as action potentials. The action potential is generated by ion gradients, involving sodium and potassium ions, which are established across the neuronal cell membrane. Lidocaine binds sodium channels and stabilizes them in their inactive state, thus impeding the inward flow of ions after an electrical stimulus and disrupting action potentials.

Lidocaine Patch. Lidocaine provides topical, localized relief of sciatica; it is not typically used to treat nonradiating CLBP. Lidocaine is available as a topical cream or gel (at both nonprescription and prescription strengths) and can be administered via infusion. However, for CLBP, lidocaine is administered as a prescription-strength 5% lidocaine patch, a 10 by 14 cm (700 mg) nonwoven polyethylene backing with a drug-containing adhesive layer. In the United States, the lidocaine patch is approved for the treatment of postherpetic neuralgia; Endo and Elan have a copromotion agreement whereby Elan promotes the drug to specialists while Endo promotes to PCPs. In Europe, Grunenthal is developing the lidocaine patch for neuropathic pain. In Japan, the patch is under development for neuropathic pain by Teikoku. (A lidocaine tape [Wyeth/Takeda Pharmaceutical's (Osaka, Japan) Penles] is available in Japan, but it is indicated only for the relief of pain when an IV catheter is inserted and is not available in a strength appropriate for chronic pain indications.)

In addition to the currently available lidocaine patch (Lidoderm), other lidocaine patch formulations are in development. Endo is developing a lidocaine patch for use in acute LBP (LidoPAIN BP) and is conducting Phase II trials in the United States and Europe. Kaken Pharmaceuticals (Tokyo, Japan) is reportedly developing a lidocaine patch for the treatment of postherpetic neuralgia in Japan (Phase II).

The lidocaine patch exerts its analgesic effect by blocking voltage-activated sodium channels on the peripheral nerves. Consequently, the rate of membrane depolarization drops, thereby increasing the threshold for electrical excitability and reducing neuronal hyperactivity. Patients generally apply up to three patches to intact skin—at the most painful site—for up to 12 hours (12 hours on, 12 hours off).

The lidocaine patch is an important alternative for patients suffering from neuropathic pain because of its lack of CNS side effects. Given that many CLBP patients receive long-term drug treatment—and patients often discontinue treatment because of systemic side effects—topical agents such as the lidocaine patch are an attractive choice for patients in whom use of orally administered therapies is contraindicated.

Although few well-designed placebo-controlled studies have been conducted in CLBP, a few open-label trials have demonstrated the lidocaine patch's ability to reduce pain for patients with this condition. A two-week, nonrandomized, prospective, open-label study ($n = 77$) of patients with postherpetic neuralgia, painful diabetic neuropathy, or LBP found that the lidocaine patch effectively treated all three conditions (Argoff CE, 2004). Inclusion criteria were partial response to gabapentin-containing analgesic regimens and moderate-to-severe pain, as measured by the Neuropathic Pain Scale (NPS). Patients were permitted to maintain existing analgesic regimens throughout the trial. The lidocaine patch was applied to the area of maximum pain (maximum of four patches, applied every 24 hours). The outcome measure was change from baseline at week 2 in four composite measures of the NPS. At study completion, patients with all three types of neuropathic pain experienced significant improvement on all four composite measures. More specifically, subgroup analyses revealed that the LBP patients had statistically significant improvements on all four NPS measures.

A second two-week, nonrandomized open-label pilot study—which assessed the effect of the lidocaine patch in combination with gabapentin (Pfizer's Neurontin, generics) on chronic pain—concluded that the lidocaine patch used in combination with gabapentin significantly relieved pain (Gimbel J, 2003a). The trial ($n = 107$) included patients with postherpetic neuralgia ($n = 11$), painful diabetic neuropathy ($n = 49$), and CLBP ($n = 47$). All patients had a partial response to gabapentin as a pain reliever before the study, but their average daily pain intensity scores at baseline were higher than 4, as measured by the BPI ($0 =$ no pain, $10 =$ intense pain). Patients were treated for two weeks with up to four lidocaine patches (applied every 24 hours) while continuing their current regimen of gabapentin. Outcome measures included pain interference with quality of life, as measured by the BPI, and global assessments of pain relief/patch satisfaction. Interim analyses of the first 50 patients (6 with postherpetic neuralgia, 13 with painful diabetic neuropathy, and 31 with CLBP) found that all patients showed significant improvements in BPI scores. A subgroup analysis of this study focused on the 47 patients with CLBP and found that combined therapy with the lidocaine patch and gabapentin significantly improved BPI pain intensity scores for this group (Speiller M, 2004).

Although, as mentioned earlier, the lidocaine patch is used primarily for sciatica (i.e., neuropathic CLBP), results from a two-week, prospective, nonrandomized, open-label, pilot study ($n = 129$) suggest that the lidocaine patch may also be effective for nonradiating (i.e., non-neuropathic) LBP (Gimbel J, 2003b). In the study, LBP patients were divided into three groups based on the duration of their pain: group 1 included patients with acute/subacute LBP lasting less than three months ($n = 20$), group 2 included patients with short-term CLBP lasting 3–12 months ($n = 33$), and group 3 included patients with long-term CLBP lasting longer than 12 months ($n = 76$). All patients maintained their analgesic regimens throughout the study. Patients received treatment with up to four lidocaine patches—applied every 24 hours—for the duration of the trial. At study completion, groups 1 and 3 experienced significant improvements in pain intensity and pain relief, as measured based on the BPI. All three groups also experienced statistically significant reductions in BPI composite scores for pain interference with quality of life and Beck Depression Inventory scores.

With regard to side effects, the lidocaine patch is fairly well tolerated when appropriately administered (i.e., 12 hours on/12 hours off). Side effects associated with the patch are generally limited to minor skin irritations (e.g., edema, burning, stinging, tenderness) at the site of application. In more severe cases, contact dermatitis or hives may occur.

Muscle Relaxants

Muscle relaxants help relieve pain attributable to muscle spasms. Drugs in this class are typically prescribed for patients with acute LBP and are not recommended for long-term therapy because they carry a risk of addiction. However, muscle relaxants are prescribed to many patients with CLBP to alleviate acute spasm attacks. In addition to relieving spasms, muscle relaxants are sedating and can therefore be beneficial to patients who have trouble sleeping because of their pain; however, muscle relaxants' sedative properties typically restrict their use to bedtime.

Availability and use of specific muscle relaxant agents vary across the major markets. In the United States, most physicians prescribe cyclobenzaprine (Johnson & Johnson's Flexeril, generics) or metaxalone (King Pharmaceutical's Skelaxin). European physicians tend to use baclofen (Novartis's Lioresal, generics), tizanidine (Novartis's Sirdalud, generics), or carisoprodol (Medpointe Pharmaceuticals [Somerset, New Jersey] Soma, generics). Commonly used muscle relaxants in Japan include eperisone (Eisai, Inc.'s [Woodcliff Lake, New Jersey] Myonal) and tizanidine.

Nonpharmacological Therapies

In addition to the pharmacological treatments discussed earlier, nonpharmacological approaches have an important place in the management of CLBP. Nonpharmacological therapies commonly used for CLBP include epidural blocks and electrical stimulation, which have a long history of use in CLBP, and artificial disc replacement, which represents a more recent form of intervention.

Epidural injections are used frequently to relieve CLBP in preoperative patients, especially those who have had pain for less than six months. Although this conservative intervention typically relieves pain only for a short time (analgesia lasts from one week to one year), the temporary reprieve allows patients to try other forms of rehabilitation.

Epidural injections work by delivering a dose of corticosteroids—which minimize the inflammation that may be responsible for the CLBP—directly onto or near the inflamed nerve root(s) in the painful region. The targeted injection limits systemic exposure and reduces the required dose of steroids, thereby lowering the potential for side effects. In general, a CLBP patient receives up to three injections per year, depending on the recurrence of pain. Although efficacy data are lacking, a meta-analysis suggests that epidural injections more than double the probability of short-term pain relief (Hession WG, 2004). Patient response appears to be enhanced if the epidural injection is used in conjunction with an integrated pharmacological and nonpharmacological treatment program.

Physicians may also use transcutaneous electronic nerve stimulation (TENS) to complement drug treatment of CLBP. Less invasive than epidural injections, TENS operates via peripherally placed electrodes that provide recurrent stimuli along the nerve pathway. A small battery-powered generator sends electricity through wires to the electrodes that are attached to the skin. An important advantage of TENS over drug therapy is that it is associated with few side effects and is therefore an important option for patients who cannot tolerate or who do not respond well to pharmacological treatment.

In cases where nerve compression is evident and more conservative measures have been unsuccessful at alleviating pain, surgery may be indicated. Historically, the surgical procedure used in cases of severe, unremitting CLBP has been discectomy and fusion. This relatively common procedure typically provides some relief for CLBP patients. However, the surgery usually limits a patient's mobility permanently, altering the biomechanics of the spine and causing further degeneration of surrounding spinal discs.

The reduced spinal mobility following discectomy and fusion has prompted device companies to develop a prosthetic disc that can be surgically implanted in place of an injured native disc. Artificial discs have been available in Europe for more than a decade, and in October 2004, the FDA granted the first U.S. approval for an artificial disc--Charité, developed by DePuy Spine, Inc. (Raynham, Massachusetts) a Johnson & Johnson company. The device is indicated for painful single-level degenerative lumbar disc disease that is unresponsive to at least six months of conservative treatment. The prosthetic disc comprises an articulating ultra-high-molecular-weight polyethylene core surrounded by concave metallic endplates; it is implanted through an abdominal incision. Less invasive alternatives to complete disc replacement are also being developed, including replacement of the injured nucleus pulposus.

Another form of electrical therapy in CLBP is spinal cord stimulation (SCS), which is often used to treat LBP following failed spinal surgery (i.e., failed back syndrome). During SCS, electrodes are inserted into the epidural space near the painful region, either percutaneously or after laminectomy (surgical removal of part of a vertebra in order to gain access to spinal cord nerves); the electrode leads are connected to an external or implanted pulse generator. Although there are few well-constructed clinical trials of SCS, a review of the literature suggests that one year after undergoing SCS, 50–60% of patients who failed back surgery experience a reduction in pain of at least 50% (Turner JA, 1995). There are no known significant long-term side effects associated with SCS.

In addition to epidural injections, SCS, and artificial disc replacement, other nondrug approaches used to treat CLBP include massage, acupuncture, psychosocial rehabilitation, and exercise therapy. They are typically used in conjunction with pharmacological treatment.

EMERGING THERAPIES

This section reviews agents in development for chronic low back pain (CLBP). It also discusses drugs that are not being studied specifically for CLBP but that are expected to be used for patients with this condition (i.e., drugs in development for other chronic pain conditions). Most emerging therapies fall into the latter category, given that few drug companies are actively testing their pain drugs in CLBP patients. In general, companies shy away from conducting clinical trials in CLBP because of the difficulties related to the design and execution of such studies. Many companies therefore seek approval in other chronic pain indications, or more generally in broader chronic pain, knowing that their drugs will still be used to treat CLBP.

Because of the large patient population, the pain markets—and the CLBP market in particular—represent an enticing commercial opportunity for drug manufacturers. Accordingly, a plethora of drug classes are under study for the treatment of CLBP (or chronic pain). This section covers drugs that will be used for nonradiating CLBP and/or chronic sciatica (i.e., CLBP of a neuropathic origin), including new selective cyclooxygenase-2 (COX-2) inhibitors, narcotic analgesics, neurotoxins, antiepileptic drugs (AEDs), antidepressants, and tumor necrosis factor inhibitors. It also provides brief overviews of nitric-oxide-releasing drugs, cannabinoid receptor modulators, and NMDA receptor antagonists. The calcium-channel blocker ziconotide (Elan's Prialt) is not discussed in detail.

Table 4 summarizes the most promising drug therapies in development for chronic pain. Table 5 lists reformulations of narcotic analgesics in development for chronic pain.

Selective Cyclooxygenase-2 Inhibitors

Overview. The success of first-to-market selective COX-2 inhibitors (e.g., Merck's rofecoxib [Vioxx], Pfizer's celecoxib [Celebrex]) was due to their reduced gastrointestinal (GI) side effects in comparison to those of NSAIDs, which suppress COX indiscriminately. Based on this success, drug manufacturers developed new COX-2 inhibitors with an even greater degree of selectivity for COX-2; developers believed that the increased specificity for COX-2 would further reduce the incidence of GI effects, thereby allowing administration at higher doses to provide superior analgesia.

However, recent concerns regarding the cardiovascular/cerebrovascular safety of COX-2 inhibitors (discussed in greater detail in "Current Therapies") have drastically lowered expectations for new COX-2 agents. Following the withdrawal of two COX-2 agents (i.e., rofecoxib, valdecoxib [Pfizer's Bextra]) from the market, it now seems unlikely that new COX-2 inhibitors will be approved. The significantly lowered sales potential associated with COX-2 inhibitors suggests that drug manufacturers will abandon development of this class. This section focuses on etoricoxib (Merck's Arcoxia) because it is the only COX-2 in development specifically for CLBP and it is already marketed in Europe. (Lumiracoxib [Novartis's Prexige] is not discussed here because it is unlikely to launch given the current regulatory environment.)

Mechanism of Action. Unlike NSAIDs, which block both COX-1 and COX-2 fairly indiscriminately, selective COX-2 inhibitors predominantly inhibit COX-2. Selective COX-2 inhibitors therefore reduce pathological inflammation caused by prostaglandins without disrupting their beneficial effects.

TABLE 4. Emerging Therapies in Development for Chronic Low Back Pain

Compound	Development Phase[a]	Marketing Company
Selective COX-2 inhibitors		
Etoricoxib (Arcoxia)		
United States	PR	Merck
Europe	—[b]	Merck
Japan	—	—
Narcotic analgesics		
Oxycodone/naltrexone (OxyTrex)		
United States	—[c]	Pain Therapeutics
Europe	—	—
Japan	—	—
Oxymorphone ER (EN-3202)		
United States	—[d]	Endo/Penwest
Europe	—	—
Japan	—	—
Neurotoxins		
Botulinum toxin type A (Botox)		
United States	III	Allergan
Europe	III	Allergan
Japan	—[e]	Allergan
Antiepileptic drugs		
Pregabalin (Lyrica)		
United States	—[f]	Pfizer
Europe	—[f]	Pfizer
Japan	—[f]	Pfizer
Lamotrigine (Lamictal)		
United States	—[g]	GlaxoSmithKline
Europe	—[g]	GlaxoSmithKline
Japan	—[h]	GlaxoSmithKline
Antidepressants		
Duloxetine (Cymbalta/Xeristar)		
United States	—[i]	Eli Lilly
Europe	—[j]	Eli Lilly/Boehringer Ingelheim
Japan	—[k]	Eli Lilly
Bicifadine		
United States	—[l]	DOV Pharmaceutical
Europe	—	—
Japan	—	—
Tumor necrosis factor inhibitors		
REN-1654		
United States	II	Renovis
Europe	—	—
Japan	—	—

[a]Development phase is for chronic low back pain (CLBP).

[b]Etoricoxib is currently marketed in Europe for osteoarthritis, rheumatoid arthritis, and acute gouty arthritis.

[c]Oxycodone/naltrexone is in Phase III trials for chronic pain in the United States.

[d]Oxymorphone ER is preregistered for cancer pain and musculoskeletal pain in the United States.

[e]Botulinum toxin type A is marketed in Japan for a variety of nonpain indications including cervical dystonia, strabismus, spasmodic torticollis, blepharospasm associated with dystonia, reduction of facial wrinkles, and primary axillary hyperhidrosis.

[f]Pregabalin is approved for painful diabetic neuropathy and postherpetic neuralgia in the United States, approved for peripheral neuropathic pain in Europe, and in Phase II trials for epilepsy in Japan.

[g]Lamotrigine is marketed for the treatment of epileptic seizures and is in Phase III trials for neuropathic pain in the United States and Europe.

[h]Lamotrigine is preregistered for epilepsy in Japan.

[i]Duloxetine is approved in the United States for the treatment of peripheral diabetic neuropathy.

[j]Duloxetine is approved in Europe for the treatment of peripheral diabetic neuropathic pain.

[k]Duloxetine is in Phase III trials for depression in Japan.

[l]Bicifadine is in Phase III trials for pain in the United States and DOV Pharmaceutical will likely pursue approval for CLBP.

PR = Preregistered.

TABLE 5. Narcotic Reformulations in Development for Chronic Pain

Compound	Company	Phase of Development[a]
Narcotic combination drugs		
Oxycodone/ibuprofen (Combunox)	Forest Laboratories	Registered
Morphine/ dextromethorphan (EN 3231; MorphiDex)	Endo Pharmaceuticals	Phase III
Hydrocodone/acetaminophen/ dextromethorphan (EN-3232; HydrocoDex)	Endo Pharmaceuticals	Phase II
Oxycodone/aspirin/dextromethorphan (OxycoDex)	Endo Pharmaceuticals	Phase II
Morphine/naltrexone (PTI-555)	Pain Therapeutics	Phase II
PTI-701 (hydrocodone/acetaminophen/naltrexone)	Pain Therapeutics	Phase II
Alvimopan (Entereg)/undisclosed narcotic analgesic drug	Adolor	Phase II
Controlled-release formulations		
Hydromorphone once-daily (Palladone XL)	Purdue	Registered
Hydromorphone once-daily (Dilaudid CR)	Abbott Laboratories/Alza	Preregistered
Hydrocodone/acetaminophen controlled-release (Vicodin CR)	Abbott Laboratories	Phase II
Transdermal patches		
Sufentanil (transdermal)	Endo Pharmaceuticals/ Durect Corporation	Phase II
Hydromorphone patch (AT-1022)	Altea Therapeutics	Phase II
Seven-day fentanyl patch	3 M/Purdue	Phase I
Subcutaneous implants		
Sufentanil implant (Chronogesic)	Durect	Phase III
Inhaled formulations		
Aero-LEF (aerosolized liposome encapsulated fentanyl)	Delex Therapeutics	Phase II

[a]Represents highest phase of development for any pain indication in the major markets (United States, France, Germany, Italy, Spain, United Kingdom, and Japan).
Note: Table includes reformulations likely to be used to treat chronic low back pain (CLBP) regardless of specific development for this indication.

Etoricoxib. Merck's second-generation COX-2 inhibitor, etoricoxib (Arcoxia) (Figure 17), was approved in the United Kingdom in April 2002 for once-daily treatment of osteoarthritis (OA), rheumatoid arthritis (RA), acute gouty arthritis (AGA), acute dental pain, dysmenorrhea, and chronic musculoskeletal pain, including CLBP. The United Kingdom acted as the reference state for approval in the rest of Western Europe. However, in August 2002, as part of the European Union's mutual recognition procedure, the licensed indications for etoricoxib were revised to include only OA, RA, and AGA. In October 2002, etoricoxib received approval for these indications in most of Europe, excluding France and Germany, where the drug met with government resistance because of its anticipated high cost. However, by 2005, etoricoxib was launched in four European markets.

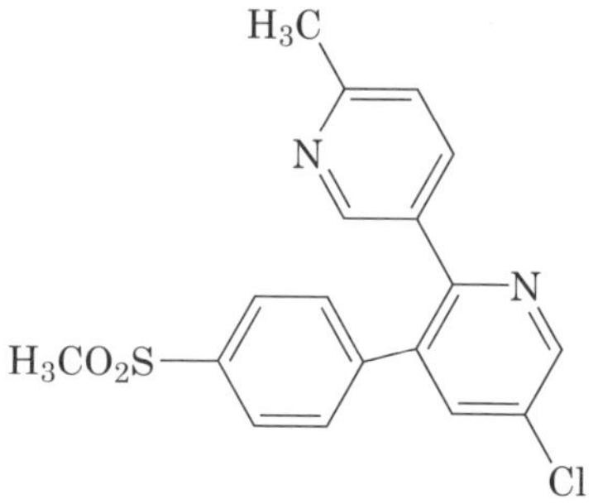

FIGURE 17. *Structure of etoricoxib.*

The U.K. launch of etoricoxib came on the heels of Merck's withdrawal of its March 2002 initial new drug application (NDA) in the United States; Merck withdrew the NDA after the FDA requested additional data on etoricoxib's efficacy for acute pain and on its cardiovascular safety. In December 2003, Merck resubmitted its revised NDA for etoricoxib that included CLBP as well as OA, RA, acute pain, dysmenorrhea, AGA, and ankylosing spondylitis. In October 2004, the FDA issued an approvable letter for etoricoxib but stated that additional safety and efficacy data would be required before the agency would grant final approval. If etoricoxib is approved, it will be the first COX-2 inhibitor to carry specific labeling for CLBP.

The primary difference between etoricoxib and first-generation selective COX-2 inhibitors is its high selectivity (COX-1/COX-2 IC50) ratio—at 344, it is the highest of all COX-2 drugs and threefold more selective than rofecoxib (Cochrane DJ, 2002). A meta-analysis showed that etoricoxib does not increase the risk of adverse GI effects (Curtis S, 2002). This analysis of ten Phase II and III comparator trials for OA, RA, and CLBP included 3142 patients who were treated once daily with etoricoxib (60 mg, 90 mg, or 120 mg) and 1828 patients who were treated daily with traditional NSAIDs (diclofenac 150 mg, ibuprofen 2400 mg, or naproxen 1000 mg). The rate of upper GI events per 100 patient-years was 1.35 and 3.42 for etoricoxib and traditional NSAIDs, respectively. The study did not report an analysis of upper GI events by drug dose. Overall, etoricoxib-treated patients developed 53% fewer GI perforations, ulcers, and bleeding than did patients receiving traditional NSAIDs. Another combined data review of 3,348 patients involved in etoricoxib trials showed that the renovascular profile of etoricoxib is comparable to that of nonselective NSAIDs, including naproxen and ibuprofen (Curtis SP, 2004), indicating that etoricoxib is no more toxic to the kidneys than traditional NSAIDs.

Unlike other COX-2s, etoricoxib has been tested in large placebo-controlled CLBP trials because it is being developed specifically for CLBP. These studies suggest that etoricoxib is effective at reducing the pain associated with this condition and at improving patient function (Birbara CA, 2003; Geba GP, 2002; Pallay RM, 2004). One double-blind, placebo-controlled trial ($n = 325$) assessed the efficacy of etoricoxib treatment in relieving CLBP over a three-month period (Pallay RM, 2004). The trial population had a mean age of 53 years (range = 19–78) and an average CLBP duration of 12 years. Patients were randomized to receive either 60 mg etoricoxib, 90 mg etoricoxib, or placebo (administered once a day, in the morning). The primary end point was improvement from baseline over four weeks, measured using an LBP intensity scale (a 100 mm visual analogue scale [VAS], where 0 = no pain and 100 = severe pain). At four weeks, both etoricoxib-treated groups experienced significant pain reduction (60 mg = −34.4, 90 mg = −32.3) compared with placebo (−19.3). The study also showed that the reduction in pain intensity values was maintained at three months (−35.1, −35.7, and −23.0, respectively).

A second double-blind, placebo-controlled CLBP study also found etoricoxib to be superior to placebo. In this trial ($n = 319$), constructed identically to the previous study, CLBP patients who had an average duration of 12 years with pain were randomized to receive once daily 60 mg etoricoxib, 90 mg etoricoxib, or placebo (Birbara CA, 2003). As in the first study, the primary outcome measure was improvement from baseline over four weeks, measured using an LBP intensity scale (a 100 mm VAS, where 0 = no pain and 100 = severe pain). At four weeks, treatment with etoricoxib (either 60 mg or 90 mg) resulted in significant improvements from baseline in pain intensity compared with placebo; patients taking 60 mg or 90 mg etoricoxib experienced mean VAS reductions of 36.13 mm and 33.48 mm, respectively, whereas patients receiving placebo experienced a mean reduction of 23.19.

Treatment with etoricoxib also improved patients' functioning, according to an analysis that reviewed the secondary end points from the two identically constructed placebo-controlled trials described earlier (Birbara CA, 2003; Pallay RM, 2004). This analysis of 644 patients found that etoricoxib (60 mg or 90 mg) significantly improved functional status after 12 weeks, as measured using the Roland-Morris Disability Questionnaire (RMDQ) (Geba GP, 2002); RMDQ scores in the 60 mg and 90 mg etoricoxib-treated groups were reduced by 6.85 points and 6.43 points, respectively, whereas scores in the placebo-treated group declined by 4.21 points. In addition, etoricoxib-treated patients exhibited significant functional improvements in standing, walking, getting dressed, and climbing steps. No difference in treatment effect was noted between the two etoricoxib treatment groups.

Given the withdrawal of both rofecoxib and valdecoxib from the market in the United States and Europe, etoricoxib's commercial future remains bleak, despite positive efficacy data from CLBP trials. Although results from the Etoricoxib Diclofenac Gastrointestinal Evaluation (EDGE) study demonstrated a mortality rate like that of diclofenac and although the two drugs showed similar overall cardiovascular thromboembolic event rates (Baraf H, 2004), the FDA said it found an increased risk for both congestive heart failure-related events and hypertension for patients receiving etoricoxib, based on its review of NDA data (FDA discloses safety reviews of Arcoxia, Prexige, and Parecoxib, 2005). However, results from the large Multinational Etoricoxib Diclofenac Arthritis Long-Term (MEDAL) cardiovascular safety study and the EDGE II study—expected in 2006—may be able to shed more light on whether etoricoxib's cardiovascular profile is more like the safer celecoxib or the other COX-2s (e.g., rofecoxib, valdecoxib).

Narcotic Analgesics

Overview. Long-term (chronic) narcotic therapy for CLBP is typically a last resort for patients with this problem. Narcotic agents are more often used for the short-term management of breakthrough pain (pain that occurs despite long-term chronic therapy with other analgesics). Narcotic analgesics are administered either as monotherapies or in conjunction with other pain-relieving agents.

Despite proven efficacy in treating chronic pain, narcotic analgesic use is limited by side effects (e.g., nausea, constipation) and the risk of tolerance and/or abuse. To reduce the risk of dependency associated with chronic therapy, physicians prefer long-acting or sustained-release agents over immediate-release formulations because these agents deliver steady pain relief with less euphoric effect. However, because long-acting narcotic analgesics are not risk-free, physicians prescribe them with caution, and generally only to patients with highly refractory pain. Chronic narcotic therapy of CLBP is usually prescribed by specialists, who are more comfortable using these drugs in this setting; PCPs generally refer patients who require chronic narcotic treatment to specialists rather than continuing this therapy on their own.

Because narcotic analgesics are effective pain relievers, many drug companies are developing agents in this class. This class is also attractive to drug developers because many popular narcotic molecules are no longer patent-protected, making them good targets for reformulations. Some drug companies are studying agents that will provide equivalent efficacy without the risk of dependence. Pain Therapeutics is developing two such agents: an abuse-resistant formulation of oxycodone (Remoxy; currently in Phase III trials) and an oxycodone/naltrexone combination drug (OxyTrex). Oxycodone/naltrexone is discussed in detail here because it is being tested in CLBP patients (Remoxy is not currently under study for CLBP).

Other companies are developing reformulations of existing narcotic agents. Reformulations, which include extended-release forms as well as a variety of delivery systems (e.g., transdermal patches, combination pills), will see some use in CLBP. The discussion of reformulations is limited to Endo/Penwest's oxymorphone ER because it is being investigated in clinical trials for CLBP and recently received an approvable letter in the United States.

Mechanism of Action. Narcotic analgesics effect analgesia via their interaction with opiate receptors in the central nervous system (CNS), primarily the mu and kappa opiate receptors. Some evidence suggests that these agents also act at the delta opioid receptors. The mu receptor has been identified in the neural tissue of areas that are part of the body's descending pain pathway, such as the periaqueductal gray area and medial thalamus area of the brain and dorsal horn of the spinal cord. Narcotic analgesics' activity at these receptors also mediates their adverse effects. The mu receptor mediates euphoria, respiratory depression, and constipation. The kappa receptor mediates sedation. The delta receptor mediates dysphoria and psychomimetic effects (i.e., hallucinations). Other common adverse effects of opioid use include urinary retention, orthostatic hypotension, constipation, and nausea and vomiting (attributable to these agents' direct stimulation of emetic chemoreceptors in the brain; these effects usually resolve after several days of therapy).

Oxycodone/Naltrexone Combination. Oxycodone/naltrexone (OxyTrex), a combination of immediate-release oxycodone and the opioid antagonist naltrexone, is in Phase III trials for the treatment of chronic pain in the United States. Pain Therapeutics is also partnering with Durect in the United States to develop a sustained-release formulation of oxycodone/naltrexone. At this time, oxycodone/naltrexone does not appear to be in development in Europe or Japan.

Oxycodone is a semisynthetic opioid that, like all narcotic analgesics, relieves pain via its interaction with opiate receptors in the CNS. Naltrexone (DuPont's ReVia/Bristol-Myers Squibb's [North Billerica, Massachusetts] Nalorex), indicated for the treatment of narcotic addiction, blocks the euphoric effects of opioids by competitive binding at opioid receptors. Pain Therapeutics believes that the combination of oxycodone with nanogram quantities of naltrexone will offer analgesia with a reduced risk of tolerance and dependence (compared with oxycodone alone); company reports of preclinical study data suggest that oxycodone/naltrexone is less prone to inducing opioid tolerance, dependence, and withdrawal effects.

Clinical human data released recently appear promising. In March 2005, Pain Therapeutics released data from a Phase III study involving ambulatory patients with moderate-to-severe CLBP. Although the primary end point of analgesic efficacy was not met, results from this trial suggest that treatment with oxycodone/naltrexone provided pain relief similar to that offered by oxycodone alone but with fewer side effects and symptoms of withdrawal effects, according to the company. In this double-blind, placebo-controlled study ($n = 719$), CLBP patients were randomized to receive oxycodone/naltrexone bid (twice daily), oxycodone/naltrexone qid (four times daily), oxycodone qid, or placebo (following a four- to ten-day washout period). Patients then entered a six-week titration period, during which dosage was increased to a maximum of 80 mg oxycodone/naltrexone or oxycodone qid (or placebo). Dose escalation ended when patients reported "adequate" pain relief (defined as <2 out of 10 on the Likert Pain Scale) or intolerable side effects. Following the titration phase, treatment was continued for three months. Patients were evaluated at the end of the study for withdrawal effects (measured using the Short Opiate Withdrawal Scale [SOWS]).

Although the oxycodone/naltrexone and oxycodone groups reported similar pain relief (approximately 45% mean reduction in pain intensity from baseline) at study completion, patients in both oxycodone/naltrexone groups required significantly less narcotic drug (35 mg per day) to achieve pain relief similar to that obtained by patients in the oxycodone group. Furthermore, oxycodone/ naltrexone bid provided pain relief equivalent to that of oxycodone qid. Opioid-related side effects were about 20% lower overall in the oxycodone/naltrexone bid group than in the oxycodone qid group; patients in the oxycodone/naltrexone bid group experienced 44% less moderate-to-severe constipation compared with patients in the oxycodone group. Pruritis and somnolence rates—although not quantified/revealed in the press release—were also reportedly lower in the oxycodone/naltrexone bid group. In addition, patients receiving oxycodone/naltrexone bid had a substantially lower mean SOWS score than did patients taking oxycodone qid (1.2 with the combination drug versus 2.6 with oxycodone) after drug discontinuation. The overall dropout rate was approximately 50%. Results from the study for oxycodone/naltrexone qid were not disclosed.

Oxycodone/naltrexone's potential to provide effective analgesia with a lower incidence of side effects (i.e., constipation) compared with other narcotic analgesics will likely be a key advantage in the CLBP market because many patients require chronic long-term treatment. CLBP patients may find the combination narcotic more tolerable than other drugs in this class and, as a result, discontinue therapy less often. In addition, physicians may be more likely to prescribe oxycodone/naltrexone because of its lower risk of dependence/tolerance. Therefore, oxycodone/naltrexone will likely gain a place as a first-line narcotic therapy for CLBP.

If confirmed in further studies, oxycodone/naltrexone's potentially superior tolerability would be an obvious commercial advantage over oxycodone and other existing narcotic agents. A likely lower risk of tolerance and dependence compared with other narcotics would be a further benefit. However, because it will probably carry a similar risk of addiction and abuse, oxycodone/naltrexone will likely be classified as a controlled substance (i.e., as a Schedule II drug) in the same manner as currently available narcotics. Nevertheless, trial results demonstrating less severe withdrawal symptoms might convince regulatory agencies to approve less restrictive labeling—albeit still with Schedule II status—and permit slightly longer-term use for oxycodone/naltrexone than for other Schedule II drugs.

Oxymorphone Extended-Release.   Endo and Penwest Pharmaceutical (Patterson, New York) are codeveloping an extended-release (ER) formulation of oxymorphone (EN-3202) (Figure 18) for the treatment of moderate-to-severe pain. In October 2003, the FDA issued an approvable letter for oxymorphone ER, but the agency requested additional clinical trials to confirm the drug's safety and efficacy. In response to this request, Endo/Penwest will conduct a 12-week Phase III trial of oxymorphone in CLBP patients with no prior narcotic treatment. Oxymorphone ER is not in development in Europe or Japan, and Endo has no plans to launch the drug outside of the United States.

Oxymorphone ER is a semisynthetic mu opioid agonist that has a more rapid onset of action and several times the analgesic potency of its parent compound morphine. The agent has been developed to provide 12 hours of continuous analgesia. The sustained-release matrix, TIMERx (Penwest Pharmaceuticals), alters

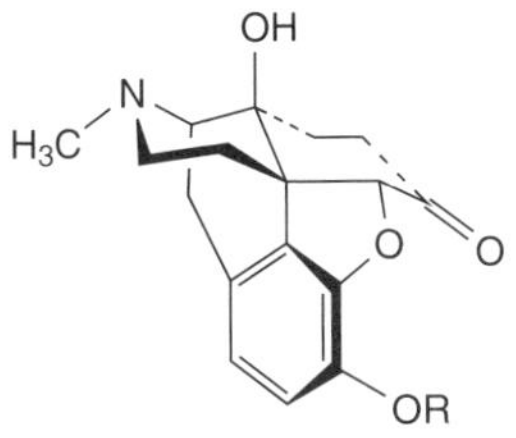

FIGURE 18. *Structure of oxymorphone (R=H).*

and delays drug dissolution and absorption from the gastrointestinal tract, thereby changing the pharmacokinetic profile relative to immediate-release drug formulations. Drug release from the sustained-release matrix is controlled by the rate of penetration of water into the hydrophilic matrix and the subsequent expansion of the gel coating. A linear dose relationship is required so that a predictable dose response of both efficacy and safety can be achieved.

An earlier Phase III trial demonstrated that CLBP patients treated with oxymorphone ER experienced pain relief similar to that of patients taking oxycodone CR (Hale ME, 2005). In this comparator study ($n = 213$), ambulatory patients with moderate-to-severe CLBP requiring opioid therapy were randomized to receive either oxymorphone ER (10–110 mg) or oxycodone CR (20–220 mg), administered every 12 hours during a 7- to 14-day dose-titration period. Patients who stabilized entered a double-blind treatment phase, during which they were re-randomized to receive their original active drug or placebo for eighteen days. The primary outcome measure was change from baseline, as measured using a 100-mm VAS. At study completion, oxymorphone ER and oxycodone CR significantly improved VAS scores compared with placebo, with no statistical significance between the two active treatment groups. Adverse events for the two narcotic drugs were also similar.

Narcotic Reformulations. The bulk of narcotic analgesic development activity focuses on reformulations of existing molecules (see Table 5 for a list of key narcotic reformulations in development for chronic pain that will likely be used for CLBP). Some drug companies (e.g., Forest Laboratories, Endo Pharmaceuticals, Adolor Corporation [Exton, Pennsylvania], Pain Therapeutics [South San Francisco, California]) are developing therapies that combine a narcotic analgesic with an NSAID, NMDA receptor antagonist, or opioid antagonist. Combination therapies are designed to reduce the risk of tolerance, ease side effects, or enhance efficacy. Other companies (e.g., Purdue, Abbott, Alza) are developing CR formulations of existing narcotic drugs. Yet another approach espoused by some companies (e.g., Altea Therapeutics [Tuker, Georgia], DURECT Corporation [Cupertino, California], 3M [St. Paul, Minnesota], Purdue, Delex Therapeutics, Inc. [Mississauga, Ontario, Canada]) is to reformulate existing narcotic molecules into non-oral delivery systems such as transdermal patches, subcutaneous implants, or inhaled formulations.

Neurotoxins

Overview. Neurotoxins are poisons that act on the nervous system. Found in many animals, neurotoxins provide protection from predators, so the effects of these compounds are of necessity highly toxic. Many neurotoxins affect neuromuscular junctions and therefore have broadly systemic effects; for example, the neuromuscular junction in skeletal muscle involves all voluntary and respiratory muscles. However, the controlled, localized application of a neurotoxin can effectively damage a single neuromuscular junction without the adverse (and sometimes fatal) side effects associated with systemic application.

Mechanism of Action. Neurotoxins work by inhibiting essential neural activity. Many bind irreversibly to ion channels, interfering with channel function, blocking channel activation, or inhibiting the flow of ions through channels, thereby disrupting normal neurotransmission. In addition, neurotoxins can block vital neurotransmitter receptors, such as glutamate and nicotinic (acetylcholine) receptors (Reisner L, 2004; Thant ZS, 2003).

Nerve injuries such as those that often contribute to CLBP can alter the dynamics of neural activity. For example, a damaged neuron can become hyperactive—in other words, its threshold for initiating an action potential drops so low that the nerve becomes overactive, sending too many messages to the brain. Overactivity of a neuron at a neuromuscular junction results in continuous muscle contraction (spasms) and pain. A locally applied neurotoxin can effectively block the activation of ion channels and stop the initiation of these action potentials.

Botulinum Toxin Type A. Botulinum toxin type A (BTX-A; Allergan, Inc.'s [Irvine, California] Botox) is marketed for cervical dystonia, strabismus (cross-eyes), spasmodic torticollis (wryneck, a twisting of the neck to one side that results in abnormal carriage of the head), blepharospasm (spasmodic blinking) associated with dystonia, reduction of facial wrinkles, and primary axillary hyperhidrosis (excessive underarm sweating). BTX-A appears to be in Phase III trials for CLBP in the United States and Europe.

BTX-A is a purified neurotoxin complex that inhibits the release of acetylcholine, resulting in the inhibition or relaxation of muscle overactivity. The drug is thought to bind irreversibly to acceptor sites on presynaptic nerve terminals, becoming internalized with the nerve terminal. Once inside the terminal, BTX-A is thought to interfere with the exocytosis of cholinergic vesicles, which contain acetylcholine, from the nerve ending. BTX-A blockage of acetylcholine release leads to chemical denervation of the muscle site, degrading it to the point that the nerve can no longer signal the muscle to contract. This denervation can result in muscle atrophy, but if injected intramuscularly, BTX-A provides an effect that is localized to the site of injury or pain and is temporary (approximately 12 weeks). Such an effect would be of benefit to CLBP patients, who can suffer from chronic spasms in muscles of the lumbar region as a result of nerve or tissue damage, resulting in pain.

Few large, well-designed clinical trials have investigated BTX-A's efficacy in CLBP. One small eight-week double-blind study ($n = 31$) showed that treatment with BTX-A provided a greater than 50% improvement in pain intensity compared with baseline levels (Foster L, 2001). Patients were randomized to receive either BTX-A injections (40 units/site of BTX-A at five lumbar paravertebral sites) or placebo (normal saline injections at the same sites). The primary outcome measure was level of pain, measured using a VAS and the Oswestry Low Back Pain Questionnaire (OLBPQ). Patients were reassessed and measured against baseline scores at three and eight weeks postinjection. At three weeks, 73.3% of BTX-A-treated patients had a greater than 50% reduction in their pain scores, versus only 25% of the placebo-treated patients. At eight weeks, 60% of the BTX-A-treated patients still had pain relief, compared with 12.5% of the placebo group. In addition, disability scores (as measured by the OLBPQ) were improved in 66.7% of the BTX-A-treated group versus 18.8% of the placebo-treated patients. Open-label trials also support BTX-A's efficacy in CLBP (Aglan M, 2003; Dunteman E, 2003; Edwards K, 2003; Edwards K, 2004; Subin B, 2003), and additional placebo-controlled studies are ongoing.

Adverse reactions with BTX-A are rare; the studies mentioned here did not report adverse events. The most common adverse effect reported during BTX-A's use in approved indications is muscle weakness in the local region of the injection. Because intramuscular injections result primarily in local effects, systemic adverse effects are reduced.

Antiepileptic Drugs

Overview. Although AEDs were originally approved for the treatment of epileptic seizures, strong similarities between the pathophysiological and biochemical mechanisms of epilepsy and neuropathic pain make them effective therapies for chronic sciatica (Backonja MM, 2002). Because older AEDs have pronounced side effects (e.g., sedation, cerebellar symptoms, hematological changes, cardiac arrhythmia, teratogenicity), second-generation AEDs are the most commonly used to treat sciatica. Of the many second-generation agents that are available, gabapentin (Pfizer's Neurontin; discussed in "Current Therapies") and pregabalin (Pfizer's Lyrica) are the only two that are approved for the treatment of neuropathic pain; gabapentin is approved for postherpetic neuralgia in the United States and peripheral neuropathic pain in Europe, and pregabalin was recently approved for painful diabetic neuropathy and postherpetic neuralgia in the United States and for peripheral neuropathic pain in Europe. Other second-generation AEDs (lamotrigine [GlaxoSmithKline's Lamictal], oxcarbazepine [Novartis's Trileptal], topiramate [Ortho-McNeil's Topamax, Janssen's Epitomax], tiagabine (Cephalon, Inc.'s [Frazer, Pennsylvania] Gabitril), zonisamide (Dainippon Pharmaceutical's [Osaka, Japan] Excegran, Eisai's Zonegran), and levetiracetam [UCB's Keppra]) are used off-label to treat various types of neuropathic pain. Pregabalin and lamotrigine are discussed in detail here.

In addition to the currently available AEDs, drug companies are investigating several compounds, including XenoPort, Inc.'s (Santa Clara, California)

XP-13512 (gabapentin pro-drug), Schwarz Pharma's (Milwaukee, Wisconsin) lacosamide (formerly known as harkoseride/SPM-927), Newron Pharmaceuticals's (Gerenzano, Italy) ralfinamide, and Icagen, Inc.'s (Durham North Carolina) ICA-69673. Based on the success of other AEDs for treating neuropathic pain, these emerging drugs may see some use in CLBP as well.

Mechanism of Action. Through various mechanisms, AEDs reduce the generation of neuronal action potentials that carry electrical signals from the pain's site of origin to the CNS. According to pain experts, similarities between the pathophysiological changes observed in epilepsy and in neuropathic pain animal models further support the role of AEDs in neuropathic pain (Carrazana E, 2003; Hansen HC, 1999). Both epilepsy and neuropathic pain processes are, in part, linked to the activation of NMDA receptors. In addition, sodium-channel antagonists effectively block neuronal transmission in animal models of both epilepsy and neuropathic pain. These preclinical observations have been borne out in positive efficacy results in clinical practice and clinical trials.

Pregabalin. Pregabalin (Figure 19) is Pfizer's follow-on to its highly successful AED gabapentin, which now faces generic competition in the United States. Like gabapentin, pregabalin will probably be prescribed for patients with chronic sciatica—approximately 14% of the total CLBP population—as opposed to CLBP patients with pain of a non-neuropathic origin. In July 2004, pregabalin was granted marketing approval in the European Union for peripheral neuropathic pain and as adjunctive therapy for partial epileptic seizures; the drug was launched in the United Kingdom, its first market, in August 2004. In Japan, pregabalin is in Phase II trials for epilepsy.

In January 2005, pregabalin received U.S. approval from the FDA for painful diabetic neuropathy and postherpetic neuralgia. However, pregabalin failed to gain approval for two additional indications in the United States; in September 2004, the FDA deemed the drug "nonapprovable" for generalized anxiety disorder and did not give final approval for use as an adjunctive therapy for partial epileptic seizures. In addition, pregabalin will be classified as a Schedule V controlled substance, based on study results suggesting that the AED produces effects similar to other controlled substances. According to the Drug Enforcement Administration (DEA) website, pregabalin's Schedule V status results from the FDA's determination that the risk of dependence or abuse is less with pregabalin than with Schedule IV drugs (i.e., benzodiazepines). Pregabalin is the only

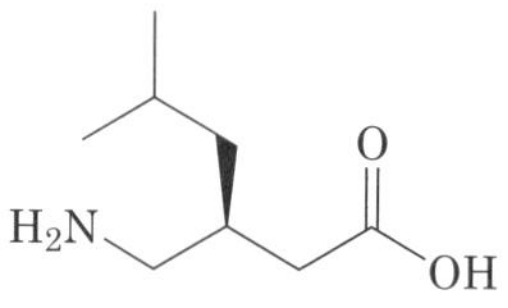

FIGURE 19. *Structure of pregabalin.*

AED to be classified as a scheduled drug and will therefore face more stringent prescribing restrictions in the United States than other agents in the class.

Like gabapentin, pregabalin is believed to exert its antiepileptic and analgesic effects by blocking voltage-gated presynaptic N- and P/Q-type calcium channels via a specific subunit called the alpha-2-delta subunit (a high-affinity binding site in neuronal membranes) (Dooley DJ, 2002; Fink K, 2002; Gee NS, 1996). Pregabalin's purported benefits over gabapentin include its higher potency and more predictable pharmacokinetics, which allow it to be administered in lower doses than gabapentin (300–600 mg/day versus 1800–2400 mg/day, respectively) and to be more rapidly titrated to an effective dose.

Although pregabalin has not been tested in large, well-designed trials with sciatica patients, it has demonstrated efficacy in other types of neuropathic pain (e.g., postherpetic neuralgia, painful diabetic neuropathy) (Dworkin RH, 2003; Rosenstock J, 2004; Sabatowski R, 2004; Strojek K, 2004). In these studies, the most common side effects associated with pregabalin treatment were somnolence, dizziness, and peripheral edema.

Lamotrigine. Lamotrigine (GlaxoSmithKline's Lamictal) (Figure 20) is approved in the United States and Europe and is preregistered in Japan for the treatment of epileptic seizures; it is also approved for the long-term maintenance treatment of bipolar disorder in the United States. Since the publication of positive trial data from small trials in patients with neuropathic pain over the past few years, physicians have begun prescribing lamotrigine for various neuropathic pain indications, including sciatica. Although GlaxoSmithKline will probably pursue supplemental approval for other neuropathic pain conditions (in particular, painful diabetic neuropathy), the company is less likely to seek specific labeling for CLBP.

If GlaxoSmithKline is successful in achieving neuropathic pain labeling for lamotrigine, the company will most certainly advance its extended-release (XR) formulation of the drug, which is reportedly in Phase I trials in the United Kingdom, to later-stage trials for neuropathic pain (lamotrigine is in Phase III trials for neuropathic pain in the United States and Europe). The XR formulation of lamotrigine allows once-daily dosing (as opposed to the twice-daily dosing required with the original formulation).

Researchers hypothesize that lamotrigine acts as an analgesic by blocking voltage-dependent sodium channels and inhibiting glutamate release (Backonja

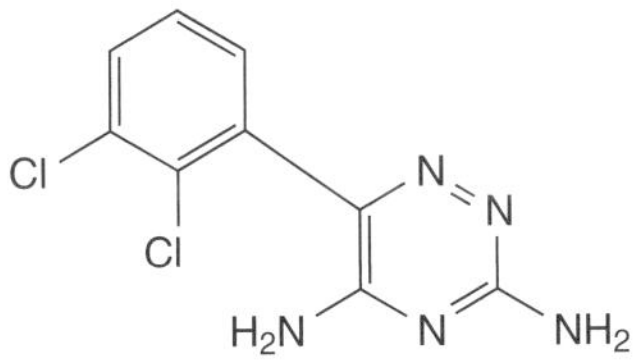

FIGURE 20. *Structure of lamotrigine.*

M, 2004; Sindrup SH, 2000). To date, lamotrigine has not been tested in large, placebo-controlled trials with CLBP (i.e., sciatica) patients, although one small open-label study ($n = 14$) found that sciatica patients treated with lamotrigine (400 mg/day) improved significantly from baseline, as measured using the Short Form McGill Pain Questionnaire (SF-MPQ), the Straight Leg Raise (SLR) test, and the range of motion of the lumbar spine (Eisenberg E, 2003). In addition, placebo-controlled studies have investigated the use of lamotrigine for other types of neuropathic pain—including painful diabetic neuropathy and HIV-related neuropathic pain—and have concluded that the drug is an effective treatment for these conditions (Eisenberg E, 2001; Simpson DM, 2000).

With regard to tolerability, many of lamotrigine's side effects (dizziness, headache, nausea, sedation) are mild and resolve without drug discontinuation. However, one potential side effect that can occur in up to 10% of patients is skin rash; very rarely, a more serious and potentially fatal reaction (toxic epidermal necrolysis) can occur.

Antidepressants

Overview. In light of the success of the older tricyclic antidepressants (TCAs) in treating neuropathic pain, investigators have tested many of the newer, more tolerable antidepressants (e.g., selective serotonin reuptake inhibitors [SSRIs], serotonergic and noradrenergic reuptake inhibitors [SNRIs]) in neuropathic pain conditions such as chronic sciatica. Drugs with antidepressant properties are particularly attractive to drug companies because of their ability to simultaneously treat pain and comorbid depression.

Although the SSRIs have demonstrated only very modest benefit, if any, in neuropathic pain, newer antidepressants with a wider range of activity appear promising for neuropathic pain; a review of antidepressant trials showed that agents with balanced activity at serotonergic/noradrenergic receptors are more effective at CLBP relief than are antidepressants with mainly serotonergic activity (i.e., SSRIs) (Fishbain D, 2000). As a result, several companies that have investigational antidepressants that act in a manner similar to that of TCAs and SNRIs have ongoing clinical programs to investigate their drugs' analgesic effects in pain syndromes.

Compounds in this drug class in development for pain include Cypress Bioscience, Inc. (San Diego, California)/Forest Laboratories' SNRI milnacipran, GlaxoSmithKline's norepinephrine/dopamine reuptake inhibitor GW-353162 (a bupropion [Wellbutrin] metabolite), DOV Pharmaceutical's (Hackensack, New Jersey) serotonin/norepinephrine transport inhibitor bicifadine, and Eli Lilly/Boehringer Ingelheim's duloxetine (Cymbalta/Xeristar). The discussion here is limited to duloxetine and bicifadine because these drugs are likely to be the most widely used for CLBP and because bicifadine is being developed specifically for this indication.

Mechanism of Action. Like the SSRIs, SNRIs (e.g., duloxetine, bicifadine) enhance the activity of neurotransmitters such as serotonin and norepinephrine; these neurotransmitters are believed to be key mediators of descending pain modulatory systems. SNRIs are considered an improvement over older TCAs because they do not affect the histamine, acetylcholine, and adrenergic receptors and therefore do not cause the severe weight gain, dry mouth, and hypotension associated with TCAs. Because SNRIs act on both serotonergic and noradrenergic systems, they are also called noradrenergic and specific serotonergic antidepressants.

Duloxetine. Eli Lilly's duloxetine received U.S. approval (as Cymbalta) for the treatment of peripheral diabetic neuropathy in September 2004 and thus became the first antidepressant officially indicated for pain. Duloxetine (Figure 21) is also approved in the United States for depression. Duloxetine was awaiting final approval for the treatment of stress urinary incontinence (SUI), but Eli Lilly withdrew its NDA for SUI in January 2005. According to an Eli Lilly press release from January 2005, the FDA was unwilling to approve duloxetine for SUI based upon the data contained in the existing NDA.

In Europe, duloxetine is approved for diabetic peripheral neuropathic pain, depression, and SUI. Eli Lilly will market the drug in the United States, and Eli Lilly and Boehringer Ingelheim will jointly market the drug throughout Europe. In Japan, Eli Lilly has licensed duloxetine to Shionogi & Co. (Osaka, Japan), which recently initiated additional Phase III trials with the drug at a higher dose than had previously been tested; the company expects to file for approval for depression in Japan in 2007.

In preclinical studies for persistent pain, duloxetine was more effective than venlafaxine, amitriptyline, and desipramine in relieving pain (Iyengar S, 2004). There is a lack, however, of published clinical data for CLBP. One analysis found that treatment with duloxetine reduced painful physical symptoms in patients with depression, indicating that duloxetine has analgesic effects (Wohlreich M, 2003). Data for the analysis were pooled from two randomized, double-blind clinical trials that evaluated duloxetine's efficacy in reducing painful physical symptoms (e.g., overall pain, back pain, headache, shoulder pain, pain while awake) in patients with major depression. Patients ($n = 495$) were randomized to receive either duloxetine (60 mg qd) or placebo for nine weeks. Efficacy was measured using a 100-mm VAS. Overall, patients receiving duloxetine experienced significantly superior mean improvements in pain (22–41%) compared with patients receiving placebo (5–18%). In addition, patients treated with duloxetine noted significant pain relief as early as one week after treatment was initiated.

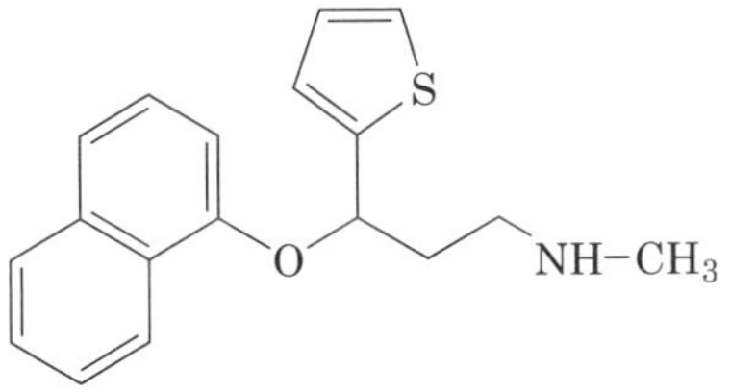

FIGURE 21. *Structure of duloxetine.*

Although duloxetine has not been studied extensively in CLBP, the drug's approval—as well as studies supporting its approval—for painful diabetic neuropathy suggests that it may be effective for other types of neuropathic pain (e.g., sciatica) that have similar pathophysiologies. Two 12-week, randomized, double-blind, placebo-controlled studies demonstrated duloxetine's efficacy in painful diabetic neuropathy (Wernicke J, 2004a). In the first study ($n = 457$), patients were randomized to receive either duloxetine (20 mg qd, 60 mg qd, 60 mg bid) or placebo; in the second study ($n = 334$), patients were randomized to receive duloxetine (60 mg qd, 60 mg bid) or placebo. The primary efficacy measure in both studies was weekly mean score of the 24-hour average pain severity on the 11-point Likert scale. Both studies reportedly showed significant improvements in patients taking duloxetine 60 mg once or twice daily compared with placebo on the primary end point, with additional evidence of rapid pain relief (noted in the first week of treatment with duloxetine). In addition, data from open-label extension studies of up to 52 weeks with duloxetine in painful diabetic neuropathy patients (presented at the 2004 annual meeting of the American Pain Society) suggest the drug is effective and well-tolerated over the long term (with rates of discontinuation due to adverse events of less than 15%) and has no negative effects on disease progression; it was also shown to improve quality-of-life measures compared with "routine care" for these patients (Raskin J, 2004; Wernicke J, 2004b).

Bicifadine. DOV Pharmaceutical is investigating bicifadine for a variety of pain indications, including CLBP. DOV originally licensed bicifadine from Wyeth in 1998. In 2002, DOV formed a business venture with Elan to develop an oral sustained-release formulation of bicifadine; however, in 2003, DOV purchased 100% of the joint venture company and is now developing bicifadine on its own. Bicifadine is in Phase III for pain in the United States and, based on its focus on CLBP in pivotal trials, will likely pursue approval for CLBP.

Bicifadine enhances and prolongs norepinephrine and serotonin activity through its inhibition of the transport proteins that terminate the actions of these neurotransmitters. Bicifadine is also a functional antagonist at a subset of excitatory glutamate receptors. Researchers believe that bicifadine's analgesic properties are a result of one or both of these biochemical behaviors.

In September 2004, DOV initiated a pivotal U.S. Phase III trial in patients with moderate-to-severe CLBP to determine bicifadine's efficacy and tolerability over three months. The double-blind, placebo-controlled study includes approximately 600 CLBP patients who will be randomized to three dose levels of bicifadine. The primary efficacy measures are changes in pain severity ratings by patients, functional disability, and patients' global impression of change. Results from this study are expected in 2006. DOV is also conducting a second U.S. pivotal CLBP trial, initiated in December 2004, designed to assess the long-term safety of bicifadine over 12 months.

Although no data have yet been released from trials of bicifadine in CLBP, results released by DOV in press releases from a Phase III study on moderate-to-severe postsurgical dental pain suggest that bicifadine is as effective as tramadol in relieving acute pain. DOV also released earlier Phase II results, which indicate that bicifadine is as effective as codeine in treating postsurgical dental pain. These studies also found bicifadine to be relatively safe and well-tolerated; nausea and emesis were the most frequently reported side effects.

Tumor Necrosis Factor Inhibitors

Overview. Tumor necrosis factor-alpha (TNF-α) inhibitors are being developed for neuropathic pain and—despite their anticipated high cost—are under study for the treatment of chronic sciatica. Several drugs in this class have been developed and launched for arthritis, including etanercept (Amgen [Thousand Oaks, California]/Wyeth's Enbrel), infliximab (Centocor, Inc. [Horsham, Pennsylvania, a Johnson & Johnson subsidiary]/Schering-Plough [Kenilworth, New Jersey]/Tanabe Seiyaku's [Osaka, Japan] Remicade), and adalimumab (Abbott's Humira). TNF-α inhibitors are of interest in sciatica because of their ability to reduce inflammation and prevent nerve damage; although direct nerve root or dorsal root ganglion compression has long been regarded as the cause of sciatica, the central role of inflammation in this condition has also been emphasized (Karppinen J, 2003). The following section discusses Renovis's REN-1654, which is in clinical trials with sciatica patients.

Mechanism of Action. TNF-α is a cytokine produced primarily by activated macrophages and T cells in response to inflammation; as a signaling molecule, TNF-α is thought to increase pain signaling and damage nerves by increasing the inflammatory response. TNF-α inhibitors are believed to ease inflammation by reducing the release of TNF-α to lessen the amount of inflammation and thus prevent nerve damage.

Receptors for TNF-α are found on the surface of most cells, including mononuclear cells and cells in the synovium. Cleavage of the membrane-bound TNF receptors yields soluble TNF receptors that retain ligand-binding ability but cannot activate cells. Two distinct types of TNF receptors have been identified: type I (p55) and type II (p75). TNF-α inhibitors reduce free, bioactive TNF-α by emulating the physiological role played by soluble TNF receptors. This action modulates the amount of circulating, bioactive TNF-α by binding to the cytokine before it can activate cell-surface receptors on mononuclear cells. Because TNF-α plays an important role in the eradication of neoplastic cells, its suppression is not without hazards—particularly as a long-term strategy. Concerns have been raised as to whether chronic immunosuppression leads to opportunistic infection, malignancies, and other complications (Alldred A, 2001; Lee JH, 2002). In October 2004, the FDA recommended that a warning regarding the risk of malignancy be added to the labeling for all TNF inhibitors. The agency cited studies that found more cases of lymphoma among patients receiving TNF-α inhibitors than among control group patients.

REN-1654. REN-1654 is an orally administered TNF-α inhibitor being developed by Renovis, Inc. (South San Francisco, California) for the treatment of sciatica. As noted previously, the compound reduces inflammation in the nervous system by reducing the release of TNF-α.

Renovis announced the completion of a U.S. Phase II trial of REN-1654 in postherpetic neuralgia in March 2005. In this trial, the compound failed to achieve statistically significant efficacy with regard to the primary end point of change in daily spontaneous pain relief. Based on these disappointing results, Renovis decided to discontinue development of REN-1654 for postherpetic neuralgia.

However, Renovis intends to continue developing REN-1654 for sciatica. In February 2005, enrollment was still ongoing for a second Phase II trial in sciatica patients; the trial is designed to include approximately 108 sciatica patients (with leg pain due to lumbosacral radiculopathy developed no more than 12 weeks prior to enrollment).

Nitric-Oxide-Releasing Drugs

Traditional NSAIDs are effective pain medications for many CLBP patients, but their use is limited by their risk of gastrointestinal (GI) toxicity (see the "Current Therapies" section for more information on NSAIDs). However, grafting nitric oxide (NO) to an NSAID (to create a "NO-NSAID") is believed to reduce the risk of GI side effects because the donation of NO may have a protective effect on the GI tract. Although selective COX-2 inhibitors also provide efficacy equivalent to that of NSAIDs, with a much lower risk of GI problems, the recent controversy over the cardiovascular safety of these drugs has made them less attractive alternatives to NSAIDs. Therefore, if NO-NSAIDs can deliver on their promise, they have the potential to become first-line pain treatment options, particularly for patients at risk for GI effects.

No companies are developing NO-NSAIDs specifically for CLBP, although compounds are in trials for other chronic pain indications. NicOx, a drug company focused on the development of NO-releasing drugs, is the furthest along in development with HCT-3012, which is in Phase II trials for osteoarthritis. If NicOx is successful, other companies will likely initiate NO programs. (Nitromed was developing a NO-releasing formulation of the COX-2 rofecoxib, but the company suspended trials when rofecoxib was withdrawn from the market in September 2004.)

Cannabinoid Receptor Modulators

Cannabinoid receptor modulators are being developed for numerous conditions (e.g., chronic pain conditions, inflammatory disorders, neurodegenerative disorders). GW Pharmaceuticals's (Salisbury, United Kingdom) Sativex (GW-1000) is the furthest along in development and is preregistered in the United Kingdom. Other companies with cannabinoid programs in earlier stages for pain include Kadmus Pharmaceuticals, Indevus, and Novartis.

The primary pain market for cannabinoid receptor modulators is likely to be cancer pain. These agents will also face significant regulatory hurdles in the United States, where the future of cannabis-based therapies is still uncertain; if cannabinoid drugs do reach the U.S. market, they will most likely be classified as controlled substances, similar to narcotic analgesics.

NMDA Receptor Antagonists

For the past decade, researchers have been trying to develop, but with little success, safe and effective NMDA receptor antagonists for the treatment of various conditions, including pain. Currently available NMDA receptor antagonists (e.g., ketamine [generics], dextromethorphan [generics]) have limited efficacy and significant dose-limiting side effects. However, researchers now have a much more advanced understanding of NMDA receptor pharmacology and are hoping to develop agents without the serious safety and tolerability issues that plagued the first generation of NMDA antagonists. Several companies (e.g., CeNes Pharmaceuticals [Histon, United Kingdom], GB Therapeutics [Mississauga, Ontario, Canada], Pfizer, Wyeth) have compounds in early-to-mid stages of development, but other manufacturers have drugs in later stages of development; among these agents are Merz Pharmaceuticals (Greensboro, North Carolina)/Forest Laboratories' memantine (Namenda/Ebixa/Axura), AVANIR Pharmaceuticals's (San Diego, California) Neurodex (dextromethorphan + quinidine), and EpiCept Corporation's (Englewood Cliffs, New Jersey) novel NP-1 (amitriptyline + ketamine) cream.

REFERENCES

Aglan M. Botulinum toxin type A injection of the iliopsoas muscle for the treatment of low back pain and sciatica. 22nd Annual Meeting of the American Pain Society; March 20, 2003; Chicago, IL. Abstract # 695.

Allan L, Kalso E. Randomized trial of transdermal fentanyl and sustained release oral morphine in chronic low back pain. EFIC Congress; September 2, 2003; Prague, Czech Republic.

Allan L, Kalso E. Response to transdermal fentanyl or sustained release oral morphine in chronic low back pain. 23rd Annual Meeting of the American Pain Society; May 6, 2004; Vancouver, BC.

Allan L, et al. Randomised crossover trial of transdermal fentanyl and sustained release oral morphine for treating chronic non-cancer pain. *BMJ*. 2001;**322**:1154–1158.

Alldred A. Etanercept in rheumatoid arthritis. *Expert Opin Pharmacother*. 2001;**2**:1137–1148.

Andersson GB. Epidemiological features of chronic low-back pain. *Lancet*. 1999;**354**:581–585.

Argoff CE, et al. Effectiveness of the lidocaine patch 5% on pain qualities in three chronic pain states: assessment with the Neuropathic Pain Scale. *Curr Med Res Opin*. 2004;**20** Suppl 2:21–28.

Atlas SJ, Nardin RA. Evaluation and treatment of low back pain: an evidence-based approach to clinical care. *Muscle Nerve*. 2003;**27**:265–284.

Backonja M. Neuromodulating drugs for the symptomatic treatment of neuropathic pain. *Curr Pain Headache Rep*. 2004;**8**:212–216.

Backonja M, et al. Gabapentin for the symptomatic treatment of painful neuropathy in patients with diabetes mellitus: a randomized controlled trial. *JAMA*. 1998;**280**:1831–1836.

Backonja MM. Use of anticonvulsants for treatment of neuropathic pain. *Neurology*. 2002;**59**:S14–S17.

Banks AT, et al. Diclofenac-associated hepatotoxicity: analysis of 180 cases reported to the Food and Drug Administration as adverse reactions. *Hepatology*. 1995;**22**:820–827.

Baraf H, et al. Tolerability and Effectiveness of Etoricoxib Compared to Diclofenac Sodium in Patients with Osteoarthritis: a Randomized Controlled Study (EDGE trial). 2004 Annual Meeting of the American College of Rheumatology; October 19, 2004; San Antonia, TX. Abstract # 832.

Bartleson JD. Low Back Pain. 2001;**3**:159–168.

Bassols A, et al. [Back pain in the general population of Catalonia (Spain). Prevalence, characteristics and therapeutic behavior]. *Gac Sanit*. 2003;**17**:97–107.

BenDebba M, et al. Persistent low back pain and sciatica in the United States: treatment outcomes. *J Spinal Disord Tech*. 2002;**15**:2–15.

Birbara CA, et al. Treatment of chronic low back pain with etoricoxib, a new cyclo-oxygenase-2 selective inhibitor: improvement in pain and disability--a randomized, placebo-controlled, 3-month trial. *J Pain*. 2003;**4**:307–315.

Biyani A, Andersson GB. Low back pain: pathophysiology and management. *J Am Acad Orthop Surg*. 2004;**12**:106–115.

Boden SD, Swanson AL. An assessment of the early management of spine problems and appropriateness of diagnostic imaging utilization. *Phys Med Rehabil Clin N Am*. 1998;**9**:411–7. viii.

Bombardier C, et al. Comparison of upper gastrointestinal toxicity of rofecoxib and naproxen in patients with rheumatoid arthritis. VIGOR Study Group. *N Engl J Med*. 2000;**343**:1520–1528.

Bresalier RS, et al. Cardiovascular events associated with rofecoxib in a colorectal adenoma chemoprevention trial. *N Engl J Med*. 2005;**352**:1092–1102.

Bressler HB, et al. The prevalence of low back pain in the elderly. A systematic review of the literature. *Spine*. 1999;**24**:1813–1819.

Brisby H. Nerve root injuries in patients with chronic low back pain. *Orthop Clin North Am*. 2003;**34**:221–230.

Carey TS, et al. Care-seeking among individuals with chronic low back pain. *Spine*. 1995;**20**:312–317.

Carragee EJ, Hannibal M. Diagnostic evaluation of low back pain. *Orthop Clin North Am*. 2004;**35**:7–16.

Carrazana E, Mikoshiba I. Rationale and evidence for the use of oxcarbazepine in neuropathic pain. *J Pain Symptom Manage*. 2003;**25**:S31–S35.

Cassidy JD, et al. The Saskatchewan health and back pain survey. The prevalence of low back pain and related disability in Saskatchewan adults. *Spine*. 1998;**23**:1860–1866.

Catella-Lawson F, et al. Cyclooxygenase inhibitors and the antiplatelet effects of aspirin. *N Engl J Med*. 2001;**345**:1809–1817.

Cedraschi C, et al. Is chronic non-specific low back pain chronic? Definitions of a problem and problems of a definition. *Br J Gen Pract*. 1999;**49**:358–362.

Cianflocco A. Common causes of back pain including athletic injuries. The Cleveland Clinic Foundation. 2001. clevelandclinic.org/health/health-info/docs/0400/0421.asp? index=4045. Accessed March 3, 2001.

Clinical Standards Advisory Group. *Epidemiology review: the epidemiology and cost of back pain. Annex to the Clinical Standards Advisory Group's Report on Back Pain.* London: Her Majesty's Stationery Office; 1994.

Cochrane DJ, et al. Etoricoxib. *Drugs*. 2002;**62**:2637–2651.

Colberg K, et al. The efficacy and tolerability of an 8-day administration of intravenous and oral meloxicam: a comparison with intramuscular and oral diclofenac in patients with acute lumbago. German Meloxicam Ampoule Study Group. *Curr Med Res Opin*. 1996;**13**:363–377.

Cole MH, Grimshaw PN. Low back pain and lifting: a review of epidemiology and aetiology. *Work*. 2003;**21**:173–184.

Coste J, et al. Clinical course and prognostic factors in acute low back pain: an inception cohort study in primary care practice. *BMJ*. 1994;**308**:577–580.

Croft PR, et al. Risk factors for neck pain: a longitudinal study in the general population. *Pain*. 2001;**93**:317–325.

Croft PR, et al. Outcome of low back pain in general practice: a prospective study. *BMJ*. 1998;**316**:1356–1359.

Currie SR, Wang J. Chronic back pain and major depression in the general Canadian population. *Pain*. 2004;**107**:54–60.

Curtis SP, et al. Renal effects of etoricoxib and comparator nonsteroidal anti-inflammatory drugs in controlled clinical trials. *Clin Ther*. 2004;**26**:70–83.

Curtis S. Fewer upper-GI perforations, ulcers, and bleeds (PUBS) with etoricoxib than with nonsteroidal anti-inflammatory drugs (NSAIDs). 2002 EULAR meeting; June 12, 2002; Stockholm, Sweden. Abstract # FR10057.

De PL, et al. The vanilloid receptor (VR1)-mediated effects of anandamide are potently enhanced by the cAMP-dependent protein kinase. *J Neurochem*. 2001;**77**:1660–1663.

Dequeker J, et al. Improvement in gastrointestinal tolerability of the selective cyclooxygenase (COX)-2 inhibitor, meloxicam, compared with piroxicam: results of the Safety and Efficacy Large-scale Evaluation of COX-inhibiting Therapies (SELECT) trial in osteoarthritis. *Br J Rheumatol*. 1998;**37**:946–951.

Deyo RA, Phillips WR. Low back pain. A primary care challenge. *Spine*. 1996;**21**:2826–2832.

Deyo RA, Tsui-Wu YJ. Descriptive epidemiology of low-back pain and its related medical care in the United States. *Spine*. 1987;**12**:264–268.

Deyo RA, Weinstein JN. Low back pain. *N Engl J Med*. 2001;**344**:363–370.

Dionne C. Low-back pain. In Crombie IK, ed. *Epidemiology of pain*. Seattle, WA: IASP Press; 1999.

Dooley DJ, et al. Preferential action of gabapentin and pregabalin at P/Q-type voltage-sensitive calcium channels: inhibition of K + -evoked [3H]-norepinephrine release from rat neocortical slices. *Synapse*. 2002;**45**:171–190.

Dooley DJ, et al. Stimulus-dependent modulation of [(3)H]norepinephrine release from rat neocortical slices by gabapentin and pregabalin. *J Pharmacol Exp Ther*. 2000;**295**:1086–1093.

Dreiser RL, et al. Relief of acute low back pain with diclofenac-K 12.5mg tablets: a flexible dose, ibuprofen 200mg and placebo-controlled clinical trial. *Int J Clin Pharmacol Ther*. 2003;**41**:375–385.

Dunteman E. Chronic low-back pain treatment with botulinum toxin type A. 22nd Annual Meeting of the American Pain Society; March 20, 2003; Chicago, IL. Abstract # 941.

Dworkin RH, et al. Pregabalin for the treatment of postherpetic neuralgia: a randomized, placebo-controlled trial. *Neurology*. 2003;**60**:1274–1283.

Edwards K. Botulinum toxin A (Botox) for refractory low-back pain. 22nd Annual Meeting of the American Pain Society; March 20, 2003; Chicago, IL. Abstract # 710.

Edwards K, Dreyer M. Botulinum toxin type A for failed back syndrome. 23rd Annual Meeting of the American Pain Society; May 6, 2004; Vancouver, BC. Abstract # 815.

Ehrlich GE. Back pain. *J Rheumatol Suppl*. 2003;**67**:26–31.

Eisenberg E, et al. Lamotrigine for intractable sciatica: correlation between dose, plasma concentration and analgesia. *Eur J Pain*. 2003;**7**:485–491.

Eisenberg E, et al. Lamotrigine reduces painful diabetic neuropathy: a randomized, controlled study. *Neurology*. 2001;**57**:505–509.

Elliott AM, et al. The epidemiology of chronic pain in the community. *Lancet*. 1999;**354**:1248–1252.

Elliott AM, et al. Changes in chronic pain severity over time: the Chronic Pain Grade as a valid measure. *Pain*. 2000;**88**:303–308.

England S, et al. PGE2 modulates the tetrodotoxin-resistant sodium current in neonatal rat dorsal root ganglion neurones via the cyclic AMP-protein kinase A cascade. *J Physiol*. 1996;**495** (Pt 2):429–440.

Farrar JT, et al. Defining the clinically important difference in pain outcome measures. *Pain*. 2000;**88**:287–294.

Farrar JT, et al. Clinical importance of changes in chronic pain intensity measured on an 11-point numerical pain rating scale. *Pain*. 2001;**94**:149–158.

FDA discloses safety reviews of Arcoxia, Prexige and Parecoxib. 2–15- 2005. http://www.fdaadvisorycommittee.com/FDC/AdvisoryCommittee/Committees/Arthritis+Drugs/021605_ cox2day1/COX2preview3.htm. Accessed April 6, 2005.

Field MJ, et al. Further evidence for the role of the alpha(2)delta subunit of voltage dependent calcium channels in models of neuropathic pain. *Br J Pharmacol*. 2000;**131**:282–286.

Fields HL. Pain modulation: expectation, opioid analgesia and virtual pain. *Prog Brain Res*. 2000;**122**:245–253.

Fink K, et al. Inhibition of neuronal Ca(2 +) influx by gabapentin and pregabalin in the human neocortex. *Neuropharmacology*. 2002;**42**:229–236.

Fishbain D. Evidence-based data on pain relief with antidepressants. *Ann Med*. 2000;**32**:305–316.

Flor H. Cortical reorganisation and chronic pain: implications for rehabilitation. *J Rehabil Med*. 2003;66–72.

Foster L, et al. Botulinum toxin A and chronic low back pain: a randomized, double-blind study. *Neurology*. 2001;**56**:1290–1293.

Frank AO, et al. A cross-sectional survey of the clinical and psychological features of low back pain and consequent work handicap: use of the Quebec Task Force classification. *Int J Clin Pract*. 2000;**54**:639–644.

Frymoyer JW, Cats-Baril WL. An overview of the incidences and costs of low back pain. *Orthop Clin North Am*. 1991;**22**:263–271.

Fuortes LJ, et al. Epidemiology of back injury in university hospital nurses from review of workers' compensation records and a case-control survey. *J Occup Med*. 1994;**36**:1022–1026.

Furberg CD, et al. Parecoxib, valdecoxib, and cardiovascular risk. *Circulation*. 2005;**111**:249.

Gammaitoni A, et al. Topical ketamine gel: possible role in treating neuropathic pain. *Pain Med*. 2000;**1**:97–100.

Gammaitoni AR, et al. Effectiveness and safety of new oxycodone/acetaminophen formulations with reduced acetaminophen for the treatment of low back pain. *Pain Med*. 2003;**4**:21–30.

Geba GP. Evaluation of chronic low-back pain therapy with etoricoxib using the Roland-Morris Disability Questionnaire. 2002 EULAR Meeting; June 12, 2002; Stockholm, Sweden. Abstract # OP0077.

Gebhart GF. Descending modulation of pain. *Neurosci Biobehav Rev*. 2004;**27**:729–737.

Gee NS, et al. The novel anticonvulsant drug, gabapentin (Neurontin), binds to the alpha2delta subunit of a calcium channel. *J Biol Chem*. 1996;**271**:5768–5776.

Gimbel J. Impact of the lidocaine patch 5% on pain interference with quality of life when used in combination with gabapentin in chronic pain. 22nd Annual Meeting of the American Pain Society; March 20, 2003a; Chicago, IL. Abstract # 882.

Gimbel J. Lidocaine patch 5% with acute/subacute and chronic low-back pain: impact on pain intensity, pain relief, and pain interference with quality of life. 22nd Annual Meeting of the American Pain Society; March 20, 2003b; Chicago, IL. Abstract # 878.

Griffin MR, et al. Nonsteroidal antiinflammatory drugs and acute renal failure in elderly persons. *Am J Epidemiol*. 2000;**151**:488–496.

Hale ME, et al. Efficacy and safety of oxymorphone extended release in chronic low back pain: Results of a randomized, double-blind, placebo- and active-controlled phase III study. *J Pain*. 2005;**6**:21–28.

Hale ME, et al. Efficacy and safety of controlled-release versus immediate-release oxycodone: randomized, double-blind evaluation in patients with chronic back pain. *Clin J Pain*. 1999;**15**:179–183.

Hansen HC. Treatment of chronic pain with antiepileptic drugs: a new era. *South Med J*. 1999;**92**:642–649.

Hawkey C, et al. Gastrointestinal tolerability of meloxicam compared to diclofenac in osteoarthritis patients. International MELISSA Study Group. Meloxicam Large-scale International Study Safety Assessment. *Br J Rheumatol*. 1998;**37**:937–945.

Hession WG, et al. Epidural steroid injections. *Semin Roentgenol*. 2004;**39**:7–23.

Hestbaek L, et al. The course of low back pain in a general population. Results from a 5-year prospective study. *J Manipulative Physiol Ther*. 2003;**26**:213–219.

Hillman M, et al. Prevalence of low back pain in the community: implications for service provision in Bradford, UK. *J Epidemiol Community Health*. 1996;**50**:347–352.

Hofmann F, et al. Low back pain and lumbago-sciatica in nurses and a reference group of clerks: results of a comparative prevalence study in Germany. *Int Arch Occup Environ Health*. 2002;**75**:484–490.

Holdcroft A, Power I. Recent developments: management of pain. *BMJ*. 2003;**326**:635–639.

Iyengar S, et al. Efficacy of duloxetine, a potent and balanced serotonin-norepinephrine reuptake inhibitor in persistent pain models in rats. *J Pharmacol Exp Ther*. 2004;**311**:576–584.

Karppinen J, et al. Tumor necrosis factor-alpha monoclonal antibody, infliximab, used to manage severe sciatica. *Spine*. 2003;**28**:750–753.

Katz N, et al. Health-related quality of life changes in chronic low back pain patients receiving either fentanyl transdermal system or oxycodone with acetaminophen. 22nd Annual Meeting of the American Pain Society; March 20, 2003; Chicago, IL.

Keeton W, et al. Long-Term, Open-Label, Efficacy & Safety Evaluation of AVINZA (Morphine Sulfate Extended-Release Capsules) in Patients with Chronic Back Pain. 2003 Annual Meeting of the American Society of Anesthesiologists; October 11, 2003; San Francisco, CA. Abstract # A979.

Kent P, Keating J. Do primary-care clinicians think that nonspecific low back pain is one condition ? *Spine*. 2004;**29**:1022–1031.

Kimmel SE, et al. The effects of nonselective non-aspirin non-steroidal anti-inflammatory medications on the risk of nonfatal myocardial infarction and their interaction with aspirin. *J Am Coll Cardiol*. 2004;**43**:985–990.

Kopec JA, et al. Predictors of back pain in a general population cohort. *Spine*. 2004;**29**:70–77.

Kosinski M, et al. Health-related quality of life of chronic low back pain patients: impact of disease and treatment effect of fentanyl transdermal system. 23rd Annual Meeting of the American Pain Society; May 6, 2004; Vancouver, BC.

Lee JH, et al. Life-threatening histoplasmosis complicating immunotherapy with tumor necrosis factor alpha antagonists infliximab and etanercept. *Arthritis Rheum*. 2002;**46**:2565–2570.

Loney PL, Stratford PW. The prevalence of low back pain in adults: a methodological review of the literature. *Phys Ther*. 1999;**79**:384–396.

Long DM. *Contemporary diagnosis and management of pain*. Newton, PA: Handbooks in Health Care Co.; 1997.

Luo X, et al. Estimates and patterns of direct health care expenditures among individuals with back pain in the United States. *Spine*. 2004;**29**:79–86.

MacDonald TM, Wei L. Effect of ibuprofen on cardioprotective effect of aspirin. *Lancet*. 2003;**361**:573–574.

Maier C, et al. Morphine responsiveness, efficacy and tolerability in patients with chronic non-tumor associated pain - results of a double-blind placebo-controlled trial (MON-TAS). *Pain*. 2002;**97**:223–233.

Maniadakis N, Gray A. The economic burden of back pain in the UK. *Pain*. 2000;**84**:95–103.

Matsui H, et al. Risk indicators of low back pain among workers in Japan. Association of familial and physical factors with low back pain. *Spine*. 1997;**22**:1242–1247.

Matsumo S, et al. Clinical evaluation of ketoprofen (Orudis) in lumbago - a double-blind comparison with diclofenac sodium. *Br J Clin Pract*. 1981;**35**:266.

Mattia C, et al. New antidepressants in the treatment of neuropathic pain. A review. *Minerva Anestesiol*. 2002;**68**:105–114.

McGorry RW, et al. The relation between pain intensity, disability, and the episodic nature of chronic and recurrent low back pain. *Spine*. 2000;**25**:834–841.

Michel A, et al. The association between clinical findings on physical examination and self-reported severity in back pain. Results of a population-based study. *Spine*. 1997;**22**:296–303.

Mukherjee D, et al. Risk of cardiovascular events associated with selective COX-2 inhibitors. *JAMA*. 2001;**286**:954–959.

Muller FO, et al. Comparison of the efficacy and tolerability of a paracetamol/codeine fixed-dose combination with tramadol in patients with refractory chronic back pain. *Arzneimittelforschung*. 1998;**48**:675–679.

Nachemson AL. Newest knowledge of low back pain. A critical look. *Clin Orthop*. 1992;8–20.

Nelemans PJ, et al. Injection therapy for subacute and chronic benign low back pain. *Spine*. 2001;**26**:501–515.

Newton W, et al. Prevalence of subtypes of low back pain in a defined population. *J Fam Pract*. 1997;**45**:331–335.

NHANES. The Third National Health and Nutrition Examination Survey, NHANES III, 1988–94 on CD-ROM. *National Center for Health Statistics, Centers for Disease Control and Prevention*. 1997; CD-ROM Series 11: No. 1.

Nyiendo J, et al. Patient characteristics and physicians' practice activities for patients with chronic low back pain: a practice-based study of primary care and chiropractic physicians. *J Manipulative Physiol Ther*. 2001;**24**:92–100.

Office of National Statistics. The Prevalence of Back Pain in Great Britain in 1998. 1999. http://www.dh.gov.uk/PublicationsAndStatistics/PressReleases/. Accessed January 18, 2005.

Ozguler A, et al. Individual and occupational determinants of low back pain according to various definitions of low back pain. *J Epidemiol Community Health*. 2000;**54**:215–220.

Pallay RM, et al. Etoricoxib reduced pain and disability and improved quality of life in patients with chronic low back pain: a 3 month, randomized, controlled trial. *Scand J Rheumatol*. 2004;**33**:257–266.

Palmer KT, et al. Back pain in Britain: comparison of two prevalence surveys at an interval of 10 years. *BMJ*. 2000;**320**:1577–1578.

Papageorgiou AC, et al. Estimating the prevalence of low back pain in the general population. Evidence from the South Manchester Back Pain Survey. *Spine*. 1995;**20**:1889–1894.

Peloso PM, et al. Analgesic efficacy and safety of tramadol/ acetaminophen combination tablets (Ultracet) in treatment of chronic low back pain: a multicenter, outpatient, randomized, double blind, placebo controlled trial. *J Rheumatol*. 2004;**31**:2454–2463.

Pheasant H, et al. Amitriptyline and chronic low-back pain. A randomized double-blind crossover study. *Spine*. 1983;**8**:552–557.

Picavet HS, Schouten JS. Physical load in daily life and low back problems in the general population-The MORGEN study. *Prev Med*. 2000;**31**:506–512.

Picavet HS, et al. Prevalence and consequences of low back problems in The Netherlands, working vs non-working population, the MORGEN-Study. Monitoring Project on Risk Factors for Chronic Disease. *Public Health*. 1999;**113**:73–77.

Pincus T, et al. A systematic review of psychological factors as predictors of chronicity/disability in prospective cohorts of low back pain. *Spine*. 2002;**27**:E109–E120.

Population Division of the Department of Economic and Social Affairs of the United Nations Secretariat. *World Population Prospects: the 2002 Revision, vol.II, the Sex and Age Distribution of Populations (United Nations publication, Sales No.E.03.XII.7).* 2003.

Pownall R, Pickvance NJ. Does treatment timing matter?--A double blind crossover study of ibuprofen 2400mg per day in different dosage schedules in treatment of chronic low back pain. *Br J Clin Pract*. 1985;**39**:267–275.

Practice guidelines for chronic pain management: A report by the American Society of Anesthesiologists Task Force on Pain Management, Chronic Pain Section. *Anesthesiology*. 1997;**86**:995–1004.

Premkumar LS, Ahern GP. Induction of vanilloid receptor channel activity by protein kinase C. *Nature*. 2000;**408**:985–990.

Raskin J. Duloxetine for patients with diabetic neuropathic pain: a six-month open label safety study. 23rd Annual Meeting of the American Pain Society; May 6, 2004; Vancouver, BC.

Raspe H. Back pain: occurrence and natural course in a one year prospective period. *British Journal of Rheumatology*. 1994a;**33**(suppl 1):119.

Raspe H, Kohlmann T. Disorders characterised by pain: a methodological review of population surveys. *J Epidemiol Community Health*. 1994b;**48**:531–537.

Ray WA, et al. Non-steroidal anti-inflammatory drugs and risk of serious coronary heart disease: an observational cohort study. *Lancet*. 2002;**359**:118–123.

Reisner L. Biologic poisons for pain. *Curr Pain Headache Rep*. 2004;**8**:427–434.

Ren XS, et al. Assessment of functional status, low back disability, and use of diagnostic imaging in patients with low back pain and radiating leg pain. *J Clin Epidemiol*. 1999;**52**:1063–1071.

Rice AS, Maton S. Gabapentin in postherpetic neuralgia: a randomised, double blind, placebo controlled study. *Pain*. 2001;**94**:215–224.

Richards P, et al. Controlled-release oxycodone relieves moderate to severe pain in a 3-month study of persistent moderate to severe back pain. *Pain Med*. 2002;**3**:176.

Rizzo JA, et al. The labor productivity effects of chronic backache in the United States. *Med Care*. 1998;**36**:1471–1488.

Rosenstock J, et al. Pregabalin for the treatment of painful diabetic peripheral neuropathy: a double-blind, placebo-controlled trial. *Pain*. 2004;**110**:628–638.

Rowbotham M, et al. Gabapentin for the treatment of postherpetic neuralgia: a randomized controlled trial. *JAMA*. 1998;**280**:1837–1842.

Ruoff GE, et al. Tramadol/acetaminophen combination tablets for the treatment of chronic lower back pain: a multicenter, randomized, double-blind, placebo-controlled outpatient study. *Clin Ther*. 2003;**25**:1123–1141.

Sabatowski R, et al. Pregabalin reduces pain and improves sleep and mood disturbances in patients with post-herpetic neuralgia: results of a randomised, placebo-controlled clinical trial. *Pain*. 2004;**109**:26–35.

Schaible HG, Grubb BD. Afferent and spinal mechanisms of joint pain. *Pain*. 1993;**55**:5–54.

Schattenkirchner M, Milachowski KA. A double-blind, multicentre, randomised clinical trial comparing the efficacy and tolerability of aceclofenac with diclofenac resinate in patients with acute low back pain. *Clin Rheumatol*. 2003;**22**:127–135.

Schaufele MK, Boden SD. Outcome research in patients with chronic low back pain. *Orthop Clin North Am*. 2003;**34**:231–237.

Schein J, et al. Activity limitations in chronic low back pain patients receiving transdermal fentanyl system: an interpretive guide to health-related quality of life. 23rd Annual Meeting of the American Pain Society; May 6, 2004; Vancouver, BC.

Schnitzer TJ, et al. Efficacy of tramadol in treatment of chronic low back pain. *J Rheumatol*. 2000;**27**:772–778.

Schochat T, Jackel WH. [Prevalence of low back pain in the population]. *Rehabilitation (Stuttg)*. 1998;**37**:216–223.

Serpell MG. Gabapentin in neuropathic pain syndromes: a randomised, double-blind, placebo-controlled trial. *Pain*. 2002;**99**:557–566.

Silverstein FE, et al. Gastrointestinal toxicity with celecoxib vs nonsteroidal anti-inflammatory drugs for osteoarthritis and rheumatoid arthritis: the CLASS study: A randomized controlled trial. Celecoxib Long-term Arthritis Safety Study. *JAMA*. 2000;**284**:1247–1255.

Simpson DM, et al. A placebo-controlled trial of lamotrigine for painful HIV-associated neuropathy. *Neurology*. 2000;**54**:2115–2119.

Simpson RK, Jr., et al. Transdermal fentanyl as treatment for chronic low back pain. *J Pain Symptom Manage*. 1997;**14**:218–224.

Sindrup SH, et al. Tramadol relieves pain and allodynia in polyneuropathy: a randomised, double-blind, controlled trial. *Pain*. 1999;**83**:85–90.

Sindrup SH, Jensen TS. Pharmacologic treatment of pain in polyneuropathy. *Neurology*. 2000;**55**:915–920.

Smith BH, et al. Factors related to the onset and persistence of chronic back pain in the community: results from a general population follow-up study. *Spine*. 2004;**29**:1032–1040.

Solomon DH. The relationship between selective COX-2 inhibitors and acute myocardial infarction. 67th Annual Meeting of the American College of Rheumatology; October 23, 2003; Orlando, FL.

Solomon SD, et al. Cardiovascular risk associated with celecoxib in a clinical trial for colorectal adenoma prevention. *N Engl J Med*. 2005;**352**:1071–1080.

Speiller M. Lidocaine patch 5% and concomitant gabapentin: rationaly polypharmacy for chronic low back pain. 2004 Meeting of the American Academy of Nurse Practitioners; June 11, 2004; New Orleans, LA.

Stein C, et al. Attacking pain at its source: new perspectives on opioids. *Nat Med*. 2003;**9**:1003–1008.

Stein D, et al. The efficacy of amitriptyline and acetaminophen in the management of acute low back pain. *Psychosomatics*. 1996;**37**:63–70.

Stranjalis G, et al. Low back pain in a representative sample of Greek population: analysis according to personal and socioeconomic characteristics. *Spine*. 2004;**29**:1355–1360.

Strojek K. Evaluation of flexible and fixed dosing of pregabalin in the management of chronic neuropathic pain. 64th Annual Meeting of the American Diabetes Association; June 4, 2004; Orlando, FL.

Subin B, et al. Treatment of chronic low back pain by local injection of botulinum toxin-a. *The Internet Journal of Anesthesiology*. 2003;**6**.

Teasell RW, White K. Clinical approaches to low back pain. Part 1. Epidemiology, diagnosis, and prevention. *Can Fam Physician*. 1994;**40**:481–485.

Thant ZS, Tan EK. Emerging therapeutic applications of botulinum toxin. *Med Sci Monit*. 2003;**9**:RA40–RA48.

Thomas E, et al. The prevalence of pain and pain interference in a general population of older adults: cross-sectional findings from the North Staffordshire Osteoarthritis Project (NorStOP). *Pain*. 2004;**110**:361–368.

Toth PP, Urtis J. Commonly used muscle relaxant therapies for acute low back pain: a review of carisoprodol, cyclobenzaprine hydrochloride, and metaxalone. *Clin Ther*. 2004;**26**:1355–1367.

Turner JA, et al. Spinal cord stimulation for chronic low back pain: a systematic literature synthesis. *Neurosurgery*. 1995;**37**:1088–1095.

Vaccaro AR, et al. Predictors of outcome in patients with chronic back pain and low-grade spondylolisthesis. *Spine*. 1997;**22**:2030–2034.

Valat JP, et al. Low back pain: risk factors for chronicity. *Rev Rhum Engl Ed*. 1997;**64**:189–194.

van Tulder MW, et al. A cost-of-illness study of back pain in The Netherlands. *Pain*. 1995;**62**:233–240.

van Tulder MW, et al. Nonsteroidal anti-inflammatory drugs for low back pain: a systematic review within the framework of the Cochrane Collaboration Back Review Group. *Spine*. 2000;**25**:2501–2513.

Volinn E. The epidemiology of low back pain in the rest of the world. A review of surveys in low- and middle-income countries. *Spine*. 1997;**22**:1747–1754.

Walker BF. The prevalence of low back pain: a systematic review of the literature from 1966 to 1998. *J Spinal Disord*. 2000;**13**:205–217.

Walker BF, et al. Low back pain in Australian adults: prevalence and associated disability. *J Manipulative Physiol Ther*. 2004;**27**:238–244.

Walsh K, et al. Low back pain in eight areas of Britain. *J Epidemiol Community Health*. 1992;**46**:227–230.

Watson DJ, et al. The upper gastrointestinal safety of rofecoxib vs. NSAIDs: an updated combined analysis. *Curr Med Res Opin*. 2004;**20**:1539–1548.

Waxman R, et al. A prospective follow-up study of low back pain in the community. *Spine*. 2000;**25**:2085–2090.

Wernicke J. Superiority of duloxetine over placebo in the treatment of diabetic neuropathic pain demonstrated in two studies. 64th Annual Meeting of the American Diabetes Association; June 4, 2004a; Orlando, FL.

Wernicke J. The safety of duloxetine in the long-term treatment of diabetic neuropathic pain. 23rd Annual Meeting of the American Pain Society; May 6, 2004b; Vancouver, BC.

Wohlreich M, et al. Treatment Efficacy of Duloxetine 60mg QD for Patients with Major Depression with Painful Physical Symptoms. 22nd Annual Meeting of the American Pain Society; March 20, 2003; Chicago, IL.

Woolf AD, Pfleger B. Burden of major musculoskeletal conditions. *Bull World Health Organ*. 2003;**81**:646–656.

World Health Organization. Three-step analgesic ladder. Cancer pain relief and palliative care: report of a WHO expert committee. *WHO Technical Support Series*. 1990;**804**:1–73.

World Health Organization. The global economic and healthcare burden of musculoskeletal disease. 2001. www.boneandjointdecade.org. Accessed April 18, 2003.

Fibromyalgia

ETIOLOGY AND PATHOPHYSIOLOGY

Introduction

Fibromyalgia is a chronic pain syndrome of unknown etiology. The American College of Rheumatology (ACR) 1990 classification criteria for fibromyalgia include a history of chronic, widespread pain for more than three months and the presence of at least 11 of 18 anatomically defined "tender points" upon physical examination (Figure 1). Fibromyalgia tender points may vary in intensity and location, but to meet ACR criteria, they must occur both above and below the waist and on both sides of the body. In addition to pain, the majority of fibromyalgia sufferers experience auxiliary symptoms: fatigue, sleep dysfunction, cognitive difficulties (e.g., memory impairment, difficulty concentrating), headache, and/or gastrointestinal upset, among others (Figure 2).

Despite recent advances, the precise pathophysiological mechanisms underlying fibromyalgia syndrome remain unclear. Nevertheless, researchers are beginning to connect various theories that may come together to help explain the symptomatology of the condition. Indeed, the potentially important role of autonomic dysregulation has recently been identified, and researchers have found that the pain in fibromyalgia is most likely centrally mediated and the result of both increased excitability of central neurons and decreased pain inhibitory mechanisms.

Wiley Handbook of Current and Emerging Drug Therapies, Volumes 5–8
Copyright © 2007 Decision Resources, Inc. Published by John Wiley & Sons, Inc.

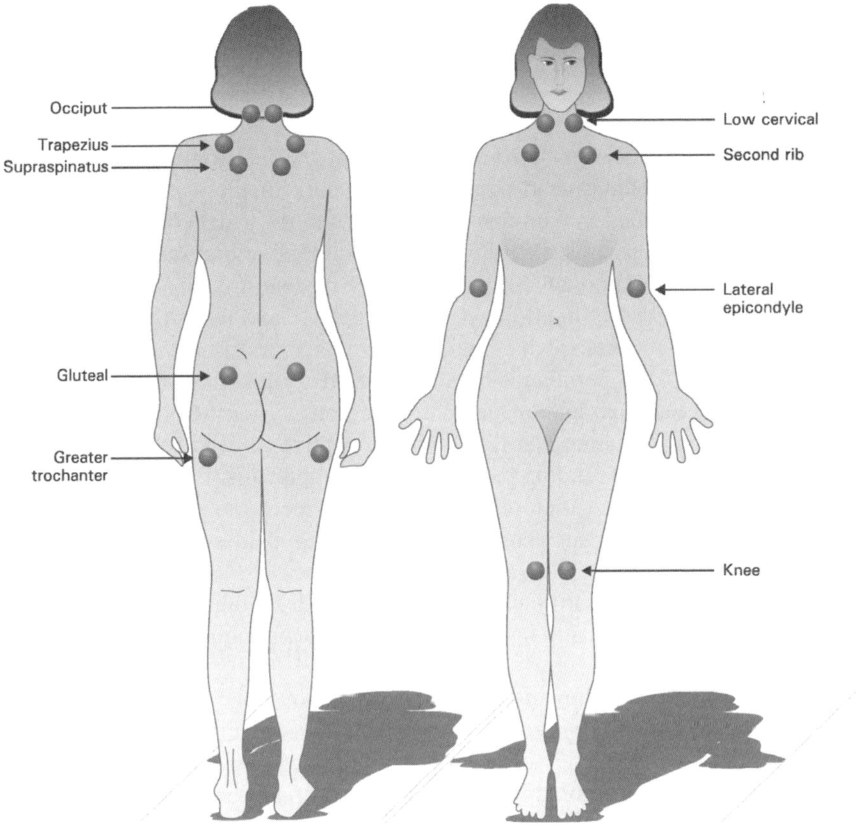

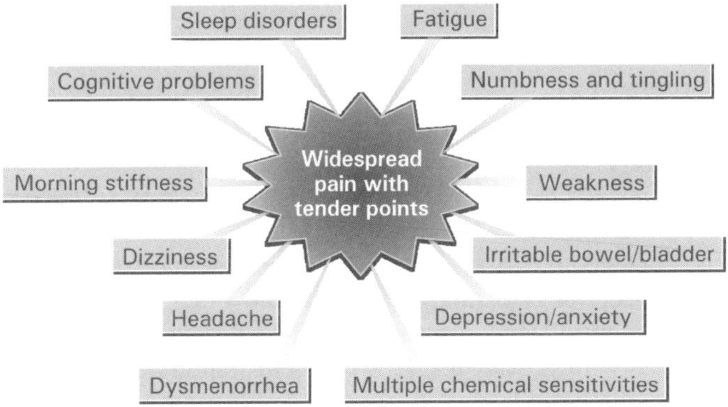

FIGURE 1. *Locations of specific tender points in fibromyalgia as defined by the American College of Rheumatology.*

FIGURE 2. *Fibromyalgia symptomatology.*

The following sections discuss the current understanding of the pathophysiology and etiology of fibromyalgia syndrome in more detail.

Pathophysiology

Pain Pathways. Although fibromyalgia patients suffer from a wide range of symptoms, chronic, widespread pain is the hallmark of the syndrome. Chronic pain is generally defined as pain that persists beyond the usual course of an acute disease, beyond a reasonable time for an injury to heal, or that recurs at intervals for months or years. Although chronic pain may present in many different forms and can vary significantly in etiology, clinical course, and response to treatment, all types of persistent, unexplained pain involve basic aberrations in somatosensory processing in the peripheral nervous system (originating, for example, in the muscles and tendons) and/or the central nervous system (CNS).

In general, pain signaling involves both nociceptive (ascending pain pathway) and antinociceptive (descending pain pathway) components. Ascending pain signals, triggered by the activation of somatic sensory receptors (nociceptors), reach the brain and result in pain perception. Descending pain signals, activated by the arrival of ascending pain signals, relay pain to various sites in the periphery and modulate further upward pain transmission. (See Figure 3.) Research implicates aberrant pain processing involving both the ascending and descending pain pathways in fibromyalgia.

More specifically, fibromyalgia sufferers seem to experience both increased sensitivity to pain, involving central neuron excitability and disturbed nociception (Coda B, 2001), and decreased activation of descending pain inhibitory systems (e.g., serotonergic, noradrenergic, opioidergic pathways) (Julien N, 2005). Researchers theorize that hypersensitivity to pain derives partly from an imbalance between the inhibitory and facilitatory impulses in the descending tracts (Henriksson KG, 2003). While the cause of such aberrant pain processing in fibromyalgia remains unclear, researchers propose the involvement of chronic psychological stressors, peripheral pain generators, and inflammatory mediators (e.g., cytokines) (Bennett R, 2004).

Central Sensitization. The neuronal excitability, or "central sensitization," theory has received much attention because this phenomenon seems to be involved in various chronic, non-inflammatory (e.g., neuropathic) pain conditions (Chen H, 2004; Essick GK, 2004; Romanelli P, 2004). Indeed, evidence suggests that sensitization of dorsal horn and brain stem neurons in response to low frequency nociceptive input that would otherwise have no effect in healthy controls plays a central role in fibromyalgia and other musculoskeletal disorders involving "referred" tenderness and pain (Arendt-Nielsen L, 2003; Staud R, 2004b). (Referred pain is pain felt in a different region, away from the source of the pain.) Researchers suspect that such sensitization results from a process called "wind up," during which repetitive nociceptive stimuli of sufficient frequency or intensity to remove the magnesium block of the N-methyl-D-aspartate

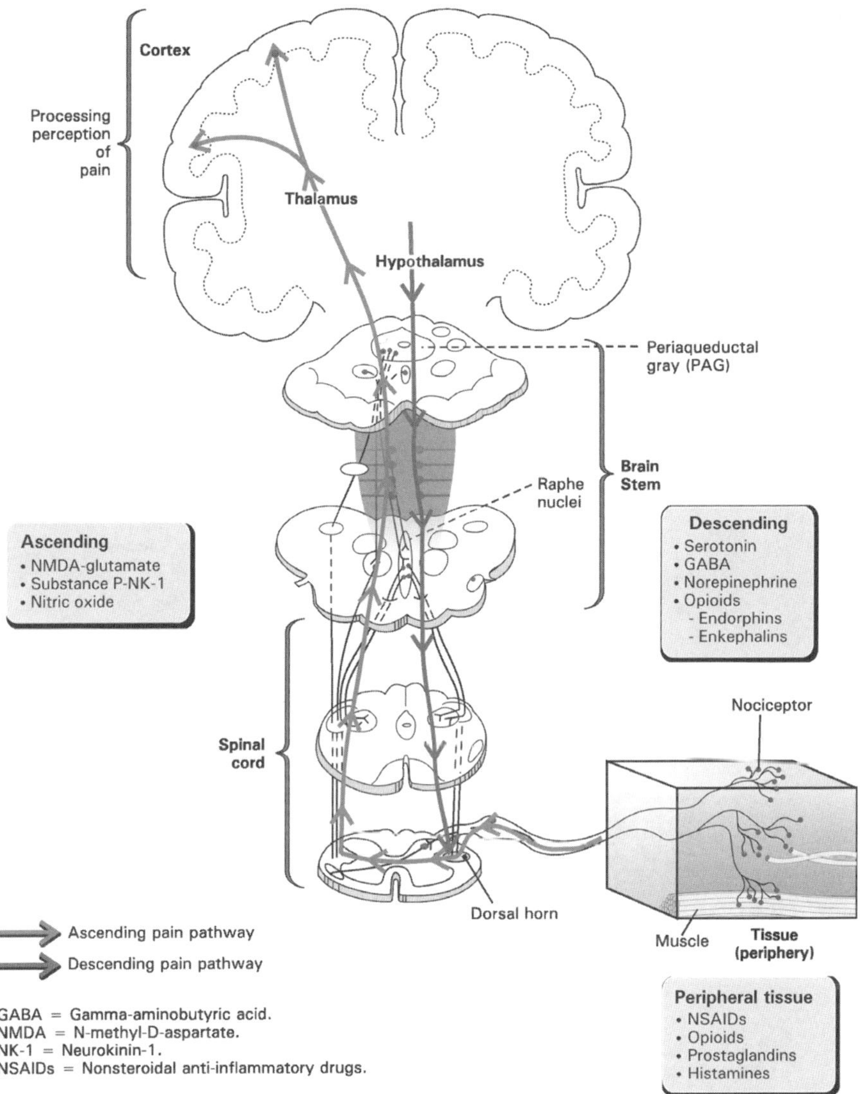

FIGURE 3. *Ascending and descending pain pathways.*

(NMDA) receptor cause cellular calcium influx that leads to the triggering of signal cascades that in turn lead to amplification of nociceptive input (Figure 4) (Price DD, 2002; Staud R, 2001; Staud R, 2003).

Central sensitization can result in hyperalgesia (heightened pain response), persistent pain (protracted pain response), and allodynia (inappropriate pain response to nonpainful stimulus). Such clinical manifestations characterize fibromyalgia pain; indeed, some fibromyalgia sufferers interpret such non-noxious stimuli as

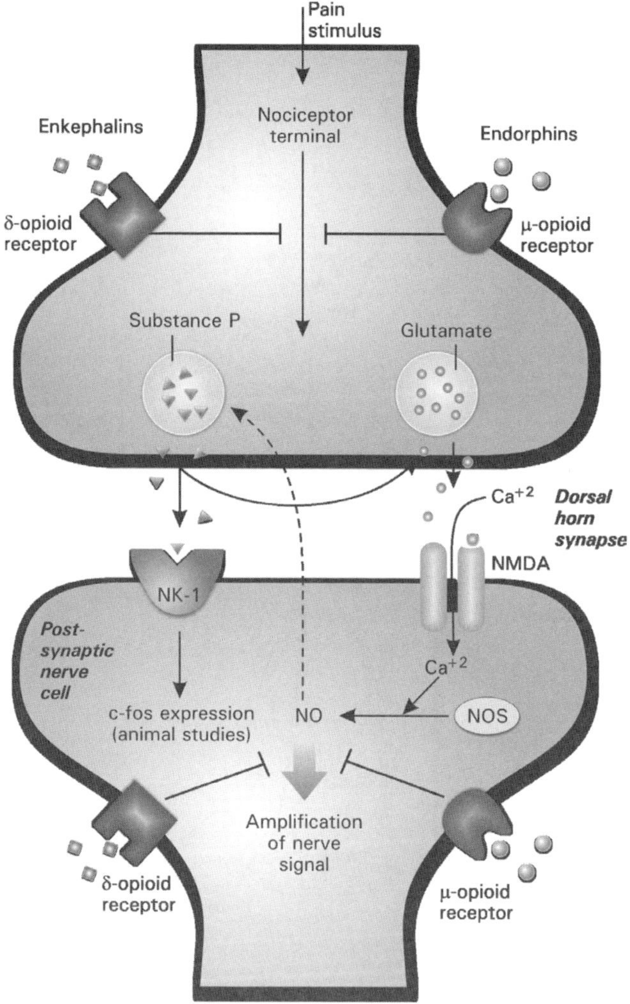

Ca^{+2} = Calcium ion.
NK-1 = Neurokinin-1.
NMDA = N-methyl-D-aspartate.
NO = Nitric oxide.
NOS = Nitric oxide synthase.

FIGURE 4. *Schematic of nociceptive and antinociceptive pathways in the dorsal horn.*

light, touch, odor, and sound as painful (much like people who suffer from migraine headaches).

As noted earlier, researchers do not yet understand what initiates such a sensitized state in fibromyalgia. The prevailing theories involve changes in the CNS (i.e., neuroplasticity) resulting from persistent nociceptive input from muscles and/or from psychological or biologic (infection, inflammation) stressors (via disordered cytokine networks). Such chronic stressors may lead to an impaired stress response involving the hypothalamic-pituitary-adrenal (HPA) axis (and impaired cortisol release) and possibly the ventral tegmental-mesolimbic dopamine system (via downregulation of dopamine secretion, resulting in hyperalgesia) (Bennett R, 2004).

Autonomic Arousal. Although central sensitization and aberrant pain processing may help to explain the chronic pain component of fibromyalgia, these phenomenon do not explain the other symptoms commonly experienced by fibromyalgia sufferers (e.g., fatigue, sleep disorders, gastrointestinal upset). Consequently, some researchers suspect a role for dysautonomia in fibromyalgia syndrome (Martinez-Lavin M, 2004). More specifically, a disruption in the sympathetic branch of the autonomic nervous system (ANS)—characterized by constant sympathetic hyperactivity—may result in the development of fibromyalgia symptoms (Kelemen J, 1998; Raj SR, 2000). Such persistent hyperactivity may eventually lead to desensitization and downregulation of adrenergic receptors. This downregulation could leave the individual incapable of responding to various stressors, which could account for some of the unrelenting fatigue and morning stiffness experienced in fibromyalgia. Chronic sympathetic hyperactivity could also contribute to such symptoms as sleep dysfunction, anxiety, and gastrointestinal upset in these patients.

Heart rate variability analyses support a role for sympathetic hyperactivity in fibromyalgia (Cohen H, 2000; Cohen H, 2001; Kooh M, 2003; Martinez-Lavin M, 1998; Raj SR, 2000). Studies have shown that fibromyalgia pain is responsive to sympathetic blockade and that such pain is also rekindled by norepinephrine injections (Bengtsson A, 1988; Martinez-Lavin M, 2002). In light of these findings, researchers are further investigating the role of dysautonomia in fibromyalgia syndrome.

Biochemical Mediators.
Serotonin and Norepinephrine. Serotonin (5-HT) and norepinephrine (NE) play an important role in pain processing (via descending inhibitory pathways), as evidenced by the analgesic properties of antidepressants that target these neurotransmitters (see "Current Therapies" and "Emerging Therapies"). Indeed, studies have shown that fibromyalgia sufferers exhibit reduced cerebrospinal fluid levels of the principal metabolites of both 5-HT and NE (Legangneux E, 2001; Russell IJ, 1992). Researchers suspect that deficits in 5-HT and NE contribute in part to the pain in fibromyalgia. Nevertheless, antidepressants that increase 5-HT- and/or NE-mediated neurotransmission (either directly or indirectly) only appear to provide pain relief in one third of fibromyalgia sufferers, reinforcing the belief that these mediators represent only one piece in a larger puzzle that leads to fibromyalgia symptomatology.

Dopamine. New findings also suggest a role for dopamine in fibromyalgia (Wood PB, 2004). The dopamine D2/D3 agonists ropinirole (GlaxoSmithKline

[Brentford, Middlesex, United Kingdom] Requip) and pramipexole (Boehringer Inhelheim's [Ingelheim, Germany] and Pfizer's [New York, New York] Mirapex/Sifrol) have been shown to provide symptom relief in severely affected fibromyalgia sufferers (Holman AJ, 2004a; Holman AJ, 2004b). While the precise role of dopamine in fibromyalgia syndrome remains unclear, researchers suspect that it may be a central component of an underlying autonomic dysfunction in these patients.

Substance P. Substance P is a neuromodulator that researchers believe plays an important role in pain transmission and, more specifically, in the process leading to central sensitization (Khasabov SG, 2002; Terman GW, 2001). Numerous studies have demonstrated elevated cerebrospinal fluid levels of substance P in fibromyalgia patients (Russell IJ, 1994; Spath M, 2003; Stratz T, 2004; Vaeroy H, 1988; Welin M, 1995), and similar findings have been reported in osteoarthritis of the hip and chronic low back pain (Clauw DJ, 2001; Ordeberg G, 2004).

Because of its role in transmitting pain and its elevated levels in individuals suffering from pain and depression, substance P has received attention as a potential therapeutic target for these conditions. However, drug development efforts to date have been disappointing; the substance P antagonists that have reached clinical development thus far have shown little efficacy in depression or pain.

Glutamate. The role of glutamate in painful conditions such as fibromyalgia is evidenced primarily through the ability of drugs that act as NMDA antagonists (e.g., dextromethorphan)—NMDA is a receptor for glutamate—to relieve chronic neurogenic pain (Clark S, 2000; Graven-Nielsen T, 2000; Sorensen J, 1995). Indeed, NMDA antagonists may help to normalize substance P-mediated neurotransmission (Eide PK, 2000; Herrero JF, 2000). Although extensive investigations have been devoted to the development of novel NMDA antagonists for conditions associated with neuronal hyperexcitability (e.g., epilepsy, central pain conditions), results to date have been disappointing because blockade of these receptors leads to numerous unwanted side effects. Nevertheless, drug companies continue to devote considerable resources to such programs in hope of developing compounds with improved tolerability and efficacy profiles. Such programs remain in early stages and include the following strategies: use of lower-affinity NMDA receptor antagonists; targeting of modulatory sites (e.g., glycine site antagonists); use of subtype-selective antagonists (e.g., NR2B-subunit selective antagonists); use of treatments that target two receptors or signaling molecules at the same pain-processing site; use of regional administration; use of peripherally limited blockers (Sang CN, 2005).

Cortisol. Some studies suggest that fibromyalgia sufferers have an impaired HPA axis response to stressors (Adler GK, 1999; Adler GK, 2002; Adler GK, 2005). (Stress is thought to be a primary trigger for fibromyalgia.) Stressful events activate the HPA axis, which releases hormones that gradually modulate circulating cortisol levels, the key compound in the stress response pathway. Cortisol is also important in regulating stress responses because it plays a role in the multiple negative feedback loops of the HPA axis (Young EA, 1991). Cortisol levels are abnormal in some fibromyalgia patients (Neeck G, 2000). Moreover, the maintenance of cortisol levels within certain boundaries is critical to proper functioning of the HPA axis; both overproduction and underproduction of cortisol in otherwise healthy people can result in symptoms common to fibromyalgia, such as fatigue, weakness, sleep disorders, muscle pain, and mood disorders (Crofford LJ, 1994; Miller DB, 2002; Sachar EJ, 1970). Such symptoms could be related to elevated cytokine levels resulting from the impaired cortisol stress response (Capuron L, 2002; Kiecolt-Glaser JK, 2003). To date, drugs affecting cortisol levels do not appear to be in development for fibromyalgia, but some companies (e.g., Bristol Myers Squibb, Neurocrine Biosciences) are investigating the potential of such compounds as corticotrophin-releasing factor (CRF) antagonists in depression and anxiety.

Sleep Disturbance. Studies have demonstrated that disruption of deep sleep in healthy volunteers results in symptoms similar to those seen in fibromyalgia, such as unrefreshed sleep, fatigue, and muscle pain (Cote KA, 1997; Moldofsky H, 1975; Moldofsky H, 2001). Moreover, polysomnographic (PSG) readings from fibromyalgia sufferers reveal an alpha-electroencephalographic (α-EEG) anomaly, or "alpha intrusion," in these patients, which investigators suspect leads to unrefreshing sleep and, ultimately, to excessive fatigue and increased pain sensitivity. Under normal conditions, the α-EEG frequency (7.5–11 Hz) occurs during light sleep, gradually disappears during deep sleep, and is replaced by slower δ frequencies (less than 3.5 Hz). The α pattern then reappears with arousals from sleep. The α-EEG anomaly seen in fibromyalgia patients is essentially due to nondiminishing alpha waves during deep sleep (Moldofsky H, 1975). These patients may not have trouble falling asleep, but, because of the continuous presence of α waves, they remain in the light, nonrestorative, and nonreplenishing phases of sleep.

Some researchers suspect that symptoms of fibromyalgia may relate to the aforementioned fragmented sleep pattern (Dauvilliers Y, 2001). Consequently, companies with sleep-enhancing drugs are now investigating their respective compounds in clinical trials for fibromyalgia. In fact, Orphan Medical's recently marketed CNS depressant sodium oxybate (used to improve sleep in narcoleptic patients) was shown to reduce alpha intrusion and simultaneously reduce pain and fatigue in fibromyalgia sufferers (Scharf MB, 2003). These data are discussed in more detail in the "Emerging Therapies" section. Importantly, these data suggest that sleep disturbance itself may be a causal contributor to fibromyalgia syndrome, rather than a symptom.

Etiology

Although fibromyalgia's etiology remains elusive, researchers hypothesize that the syndrome results from precipitating events ("stress triggers"), such as physical or emotional trauma, infection, sleep disorders, various physiological dysfunctions, and pathological activation of the immune system. Gender (i.e., being female) and age (i.e., 35–55 years of age) also appear to be relevant risk factors, and some suspect that genetic predisposition plays an important role as well. Expert consensus is that fibromyalgia emerges when a genetically predisposed person is exposed to various stressors that, in turn, cause a complex, multisystem syndrome (Staud R, 2004a).

CURRENT THERAPIES

Given that there is no universally accepted pathophysiological mechanism that underlies fibromyalgia syndrome, pharmacological treatment remains largely empiric. Indeed, no drugs have yet achieved official regulatory approval for the treatment of this condition in any of the major pharmaceutical markets (United States, France, Germany, Italy, Spain, United Kingdom, and Japan). Consequently, physicians prescribe a wide variety of drugs to treat the syndrome, with particular emphasis on pain control and improvements in sleep and mood. Many patients find the currently available agents—all of which are used off-label for this indication—either insufficient to control their symptoms or difficult to tolerate; as a result, patient satisfaction with current treatments is low.

Table 1 summarizes the leading pharmacological therapies used to treat fibromyalgia. Table 2 compares the advantages and disadvantages of the respective therapies. Table 3 reviews the clinical end points used to determine drug efficacy in clinical trials for fibromyalgia.

Antidepressants

Overview. Antidepressants—particularly the older tricyclic antidepressants (TCAs) such as amitriptyline (AstraZeneca's [Wilmington, Delaware], Elavil, Roche's [Basel, Switzerland] Laroxyl, generics)—are standard first-line pharmacological therapies for fibromyalgia. In addition to these agents' proven benefits in mood disorders such as anxiety and depression—both of which are very common in fibromyalgia patients—antidepressants have been shown to reduce the pain and fatigue associated with fibromyalgia. Whether this reduction in pain and fatigue is simply a by-product of such agents' mood-enhancing effects has been an area of controversy among physicians; however, recent findings involving functional imaging of the brains of fibromyalgia sufferers with depression support the widely held belief of most pain experts that these two pathways function independently (Giesecke T, 2005). Indeed, such findings help explain why some narrowly acting antidepressants provide only mood-enhancing effects in fibromyalgia while other, broader-acting antidepressants provide both mood-enhancing and analgesic effects (or even analgesic effects only). The mechanisms governing such effects seem to be similar but separate.

TCAs are the mainstay of antidepressant treatment for fibromyalgia—despite the availability of more tolerable antidepressants such as the selective serotonin reuptake inhibitors (SSRIs) and the serotonergic and noradrenergic reuptake

TABLE 1. Current Therapies Used to Treat Fibromyalgia

Agent	Company/Brand	Average Daily Dose	Availability
Antidepressants			
Amitriptyline	AstraZeneca's Elavil, Roche's Laroxyl, generics	10–25 mg	US, F, G, I, S, UK, J
Fluoxetine	Eli Lilly's Prozac, generics	20 mg	US, F, G, I, S, UK
Venlafaxine	Wyeth's Effexor/Effexor XR	75–150 mg	US, F, G, I, S, UK
Muscle relaxants			
Cyclobenzaprine	Alza's Flexeril, generics	5–10 mg	US, I, S
NSAIDs			
Ibuprofen	Pfizer's Motrin, Knoll's Brufen, generics	1,200–2,400 mg	US, F, G, I, S, UK, J
Celecoxib	Pfizer's Celebrex	100–200 mg	US, F, G, I, S, UK
Sedative hypnotics			
Temazepam	Mallinckrodt's Restoril, generics	30 mg	US, F, G, I, UK
Zolpidem	Sanofi-Aventis's Ambien, generics	10 mg	US, F, G, I, S, UK, J
Narcotic analgesics			
Codeine	Multiple brands and generics	60–120 mg	US, F, G, I, S, UK, J
Fentanyl	Janssen/Alza's Duragesic/ Durogesic	25–300 mcg/hour patch (replaced every 3 days)	US, F, G, I, S, UK, J
Other analgesics			
Paracetamol	Multiple brands and generics	4 g	F, G, I, S, UK, J
Tramadol	Ortho-McNeil's Ultram/Ultracet[a]	150–200 mg	US, F, G, I, S, UK
Antiepileptic drugs			
Clonazepam	Roche's Klonopin, generics	1.5 mg	US, F, G, I, S, UK, J
Gabapentin	Pfizer's Neurontin, generics	900–1,800 mg	US, F, G, I, S, UK

[a]Ortho-McNeil's Ultracet is a fixed combination of tramadol + acetaminophen.
US = United States; F = France; G = Germany; I = Italy; S = Spain; UK = United Kingdom; J = Japan.
NSAIDs = Nonsteroidal anti-inflammatory drugs.

inhibitors (SNRIs)—because these older agents have been more thoroughly studied, clinically speaking, than the newer agents, and because they have a relatively long history of use in treating fibromyalgia. SSRIs and SNRIs, on the other hand, have a relatively short history of use in fibromyalgia and have few reliable data to support their efficacy in treating this population. Nevertheless, physicians often prescribe these newer antidepressants for fibromyalgia patients in an attempt to avoid the tolerability issues that plague the TCAs (e.g., anticholinergic effects, weight gain, sedation).

TABLE 2. Comparison of Current Therapies Used to Treat Fibromyalgia

Class/Compound	Advantages	Disadvantages
Antidepressants	• Demonstrated efficacy in well-controlled fibromyalgia trials (amitriptyline, fluoxetine) • Improve pain, mood, and sleep • Treat comorbid depression and/or anxiety • Affordable (if generically available) • Simple dosing (usually at bedtime)	• Unpredictable patient response • Not well tolerated in some patients • High occurrence of sexual dysfunction • Stigma associated with "antidepressant" use • No evidence for long-term efficacy in fibromyalgia
Muscle relaxants	• Demonstrated efficacy in well-controlled fibromyalgia trials (cyclobenzaprine) • Improve sleep • Affordable • Simple dosing (at bedtime)	• Unpredictable patient response • Sedating • Minimal effect on pain • No mood-enhancing properites • No evidence for long-term efficacy in fibromyalgia
NSAIDs	• Physician familiarity and ease of use • Well-tolerated • Affordable (if generically available)	• No evidence for efficacy in fibromyalgia • Can cause gastrointestinal damage with long-term use • Increased risk for cardiovascular events with long-term use
Sedative hypnotics	• Demonstrated efficacy for insomnia • Well-tolerated • Simple dosing (at bedtime)	• No evidence for efficacy in fibromyalgia • No analgesic properties • No mood-enhancing properties • Physician reluctance to prescribe chronically
Narcotic analgesics	• Demonstrated efficacy in moderate-to-severe pain • Relatively well-tolerated • Affordable (if generically available) • Rapid-acting	• No evidence for efficacy in fibromyalgia • Unpredictable patient response • Risk for tolerance and dependence • Regulatory restrictions on use ("controlled substances") • Stigma associated with "narcotic" use
Tramadol	• Demonstrated efficacy in well-controlled fibromyalgia trials • Relatively well-tolerated • Rapid-acting	• Unpredictable patient response • No mood-enhancing properties • Minimal sleep benefit • No evidence for long-term efficacy in fibromyalgia
Antiepileptic drugs (AEDs)	• Proven efficacy in centrally-mediated pain syndromes (neuropathic pain) • Relatively well-tolerated (gabapentin)	• No evidence for efficacy in fibromyalgia • Unpredictable patient response • No mood-enhancing properties • Complicated dosing

TABLE 3. Standard Clinical End Points Used In Fibromyalgia Trials

Assessment of Pain
Visual Analog Scale (VAS)-Pain
Gracely Pain Scale
Fibromyalgia Impact Questionnaire (FIQ)-Pain VAS and Stiffness VAS
Brief Pain Inventory (BPI)
McGuill Pain Questionnaire (MPQ)
Tender Point Index (TPI)/ Tender Point Count (TPC)
Likert Pain Scale (LPS)

Assessment of Sleep/Fatigue
VAS-Sleep
FIQ-Fatigue VAS and Morning Tiredness VAS
Medical Outcomes Study (MOS)-Sleep
Chalder Fatigue Rating Scale
Pittsburgh Sleep Quality Index
Sleep Interference Diary
Jenkins Sleep Scale
Multidimensional Assessment of Fatigue
Polysomnography (PSG)

Assessment of Mood
Montgomery-Asberg Depression Rating Scale (MADRS)
Beck Depression Inventory (BDI)
FIQ-Depression VAS and Anxiety VAS
Quality of Life in Depression Scale
Arthritis Impact Measurement Scales (AIMS)-Anxiety and Depression
Profile of Mood States (POMS)

Assessment of Disability/Quality of Life
MOS Short Form 36 (SF-36)
Nottingham Health Profile
Sheehan Disability Scale
VAS-General Health
FIQ-Domains (physical function, feel good, missed work, job ability)
Health Utility Index (HUI)
Quality of Life Index
Quality of Life Survey
Sickness Impact Profile (SIP)

Assessment of Global Outcomes
FIQ-Total
Clinical Global Impression (CGI)[a]
Patient Global Impression (PGI)[a]
Clinical Health Assessment Questionnaire (CLINHAQ)

[a]Measures severity, change, and improvement.

Mechanism of Action. Antidepressants are believed to elicit their mood-enhancing and analgesic effects primarily by blocking the synaptic reuptake of two neurotransmitters—serotonin (5-HT) and norepinephrine (NE)—both of which are functionally inhibitory on pain transmission (via the descending pain pathway). While other purported antidepressant mechanisms such as potassium-channel modulation and N-methyl-D-aspartate (NMDA) receptor antagonism may also play a role in pain modulation, the relative importance of these mechanisms in pain control remains unclear (Lawson K, 2002).

TCAs, which are the most broadly acting antidepressants (i.e., they block muscarinic, α1-adrenergic, cholinergic, and histaminergic receptors in addition to their activity on 5-HT and NE), boast the most evidence for efficacy in painful conditions such as fibromyalgia. SSRIs, which are the most narrowly acting antidepressants (i.e., they are very selective for 5-HT), have the least evidence for efficacy in such conditions. SNRIs, which fall somewhere in the middle in the sense that they provide clinically meaningful reuptake inhibition of both 5-HT and NE, are slowly gaining momentum when it comes to the treatment of pain, largely because of the positive data that has recently emerged for both Cypress Bioscience, Inc. (San Diego, California)/Forest Laboratories (New York, New York) milnacipran and Eli Lilly and Company's (Indianapolis, Indiana) new SNRI duloxetine (see "Emerging Therapies"). This apparent spectrum of efficacy within the antidepressant class of drugs suggests that multiple neurotransmitters are involved in the analgesic effects of these agents (Arnold LM, 2000; O'Malley PG, 2000).

Amitriptyline. Amitriptyline (AstraZeneca's Elavil, Roche's Laroxyl, generics) (Figure 5) was approved in the United States more than 40 years ago for the treatment of depression and has since reached every other major market. Although the drug never received supplemental approval for any pain condition, a wealth of positive data from small clinical trials in which amitriptyline was administered to treat chronic pain has elevated the drug to the level of first-line treatment for various chronic pain conditions (e.g., fibromyalgia) in which patients have few effective alternatives. Researchers suspect that amitriptyline relieves pain primarily by blocking the synaptic uptake of 5-HT and NE.

In one 12-week study, amitriptyline improved quality of life and disability in fibromyalgia patients (Hannonen P, 1998). In this two-part multicenter study, 130 female patients with fibromyalgia were randomized to receive amitriptyline 25 mg, moclobemide 450 mg, or placebo for six weeks, followed by amitriptyline 37.5 mg, moclobemide 600 mg, or placebo for the remaining six weeks. (Moclobemide [Roche's Aurorix/Maclamine/Manerix] is an antidepressant that acts as a reversible monoamine oxidase-type A inhibitor.) At the end of the study period, amitriptyline conferred significant pain relief in 74% of patients, compared with 54% and 49% for moclobemide and placebo, respectively, as measured using the 0–100 mm visual analogue score (VAS), a commonly used and well-validated method for measuring the severity of pain. The amitriptyline-treated patients also showed significant improvements in general health, sleep

$$CH(CH_2)_2N(CH_3)_2$$

FIGURE 5. *Structure of amitriptyline.*

quality and quantity, and fatigue on the Nottingham Health Profile (a quality-of-life measure that evaluates emotional, social, and physical distress) and the Sheehan Functional Disability Scale (a measure of psychiatric impairment).

In a separate six-month trial in which fibromyalgia patients ($n = 208$) were randomized to receive either amitriptyline, cyclobenzaprine (a muscle relaxant that has a tricyclic structure similar to that of amitriptyline; see the later section "Muscle Relaxants"), or placebo (Carette S, 1994), study investigators recorded an initial improvement in patients taking drug therapy compared to placebo; however, by the six-month time point, the difference in improvement between drug-treated and placebo-treated patients was no longer significant. Experts in the field say that these findings reflect either a loss of response to the drugs over time (i.e., tachyphylaxis) or, more likely, a study design that was underpowered and/or not designed to give optimal doses of the drugs (Clauw DJ, 2003). Nevertheless, these data underscore the difficulty in effectively treating fibromyalgia patients.

Because so few drugs have shown efficacy in fibromyalgia, even a small degree of improvement—such as that seen in clinical trials with amitriptyline—is an important finding. However, that amitriptyline has its own host of tolerability issues, which make it a less than ideal treatment option for many patients. Even at the low doses administered for fibromyalgia (10–25 mg at bedtime), many patients cannot tolerate the drug's anticholinergic effects (e.g., dry mouth, constipation, blurred vision, urinary retention, cognitive impairment).

Fluoxetine. Fluoxetine (Eli Lilly's Prozac, generics) (Figure 6) has been marketed for depression in the United States and Europe since 1988 and has since achieved supplemental approvals for obsessive-compulsive disorder (OCD), bulimia, and panic disorder. In Japan, fluoxetine had reached Phase III development for depression before Chugai Pharmaceutical (Tokyo, Japan) and Eli Lilly terminated their codevelopment deal for the drug.

Fluoxetine is the least selective SSRI and has the longest half-life (seven to ten days for its active metabolite norfluoxetine). The drug's extended half-life allows for missed doses without the loss of effect associated with some other SSRIs. However, the drug's relatively long time to elimination necessitates an extended washout period (two to five weeks) after discontinuation of therapy—a drawback when a patient needs to be switched to another agent. Enteric-coated, delayed-release fluoxetine (Prozac Weekly) is also available for patients who have been stabilized on immediate-release fluoxetine and who want weekly instead of daily administration.

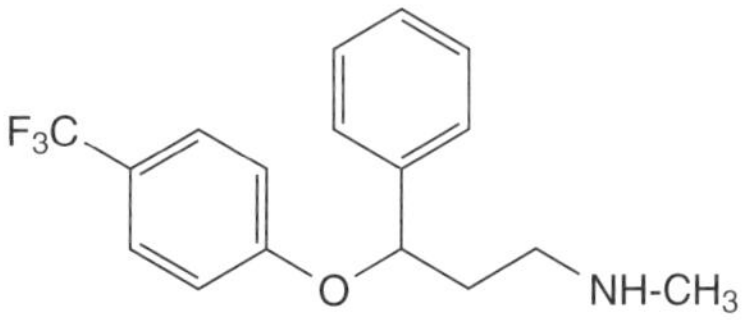

FIGURE 6. *Structure of fluoxetine.*

Clinical results with fluoxetine for fibromyalgia have been mixed. In one six-week, placebo-controlled study involving 42 female fibromyalgia patients, fluoxetine 20 mg daily was no more effective than placebo at reducing the symptoms of fibromyalgia (Wolfe F, 1994). However, in a more recent 12-week, placebo-controlled study involving 60 female fibromyalgia patients, fluoxetine (10–80 mg daily; mean dose 45 ± 25 mg) was shown to be superior to placebo in reducing pain and other fibromyalgia symptoms, as measured by the Fibromyalgia Impact Questionnaire (FIQ) (Arnold LM, 2002). In this study, fluoxetine-treated patients showed significant improvements in the primary outcome measures of FIQ-total score (difference of -12 compared with placebo) and FIQ-pain score (difference of -2.2 compared with placebo), as well as in the FIQ-fatigue and depression scores and the McGill Pain Questionnaire; differences in the number of tender points and total myalgic scores were not statistically significant, although there was a trend toward more improvement in fluoxetine-treated patients. Additional data from studies in which fluoxetine was administered in combination with either amitriptyline or cyclobenzaprine reveal that these drug combinations provide effective symptom relief in many fibromyalgia sufferers (Cantini F, 1994; Goldenberg D, 1996).

Venlafaxine. Venlafaxine (Wyeth's [Madison, New Jersey] Effexor/Effexor XR) (Figure 7) is approved for depression, generalized anxiety disorder, and social phobia. It is available in all the major markets except Japan, in both immediate- and extended-release (XR, or once-daily) formulations; it is in Phase III trials for depression in Japan. Wyeth has also conducted clinical trials for painful conditions, including fibromyalgia, in the United States and Europe (Grothe DR, 2004).

Venlafaxine blocks the uptake of 5-HT and NE almost equally and has little effect on muscarinic, cholinergic, histaminergic, and noradrenergic receptors. It also has some dopaminergic activity, but whether this activity is clinically meaningful at therapeutic doses is unclear. Venlafaxine's NE reuptake inhibition is like that of the TCAs, whereas its side-effect profile is more like that of the SSRIs. Because venlafaxine can be difficult to tolerate initially (owing to side effects such as nausea, headache, and dizziness), slow titration to a therapeutic dose is usually necessary. At doses greater than 200 mg/day, patients may experience sustained, dose-dependent increases in blood pressure; consequently, patients taking the higher doses require careful monitoring.

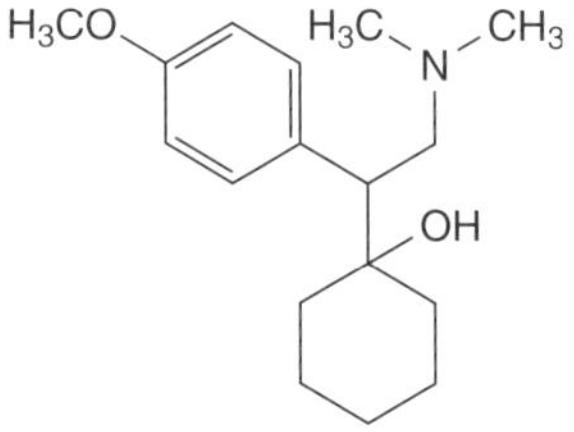

FIGURE 7. *Structure of venlafaxine.*

Results from the only placebo-controlled study conducted with venlafaxine in fibromyalgia patients to date revealed that the 75 mg dose of the drug was not effective at relieving symptoms of the condition (Zijlstra TR, 2002). In this study, 90 patients were randomized to receive venlafaxine 75 mg daily or placebo for six weeks. The primary end point was pain reduction, as measured using the VAS and the McGill Pain Questionnaire (MPQ). Secondary end points included reduction in the number of tender points and improvement in general health, including depression and sleep; these were measured using the FIQ, the Beck Depression Inventory (BDI), the VAS-general health, and the VAS-sleep. Patients were assessed at zero, two, four, and six weeks of treatment. At study completion, treatment with both venlafaxine and placebo resulted in a 10% improvement in the VAS and MPQ pain scores; similar results were observed on the secondary end points.

Other small, open-label studies in fibromyalgia patients have shown more positive results for venlafaxine (Borman P, 2004; Dwight MM, 1998; Sayar K, 2003). However, the uncontrolled nature of these studies renders these data less than reliable.

Muscle Relaxants

Overview. Muscle relaxants, which are most commonly prescribed to relieve the pain and discomfort associated with muscle injury or spasm, include a heterogeneous mixture of agents that differ greatly in their chemical, pharmacological, and pharmacokinetic properties. In the treatment of fibromyalgia, the muscle relaxant cyclobenzaprine (ALZA Corporation's [Mountain View, California] Flexeril, generics) provides modest pain relief. The following section discusses cyclobenzaprine in more detail because this agent is the only muscle relaxant that has been studied in well-controlled fibromyalgia trials.

Mechanism of Action. Most muscle relaxants modify pain perception via multiple mechanisms of action. Cyclobenzaprine, in particular, inhibits NE and 5-HT reuptake while also inhibiting gamma and alpha motor neurons within the brain stem.

Cyclobenzaprine. Cyclobenzaprine (Alza's Flexeril, generics) (Figure 8) was introduced in the United States more than 25 years ago as an adjunctive therapy for the treatment of muscle spasm associated with acute, painful musculoskeletal

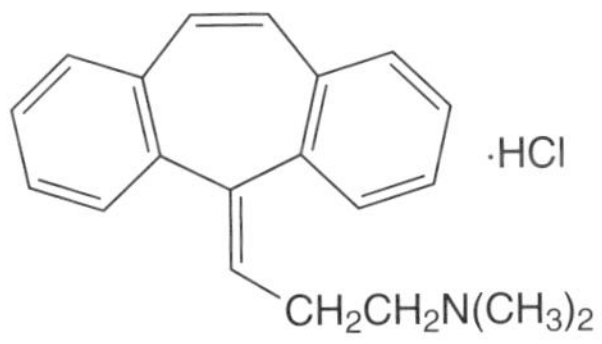

FIGURE 8. *Structure of cyclobenzaprine hydrochloride.*

conditions. Since its launch, cyclobenzaprine has become the most commonly prescribed therapy for the treatment of muscle spasms in the United States (it is also available in some European Union countries, including Italy and Spain). In 2003, McNeil Consumer & Specialty Pharmaceuticals (Fort Washington, Pennsylvania) introduced a new low-dose form of cyclobenzaprine (Flexeril 5 mg) that was shown to be comparable to the standard 10 mg dose in terms of pain relief (in patients with muscle spasm associated with acute, painful musculoskeletal conditions), but less sedating. This low-dose form of the drug is an attractive alternative for fibromyalgia patients, whose fatigue can be exacerbated by highly sedating drugs such as cyclobenzaprine.

Cyclobenzaprine has a tricyclic structure similar to that of amitriptyline. It has anticholinergic, antihistaminic, and sedative properties but negligible antidepressant activity because it only weakly inhibits NE and 5-HT reuptake. In several small, well-controlled clinical trials, cyclobenzaprine has been shown to improve the symptoms of fibromyalgia (Bennett RM, 1988; Cantini F, 1994; Reynolds WJ, 1991; Santandrea S, 1993). Cyclobenzaprine is prescribed primarily as an adjunct to other medications for the treatment of fibromyalgia.

Nonsteroidal Anti-Inflammatory Drugs

Overview. There is currently no evidence that nonsteroidal anti-inflammatory drugs (NSAIDs)—including traditional NSAIDs and selective COX-2 inhibitors—are effective in the treatment of fibromyalgia. Nevertheless, both the traditional agents, such as ibuprofen (Pfizer's Motrin, Knoll Pharmaceutical's [Mount Olive, New Jersey] Brufen, generics) and naproxen (Roche's Naprosyn, generics), and the newer COX-2-selective agents, such as celecoxib (Pfizer's Celebrex) and (up until it was withdrawn from the market in late 2004) rofecoxib (Merck's [Whitehouse Station, New Jersey] Vioxx), are regularly prescribed by physicians for the treatment of this condition.

Mechanism of Action. Although the mechanism of NSAID action is not fully understood, these drugs are known to block the arachidonic acid pathway at an early stage. Arachidonic acid is the major fatty acid incorporated into cell membranes; its metabolites serve as precursors to the synthesis of inflammatory mediators known as prostanoids. The enzyme cyclooxygenase (COX) initially converts arachidonic acid into intermediary cyclic endoperoxides, which, in turn, are converted into prostanoids. Prostanoid inflammatory mediators (especially PGE_2) cause inflammation by increasing the vascular permeability of the blood vessels. Nonselective NSAIDs inhibit the activity of COX, thereby preventing the production of prostanoids. COX-2-selective NSAIDs inhibit the activity of COX-2 but not that of COX-1, affording them a better gastrointestinal (GI) profile (because COX-1 has been found to be protective against GI damage).

Ibuprofen. Ibuprofen (Pfizer's Motrin, Knoll's Brufen, generics) (Figure 9) has been on the market for more than 30 years and is available in both prescription

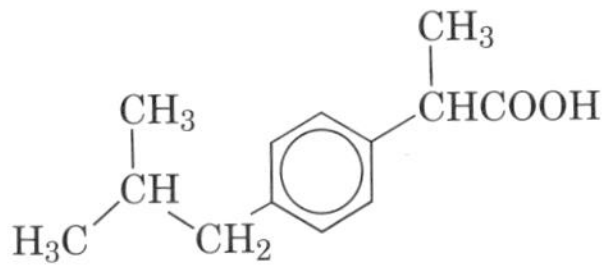

FIGURE 9. Structure of ibuprofen.

and nonprescription strengths. Even though ibuprofen is a relatively old drug, it is still one of the most commonly prescribed NSAIDs for fibromyalgia.

No well-controlled clinical studies have evaluated the efficacy of ibuprofen in fibromyalgia. However, because of physician familiarity with the drug and its efficacy in treating other types of chronic pain (e.g., osteoarthritis [OA], chronic low back pain), physicians frequently prescribe ibuprofen for fibromyalgia. The drug's minimal expense and physicians' comfort with prescribing it in combination with other drug therapies have contributed to ibuprofen's continuing popularity. Nevertheless, physicians may become much more conservative in prescribing NSAIDs such as ibuprofen for chronic conditions in the future, because all drugs from this class now have warnings about their potential to cause life-threatening cardiovascular events with long-term use.

Only minimal data from scattered small trials in which the drug was administered in combination with other fibromyalgia therapies suggest that ibuprofen provides any benefit for fibromyalgia sufferers (Fossaluzza V, 1992; Russell IJ, 1991). In addition, nonspecific NSAIDs such as ibuprofen can cause potentially serious GI complications (e.g., gastritis, mucosal damage, peptic erosions, ulcers, and bleeding) when administered over the long term.

Celecoxib. Celecoxib (Pfizer's Celebrex) (Figure 10) is currently marketed for OA, rheumatoid arthritis (RA), familial adenomatous polyposis (FAP), and the management of acute pain and primary dysmenorrhea. Pfizer markets celecoxib in all of the major markets except Japan, where Yamanouchi Pharmaceutical (Tokyo, Japan) is currently developing the drug. Celecoxib works by the same mechanism of action as other selective COX-2 inhibitors, inhibiting predominantly COX-2 while having little effect on COX-1.

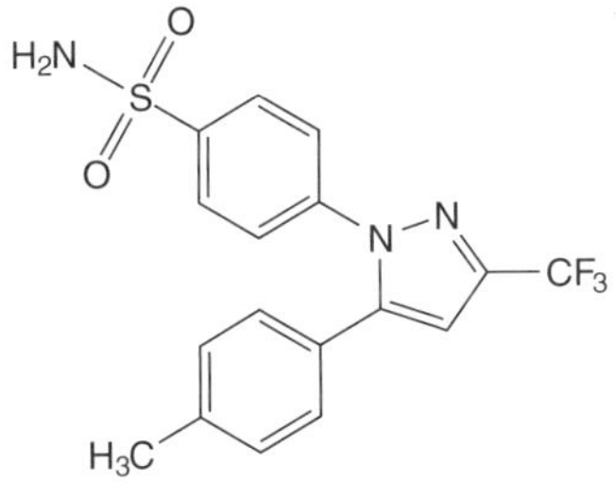

FIGURE 10. Structure of celecoxib.

No studies have been published on the effects of celecoxib in fibromyalgia; the numerous trials of celecoxib have been designed primarily to show that its efficacy in OA and RA patients is comparable to (or better than) that of other NSAIDs while highlighting the absence of significant GI toxicity. One Phase III trial compared celecoxib (100, 200, or 400 mg daily) with naproxen (1000 mg daily) in 1004 OA patients. At the end of the 12-week trial, patients' functional status was measured by the Western Ontario and McMaster Universities (WOMAC) OA Index, a composite questionnaire that measures pain, stiffness, and functional levels in OA. The group receiving 200 mg celecoxib daily showed a 23.7% improvement in their composite WOMAC scores (pain, stiffness, and physical functioning), compared with a 21.4% improvement for the naproxen group (Zhao SZ, 1999).

Sedative Hypnotics

Overview. Sedative hypnotics, such as the traditional benzodiazepines (BZDs) (e.g., temazepam [Mallinckrodt, Inc.'s (Hazelwood, Missouri) Restoril, generics]) and the newer non-BZD sedative hypnotics (e.g., zolpidem [Sanofi-Aventis's (Tokyo, Japan) Ambien/Stilnox, Fujisawa's (Osaka, Japan) Myslee]), hold an important place in the treatment of sleep difficulties in fibromyalgia patients. These agents are often prescribed on an "as needed" basis for fibromyalgia patients who do not derive sleep benefits from other standard treatments (e.g., antidepressants). Although none of the marketed agents has been studied in fibromyalgia, their proven efficacy in treating insomnia has led physicians to prescribe them on a regular basis for patients with fibromyalgia. The two newest non-BZD sedative hypnotics are Sepracor, Inc.'s (Marlborough, Massachusetts) eszopiclone (Lunesta) and Neurocrine and Pfizer's indiplon (discussed in "Emerging Therapies").

Mechanism of Action. Traditional BZDs act nonselectively at two central receptor binding sites—BZD type-1 (or omega 1) and BZD type-2 (or omega 2)—located on the GABA-A receptor complex (but in different areas of the central nervous system). Activation of these receptors facilitates the binding of the endogenous transmitter gamma-aminobutyric acid (GABA) and the subsequent opening of chloride channels. GABA-A activation results in increased inhibition of activating neuronal inputs to the ascending reticular activating system. Researchers suspect that the hypnosedative action of traditional BZDs results from their activity at BZD-1 receptors and that these agents' action at BZD-2 receptors mediates their negative effects on psychomotor performance and memory, as well as their habit-forming effects. Non-BZD sedative hypnotics, by contrast, interact preferentially with BZD-1 receptors, which affords them sleep-enhancing properties without the BZD-2 associated side effects.

Zolpidem. Zolpidem (Sanofi-Aventis's Ambien/Stilnox, Fujisawa's Myslee, generics) (Figure 11) has been marketed for the short-term treatment of insomnia

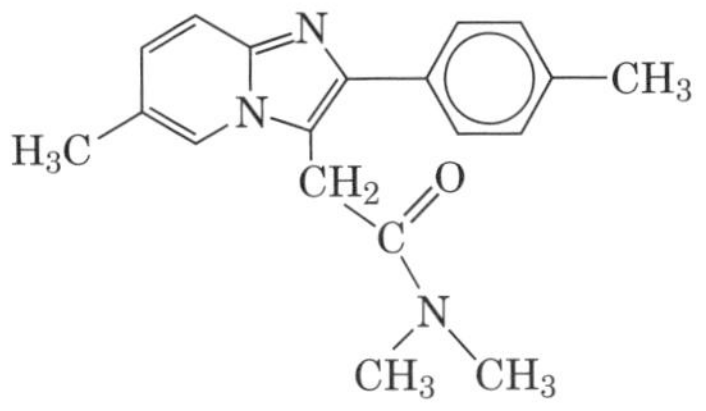

FIGURE 11. *Structure of zolpidem.*

in Europe since 1988 and in the United States since 1993. (Note: Sanofi-Synthélabo [now Sanofi-Aventis] acquired sole rights to the compound from Pharmacia (Bridgewater, New Jersey) [formerly Searle] in 2002). In Japan, the drug was launched (as Myslee) by its Japanese licensee Fujisawa in late 2000.

Zolpidem has a rapid onset of action and a short elimination half-life (approximately 2.5 hours). The drug elicits its hypnotic effects via selective binding to the BZD-1 subtype of the BZD receptor located on the alpha subunit of the GABA-A receptor complex. Unlike traditional BZDs, zolpidem has little activity at the BZD-2 subtype of the BZD receptor; researchers suspect that this lack of activity may explain zolpidem's apparent lack of myorelaxant and anticonvulsant effects commonly associated with the less selective BZDs. Also unlike the traditional BZDs, zolpidem does not appear to disturb normal sleep architecture (Dujardin K, 1998; Nicholson AN, 1986).

More than 15 years of postmarketing experience supports zolpidem's efficacy and safety as a hypnotic agent. The drug has been shown to effectively decrease sleep latency and increase total sleep time in patients with chronic insomnia while bringing a low occurrence of side effects and minimal effects on memory and next-day functioning. The most common side effects associated with zolpidem are nausea, dizziness, malaise, nightmares, agitation, and headache (occurring in less than 10% of patients). The drug has also been shown to have a lower propensity than traditional BZDs to induce tolerance, dependence, and rebound insomnia.

Narcotic Analgesics

Because of their powerful ability to control pain, narcotic analgesics (i.e., "opioids") are frequently used to treat severe chronic pain conditions. However, the use of narcotic analgesics remains controversial among fibromyalgia experts, in part because there is no evidence to support their use in this patient population and in part because of these agents' tendency to lead to tolerance and dependence with long-term use. Nevertheless, narcotic analgesics are sometimes prescribed for fibromyalgia patients who suffer from severe symptoms that are unresponsive to other medications.

Narcotic analgesics relieve pain via agonist activity, primarily at opiate receptors (mostly the mu and kappa receptors) in the CNS; these agents are classified as either full or partial agonists by their activity at opiate receptors. Clinically, mu opioid receptor agonists are used more often than kappa agonists because they are full rather than partial agonists (Holdcroft A, 2003) and are therefore more effective (the analgesic potency of opioids is believed to correlate directly with their affinity for the mu receptor). Activity at these receptors also mediates the adverse effects associated with narcotic analgesics (e.g., euphoria, respiratory depression, constipation, sedation).

When narcotic analgesics are in fact used to treat fibromyalgia, the most frequently prescribed agents include codeine, propoxyphene, hydrocodone, and oxycodone—all of which are available with or without acetaminophen in multiple brand and generic formulations—as well as transdermal fentanyl (Janssen [Titusville, New Jersey]/ALZA's Duragesic/Durogesic). Although there are no data from well-controlled trials of narcotic analgesics in fibromyalgia, these agents' proven efficacy in treating other types of severe pain leads physicians to prescribe them when other treatment options have failed.

Other Analgesics

Overview. The following discussion focuses primarily on tramadol (Ortho-McNeil Pharmaceutical, Inc.'s [Raritan, New Jersey] Ultram), which is one of the few drugs to have shown efficacy in well-controlled fibromyalgia trials. Paracetamol (acetaminophen)—the other drug that falls into this category—is widely prescribed in Europe for patients with fibromyalgia, but there is no evidence to support paracetamol's efficacy in this patient population.

Mechanism of Action. Tramadol, a synthetic analogue of codeine, is classified by the U.S. FDA as a non-narcotic analgesic because, despite binding to opioid receptors (albeit weakly, at 6000 times lower affinity than morphine), its analgesic activity is only partially inhibited by the opioid antagonist naloxone. This fact suggests that tramadol derives at least some of its pain-relieving properties from a separate, nonopioid mechanism (i.e., 5-HT/NE reuptake inhibition), indicating a dual mechanism of action and earning the drug a non-narcotic classification.

Tramadol. Tramadol (Figure 12) has been marketed for the short-term treatment of moderate to moderately severe pain in Europe for more than two decades and in the United States since the mid-1990s; in Japan, the oral tablet formulation of tramadol is in Phase II trials for pain. Several companies—including Purdue Pharma

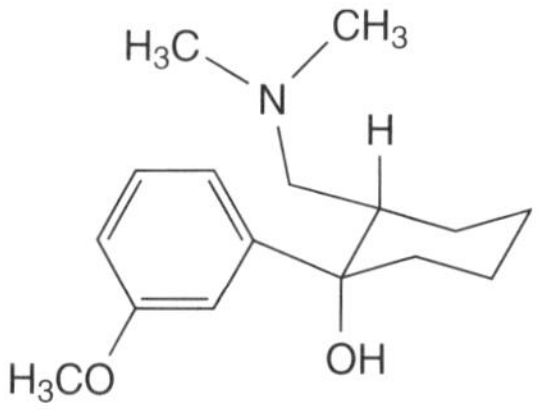

FIGURE 12. *Structure of tramadol.*

(Cranbury, New Jersey), Biovail Corporation (Mississauga, Ontario, Canada), and Labopharm (Laval, Quebec, Canada)—have developed once-daily formulations of the drug (the original formulation requires dosing three or four times daily), one of which (Biovail's Ralivia ER) is expected to launch in the United States in 2006. Tramadol is also available in combination with acetaminophen (Ortho-McNeil's Ultracet); this combination is thought to have a faster onset of action and a longer duration of pain relief than tramadol alone.

Tramadol initially showed potential efficacy in fibromyalgia in a small, double-blind, crossover trial in 12 fibromyalgia patients who received the drug intravenously (Biasi G, 1998). In this trial, tramadol-treated patients showed improvement in spontaneous pain on the VAS. Further results from larger controlled trials using the oral tablet form of the drug have confirmed the drug's efficacy in relieving pain in fibromyalgia (Bennett RM, 2003; Russell J, 2000). In a recent trial (Bennett RM, 2003), 315 patients (94% female) with fibromyalgia were randomized to receive a fixed combination of 37.5 mg tramadol/325 mg acetaminophen (Ultracet) or placebo for three months. The primary outcome measure of the trial was cumulative time to discontinuation (Kaplan-Meier analysis); secondary outcomes included pain, pain relief, total tender points, myalgia, health status, and FIQ scores.

At study completion, 48% of tramadol-treated patients had discontinued for any reason, compared with 62% in the placebo group. (Note: Discontinuation due to lack of efficacy was also significantly lower in tramadol- than in placebo-treated patients [29% versus 51%, respectively]). Tramadol-treated patients also had significantly less pain than did placebo-treated patients (53 ± 32 versus 65 ± 29, respectively, on a VAS scale of 0–100), as well as better pain relief (1.7 ± 1.4 versus 0.8 ± 1.3, respectively, on a scale of −1 to 4). When investigators looked at the percentage of patients with at least a 30% or 50% reduction in pain score, results also favored tramadol (42% of tramadol- versus 24% of placebo-treated patients had at least 30% pain reduction and 35% versus 18% had at least 50% pain reduction, respectively). Discontinuation due to adverse events (AEs) in this study occurred in 19% of tramadol-treated patients and 12% of placebo-treated patients; the most common AEs associated with tramadol were nausea, dizziness, somnolence, and constipation.

Antiepileptic Drugs

Overview. Despite a paucity of evidence for efficacy in fibromyalgia, antiepileptic drugs (AEDs, also called anticonvulsants) hold an important place in the treatment of this syndrome. Specifically, physicians prescribe AEDs such as gabapentin (Pfizer's Neurontin, generics) and clonazepam (Roche's Klonopin, generics) for fibromyalgia patients who fail to respond to standard first-line therapies (e.g., antidepressants). This class of drugs is expected to experience growing use for fibromyalgia in the future for two reasons: (1) there is mounting evidence for efficacy of several AEDs in treating other related pain syndromes (e.g., neuropathic pain), and (2) Pfizer's new AED pregabalin (Lyrica) will likely be one of the first drugs to achieve official regulatory approval for fibromyalgia (see "Emerging Therapies").

Mechanism of Action. Although AEDs' exact mechanism of action in pain management is unknown, research suggests that drugs in this class work through several neuronal pathways. Some shared mechanisms of AEDs that may contribute to their analgesic properties include blockade of neuronal sodium and/or calcium channels, inhibition of the excitatory effects of glutamate, and potentiation of the inhibitory effects of gamma-aminobutyric acid (GABA).

Gabapentin. Gabapentin (Figure 13) is currently approved for the treatment of epilepsy and postherpetic neuralgia (PHN) in the United States and for epilepsy and peripheral neuropathic pain in Europe. In Japan, where gabapentin was originally licensed to Fujisawa (which became Astellas Pharma in 2005 following a merger with Yamanouchi), the agent is in Phase III development for the treatment of epilepsy.

Despite much research, gabapentin's precise mechanism of action remains unknown. Studies suggest that the drug binds to the alpha-2-delta subunit of voltage-dependent calcium channels (VDCCs), a high-affinity binding site in neuronal membranes. This subunit has been implicated in the maintenance of mechanical hypersensitivity in models of neuropathic pain. Calcium ions enable neurotransmitters to bind vesicles at the presynaptic membrane terminal; thus, it has been hypothesized that gabapentin exerts its therapeutic effect by blocking calcium influx via the alpha-2-delta receptor and reducing the release of neurotransmitters that transmit nociceptive signals between neurons. Specifically, in vitro findings suggest that gabapentin may decrease the presynaptic release of excitatory neurotransmitters such as glutamate and norepinephrine.

Gabapentin is one of only two available AEDs that is approved for the treatment of pain (the other is carbamazepine [Novartis's (Basel, Switzerland) Tegretol, generics], which is approved to treat trigeminal neuralgia in the United States). In addition, gabapentin has been shown in a small placebo-controlled trial to improve sleep in individuals who suffer from restless legs syndrome (RLS) (Garcia-Borreguero D, 2002), a condition that frequently affects fibromyalgia sufferers.

The U.S. National Institute of Arthritis and Musculoskeletal and Skin Diseases (NIAMS) is currently conducting a randomized, placebo-controlled study—called GIFT (Gabapentin in Fibromyalgia Trial)—to examine the efficacy of gabapentin

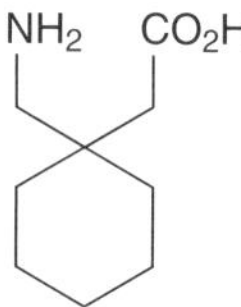

FIGURE 13. *Structure of gabapentin.*

in treating the symptoms of fibromyalgia. In this trial, investigators will evaluate the three-month efficacy of gabapentin versus placebo in 150 fibromyalgia sufferers using such scales as the Brief Pain Inventory (BPI), the FIQ, the Clinical Global Impression (CGI)-Severity, the SF-36, the Montgomery-Asberg Depression Rating Scale (MADRS), and the Medical Outcomes Study (MOS)-Sleep, among others (see Table 5 for descriptions of clinical scales). This study is scheduled for completion in March 2006.

The results from the GIFT trial will likely determine whether gabapentin will continue to hold a place in the treatment of fibromyalgia. Indeed, with the expected approval of Pfizer's follow-on to gabapentin—pregabalin (Lyrica)—for fibromyalgia in the near future (see "Emerging Therapies"), gabapentin (now generically available in most markets) will need to show results at least as good as those of pregabalin if it is to compete with the newer drug.

Nonpharmacological Approaches

Nonpharmacological therapies are an integral part of the treatment regimen for fibromyalgia patients. Therapy options range from relatively simple programs like exercise and physical therapy to more detailed programs such as psychological counseling and cognitive behavioral therapy (CBT).

The benefit of low-impact aerobic exercise seems to derive from its systemic effects rather than from a direct effect on the exercised muscles. Examples of low-impact aerobic exercise include walking and stationary cycling, although water aerobics may be best tolerated because it is void of any weight-bearing activity. Relaxation techniques such as massage are also commonly used to ease muscle tension and anxiety.

Recent studies demonstrate that when fibromyalgia patients increase their psychological capacity to deal with their disease, they are more likely to experience physical improvement. CBT is an example of an educational program that allows fibromyalgia patients to gain control over their symptoms and to learn behaviors to deal with them. This program is based on the theory that pain is the result of a complex integration of pathophysiology, cognition, affect, and behavior.

EMERGING THERAPIES

No drugs are yet approved to treat fibromyalgia (see "Current Therapies"). Even so, only a small number of compounds are currently in development for the condition. Reasons for the sparsely populated pipeline include a poor understanding of the pathophysiology of fibromyalgia, the difficulty in achieving good drug efficacy in such a heterogeneous patient population, the prominent place of nonpharmacological treatments in management of the condition, and physicians' continuing reticence to accept fibromyalgia as a serious medical condition, among others. In fact, nearly all of the companies conducting clinical trials in fibromyalgia are looking at this patient population as secondary to other conditions for which their respective compounds have already been approved. More specifically, fibromyalgia trials tend to come on the heels of initial approvals for depression, sleep disorders, or other, painful conditions (e.g., neuropathic pain), which represent more potentially lucrative markets than fibromyalgia.

In spite of the less than dynamic pipeline, the current clinical activity in the fibromyalgia arena represents a major advance in drug companies' historical interest in this condition. Indeed, the only valid data that had emerged from well-controlled trials in fibromyalgia prior to the past five years had been that for older, generically available drugs like amitriptyline and cyclobenzaprine—drugs for which no company was going to pursue supplemental regulatory approval for a condition such as fibromyalgia. Consequently, clinical data released in recent years from well-controlled fibromyalgia trials with new compounds such as Cypress Bioscience's and Forest Laboratories's antidepressant milnacipran and Eli Lilly's duloxetine, among others, represent a major step forward in the evidence-based treatment of this highly underrecognized condition.

Drugs in clinical development for fibromyalgia are shown in Table 4.

Antidepressants

Overview. As noted in the "Current Therapies" section, tricyclic antidepressants (TCAs)—most notably amitriptyline (AstraZeneca's Elavil, Roche's Laroxyl, generics)—are the mainstay of antidepressant treatment for fibromyalgia, primarily because, until now, few other antidepressants have shown efficacy in well-controlled clinical trials for fibromyalgia. In the past year, positive data have been released for Eli Lilly's duloxetine and Forest/Cypress Bioscience's milnacipran, both of which are marketed antidepressants that target serotonin (5-HT) and norepinephrine (NE). These data will likely support the near-term approval of these two agents for fibromyalgia, making dual-action serotonergic and noradrenergic antidepressants the first class of drugs to gain regulatory approval for the treatment of fibromyalgia.

Doxepin, another older TCA that is sometimes prescribed off-label to treat fibromyalgia, is currently being investigated at very low doses in clinical trials for insomnia by Somaxon Pharmaceuticals, Inc. (San Diego, California). Somaxon recently released promising results from Phase II trials in elderly patients with primary sleep maintenance insomnia. While it is unclear whether the company will expand its investigations to include fibromyalgia, low-dose doxepin, if approved for insomnia, may see off-label use for fibromyalgia.

Other investigational-stage antidepressants may have clinical potential in fibromyalgia but are not in formal trials for the indication. These agents include DOV Pharmaceutical's (Hackensack, New Jersey) triple reuptake inhibitors, which target 5-HT, NE, and dopamine, and are currently under investigation for depression, anxiety, drug and alcohol dependence, and smoking cessation, and Wyeth's follow-on to venlafaxine (Effexor), desvenlafaxine, which is a serotonergic and noradrenergic reuptake inhibitor (SNRI). These compounds have activity at neurotransmitters involved in pain processing and are similar to other antidepressants that have shown efficacy in fibromyalgia. However, because

TABLE 4. Emerging Therapies in Development for Fibromyalgia

Compound	Development Phase[a]	Marketing Company
Antidepressants		
Duloxetine (Cymbalta)		
United States	III	Eli Lilly
Europe	—	Eli Lilly/Boehringer Ingelheim
Japan	—	Shionogi
Milnacipran		
United States	III	Cypress Bioscience/Forest Labs
Europe	—	Pierre-Fabre
Japan	—	Asahi Kasei/Janssen Pharmaceutical KK
Radafaxine		
United States	—	—
Europe	I	GlaxoSmithKline
Japan	—	—
AD-337		
United States	—	—
Europe	I	Arakis
Japan	—	—
Sedative hypnotics		
Eszopiclone (Lunesta)		
United States	Clinical	Sepracor
Europe	—	—
Japan	—	—
Sodium oxybate (Xyrem)		
United States	II	Orphan Medical
Europe	—	UCB Pharma
Japan	—	—
Antiepileptic drugs (AEDs)		
Pregabalin (Lyrica)		
United States	II	Pfizer
Europe	—	Pfizer
Japan	—	Pfizer
5-HT2 antagonists		
Eplivanserin		
United States	—	—
Europe	II	Sanofi-Aventis
Japan	—	—
Dopamine agonists		
Ropinirole (Requip)		
United States	—	GlaxoSmithKline
Europe	II	GlaxoSmithKline
Japan	—	GlaxoSmithKline

[a]Development phase is for fibromyalgia.

fibromyalgia does not yet appear on the list of potential areas of therapeutic interest for these drugs (suggesting that clinical data supporting their use in fibromyalgia will not be available anytime soon), and because several other emerging therapies will likely have a more near-term impact on the fibromyalgia market, they are not discussed further here. More detailed information is provided for two similar compounds—GlaxoSmithKline's radafaxine and Arakis's AD 337—because these drugs are officially under investigation (albeit very early investigation) for fibromyalgia.

Mechanism of Action. Antidepressants are believed to elicit their mood-enhancing and analgesic effects primarily by blocking the synaptic reuptake of two neurotransmitters—serotonin (5-HT) and norepinephrine (NE)—both of which are functionally inhibitory on pain transmission (via the descending pain pathway). While other purported antidepressant mechanisms, such as potassium-channel modulation and N-methyl-D-aspartate (NMDA) receptor antagonism, may also play a role in pain modulation, the relative importance of these mechanisms in pain control remains unclear (Lawson K, 2002).

Duloxetine. Eli Lilly's SNRI duloxetine (Cymbalta) (Figure 14) was recently approved in the United States for the treatment of depression and peripheral diabetic neuropathic pain (NP); the drug was also awaiting final U.S. approval for the treatment of stress urinary incontinence (SUI), but Lilly withdrew its application for this condition in early 2005. Based on recently released Phase II results from fibromyalgia trials in which duloxetine was shown to reduce pain and improve overall quality of life in this patient population, Lilly has initiated a Phase III program with the drug for fibromyalgia.

In Europe, duloxetine is jointly marketed by Lilly and Boehringer Ingelheim for SUI (as Yentreve/Ariclaim) and depression (as Cymbalta) and, most recently, by Lilly for peripheral diabetic NP (as Cymbalta). In Japan, Lilly has licensed duloxetine to Shionogi, which recently initiated Phase III depression trials with the drug at a higher dose than had previously been tested; the company expects to file for approval for depression in Japan in 2007. Shionogi is also investigating duloxetine in Phase II SUI trials.

As noted, researchers suspect that duloxetine elicits its analgesic effects via 5-HT/NE reuptake inhibition. More specifically, they consider duloxetine's greater relative activity at NE versus 5-HT (1:8)—compared with that of other marketed antidepressants, such as venlafaxine (1:30) and fluoxetine (1:55)—to be a key component of the newer drug's analgesic activity.

Data supporting duloxetine's efficacy in fibromyalgia were first published in 2004 in the journal *Arthritis and Rheumatism* (Arnold LM, 2004). In this study, 207 fibromyalgia patients (89% female) were randomly assigned to receive either

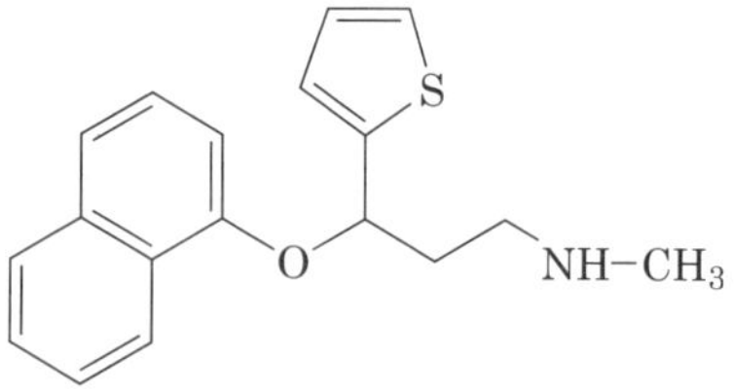

FIGURE 14. *Structure of duloxetine.*

duloxetine 60 mg twice daily (bid) or placebo for 12 weeks. Thirty-eight percent of patients in the study had current major depression. The primary outcome measures were Fibromyalgia Impact Questionnaire (FIQ) total score (0–80, with 0 indicating no impact) and FIQ pain score (0–10). Secondary outcome measures included mean tender point pain threshold, number of tender points, FIQ fatigue, tiredness on awakening and stiffness scores, Clinical Global Impression of Severity (CGI-Severity) and Patient Global Impression of Improvement (PGI-Improvement), Brief Pain Inventory (BPI) short form, Medical Outcomes Study Short Form 36 (MOS-SF-36), Quality of Life (QOL) in Depression Scale, and Sheehan Disability Scale (SDS). One hundred and twenty-four patients successfully completed the trial; reasons for discontinuation did not differ significantly between the two groups.

At study completion, duloxetine-treated patients showed significantly greater improvement than placebo-treated patients in the FIQ total score (-13.46 ± 1.82 versus -7.93 ± 1.73, respectively) but not in the FIQ pain score (-1.98 ± 0.3 versus -1.35 ± 0.29, respectively). Response rates—defined as a reduction of at least 50% in the FIQ pain score at end point—were 27.7% and 16.7% for the duloxetine and placebo groups, respectively. When female subjects were analyzed as a group, duloxetine-treated patients showed significant improvements over placebo on both primary end points, and response rates were 30.3% versus 16.5%, respectively (duloxetine-treated male subjects failed to improve significantly on any efficacy measure). Overall improvements were also noted for duloxetine-treated subjects on most secondary end points, including BPI severity and interference scores, number of tender points, FIQ stiffness score, mean tender point threshold, and CGI-Severity and PGI-Improvement scores, as well as on several QOL measures. Study investigators concluded that improvements in pain reduction with duloxetine were independent of the drug's effect on mood or anxiety (suggesting that duloxetine provides analgesia through a mechanism other than its mood-enhancing mechanism).

Additional trial data presented at the 2004 meeting of the American College of Rheumatology provide further support for duloxetine in the treatment of fibromyalgia. In this study (Wernicke J, 2004), 354 fibromyalgia sufferers with or without current major depressive disorder were randomized to receive duloxetine 60 mg once daily (qd), duloxetine 60 mg twice daily (bid), or placebo for a period of 12 weeks, followed by a one-week discontinuation phase. The primary outcome measure in this study was the BPI 24-hour average pain severity score (0–10, with 0 being no pain). Treatment response was defined as a 30% reduction in the BPI 24-hour score; secondary outcomes included remaining BPI pain and interference scores, FIQ, number of tender points, tender point pain threshold, CGI-Severity and PGI-Improvement, and the 17-item Hamilton Rating Scale for Depression (HAM-D), as well as several QOL measures.

At study completion, duloxetine-treated subjects showed significant improvements on the primary end point of 24-hour BPI average pain score compared with placebo (difference of -1.23 and -1.24 for duloxetine qd and duloxetine bid, respectively; $p < 0.001$). The proportions responding (i.e., at least a 30%

reduction in BPI score) for duloxetine qd, duloxetine bid, and placebo were 55%, 54%, and 33%, respectively. When investigators looked at the more stringent criteria of 50% reduction in BPI score, they noted a 41% response rate for duloxetine-treated patients and a 23% response rate for placebo-treated patients.

Improvements with both doses of duloxetine were also reported for several secondary measures, including the CGI-Severity and PGI-Improvement, BPI 24-hour average pain AUC, FIQ total score, and all other BPI pain and interference scores, as well as most health outcome measures. Duloxetine bid also showed superiority over placebo on measures of mean tender point threshold and number of tender points. As was the case in the previously discussed trial, study investigators determined that duloxetine's effect on pain reduction was independent of the drug's effect on mood. Commonly reported AEs with both doses of duloxetine were nausea, dry mouth, constipation, diarrhea, decreased appetite, nasopharyngitis, increased sweating, and anorexia; these AEs contributed to a higher discontinuation rate among duloxetine-treated patients (21.2%, 23.3%, and 11.7% for duloxetine qd, bid, and placebo, respectively). Sleepiness and feeling jittery were also commonly reported by patients taking duloxetine bid.

Milnacipran. Pierre Fabre (Castres, France) launched its SNRI milnacipran (Ixel/Dalcipran) in France for the treatment of depression in 1997 and subsequently outlicensed the drug to Sanofi-Synthelabo (New York, New York, now Sanofi-Aventis) for marketing in the rest of Europe (where it has launched in numerous markets, but not in Germany, Italy, Spain, or the United Kingdom). In Japan, where milnacipran is a leading antidepressant, Asahi Kasei Corporation (Tokyo, Japan) and Janssen Pharmaceutical KK copromote the drug (as Toledomin) for depression. In the United States, where the drug is not yet marketed, Cypress Bioscience (the drug's original U.S. licensee) has licensed development and marketing rights for fibromyalgia to Forest Labs. Cypress initiated the first Phase III trial with milnacipran in fibromyalgia in October 2003; enrollment was completed in December 2004, and this six-month trial was completed in mid-2005. The Preliminary top-line results of the study support the continued development of milnacipran as a treatment for fibromyalagia. Although the results did not achieve statistical significance, the planned development program for milnacipran, which includes an ongoing Phase III study and an additional third Phase III study, to be initiated by Forest Laboratories, will continue.

A second Phase III trial initiated by both Cypress and Forest is currently enrolling patients (as of May 2005). Results from the Phase III program are expected in 2006. Cypress is also reportedly investigating the potential for use of milnacipran in irritable bowel syndrome (IBS), a condition that is frequently reported by fibromyalgia sufferers.

Like duloxetine and venlafaxine, milnacipran inhibits the reuptake of 5-HT and NE. However, unlike the two previously mentioned agents (and similar to amitriptyline), milnacipran shows a slight preference for inhibition of NE over 5-HT (approximately 2.5:1). The drug also binds to NMDA receptors; although the clinical relevance of this activity remains unclear, researchers have long suspected that the glutamate-NMDA receptor axis plays an important role in pain transmission.

Cypress initiated its Phase III clinical program with milnacipran based on positive results from a 125-patient trial in which milnacipran was shown to relieve the symptoms of fibromyalgia (Vitton O, 2004). In this double-blind, flexible-dose trial, fibromyalgia sufferers (mostly women) were randomized to receive either milnacipran or placebo for four weeks of dose escalation (up to 200 mg/day) followed by eight weeks at a constant dose. Patients were assigned to one of three dosing groups: placebo in the morning and evening, milnacipran in the morning and placebo in the evening (qd group), or milnacipran in the morning and milnacipran in the evening (bid group). The primary outcome measure was percentage change from baseline (i.e., magnitude of improvement) in patient reported pain score (using an electronic diary), as measured by the VAS and the Gracely logarithmic scale (Gracely RH, 1988); average pain scores from the two-week baseline period were compared to average pain scores from the final two weeks of the study. A binary responder analysis was also implemented using a 30% and 50% reduction in pain as a definition. Secondary end points included PGI-Change, FIQ, SF-36, Beck depression inventory, Jenkins sleep scale, Arizona sexual experience scale, and other QOL measures. Seventy-two percent of patients completed the study, and there were no significant differences in dropout rates across the three groups.

At study completion, patients taking bid milnacipran showed statistically significant improvements in pain on all but one measure (e-diary pain score collected daily); patients taking qd milnacipran, as well as pooled milnacipran-treated patients (i.e., both qd and bid groups), showed significant improvements in three of ten measures. In the responder analysis, bid-treated milnacipran patients again showed the most improvement, with 37% reporting at least a 50% reduction in pain intensity, compared with 14% of placebo-treated patients (and 22% in the qd milnacipran group). On the secondary measure of PGI, 70% of patients treated with milnacipran versus 38% of placebo-treated patients reported improvement. In contrast, milnacipran treatment did not result in statistically significant differences in the total FIQ scores; however, significant improvements were noted on the individual domains of "physical function" and "feel good." Milnacipran-treated patients also showed significant improvements on the FIQ VAS scores of pain, fatigue, and morning stiffness (but not on depression or anxiety).

With regard to tolerability, bid milnacipran appeared to be better tolerated than qd milnacipran. Study investigators reported a higher incidence of nausea, abdominal pain, headache, dizziness, flushes, and palpitations in the 200 mg qd group compared with the 200 mg bid group. Nevertheless, investigators reported that approximately 87% of milnacipran-treated patients who completed the trial tolerated dose escalation to the maximum allowed stable dose of 200 mg/day (92% in the bid group and 81% in the qd group). Overall, 14%, 22%, and 4% of patients in the bid, qd, and placebo groups, respectively, withdrew from the study because of AEs.

Radafaxine. GlaxoSmithKline's novel noradrenergic/dopaminergic reuptake inhibitor radafaxine is reportedly in Phase I development for fibromyalgia and neuropathic pain and in Phase II development for depression and restless legs syndrome (RLS). It is unclear whether radafaxine will be effective in the treatment of fibromyalgia, as no data are yet available from fibromyalgia trials. Nevertheless, recent evidence supports an underlying role for dopamine in some fibromyalgia sufferers (evidenced by the efficacy of dopamine agonists; see the "Dopamine Agonists" section).

AD-337. Arakis's (Babraham, United Kingdom) AD-337, a single-isomer formulation of an undisclosed SNRI, is currently in Phase I development for fibromyalgia and chemotherapy-induced emesis. The absence of clinical data for this compound precludes an evaluation of its clinical potential in fibromyalgia.

Sedative Hypnotics

Overview. Because sleep disorders and daytime fatigue are so common among fibromyalgia sufferers, physicians sometimes prescribe sedative hypnotics to these patients in an attempt to improve their sleep and, in turn, their daytime functioning. However, no currently marketed sedative hypnotics have been proven safe and effective for the long-term treatment of sleep dysfunction in fibromyalgia. Indeed, currently marketed agents are restricted by their potential to induce tolerance and dependence with long-term use and—in the case of the traditional benzodiazepines (BZDs)—their negative effects on sleep architecture, memory, coordination, and respiratory function (in those with preexisting respiratory conditions). Consequently, all available BZD and non-BZD hypnotics (except the newly marketed eszopiclone; see next section) are labeled only for the short-term (i.e, less than 30 days) treatment of insomnia. This situation leaves much room for improvement for sleep drugs—specifically, for drugs that can be safely taken on a chronic basis with no negative effects on sleep architecture.

A new batch of sedative hypnotics may help to address the aforementioned need. Indeed, Sepracor's eszopiclone (Lunesta)—the newest non-BZD sedative hypnotic to reach the U.S. market (in 2005) and the only one with no restrictions on duration of use—is reportedly in clinical trials in the United States for insomnia related to chronic pain (including fibromyalgia). Other new sedative hypnotics that have yet to reach the market but that may have similar labeling to eszopiclone include Neurocrine/Pfizer's indiplon (both immediate- and modified-release formulations), Takeda Pharmaceutical's (Osaka, Japan) TAK-375 (Ramelteon), and Merck's gaboxadol. When launched, these agents will boast a wealth of safety and efficacy data from long-term (6- to 12-month) trials in chronic insomnia.

Another hypnotic agent that may prove useful in fibromyalgia is Orphan Medical, Inc.'s (Minnetonka, Minnesota) narcolepsy drug Xyrem (sodium oxybate, a commercial form of the naturally occurring CNS depressant gamma-hydroxybutyrate [GHB]). Orphan Medical is currently investigating Xyrem in a proof-of-principle trial in fibromyalgia. Although Xyrem is a Schedule III controlled substance (previously discussed sedative hypnotics are classified as Schedule IV drugs, a less restrictive category), recently released clinical data may support this drug's use in fibromyalgia patients who suffer from nonrestorative sleep.

Mechanism of Action. Most currently marketed sedative hypnotics elicit their sleep-enhancing effects via central activity at BZD-1 and/or BZD-2 receptors located on the GABA-A receptor complex (but in different areas of the CNS). Older, traditional BZDs act nonselectively at these two receptors, whereas newer, "non-BZD" hypnotics interact preferentially with BZD-1 receptors. Researchers suspect that activity at BZD-1 receptors is responsible for these agents' sedative effects, whereas activity at BZD-2 receptors mediates their negative effects on psychomotor performance and memory, as well as their habit-forming effects.

Eszopiclone. Sepracor received FDA approval in December 2004 for its non-BZD hypnotic eszopiclone (Lunesta) for the treatment of insomnia. The approval was for the 2 mg and 3 mg tablets for insomnia characterized by difficulty falling asleep and/or difficulty maintaining sleep during the night and early morning for adult and elderly patients and for the 1 mg tablet for elderly patients whose primary complaint is difficulty falling asleep. Labeling that includes "sleep maintenance" and no restrictions on duration of use differentiates eszopiclone from its primary competitors in the U.S. market—zolpidem (Sanofi-Aventis's Ambien) and zaleplon (Wyeth/King Pharmaceuticals's [Bristol, Tennessee] Sonata)—because these two marketed non-BZD hypnotics are indicated only for sleep onset (i.e., difficulty falling asleep), not sleep maintenance, and are restricted by short-term (i.e., 7- to 10-day) prescribing limits. Sepracor is reportedly conducting other trials with eszopiclone in patients with secondary insomnia, including those suffering from depression, rheumatoid arthritis (RA), and symptoms of perimenopause.

Eszopiclone is the (S)-enantiomer of the cyclopyrrolone hypnotic zopiclone (Sanofi-Aventis's Imovane/Amoban, Chugai's Amban, generics), which has been marketed in Europe for insomnia for more than 15 years. Eszopiclone has a 50-fold greater affinity for GABA-A receptors than the (R)-enantiomer of zopiclone, and investigators believe that eszopiclone is mainly responsible for the hypnotic effects of zopiclone (Sepracor, 2003). Like its predecessor zopiclone, eszopiclone is rapidly absorbed after oral administration and has a half-life of approximately five to seven hours. Unlike its predecessor, eszopiclone has been shown to be safe and effective with minimal potential for tolerance or dependence in long-term (6- to 12-month) trials in chronic insomniacs.

In a clinical program involving nearly 5000 insomnia sufferers, eszopiclone produced sustained improvements in sleep onset, duration of sleep, and maintenance of sleep compared with placebo with no evidence of tolerance when administered at the 2 mg and 3 mg doses (2 mg in the elderly and 3 mg in nonelderly adults) (Erman M, 2004; Krystal A, 2003; Roth T, 2004; Scharf M, 2004; Wessel T, 2004; Zammit G, 2003). The drug was also shown to improve next-day functioning in both elderly and nonelderly adults; in a comparison of data from three studies, investigators found that patients consistently reported improvements in measures of daytime functioning, including daytime alertness, morning sleepiness, sense of well-being, and daytime ability to function (Scharf M, 2004).

Investigators also conducted a subgroup analysis of six-month trial data from nonelderly adults ($n = 788$) to evaluate whether eszopiclone is effective in those with substantial sleep maintenance problems and to estimate the effects of eszopiclone in patients with difficulties in staying asleep (Krystal A, 2004). Two subgroups were defined by baseline wake time after sleep onset (WASO): Group one ($n = 336$) was the low-WASO group (<60 minutes of wake time after sleep onset) and group two ($n = 340$) was the high-WASO group ($\geq$60 minutes of wake time after sleep onset). Final six-month analysis revealed statistically significant differences in WASO between eszopiclone-treated and placebo-treated patients in both groups (19 versus 30 minutes in the low-WASO group and 39 versus 60 minutes in the high-WASO group for eszopiclone versus placebo, respectively).

Data from the six-month open-label extension of the initial six-month trial in nonelderly adults with chronic insomnia provided additional support for eszopiclone's safety and efficacy when used over the long term (i.e., 12 months) (Roth T, 2004). In the six-month extension, 471 patients (111 who had been treated with placebo and 360 who had been treated with eszopiclone) received 3 mg eszopiclone nightly; at the end of the six-month extension, 86 of the original 111 placebo-treated patients and 296 of the original 360 eszopiclone-treated patients who had entered the extension phase of the trial had received eszopiclone for 6 months or 12 months, respectively. Overall, eszopiclone was well tolerated, and there was no evidence of tolerance or adverse withdrawal effects upon discontinuation. In addition, patients switched from placebo to eszopiclone reported rapid and significant improvement in sleep and daytime functioning that persisted throughout the six-month duration of the extension phase. The most common side effects associated with eszopiclone were unpleasant taste, headache, and dry mouth.

Based on the robustness of the Phase III clinical data to support eszopiclone's safety and efficacy in chronic insomnia, this drug is likely to find a place in the fibromyalgia market. More specifically, the drug's relaxed prescribing restrictions will allow physicians to use it more freely for fibromyalgia patients who require chronic treatment for sleep difficulties.

Sodium Oxybate. Sodium oxybate (Xyrem), from Jazz Pharmaceuticals, Inc. (Palo Alto, California, formerly Orphan Medical), is a CNS depressant marketed in the United States since 2002 for narcolepsy associated cataplexy (sudden loss of muscle control, typically during episodes of emotional stimulation); UCB Pharma (Brussels, Belgium) has licensed the drug from Jazz Pharmaceuticals and received approval to market Xyrem for this condition in Europe. The drug received regulatory in the United States for reduction of excessive daytime sleepiness (EDS) and improvement in fragmented sleep in narcolepsy patients in 2006. Initial results from a U.S.-based Phase II trial involving more than 150 fibromyalgia patients were expected in mid-2005.

Sodium oxybate is a commercial form of gamma-hydroxybutyrate (GHB), a naturally occurring CNS depressant that is found in high concentrations in the hypothalamus and basal ganglia. Although the compound has been shown to improve sleep in subjects with sleep disorders, it has also gained a reputation as being a "date rape" drug. (The agent is both odorless and tasteless and, when added to alcohol, creates a sense of amnesia along with its soporific effects, making it an ideal substance for such illicit use.) In the United States, the drug is classified as a Schedule III controlled substance (this classification includes anabolic steroids and some low-potency narcotics); this category is more restrictive than that of the BZD and non-BZD sedative hypnotics, which are classified as Schedule IV drugs (see the "Overview" section).

The exact mechanism by which sodium oxybate works is not entirely clear, but researchers suspect that its sedative, anxiolytic, and euphoric effects may be due to GHB-induced potentiation of cerebral GABAergic, dopaminergic, and possibly serotonergic activities. It has also been shown to cause dose-related increases in slow-wave (i.e., restorative) sleep and growth hormone levels (Van CE, 1997); research suggests that up to 80% of adult growth hormone is secreted during slow-wave sleep.

Data from a small clinical trial in which sodium oxybate was administered to fibromyalgia sufferers suggest that the drug improves both sleep quality and the clinical symptoms of pain and fatigue in these patients (Scharf MB, 2003). In this double-blind, randomized, crossover study, 24 female fibromyalgia patients were randomized to receive either 6 g of sodium oxybate solution or placebo in two nightly divided doses (one at bedtime and one four hours later) over a 10–12 week timeframe. The study consisted of five periods: a two- to four-week baseline period, three nights of pretreatment polysomnographic (PSG) evaluation, treatment phase I (32 days), a two-week withdrawal/washout period, and treatment phase II (32 days). The primary efficacy measures were change from baseline for the tender point index (TPI) and subjective assessments of pain and fatigue; secondary efficacy analyses included change from baseline for alpha intrusion (% of non-REM epochs with alpha rhythm), total sleep time (TST), sleep latency (SL), time to wake after sleep onset (WASO), sleep efficiency (SE) index, and number of awakenings.

At study completion, TPI was decreased significantly from baseline with sodium oxybate (−8.5), whereas placebo-treated patients experienced an increase from baseline (+0.4). In addition, all pain and fatigue scores (i.e., overall pain, pain at rest, pain during movement, end-of-day fatigue, overall fatigue, morning fatigue) except daily pain (which was based on a comparison with usual daily pain levels) were significantly improved with sodium oxybate compared with placebo. In the secondary analyses, sodium oxybate significantly decreased PSG variables of SL, alpha intrusion, and REM sleep and significantly increased percentage of slow-wave (Stage 3/4) sleep compared with placebo after four weeks of treatment. These findings corresponded with improvements on two of five subjective sleep measures (morning alertness and quality of sleep the previous night).

The most common AEs associated with sodium oxybate are dizziness, headache, nausea, and urinary incontinence. Large doses of sodium oxybate can also cause a number of more serious AEs, ranging from seizure to a pronounced depression of CNS activity that can result in a coma-like state or even death. Indeed, because of the potential for serious AEs, sodium oxybate is available only through restricted distribution, which requires signed documentation stating that both the physician and the patient have read the educational materials and are aware of the dangers. The treatment program also includes provisions for detailed surveillance that requires that the patient be seen by a physician no less often than every three months.

While efficacy data from the aforementioned trial look promising, larger-scale trials are necessary before it becomes clear whether sodium oxybate offers a favorable risk/benefit profile for the treatment of fibromyalgia. Although physicians currently prescribe agents with similarly restrictive labeling (i.e., narcotic analgesics) to fibromyalgia patients, they are generally unwilling to use these agents over the long term. Additionally, GHB's association with illicit use may be a red flag to many physicians who do not want to take any chances with such a drug; these physicians will likely opt for the less risky alternative of one of the newer non-BZD sedative hypnotics. Not only are these agents safer (relatively speaking), they allow for easier dosing (i.e., one pill at bedtime)—in the aforementioned trial, sodium oxybate required administration both at bedtime and four hours later.

Antiepileptic Drugs

Overview. Nearly all of the antiepileptic drugs (AEDs) marketed over the past ten years are now under investigation for their analgesic properties in chronic pain conditions, particularly neuropathic pain. Accordingly, some AED marketers have recently turned their attention to fibromyalgia, because this condition is characterized by chronic, widespread pain, the origin of which is not fully understood but which most pain experts believe involves both central and peripheral pain mechanisms. Pfizer's pregabalin (Lyrica), the company's follow-on to gabapentin, is the most extensively studied AED for fibromyalgia.

Mechanism of Action. Although AEDs' exact mechanism of action in pain management is unknown, research suggests that drugs in this class tend to work through several neuronal pathways. Some mechanisms that are common to many AEDs and that may contribute to their analgesic properties include blockade of neuronal sodium and/or calcium channels, inhibition of the excitatory effects of glutamate, and potentiation of the inhibitory effects of gamma-aminobutyric acid (GABA).

Pregabalin. Pregabalin (Lyrica) (Figure 15) is Pfizer's follow-on to its highly successful AED gabapentin (Neurontin), which is now generically available in the United States and Europe. Pregabalin was granted marketing approval in the

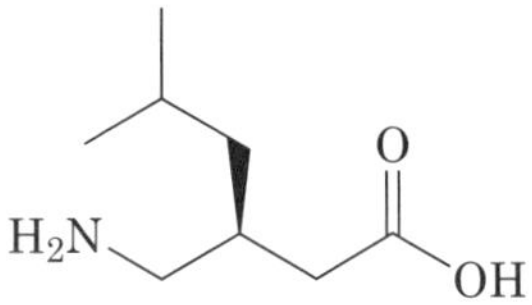

FIGURE 15. Structure of pregabalin.

European Union for peripheral neuropathic pain (NP) and as adjunctive therapy for partial epileptic seizures in mid 2004 and was launched in its first market (the United Kingdom) in August 2004. In the United States, the drug achieved FDA approval for the treatment of postherpetic neuralgia (PHN) and peripheral NP associated with diabetes in January 2005, but with the added labeling restriction that the drug be classified as a Schedule V controlled substance (the least restrictive category for controlled substances). At that time, the FDA did not grant marketing approval for the two other indications for which pregabalin was submitted—generalized anxiety disorder (GAD) and adjunctive therapy for partial epileptic seizures; however, approval for the epilepsy indication was subsequently achieved in June 2005. In Japan, pregabalin is in Phase II trials for epilepsy.

Like gabapentin, pregabalin is believed to exert its anticonvulsant and analgesic effects by blocking voltage-gated presynaptic N- and P/Q-type calcium channels via a specific subunit called the alpha-2-delta subunit (a high-affinity binding site in neuronal membranes) (Dooley DJ, 2002; Field M, 2004; Fink K, 2002). Pregabalin's purported benefits over gabapentin include its higher potency and more predictable pharmacokinetics, which allow it to be administered in lower doses than gabapentin (300–600 mg/day versus 1800–2400 mg/day, respectively) and to be more rapidly titrated to an effective dose.

Data from a double-blind, eight-week trial in which 529 fibromyalgia patients were randomized to receive either placebo or 150, 300, or 450 mg of pregabalin per day (split into three daily doses) revealed that the 450 mg/day dose of the drug provided significant improvements compared with placebo in pain, sleep, and fatigue scores, whereas the 150 and 300 mg doses did not (Crofford LJ, 2002). However, while results favored pregabalin with regard to "% responders" (i.e., patients with a 50% reduction in pain from baseline), the data for pregabalin were not highly impressive (29% for pregabalin versus 13% for placebo). The most commonly reported AEs associated with pregabalin in this trial were dizziness and somnolence; 9% of patients ($n = 48$) withdrew from the trial because of AEs and 8% ($n = 44$) withdrew because of lack of efficacy.

Further data from a separate open-label, long-term (15-month) follow up of 25 fibromyalgia patients who were refractory to therapy with TCAs (≥ 75 mg/day), gabapentin (≥ 1800 mg/day), and third-line analgesics (e.g., other AED, opioid, tramadol, SSRI, SNRI, NSAID/COX-2, topical lidocaine, or mexiletine) and who were taking 150–600 mg/day pregabalin were reported at the 2005 annual meeting of the American Pain Society (Dworkin RH, 2005). To ascertain patients' ongoing level of pain (and consequent need for treatment) throughout the study, investigators conducted quarterly drug holidays (mean duration = three days); patients whose pain became moderately, much, or very much worse during these drug holidays were kept in the trial. Study investigators found that 50% of fibromyalgia patients reported $\geq$50% reduction in pain relief at 3 months and 38% reported similar reductions at 15 months. These data suggest that pregabalin may be an effective treatment alternative for fibromyalgia patients who experience inadequate pain relief and/or who suffer from intolerable side effects with standard first-line fibromyalgia therapies.

5-HT2 Antagonists

Overview. Because drugs that act as 5-HT2A and/or 5-HT2 C antagonists have exhibited sleep-enhancing effects when used as treatments for anxiety and depression, several drug companies—including Sanofi-Aventis, Merck KGaA (Darmstadt, Germany) in collaboration with Eli Lilly, and Sepracor in collaboration with Acadia—are investigating such compounds for the treatment of insomnia. As is the case with the sedative hypnotics (discussed earlier), these agents' (purported) sleep-enhancing effects could translate into a broader therapeutic effect in fibromyalgia, because improvements in sleep in fibromyalgia patients often lead to improvements in daytime functioning related to pain and fatigue.

Mechanism of Action. Investigators suspect that 5-HT2 antagonists exert their sedative effects by enhancing slow wave sleep. In particular, 5-HT2 antagonists may tone down serotonin-induced arousal, which is part of the sleep-wake cycle.

Eplivanserin. Sanofi-Aventis is currently the only company investigating a 5-HT2 antagonist in clinical trials for fibromyalgia. The company's compound, called eplivanserin, is reportedly in Phase IIb trials for fibromyalgia in France; however, no data are available with which to further evaluate this compound for fibromyalgia.

Dopamine Agonists

Dopamine agonists are used primarily to treat Parkinson's disease (PD) and, more recently, restless legs syndrome (RLS). (RLS is a common cause of sleep dysfunction in fibromyalgia sufferers.) Data from two small, randomized, placebo-controlled fibromyalgia trials in which investigators used the dopamine D2/D3 agonists ropinirole (GlaxoSmithKline's Requip) or pramipexole (Boehringer Ingelheim/Pfizer's Mirapex/Sifrol) suggest that these agents also provide therapeutic benefit in treatment-refractory fibromyalgia patients who suffer from a high level of disability (Holman AJ, 2004a; Holman AJ, 2004b). In these studies, patients treated with dopamine agonists reportedly experienced notable reductions in pain as well as overall improvements in function and fatigue. The most commonly reported side effects were weight loss (with pramipexole) and nausea (reported with both compounds).

While dopamine agonists may in fact address what some researchers believe is an underlying autonomic dysfunction in fibromyalgia, these drugs must be investigated in larger-scale trials in the broader fibromyalgia population; studies to date have been limited to the most severely affected, treatment-refractory patients. (Note: Many patients in these trials were also taking concomitant medications, including narcotic analgesics.) Nevertheless, dopamine agonists may find a place in the treatment of fibromyalgia in the future, even if it is only for the most severely affected patients. These agents' apparent ability to improve sleep in RLS sufferers (Allen R, 2004; Stiasny-Kolster K, 2004) may afford them a fairly smooth transition into the treatment of fibromyalgia, because RLS is a fairly common comorbidity with fibromyalgia. Although Boehringer Ingelheim reportedly has little interest in pursuing approval for pramipexole for the treatment of fibromyalgia (at least at the present time), GlaxoSmithKline has initiated a 300-patient proof-of-principle trial in Europe to determine whether ropinirole represents an effective treatment alternative for difficult-to-treat fibromyalgia sufferers.

CNS Stimulants

Anecdotal reports suggest that the CNS stimulant modafinil (Cephalon, Inc.'s [Frazer, Pennsylvania] Provigil) reduces fatigue and improves daytime functioning in fibromyalgia sufferers (Schaller JL, 2001). Although no well-controlled trials have been initiated to examine this effect further, modafinil—and possibly Cephalon's single-isomer follow-on to modafinil, Nuvigil (R-modafinil), which is undergoing FDA review for the treatment of excessive daytime sleepiness—may find a niche in the fibromyalgia market for patients who suffer from excessive daytime fatigue.

5-HT3 Antagonists

5-HT3 antagonists are widely prescribed for the treatment of chemotherapy-induced nausea and vomiting. These agents appear to elicit their therapeutic effects via antagonism of 5-HT3 receptors in both the peripheral and central nervous systems. Based on the purported role of serotonin in fibromyalgia, a group of German investigators have conducted several clinical trials of varying designs with the 5-HT3 antagonist tropisetron (Novartis's Novaban) in patients with fibromyalgia. However, results to date have been difficult to interpret because of the various dosing parameters employed and the short duration and uncontrolled nature of many of the trials (Spath M, 2004).

REFERENCES

Adler GK, Geenen R. Hypothalamic-pituitary-adrenal and autonomic nervous system functioning in fibromyalgia. *Rheum Dis Clin North Am*. 2005;**31**:187–202.

Adler GK, et al. Reduced hypothalamic-pituitary and sympathoadrenal responses to hypoglycemia in women with fibromyalgia syndrome. *Am J Med*. 1999;**106**:534–543.

Adler GK, et al. Neuroendocrine abnormalities in fibromyalgia. *Curr Pain Headache Rep*. 2002;**6**:289–298.

Allen R, et al. Ropinirole decreases periodic leg movements and improves sleep parameters in patients with restless legs syndrome. *Sleep*. 2004;**27**:907–914.

Allison TR, et al. Musculoskeletal pain is more generalised among people from ethnic minorities than among white people in Greater Manchester. *Ann Rheum Dis*. 2002;**61**:151–156.

Andrade L, et al. The epidemiology of major depressive episodes: results from the International Consortium of Psychiatric Epidemiology (ICPE) Surveys. *Int J Methods Psychiatr Res*. 2003;**12**:3–21.

Angst J, et al. Gender differences in depression. Epidemiological findings from the European DEPRES I and II studies. *European Archives of Psychiatry and Clinical Neuroscience*. 2002;**252**:201–209.

Arendt-Nielsen L, Graven-Nielsen T. Central sensitization in fibromyalgia and other musculoskeletal disorders. *Curr Pain Headache Rep*. 2003;**7**:355–361.

Arnold LM, et al. A randomized, placebo-controlled, double-blind, flexible-dose study of fluoxetine in the treatment of women with fibromyalgia. *Am J Med*. 2002;**112**:191–197.

Arnold LM, et al. Antidepressant treatment of fibromyalgia. A meta-analysis and review. *Psychosomatics*. 2000;**41**:104–113.

Arnold LM, et al. A double-blind, multicenter trial comparing duloxetine with placebo in the treatment of fibromyalgia patients with or without major depressive disorder. *Arthritis Rheum*. 2004;**50**:2974–2984.

Bengtsson A, Bengtsson M. Regional sympathetic blockade in primary fibromyalgia. *Pain*. 1988;**33**:161–167.

Bennett R. Fibromyalgia, chronic fatigue syndrome, and myofascial pain. *Curr Opin Rheumatol*. 1998;**10**:95–103.

Bennett R. Fibromyalgia: present to future. *Curr Pain Headache Rep*. 2004;**8**:379–384.

Bennett RM, et al. A comparison of cyclobenzaprine and placebo in the management of fibrositis. A double-blind controlled study. *Arthritis Rheum*. 1988;**31**:1535–1542.

Bennett RM, et al. Tramadol and acetaminophen combination tablets in the treatment of fibromyalgia pain: a double-blind, randomized, placebo-controlled study. *Am J Med*. 2003;**114**:537–545.

Biasi G, et al. Tramadol in the fibromyalgia syndrome: a controlled clinical trial versus placebo. *Int J Clin Pharmacol Res*. 1998;**18**:13–19.

Borman P, et al. The efficacy of venlafaxine in treatment of fibromyalgia. EULAR, European League Against Rheumatism; June 9, 2004; Berlin, Germany. Abstract # SAT0191.

Breau LM, et al. Review of juvenile primary fibromyalgia and chronic fatigue syndrome. *J Dev Behav Pediatr*. 1999;**20**:278–288.

Cantini F, et al. [Fluoxetin combined with cyclobenzaprine in the treatment of fibromyalgia]. *Minerva Med*. 1994;**85**:97–100.

Capuron L, et al. Treatment of cytokine-induced depression. *Brain Behav Immun*. 2002;**16**:575–580.

Carette S, et al. Comparison of amitriptyline, cyclobenzaprine, and placebo in the treatment of fibromyalgia. A randomized, double-blind clinical trial. *Arthritis Rheum*. 1994;**37**:32–40.

Carmona L, et al. The burden of musculoskeletal diseases in the general population of Spain: results from a national survey. *Ann Rheum Dis*. 2001;**60**:1040–1045.

Chen H, et al. Contemporary management of neuropathic pain for the primary care physician. *Mayo Clin Proc*. 2004;**79**:1533–1545.

Cimmino MA, et al. [Methodology of an epidemiologic prevalence study in rheumatology: the Chiavari study]. *Reumatismo*. 2002;**54**:40–47.

Clark S, Bennett R. Supplemental dextromethorphan in the treatment of fibromyalgia: a double-blind, placebo-controlled study of efficacy and side-effects. *Arthritis Rheum*. 2000;**43**:S333.

Clauw DJ. Fibromyalgia. In Ruddy S, et al., eds. *Kelly's Textbook of Rheumatology*; Philadelphia: W.B. Saunders Company, 2001.

Clauw DJ, Crofford LJ. Chronic widespread pain and fibromyalgia: what we know, and what we need to know. *Best Pract Res Clin Rheumatol*. 2003;**17**:685–701.

Coda B, Bonica J. General considerations of acute pain. In Loeser J, et al, eds. *Bonica's management of pain*; Philadelphia, PA: Lippincott Williams & Wilkins, 2001.

Cohen H, et al. Abnormal sympathovagal balance in men with fibromyalgia. *J Rheumatol*. 2001;**28**:581–589.

Cohen H, et al. Autonomic dysfunction in patients with fibromyalgia: application of power spectral analysis of heart rate variability. *Semin Arthritis Rheum*. 2000;**29**:217–227.

Cote KA, et al. Sleep, daytime symptoms, and cognitive performance in patients with fibromyalgia. *J Rheumatol*. 1997;**24**:2014–2023.

Crofford LJ, et al. Pregabalin improves pain associated with fibromyalgia syndrome in a multicenter, randomized, placebo-controlled monotherapy trial. *Arthritis Rheum*. 2002;**46**:S613.

Crofford LJ, et al. Hypothalamic-pituitary-adrenal axis perturbations in patients with fibromyalgia. *Arthritis Rheum*. 1994;**37**:1583–1592.

Croft P, et al. More pain, more tender points: is fibromyalgia just one end of a continuous spectrum? *Ann Rheum Dis*. 1996;**55**:482–485.

Croft P, et al. The prevalence of chronic widespread pain in the general population. *J Rheumatol*. 1993;**20**:710–713.

Croft P, et al. Population study of tender point counts and pain as evidence of fibromyalgia. *BMJ*. 1994;**309**:696–699.

Dauvilliers Y, Touchon J. [Sleep in fibromyalgia: review of clinical and polysomnographic data]. *Neurophysiol Clin*. 2001;**31**:18–33.

Deluze C, et al. Electroacupuncture in fibromyalgia: results of a controlled trial. *BMJ*. 1992;**305**:1249–1252.

DeWalt DA, et al. Further clues to recognition of patients with fibromyalgia from a simple 2-page patient multidimensional health assessment questionnaire (MDHAQ). *Clin Exp Rheumatol*. 2004;**22**:453–461.

Dooley DJ, et al. Preferential action of gabapentin and pregabalin at P/Q-type voltage-sensitive calcium channels: inhibition of K+-evoked [3H]-norepinephrine release from rat neocortical slices. *Synapse*. 2002;**45**:171–190.

Dujardin K, et al. Comparison of the effects of zolpidem and flunitrazepam on sleep structure and daytime cognitive functions. A study of untreated unsomniacs.. *Pharmacopsychiatry*. 1998;**31**:14–18.

Dwight MM, et al. An open clinical trial of venlafaxine treatment of fibromyalgia. *Psychosomatics*. 1998;**39**:14–17.

Dworkin RH, et al. Long-term treatment of neuropathic pain and fibromyalgia syndrome with pregabalin in treatment-refractory patients. 24th Annual Meeting of the American Pain Society; March 30, 2005; Boston, MA.

Eide PK. Wind-up and the NMDA receptor complex from a clinical perspective. *Eur J Pain*. 2000;**4**:5–15.

Erman M, et al. Polysomnographic and patient-reported evaluation of the efficacy and safety of eszopiclone in elderly subjects with chronic insomnia. *Sleep*. 2004;**27**(abstract suppl):L577.

Essick GK. Psychophysical assessment of patients with posttraumatic neuropathic trigeminal pain. *J Orofac Pain*. 2004;**18**:345–354.

Farooqi A, Gibson T. Prevalence of the major rheumatic disorders in the adult population of north Pakistan. *Br J Rheumatol*. 1998;**37**:491–495.

Field M, et al. The analgesic actions of pregabalin are mediated through its binding to the alpha-2-delta subunit. 2nd Joint Scientific Meeting of the American Pain Society and the Canadian Pain Society; May 6, 2004; Vancouver, BC.

Fink K, et al. Inhibition of neuronal Ca(2+) influx by gabapentin and pregabalin in the human neocortex. *Neuropharmacology*. 2002;**42**:229–236.

Forseth KO, Gran JT. The prevalence of fibromyalgia among women aged 20–49 years in Arendal, Norway. *Scand J Rheumatol*. 1992;**21**:74–78.

Fossaluzza V, De VS. Combined therapy with cyclobenzaprine and ibuprofen in primary fibromyalgia syndrome. *Int J Clin Pharmacol Res*. 1992;**12**:99–102.

Garcia del Rio J. Prevalence of widespread pain and fibromyalgia among women. *Atencion Primaria*. 2000;**1**.

Garcia-Borreguero D, et al. Treatment of restless legs syndrome with gabapentin [neurontin]: a double-blind, cross-over study. *Neurology*. 2002;**59**:1573–1579.

Giesecke T, et al. The relationship between depression, clinical pain, and experimental pain in a chronic pain cohort. *Arthritis and Rheumatism*. 2005;**52**:1577–1584.

Goldenberg D, et al. A randomized, double-blind crossover trial of fluoxetine and amitriptyline in the treatment of fibromyalgia. *Arthritis Rheum*. 1996;**39**:1852–1859.

Goldenberg DL, et al. High frequency of fibromyalgia in patients with chronic fatigue seen in a primary care practice. *Arthritis Rheum*. 1990;**33**:381–387.

Gracely RH, Kwilosz DM. The descriptor differential scale: applying psychophysical principles to clinical pain assessment. *Pain*. 1988;**35**:279–288.

Graven-Nielsen T, et al. Ketamine reduces muscle pain, temporal summation, and referred pain in fibromyalgia patients. *Pain*. 2000;**85**:483–491.

Grothe DR, et al. Treatment of pain syndromes with venlafaxine. *Pharmacotherapy*. 2004;**24**:621–629.

Hannonen P, et al. A randomized, double-blind, placebo-controlled study of moclobemide and amitriptyline in the treatment of fibromyalgia in females without psychiatric disorder. *Br J Rheumatol*. 1998;**37**:1279–1286.

Harkness EF, et al. Is musculoskeletal pain more common now than 40 years ago?: two population-based cross-sectional studies. *Rheumatology (Oxford)*. 2005.

Henriksson KG. Hypersensitivity in muscle pain syndromes. *Curr Pain Headache Rep*. 2003;**7**:426–432.

Herrero JF, et al. Wind-up of spinal cord neurones and pain sensation: much ado about something? *Prog Neurobiol*. 2000;**61**:169–203.

Holdcroft A, Power I. Recent developments: management of pain. *BMJ*. 2003;**326**:635–639.

Holman AJ. Treatment of fibromyalgia with the dopamine agonist pramipexole: a double-blind, randomized, placebo controlled 14-week trial. Late-breaking abstract. Annual Meeting of the American College of Rheumatology; October 16, 2004a; San Antonio, TX.

Holman AJ. Treatment of fibromyalgia with the dopamine agonist ropinirole: a 14-week double-blind pilot randomized controlled trial with 14-week blinded extension. Annual Meeting of the American College of Rheumatology; October 16, 2004b; San Antonio, TX.

Jacobsson L, et al. The commonest rheumatic complaints of over six weeks' duration in a twelve-month period in a defined Swedish population. Prevalences and relationships. *Scand J Rheumatol*. 1989;**18**:353–360.

Jason LA, et al. Chronic fatigue syndrome, fibromyalgia, and multiple chemical sensitivities in a community-based sample of persons with chronic fatigue syndrome-like symptoms. *Psychosom Med*. 2000;**62**:655–663.

Julien N, et al. Widespread pain in fibromyalgia is related to a deficit of endogenous pain inhibition. *Pain*. 2005;**114**:295–302.

Katz RS, Wolfe F. Somatization and its discontents: rates, predictors and correlates of somatic symptoms in rheumatic disease patients. American College of Rheumatology Annual Meeting; October 17, 2004; San Antonio, TX. Abstract # 1249.

Kelemen J, et al. Orthostatic sympathetic derangement of baroreflex in patients with fibromyalgia. *J Rheumatol*. 1998;**25**:823–825.

Kessler RC, et al. The epidemiology of major depressive disorder:results from teh National Comorbidity Survey Replication (NCS-R). *JAMA*. 2003;**289**:3095–3105.

Khasabov SG, et al. Spinal neurons that possess the substance P receptor are required for the development of central sensitization. *J Neurosci*. 2002;**22**:9086–9098.

Kiecolt-Glaser JK, et al. Chronic stress and age-related increases in the proinflammatory cytokine IL-6. *Proc Natl Acad Sci U S A*. 2003;**100**:9090–9095.

Kooh M, et al. Simultaneous heart rate variability and polysomnographic analyses in fibromyalgia. *Clin Exp Rheumatol*. 2003;**21**:529–530.

Krystal A, et al. Sustained efficacy of eszopiclone over 6 months of nightly treatment: results of a randomized, double-blind, placebo-controlled study in adults with chronic insomnia. *Sleep*. 2003;**26**:793–799.

Kurtze N, Svebak S. Fatigue and patterns of pain in fibromyalgia: correlations with anxiety, depression and co-morbidity in a female county sample. *Br J Med Psychol*. 2001;**74**:523–537.

Lawrence RC, et al. Estimates of the prevalence of arthritis and selected musculoskeletal disorders in the United States. *Arthritis Rheum*. 1998;**41**:778–799.

Lawson K. Tricyclic antidepressants and fibromyalgia: what is the mechanism of action? *Expert Opin Investig Drugs*. 2002;**11**:1437–1445.

Legangneux E, et al. Cerebrospinal fluid biogenic amine metabolites, plasma-rich platelet serotonin and [3H]imipramine reuptake in the primary fibromyalgia syndrome. *Rheumatology (Oxford)*. 2001;**40**:290–296.

Lepine JP. Depression in the community: the first pan-European study DEPRES (Depression Research in European Society). *International Clinical Psychopharmacology*. 1997;**12**:19–29.

Lindell L, et al. Prevalence of fibromyalgia and chronic widespread pain. *Scand J Prim Health Care*. 2000;**18**:149–153.

Macfarlane GJ. Fibromyalgia and chronic widespread pain. In Crombie IK e, ed. *Epidemiology of Pain*; Seattle: IASP Press: 1999a.

Macfarlane GJ. Generalized pain, fibromyalgia and regional pain: an epidemiological view. *Baillieres Best Pract Res Clin Rheumatol*. 1999b;**13**:403–414.

Makela M, Heliovaara M. Prevalence of primary fibromyalgia in the Finnish population. *BMJ*. 1991;**303**:216–219.

Makela MO. Is fibromyalgia a distinct clinical entity? The epidemiologist's evidence. *Baillieres Best Pract Res Clin Rheumatol*. 1999;**13**:415–419.

Martinez-Lavin M. Fibromyalgia as a sympathetically maintained pain syndrome. *Curr Pain Headache Rep*. 2004;**8**:385–389.

Martinez-Lavin M, et al. Circadian studies of autonomic nervous balance in patients with fibromyalgia: a heart rate variability analysis. *Arthritis Rheum*. 1998;**41**:1966–1971.

Martinez-Lavin M, et al. Norepinephrine-evoked pain in fibromyalgia. A randomized pilot study [ISRCTN70707830]. *BMC Musculoskelet Disord*. 2002;**3**: 2.

Miller DB, O'Callaghan JP. Neuroendocrine aspects of the response to stress. *Metabolism*. 2002;**51**:5–10.

Moldofsky H. Sleep and pain. *Sleep Med Rev*. 2001;**5**:385–396.

Moldofsky H, et al. Musculoskeletal symptoms and non-REM sleep disturbance in patients with "fibrositis syndrome" and healthy subjects. *Psychosom Med*. 1975;**37**:341–351.

Neeck G. Neuroendocrine and hormonal perturbations and relations to the serotonergic system in fibromyalgia patients. *Scand J Rheumatol Suppl*. 2000;**113**:8–12.

Nicholson AN, Pascoe PA. Hypnotic activity of an imidazo-pyridine (zolpidem). *Br J Clin Pharmacol*. 1986;**21**:205–211.

O'Malley PG, et al. Treatment of fibromyalgia with antidepressants: a meta-analysis. *J Gen Intern Med*. 2000;**15**:659–666.

Okifuji A, et al. Evaluation of the relationship between depression and fibromyalgia syndrome: why aren't all patients depressed? *J Rheumatol*. 2000;**27**:212–219.

Ordeberg G. Characterization of joint pain in human OA. *Novartis Found Symp*. 2004; **260**:105–115.

Picavet HS, Hazes JM. Prevalence of self reported musculoskeletal diseases is high. *Ann Rheum Dis*. 2003;**62**:644–650.

Population Division. *Population Division of the Department of Economic and Social Affairs of the United Nations Secretariat. World Population Prospects: The 2002 Revision, vol. II, The Sex and Age Distribution of Populations*, 2003.

Prescott E, et al. Fibromyalgia in the adult Danish population: I. A prevalence study. *Scand J Rheumatol*. 1993;**22**:233–237.

Prescott EE, et al. Red blood cell magnesium and fibromyalgia. *Scand J Rheumatol*. 1992;**94**:31.

Price DD, et al. Enhanced temporal summation of second pain and its central modulation in fibromyalgia patients. *Pain*. 2002;**99**:49–59.

Raj SR, et al. Dysautonomia among patients with fibromyalgia: a noninvasive assessment. *J Rheumatol*. 2000;**27**:2660–2665.

Raspe H. The epidemiology of the fibromyalgia syndrome in a German town. *Scand J Rheumatol*. 1992;**94**:8.

Rau CL, Russell IJ. Is fibromyalgia a distinct clinical syndrome? *Curr Rev Pain*. 2000;**4**:287–294.

Reisine S, et al. The expression and experience of pain among women with fibromyalgia (FM) and controls with chronic pain using the McGill Pain Questionnaire (MPQ). American College of Rheumatology Annual Meeting; October 17, 2004; San Antonio, TX. Abstract # 1821.

Reynolds WJ, et al. The effects of cyclobenzaprine on sleep physiology and symptoms in patients with fibromyalgia. *J Rheumatol*. 1991;**18**:452–454.

Romanelli P, Esposito V. The functional anatomy of neuropathic pain. *Neurosurg Clin N Am*. 2004;**15**:257–268.

Roth T, et al. Twelve months of nightly eszopiclone treatment in patients with chronic insomnia: assessment of long-term efficacy and safety. *Sleep*. 2004;**27**(abstract suppl):L584.

Russell J, et al. Efficacy of tramadol in the treatment of fibromyalgia. *J Clin Rheumatol*. 2000;**6**:250–257.

Russell IJ, et al. Treatment of primary fibrositis/fibromyalgia syndrome with ibuprofen and alprazolam. A double-blind, placebo-controlled study. *Arthritis Rheum*. 1991;**34**:552–560.

Russell IJ, et al. Elevated cerebrospinal fluid levels of substance P in patients with the fibromyalgia syndrome. *Arthritis Rheum*. 1994;**37**:1593–1601.

Russell IJ, et al. Cerebrospinal fluid biogenic amine metabolites in fibromyalgia/fibrositis syndrome and rheumatoid arthritis. *Arthritis Rheum*. 1992;**35**:550–556.

Sachar EJ, et al. Cortisol production in depressive illness. A clinical and biochemical clarification. *Arch Gen Psychiatry*. 1970;**23**:289–298.

Sang CN. Challenges in clinical translational pain research: NMDA glutamate receptor antagonists in neuropathic pain. American Pain Society Annual Meeting; April 2, 2005; Boston, MA.

Santandrea S, et al. A double-blind crossover study of two cyclobenzaprine regimens in primary fibromyalgia syndrome. *J Int Med Res*. 1993;**21**:74–80.

Sayar K, et al. Venlafaxine treatment of fibromyalgia. *Ann Pharmacother*. 2003;**37**:1561–1565.

Schaller JL, Behar D. Modafinil in fibromyalgia treatment. *J Neuropsychiatry Clin Neurosci*. 2001;**13**:530–531.

Scharf M, et al. Eszopiclone efficacy and daytime functioning in non-elderly and elderly patients with chronic insomnia. *Sleep*. 2004;**27**(abstract suppl):L578.

Scharf MB, et al. The effects of sodium oxybate on clinical symptoms and sleep patterns in patients with fibromyalgia. *J Rheumatol*. 2003;**30**:1070–1074.

Senna ER, et al. Prevalence of rheumatic diseases in Brazil: a study using the COPCORD approach. *J Rheumatol*. 2004;**31**:594–597.

Sepracor. Eszopiclone. *Drugs of the Future*. 2003;**28**:640–646.

Sim J, Adams N. Systematic review of randomized controlled trials of nonpharmacological interventions for fibromyalgia. *Clin J Pain*. 2002;**18**:324–336.

Sorensen J, et al. Pain analysis in patients with fibromyalgia. Effects of intravenous morphine, lidocaine, and ketamine. *Scand J Rheumatol*. 1995;**24**:360–365.

Spath M. [What's new in the therapy of fibromyalgia?]. *Schmerz*. 2003;**17**:437–440.

Spath M, et al. Treatment of fibromyalgia with tropisetron--dose and efficacy correlations. *Scand J Rheumatol Suppl*. 2004;63–66.

Stahl SM. Fibromyalgia: the enigma and the stigma. *J Clin Psychiatry*. 2001;**62**:501–502.

Staud R. Fibromyalgia pain: do we know the source ? *Curr Opin Rheumatol*. 2004a;**16**:157–163.

Staud R, et al. Temporal summation of pain from mechanical stimulation of muscle tissue in normal controls and subjects with fibromyalgia syndrome. *Pain*. 2003;**102**:87–95.

Staud R, et al. Maintenance of windup of second pain requires less frequent stimulation in fibromyalgia patients compared to normal controls. *Pain*. 2004b;**110**:689–696.

Staud R, et al. Abnormal sensitization and temporal summation of second pain (wind-up) in patients with fibromyalgia syndrome. *Pain*. 2001;**91**:165–175.

Stiasny-Kolster K, et al. Restless legs syndrome--new insights into clinical characteristics, pathophysiology, and treatment options. *J Neurol*. 2004;**251** Suppl 6:VI/39-VI/43.

Stratz T, et al. Influence of tropisetron on the serum substance P levels in fibromyalgia patients. *Scand J Rheumatol Suppl*. 2004;41–43.

Terman GW, et al. Mu opiates inhibit long-term potentiation induction in the spinal cord slice. *J Neurophysiol*. 2001;**85**:485–494.

Thomas E, et al. Fibromyalgia as a national issue: the French example. *Baillieres Best Pract Res Clin Rheumatol*. 1999;**13**:525–529.

Vaeroy H, et al. Elevated CSF levels of substance P and high incidence of Raynaud phenomenon in patients with fibromyalgia: new features for diagnosis. *Pain*. 1988;**32**:21–26.

Van CE, et al. Simultaneous stimulation of slow-wave sleep and growth hormone secretion by gamma-hydroxybutyrate in normal young Men. *J Clin Invest*. 1997;**100**:745–753.

Vitton O, et al. A double-blind placebo-controlled trial of milnacipran in the treatment of fibromyalgia. *Hum Psychopharmacol*. 2004;**19** Suppl 1:S27-S35.

Welin M, et al. Elevated substance P levels are contrasted by a decrease in metenkephalin-arg-phe levels in CSF from fibromyalgia patients. *Journal of Musculoskeletal Pain*. 1995;**3**(suppl 1): 4.

Wernicke J, et al. Duloxetine in the treatment of fibromyalgia. American College of Rheumatology Annual Scientific Meeting; 2004; San Antonio, TX. Abstract # 1867.

Wessel T, et al. Eszopiclone improves next day function of elderly patients with chronic insomnia. 56th Annual Meeting of the American Academy of Neurology; April 24, 2004; San Francisco, CA.

Wessely S, Hotopf M. Is fibromyalgia a distinct clinical entity? Historical and epidemiological evidence. *Baillieres Best Pract Res Clin Rheumatol*. 1999;**13**:427–436.

White KP, Harth M. Classification, epidemiology, and natural history of fibromyalgia. *Curr Pain Headache Rep*. 2001;**5**:320–329.

White KP, et al. Chronic widespread musculoskeletal pain with or without fibromyalgia: psychological distress in a representative community adult sample. *J Rheumatol*. 2002;**29**:588–594.

White KP, et al. The London Fibromyalgia Epidemiology Study: the prevalence of fibromyalgia syndrome in London, Ontario. *J Rheumatol*. 1999;**26**:1570–1576.

Wolfe F. The relation between tender points and fibromyalgia symptom variables: evidence that fibromyalgia is not a discrete disorder in the clinic. *Ann Rheum Dis*. 1997a;**56**:268–271.

Wolfe F, et al. A prospective, longitudinal, multicenter study of service utilization and costs in fibromyalgia. *Arthritis Rheum*. 1997b;**40**:1560–1570.

Wolfe F, et al. A double-blind placebo controlled trial of fluoxetine in fibromyalgia. *Scand J Rheumatol*. 1994;**23**:255–259.

Wolfe F, et al. The prevalence and characteristics of fibromyalgia in the general population. *Arthritis Rheum*. 1995;**38**:19–28.

Wolfe F, et al. The American College of Rheumatology 1990 Criteria for the Classification of Fibromyalgia. Report of the Multicenter Criteria Committee. *Arthritis Rheum*. 1990;**33**:160–172.

Wood PB. Stress and dopamine: implications for the pathophysiology of chronic widespread pain. *Med Hypotheses*. 2004;**62**:420–424.

Young EA, et al. Loss of glucocorticoid fast feedback in depression. *Arch Gen Psychiatry*. 1991;**48**:693–699.

Zammit G, et al. Eszopiclone, a novel non-benzodiazepine anti-insomnia agent: a six-week efficacy and safety study in adult patients with chronic insomnia. *Sleep*. 2003;**26**(abstract suppl):A0747.L.

Zhao SZ, et al. Evaluation of the functional status aspects of health-related quality of life of patients with osteoarthritis treated with celecoxib. *Pharmacotherapy*. 1999;**19**:1269–1278.

Zijlstra TR, et al. Venlafaxine in fibromyalgia: results of a randomized, placebo-controlled, double-blind trial. *Arthritis Rheum*. 2002;**45**(suppl 9): 105.

RESPIRATORY

Chronic Obstructive Pulmonary Disease

ETIOLOGY AND PATHOPHYSIOLOGY

Anatomy

The bronchial tree consists of two branched airways—the right and left bronchus—leading from the trachea to microscopic air sacs in the lungs (Figure 1). Each bronchus, accompanied by large blood vessels, enters its respective lung. A short distance from the origin of the bronchus, the bronchial tree divides into secondary bronchi, which in turn branch into progressively smaller airways called bronchioles. The bronchioles continue to divide, giving rise to very thin tubes called alveolar ducts. These ducts terminate in masses of microscopic air sacs called alveoli, which are surrounded by a net of capillaries.

The branches of the bronchial tree serve as air passages, distributing inhaled air to alveoli throughout the lungs. The alveoli, in turn, provide a large surface area for gas exchange. During these exchanges, oxygen diffuses through the alveolar walls and enters the blood in nearby capillaries, while carbon dioxide diffuses from the blood through these walls and enters the alveoli.

The amount of air entering the lungs during a normal, quiet inspiration is about 600 cc in men and 450 cc in women—approximately the same volume that leaves during a normal expiration. This volume is called the tidal volume. During forced inspiration, a quantity of air in addition to the tidal volume enters the lungs.

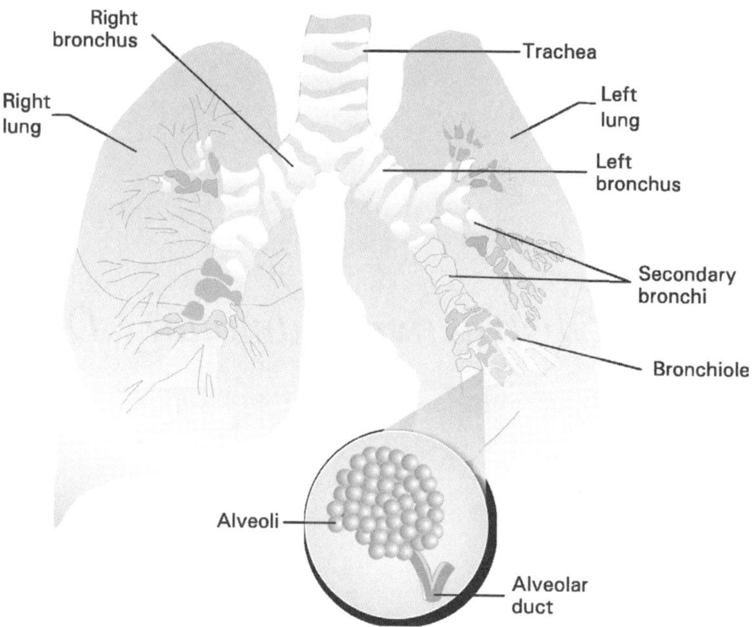

FIGURE 1. The bronchial tree.

This additional volume is called the inspiratory reserve volume, and it equals approximately 3000 cc in men and 1950 cc in women. During forced expiration, about 1200 cc of air for men and 800 cc of air for women in addition to the tidal volume can be expelled from the lungs. This quantity is called the expiratory reserve volume. Even after the most forceful expiration, approximately 1200 cc of air for men and 1000 cc of air for women—the residual volume—remains in the lungs. As air is inhaled, it mixes with the residual volume, preventing oxygen and carbon dioxide concentrations in the lungs from fluctuating excessively with each breath. The expiratory reserve volume plus the residual volume constitute the functional residual capacity, the volume of air in the lungs at the end of a normal expiration, when all respiratory muscles are relaxed.

Vital capacity refers to the sum of the inspiratory reserve volume plus the tidal volume and the expiratory reserve volume. This volume, totaling approximately 4800 cc in men and 3200 cc in women, is the maximum amount of air a person can slowly exhale after taking the deepest possible breath. A measure of vital capacity is commonly used in the clinical setting to assess pulmonary function. Vital capacity plus residual volume equal the total lung capacity, which is approximately 6000 cc in men and 4200 cc in women, depending on age and body size.

Some of the air that enters the respiratory tract during breathing fails to reach the alveoli. This volume, approximately 150 cc, remains in the passageways of the trachea, bronchi, and bronchioles.

Disease Definition

No consensus has been reached on the operational definition of chronic obstructive pulmonary disease (COPD). The American Thoracic Society (ATS) Standards for the Diagnosis and Care of Patients with Chronic Obstructive Pulmonary Disease defines COPD as a disease process featuring progressive and, in some cases, partly reversible airflow obstruction caused by emphysema, chronic bronchitis, or both (American Thoracic Society, 1995). The European Respiratory Society (ERS) defines COPD as "reduced maximum expiratory flow and slow forced emptying of the lungs, which is slowly progressive and mostly irreversible to present medical treatment" (Siafakas NM, 1995). Finally, the definition of COPD published in the Global Initiative for Chronic Obstructive Lung Disease (GOLD) Workshop Report (2003) underscores the role of inflammation in the pathophysiology of the disease: "a disease state characterized by airflow limitation that is not fully reversible. The airflow limitation is usually both progressive and associated with an abnormal inflammatory response of the lungs to noxious particles or gases." In focusing on lung function, the GOLD description is a departure from earlier descriptions, which focused on the phenotypic distinctions of emphysema and chronic bronchitis. These definitions differ in the extent of airflow limitation and reversibility used to diagnose COPD (Mannino DM, 2002).

Generally excluded from these definitions is asthma. Although asthma may have the same symptoms as COPD and, in some cases, may be difficult to distinguish from COPD, the airflow characteristics, response to therapy, and long-term outcome of the two diseases differ. Table 1 examines clinical and pathological characteristics of COPD and asthma. COPD may coexist with asthma, but the inflammation characteristic of COPD differs from that of asthma.

TABLE 1. Comparison of the Clinical and Pathological Characteristics of Chronic Obstructive Pulmonary Disease and Asthma

	COPD	Asthma
Cause	Smoking	Immune
Airflow obstruction	Progressive, largely irreversible	Largely reversible
Clinical manifestations	Dyspnea, cough, sputum production	Wheeze, breathlessness, chest tightness, cough
Diagnosis	History, symptoms FEV_1/FVC <70%	FEV_1/FVC <75% Acute response to bronchodilators (FEV_1 increase of 12–15%)
Inflammatory cells	Macrophages, neutrophils, T cells	Eosinophils, T cells
Inflammatory mediators	IL-8, TNF-α, leukotriene B_4	Interleukins 3, 4, 5, 13; leukotrienes C_4, D_4, E_4
Response to glucocorticoids	Variable	Significant
Treatments	Beta$_2$ agonists, anticholinergics	Beta$_2$ agonists, corticosteroids, leukotriene antagonists

[a]COPD = Chronic obstructive pulmonary disease; FEV_1 = Forced expiratory volume in one second; FVC = Chronic vital capacity; IL-8 = Interleukin-8; TNF-α = Tumor necrosis factor-α.

Another factor hindering understanding of COPD etiology and pathophysiology is that COPD is a complex disease, often considered to encompass a collection of conditions. The GOLD description addresses the struggle to uniformly define disorders associated with airflow limitation. Physicians still sometimes have difficulty differentiating COPD—chronic bronchitis and/or emphysema—from unremitting asthma. Because the definitions are based primarily on outcome measures (airflow limitation), determining which conditions are considered COPD is confusing. This confusion over the breadth of COPD complicates research into the pathophysiological processes underlying the disease and assessment of treatment efficacy.

Although COPD is widely accepted to include emphysema (considered by GOLD to be a pathological state) and chronic bronchitis, the definition of COPD in some countries is frequently expanded to include asthma and other diseases of airflow obstruction such as bronchiectasis (chronic dilation of bronchi or bronchioles from inflammatory disease or obstruction) and bronchiolitis obliterans (obstruction of bronchioles and alveolar ducts by fibrous granulation tissue induced by mucosal ulceration). In the United States, smokers with asthma who develop chronic bronchitis may be said to have "chronic asthmatic bronchitis." Some physicians maintain that irreversible airflow obstruction is the defining feature of COPD; others see the disease as having a reversible component (i.e., airflow obstruction and symptoms such as a productive cough, varying wheeze, and exertional dyspnea may reverse significantly in response to bronchoactive drugs such as bronchodilators and corticosteroids). Finally, some clinicians believe only smokers can develop COPD (the reason COPD is sometimes referred to as "smoker's cough"), and these clinicians refuse to classify airflow obstruction in nonsmokers as COPD. Although COPD is associated primarily with chronic smokers, only a relatively small fraction of smokers develop COPD. The commonly referenced estimate for the percentage of smokers who develop the disease is 15–20%; however, GOLD guidelines iterate that this commonly cited figure is likely an underestimate, due largely to the fact that COPD is underdiagnosed. Researchers have been unable to identify host factors that make a proportion of chronic smokers susceptible to COPD.

Emphysema. Emphysema is defined pathologically as abnormal and permanent alveolar enlargement. As the alveoli stretch beyond normal limits, their walls break down. Once the walls' tethering function diminishes, the grapelike clusters of alveoli merge, forming larger chambers and reducing the surface area for gas exchange. Over time, alveolar damage reduces elastic recoil of the lungs and can cause the bronchioles to collapse, thus increasing airway resistance and reducing the efficiency of expiration.

Chronic Bronchitis. Chronic bronchitis is persistent and recurring inflammation of the bronchi—clinically defined by a chronic cough, mucus production, or both—persisting for at least three months and occurring in at least two successive years during which other causes of chronic cough have been excluded. Over time, the pathophysiological components of bronchial inflammation—mucosal inflammation, mucous gland enlargement, overgrowth of goblet (mucus-producing) cells in the lungs, and infiltration by inflammatory cells (white blood cells/leukocytes)—cause thickening of the bronchial walls, thereby constricting or narrowing the airways and obstructing airflow. As damage increases, airways become more susceptible to infection, leading to the increased cough, sputum volume, purulence, dyspnea, and diminished gas exchange that often mark acute exacerbations of chronic bronchitis (AECB), which are especially common during winter when cold, dry air can be particularly irritating to the airways.

Airflow Obstruction. Both emphysema and chronic bronchitis are characterized by reduced expiratory airflow and slow, forced emptying of the lungs. The often overlapping conditions of emphysema and chronic bronchitis differ in their pathophysiology, which is described in detail in the "Pathophysiology" section. Because differentiating between emphysema or chronic bronchitis and unremitting asthma is often impossible, patients with this form of asthma are classified as having COPD; patients with a reversible component to their asthma—the majority of asthmatics—are excluded from a COPD diagnosis.

To determine the level of airflow obstruction, spirometric testing is used. Spirometry measures the volume of air exhaled during various points in time: at one second (forced expiratory volume-1, or FEV_1), at three seconds (forced expiratory volume-3, or FEV_3), or at the volume of exhalation after a maximal inspiration (forced vital capacity, or FVC). The spirometric values typically used in the diagnosis of COPD are FEV_1 and FVC. Beginning at approximately age 35, FEV_1 in nonsmokers without respiratory disease declines by 25–30 mL per year. This rate of decline is accelerated in smokers, with significant reductions in FEV_1—often surpassing 80 mL annually—strongly suggestive of COPD. An FEV_1 of less than 70% of predicted volume (adjusted for height, age, and gender) is a generally accepted indicator of airflow obstruction.

The FEV_1 value often is presented as a percentage of the predicted FVC volume to indicate the degree of lung obstruction. In normal lungs, FEV_1/FVC is typically 80%. In a patient with COPD, airflow obstruction may reduce this ratio to 70% or less. FEV_1 has been shown to be the single best predictor of survival in COPD patients, with FEV_1 and FEV_1/FVC values used to stage COPD from mild to very severe (Figure 2).

Etiology

Risk Factors.

Smoking. Cigarette use is unquestionably the most significant risk factor for the development and progression of COPD. Smoking is responsible for 90% of COPD cases and 80–90% of COPD deaths. By contrast, COPD is relatively uncommon in those who have never smoked. Pipe and cigar smokers also have

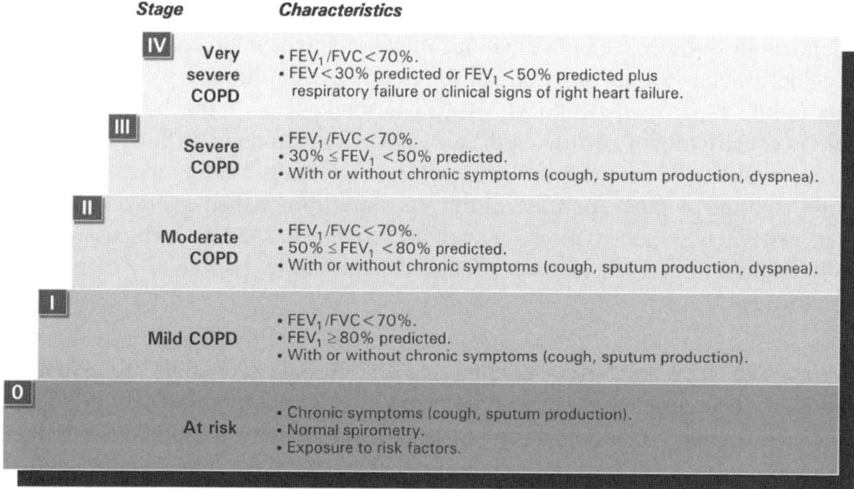

FEV$_1$ = Forced expiratory volume in one second.
FVC = Forced vital capacity.

FIGURE 2. *Chronic obstructive pulmonary disease severity definitions.*

higher COPD morbidity and mortality rates than do nonsmokers, but these rates are lower than those for cigarette smokers.

On average, smokers lose lung function at two to five times the rate normally associated with aging. A dose-response relationship exists between cumulative cigarettes smoked and the rate of lung function decline, with COPD symptoms typically arising after a cumulative cigarette exposure of 20 cigarettes/day for 20 years (i.e., 20 pack-years). Only 15–20% of heavy smokers develop clinically important chronic airflow obstruction. Why this subpopulation is susceptible to lung injury from tobacco is unknown (Silverman EK, 1996; Chen Y, 1999; Laurell CB, 1963; Hubbard RC, 1991; McElvaney NG, 1997).

Environmental Factors. Intense or prolonged exposure to particulate dusts (e.g., coal) and chemical fumes encountered in an occupational setting (e.g., in the grain or solvent industries) is associated with the development of COPD, independent of cigarette use.

Respiratory symptoms and reduced pulmonary function are more common in urban populations, suggesting a link between air pollution and COPD. Some researchers suspect that pollution reduces lung function directly or increases the risk of childhood respiratory infection, which itself may be a COPD risk factor. Specific damaging pollutants remain unidentified, however, and the overall culpability of air pollutants in COPD is unknown.

The effect of passive exposure to tobacco smoke on the development of COPD has been studied but remains to be determined (Buist AS, 1994; Leuenberger P, 1994; Dayal HH, 1994). Research has shown, however, that childhood and workplace exposure to passive smoke are associated with more frequent respiratory infections (Dhala A, 2004; Gurkan F, 2000; McConnochie KM, 1986; Morkjaroenpong V, 2002).

Childhood Respiratory Infections. Many epidemiological studies have implicated childhood respiratory infections as an independent risk factor for the subsequent development of COPD (Tager IB, 1988; Petty TL, 2003). Evidence suggests that these acute illnesses, typically viral in nature, impair lung growth and reduce the level of pulmonary function achieved in adulthood. Nonetheless, a causal relationship between acute childhood respiratory infections and COPD has not been definitively established.

Genetic Factors. Alpha1-antitrypsin (AAT) deficiency is the only known genetic abnormality linked to the development of COPD, accounting for 1–3% of all cases. AAT is a serum glycoprotein encoded on chromosome 14, produced by the liver, and found in the lungs. When present in sufficient quantities, this protein inhibits the activity of enzymes implicated in emphysema (this topic is discussed in detail in the "Pathophysiology" section).

One gene (with approximately 75 genetic alleles) is involved in AAT production (Bartolome R, 1995). Depending on which alleles are expressed, AAT production may be normal, with expected serum AAT levels; deficient, with below-normal AAT serum levels; null, with nondetectable AAT serum levels; or dysfunctional, with AAT failing to function correctly. Normal serum AAT levels are 20–48 µM, while the minimum protective level is believed to be 11 µM, or 35% of normal (Bartolome R, 1995). Genetic abnormalities in AAT were thought to be almost exclusively limited to Caucasians, but a recent epidemiological study casts doubt on this assumption (de Serres FJ, 2002).

AAT deficiency is associated with the development of emphysema as well as bronchiectasis, a non-COPD condition in which the bronchi are distorted or stretched and their lining is damaged. Although AAT-deficient people with clinically defined COPD usually are younger than the typical COPD patient, their disease differs from that induced by smoking only in that it results from an inherited, rather than acquired, defect. Not surprisingly, smoking significantly exacerbates and accelerates pulmonary disease in AAT-deficient patients: The median age of dyspnea onset is 40 years in AAT-deficient smokers compared with 53 years in AAT-deficient nonsmokers (Bartolome R, 1995).

Many people with AAT deficiency do not develop COPD, or they develop the disease with varying degrees of severity, indicating that other factors are involved in the pathogenesis of this disease.

Other Potential Genetic Factors. Other heritable factors may predispose a person to COPD. Investigators have observed a clustering of the disease in families, even when data are adjusted for confounding environmental factors and smoking (DeMeo DL, 2003). In addition to AAT, the genes for alpha1-antichymotrypsin, alpha2-macroglobulin, vitamin-D-binding protein, and certain blood-group antigens have been researched as possible genetic factors. Variants of the cystic fibrosis transmembrane regulator gene have been implicated as risk factors for disseminated bronchiectasis, which, although not a COPD component, may point to the involvement of the gene in COPD as well. Although association between several genes and susceptibility to COPD has been proposed, study data are inconsistent. Eventually, genes will likely be implicated in the pathophysiology of COPD.

Airway Hyperreactivity and Allergies. A genetic or constitutional predisposition to airway hyperreactivity (AHR), also called airway hyperresponsiveness, and allergies may play a role in COPD development. Many COPD patients exhibit an increased tendency toward bronchial constriction in reaction to exogenous stimuli. AHR and allergic sensitization also are salient features of asthma. This commonality between COPD and asthma led to the "Dutch hypothesis," postulated in 1961, which proposes that asthma, chronic bronchitis, and emphysema are expressions of a single, chronic, nonspecific lung disease (Orie NGM, 1961). Noting that environmental, genetic, and other factors determine which pathological components are expressed in an individual patient, the theory states that AHR and allergic sensitization are essential risk factors in disease development. If true, the Dutch hypothesis might explain both family clustering as well as the variation in COPD susceptibility among smokers.

Several multicenter, longitudinal studies, including the Lung Health Study (LHS) sponsored by the Division of Lung Diseases of the U.S. National Heart, Lung, and Blood Institute (NHLBI), have found compelling evidence linking AHR to accelerated decline in lung function. Yet other trials suggest that increased AHR may be an effect, rather than a cause, of existing airflow obstruction in COPD patients. Although most experts agree that AHR is a component of many COPD cases, they remain divided on the validity of the Dutch hypothesis. Debate will continue until researchers identify and confirm specific genetic factors for COPD (in addition to AAT deficiency) and their interactions with smoking and environmental risk factors.

Age. COPD risk increases with age—the result of cumulative damage from decades of smoking and/or exposure to environmental toxins/pollutants coupled with the natural reduction in pulmonary function that occurs with aging. Peak COPD incidence is observed in people aged 65 or older.

Pathophysiology

The pathophysiological changes associated with COPD occur in the central airways (bronchi), the small airways (bronchioles), and the lung tissue (parenchyma). As the disease progresses, it affects the pulmonary circulation, heart, and respiratory muscles. The primary cause of all these changes is chronic inflammation. Oxidative stress and an imbalance of proteases and protease inhibitors are also thought to contribute to lung damage and subsequent airflow restriction observed in patients with COPD.

Inflammation. The inflammatory response is a protective mechanism intended to neutralize or destroy toxins, bacteria, or other body "invaders." When this response is successful and any resultant tissue damage is repaired, function is preserved. In some situations, however, these protective efforts disrupt normal tissue and contribute to tissue injury. According to the GOLD guidelines (GOLD, 2003), chronic inflammation induced by cigarette smoke or other irritants is the driving force behind the development of airway abnormalities and the progressive, largely irreversible decline in lung function in patients with COPD.

Lung inflammation caused by the inhalation of cigarette smoke leads to the destruction or remodeling of lung tissue and consequent airflow limitation. The degree of inflammation and the cellular involvement differ with disease severity. In general, the lungs of COPD patients have increased numbers of neutrophils, macrophages, and T lymphocytes (also termed T cells). Cigarette smoke causes alveolar macrophages to release soluble mediators (e.g., tumor necrosis factor-alpha [TNF-α], interleukin-8 [IL-8], leukotriene B4 [LTB4]) that promote neutrophil inflammation. Airway and alveolar epithelial cells may also play a role in recruiting neutrophils in response to noxious agents by secreting proinflammatory mediators and increasing the expression of adhesion molecules, thereby facilitating the binding of neutrophils.

Lung neutrophils and macrophages secrete proteolytic (i.e., protein-degrading) enzymes, also known as proteases or proteinases, to aid in their digestion of foreign substances. Among these proteases are elastases—enzymes that break down elastin, a protein that gives lungs and other tissues their elastic quality (elastin allows tissue fibers to stretch up to 1.5 times their resting length). In addition to neutrophil elastase, neutrophils release cathepsin G, matrix metalloproteinases (MMPs), and proteinase-3. Macrophages release MMPs and cathepsins B, S, and L. These proteases damage lung tissue and induce mucus hypersecretion. To protect the delicate, nonregenerative architecture of the lung from injury by these proteolytic enzymes, the body releases protease inhibitors (antiproteases). The most important of these inhibitors is AAT, which neutralizes neutrophil elastase. In other words, during a normal lung inflammatory response, AAT and other protease inhibitors counteract the activity of elastase and other proteases.

After years of lung tissue degradation mediated by neutrophils and macrophages, other leukocytes involved in the inflammatory response—T cells—become prominent at the inflammation site. As COPD progresses, both macrophages and T cells increase in number, suggesting their partnership in promoting lung damage. T cells also may recruit even more neutrophils as well as eosinophils (another white blood cell) to the inflamed area. Thus, it appears that the various inflammatory cells work together to produce airway abnormalities, lung destruction, and, eventually, COPD.

Frequent or prolonged lung inflammation can cause enlargement of the mucous glands, dilation of gland ducts, increased numbers of mucus-secreting goblet cells, growth of bronchial smooth muscles, and fibrosis of airway walls. The resultant bronchial remodeling may lead to the formation of airway lesions. By obstructing airflow and increasing mucus production, these lesions contribute both to the chronic productive cough that typifies COPD and, possibly, to AHR.

A recent study provides new information on the role of small airways in the progression and severity of COPD (Hogg JC, 2004). In this study, the investigators surgically resected lung tissue from 159 patients at various stages of severity of COPD with a goal of quantifying the histological changes in small airways at the various COPD stages and relating the changes to impairment in FEV_1. The researchers report that COPD progression was strongly associated with an increase in the volume of tissue in the wall and the accumulation of inflammatory mucous exudates in the lumen of the small airways. Additionally, increases in the percentage of airways that contained various inflammatory cells (e.g., neutrophils, macrophages, lymphocytes) and, in some cases, the volume of the cells themselves were seen with COPD progression. Airway wall infiltration occurred via immune cells that form lymphoid follicles, a phenomenon that accompanies the remodeling process previously reported in wall thickening.

In a related editorial, P.J. Barnes notes that the presence of lymphoid follicles composed of B lymphocytes and T lymphocytes suggests an acquired immune response, possibly to chronic exposure to bacteria seen in COPD, in patients with the most severe disease (Barnes PJ, 2004); thus, Barnes postulates that immunosuppressants or novel anti-inflammatory therapies that target both small airways and lung parenchyma may be helpful in treating COPD. COPD patients appear to have an amplified inflammatory response to airway irritants, possibly due to gene polymorphisms that may be elucidated by further investigation, and persistent inflammatory response (at least in severe COPD patients) despite cessation of smoking.

Protease-Antiprotease Imbalance. One prevailing theory of the pathogenesis of COPD patients with emphysema is that the protease-antiprotease balance shifts in favor of proteolysis (i.e., protein breakdown), resulting in unchecked protease activity that degrades the elastin and collagen in the alveolar walls. This tissue breakdown causes air sac merging, leading to bronchiole collapse, reduced lung elasticity, airflow obstruction, and impaired expiration (Rennard SI, 2003; Shapiro SD, 1995.

The protease-antiprotease imbalance can result from one or both of the following factors:

- *Increased proteolytic activity.* Smoking disrupts both protease and antiprotease activity. The inflammatory response triggered by tobacco smoke causes the migration of neutrophils and macrophages to the lungs, where they release elastases. At the same time, oxygen free radicals (oxidants) derived from both smoke and neutrophils inhibit AAT activity, allowing unimpeded elastase activity that damages the lungs.
- *Reduction or inactivation of protease inhibitors.* The best example is inherited AAT deficiency, characterized by the reduced ability to inhibit neutrophil elastase. When the protease inhibitor component of the protease-antiprotease

balance falls below protective levels, unchecked alveolar break down and parenchymal destruction can occur.

Oxidative Stress. Oxidative stress causes the production of biological markers (e.g., hydrogen peroxide, nitric oxide [NO], isoprostane F2α III [prostaglandin isomer]) that are detectable in the breath and urine of patients with COPD. Oxidative stress may trigger lung damage by inducing inflammation, damaging various cellular or extracellular matrix molecules, inactivating antiproteases, and constricting airways. Increasing evidence suggests that oxidative stress is an important contributor to the pathogenesis of COPD (Barnes PJ, 2000; GOLD, 2003).

Direct Airway Damage. In addition to eliciting an inflammatory response, cigarette smoking directly damages airways. Smoke disables cilia, the waves of tiny hairs that line the respiratory tract and normally push mucus-trapped microorganisms, other cells, and debris toward the nose and throat, allowing the debris to be eliminated by coughing or sneezing. Without effective mucociliary clearance, thick plugs of lung secretions accumulate in the bronchioles and bronchi, intensifying inflammation and increasing the risk of bacterial and viral infection. Infection causes additional inflammation, part of a vicious cycle leading to further neutrophil recruitment and elastase release into the airways.

COPD Progression. Inefficient respiration associated with advanced COPD places enormous stress on the respiratory and circulatory systems. Patients are more susceptible to pneumonia and other respiratory infections, leading to acute COPD exacerbations that are further disabling. The pathophysiology of exacerbations is not fully understood. What is known is that in more severe exacerbations, the primary physiological change revolves around a cyclical process that starts with a worsening of gas exchange (i.e., ventilation-perfusion mismatching, where there is an imbalance in ventilation and pulmonary blood flow), causing increases in the demand on respiratory muscles and oxygen consumption (Barbera JA, 1997). Worsening gas exchange may be caused by airway inflammation and edema, mucus hypersecretion, and bronchoconstriction, which may contribute to changes in the distribution of ventilation; hypoxemia (low blood oxygen), a result of damaged air sacs in the lung, can modify perfusion. Hypercarbia or hypercapnia—when carbon dioxide in the blood is high—may also occur.

Other complications associated with severe COPD include cor pulmonale (enlargement and strain or failure of the right side of the heart due to increased blood flow resistance through damaged lungs), heart arrhythmias, and pulmonary embolism (a potentially life-threatening blockage of the pulmonary artery by a blood clot that has traveled to the lungs). Roughly 30–40% of COPD patients experience acute respiratory insufficiency; 10% suffer from acute respiratory failure.

CURRENT THERAPIES

Apart from smoking cessation, no treatment options affect the rate of decline in lung function and the inexorable disease progression seen with chronic obstructive pulmonary disease (COPD). Consequently, pharmacological and nonpharmacological treatment strategies for stable and occasional mild exacerbations of COPD focus on improving symptoms, pulmonary function, performance in the activities of daily living, and quality of life (QOL), as well as preventing acute exacerbations. (Acute exacerbations of chronic bronchitis [AECB] are treated with antibiotics and are not discussed here.) Increasingly, physicians recognize the need for a multifaceted approach to COPD management that incorporates the concurrent use of both drug and nondrug therapies. Table 2 summarizes the leading pharmacological therapies available to treat COPD.

Short-Acting Beta$_2$ Agonists

Overview. Short-acting beta$_2$ agonists quickly relieve bronchospasm—usually within minutes. These drugs are most appropriate as rescue agents in patients with acute symptoms, although the short-acting agents are also used alone or in combination with an anticholinergic (discussed in detail in the "Anticholinergic/Beta$_2$ Agonist Combination Products" section) for chronic therapy. In addition to the frequently prescribed short-acting beta$_2$ agonists described in detail in this section, several other short-acting agents are prescribed in some of the major pharmaceutical markets to treat COPD: levalbuterol (Sepracor, Inc.'s [Marlborough, Massachusetts] Xopenex, and now Xopenex HFA, a metered-dose inhaler [MDI] formulation that contains nonchlorofluorocarbon [non-CFC] propellants), clenbuterol (Teijin Pharma's [Tokyo, Japan] Spiropent), procaterol (Otsuka's [Tokyo, Japan] Pro-air), tulobuteral (Abbott Japan's Hokunalin), oral and inhaled formulations of terbutaline (AstraZeneca's [Wilmington, Delaware] Bricanyl, Novartis's [Basel, Switzerland] Brethine/Brethaire), and the inhaled and nebulizer formulations of fenoterol (Boehringer Ingelheim's [Ingelheim, Germany] Berotec). The discussion here is limited to short-acting beta$_2$ agonists to albuterol/salbuterol/salbutamol because the use of this drug predominates in COPD.

Concerns that the regular use of short-acting beta$_2$ agonists, particularly at high doses, might increase underlying COPD morbidity and mortality led to U.S. and international management guidelines recommending that these agents be used to relieve intermittent or worsening symptoms (as opposed to persistent symptoms). For continuous bronchodilation, long-acting beta$_2$ agonists are preferred to short-acting agents.

Mechanism of Action. Epinephrine and norepinephrine, neurotransmitters released by the sympathetic nervous system, increase heart rate and dilate airways as well as blood vessels by stimulating two types of beta-adrenergic receptors: beta$_1$ receptors, found in the heart, and beta$_2$ receptors, found mainly in the lungs, blood vessels, and other tissues. Beta$_2$ agonists selectively activate beta$_2$

TABLE 2. Current Therapies Used for Chronic Obstructive Pulmonary Disease

Agent	Company/Brand	Dose	Availability
Bronchodilators			
Short-acting beta$_2$ agonists			
Albuterol/ salbutamol	GlaxoSmithKline's Ventolin/Ventoline/Sultanol, Schering-Plough's Proventil, generics	1–2 puffs (100–200 μg total) as needed for acute symptom relief; 1–2 puffs tid or qid for maintenance therapy	US, F, G, I, S, UK, J
Long-acting beta$_2$ agonists			
Salmeterol	GlaxoSmithKline's Serevent/ Aeromax	1 puff (50 μg total) bid	US, F, G, I, S, UK
Formoterol	Yamanouchi/Novartis's Foradil, AstraZeneca's Oxis Turbuhaler; Yamanouchi/Aventis's Atock	1 puff (12 μg total) bid	US, F, G, I, S, UK
Anticholinergics			
Ipratropium bromide	Boehringer Ingelheim/Teijin's Atrovent, generics	1–2 puffs (18–36 μg total) qid	US, F, G, I, S, UK, J
Tiotropium	Boehringer Ingelheim/Pfizer's Spiriva	18 mcg qd	US, G, I, S, UK, J
Beta$_2$ agonist/anticholinergic combination products			
Ipratropium/ albuterol	Boehringer Ingelheim's Combivent, Merck KGaA/Dey's Duoneb, Valeas's Breva	2 puffs (18 μg ipratropium + 100 μg albuterol total) tid	US, F, I, S, UK
Ipratropium/ fenoterol	Boehringer Ingelheim's Duovent/Berodual/ Bronchodual	1–2 puffs (50–100 μg fenoterol + 21–42 μg ipratropium total) tid	F, G, I, S
Inhaled corticosteroids			
Fluticasone propionate	GlaxoSmithKline's Flovent/Flixotide/Atemur/ Flutide	2 puffs (440 μg total) bid	US, F, G, I, S, UK, J
Budesonide	AstraZeneca's Pulmicort/ Pulmaxan, Novartis's Miflonide	2–4 puffs (200–800 μg total) bid	US, F, G, I, S, UK
Triamcinolone acetonide	Aventis's Azmacort, Wyeth's Delphicort, Bristol-Myers Squibb's Volon	2 puffs (200 mcg total) bid or tid; or 4 puffs (400 μg total) bid	US
Corticosteroid/beta$_2$ agonist combination products			
Fluticasone/ salmeterol	GlaxoSmithKline's Seretide/Advair/Advair Diskus/Atmadisc/Viani	1 puff (100, 250, or 500 μg fluticasone + 50 μg salmeterol total) bid	US, F, G, I, S, UK

(continued overleaf)

TABLE 2. (*continued*)

Agent	Company/Brand	Dose	Availability
Budesonide/ formoterol	AstraZeneca's Symbicort	1–2 puffs (4.5 µg formoterol + 160 µg budesonide total) bid	F, G, I, UK
Methylxanthines			
Theophylline	Various manufacturers and generics	(300 mg bid po) 6–20 mg/kg (serum levels should be maintained in the range of 10–15 µg/mL)	US, F, G, I, S, UK, J
Mucolytic agents			
N-acetylcysteine	Various manufacturers and generics	3–5 mL of 20% solution or 6–10 mL of 10% solution (100–200 mg/mL) via nebulizer tid or qid	US, F, G, I, S, J
Alpha1-antitrypsin (AAT) augmentation			
Partially purified human AAT	Bayer's Prolastin	60 mg/kg per week, IV	US, G, I, S

bid = Twice daily; po = Administered orally; IV = Administered intravenously; qd = Once daily; qid = Four times daily; sid = Six times daily; tid = Three times daily.
US = United States; F = France; G = Germany; I = Italy; S = Spain; UK = United Kingdom; J = Japan.

receptors, resulting in relaxation of the bronchial smooth muscles and reduced mucus secretion.

At the molecular level, $beta_2$ agonists bind to active $beta_2$ receptors (i.e., receptors associated with active G proteins). These G proteins initiate an intracellular signal transduction cascade (involving activation of adenylyl cyclase and the subsequent generation of cyclic adenine monophosphate [cAMP]) that results in reduced free intracellular calcium, which induces smooth-muscle relaxation and improves breathing in COPD patients (Johnson M, 1998). Several other effects of $beta_2$ agonists have been observed experimentally: blockade of mast-cell release of leukotrienes and histamine in the lungs; microvascular permeability and mucus production declines; mucociliary function increase; and possibly inhibition of the activity of phospholipase A_2, a key enzyme in the proinflammatory arachidonic acid pathway.

Formulation. Short-acting $beta_2$ agonists come in a variety of formulations (inhalers, tablets, capsules, syrups, patches, and respirator solutions), but metered-dose inhalers (MDIs) and dry-powder inhalers (DPIs) are the formulations most commonly used to treat respiratory disorders, including COPD.

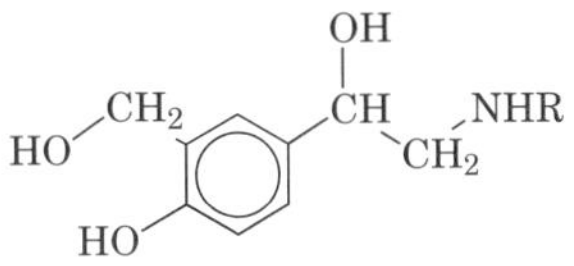

FIGURE 3. *Structure of albuterol (R = C(CH3)3).*

Albuterol. Albuterol (GlaxoSmithKline's [Brentford, Middlesex, United Kingdom] Ventolin/Ventoline/Sultano; Schering-Plough's [Kenilworth, New Jersey] Proventil/Repetabs; generics) (Figure 3) has been available in nearly all major markets for COPD and asthma management for more than two decades. In the United States, the agent is known as albuterol/salbuterol; elsewhere, it is known as salbutamol.

Like other short-acting $beta_2$ agonists, albuterol activates adenylyl cyclase and cAMP, resulting in bronchodilation. Albuterol interacts with the extracellular active site of the $beta_2$ receptor, enabling direct and rapid receptor activation (Johnson M, 1983). However, the interaction is short-lived and the receptor returns to an inactive, unbound state within four to six hours. This time frame reflects the short-acting bronchodilatory effects of albuterol.

Many studies have examined the efficacy of albuterol in relieving symptoms of COPD. In a double-blind, dose-ranging study involving 30 patients with COPD, inhaled albuterol improved airflow over a range of doses (Vathenen AS, 1988). Each patient randomly received each treatment (placebo or albuterol [0.4, 1, 2, or 4 mg]) once via inhaler over the course of five single-dose study periods. The 1 mg dose provided good efficacy, including increased forced expiratory volume (FEV) measurements. Higher doses were associated with lower blood oxygenation levels and increased side effects, such as headache, tremor, and increased heart rate.

A meta-analysis of 13 controlled trials involving the administration of inhaled short-acting $beta_2$ agonists (including 7 trials utilizing albuterol) in COPD patients echoes the results of the Vathenen trial (Ram FS, 2003). The meta-analysis examined controlled trials that utilized inhaled $beta_2$ agonists for a treatment period ranging from one to eight weeks (six trials employed 200 µg of inhaled albuterol administered four times daily; one trial involved doses of 5 mg of inhaled albuterol administered four times daily). The authors determined that treatment with short-acting $beta_2$ agonists for at least seven days was effective and associated with improved lung function. The efficacy of different doses was not addressed. The weighted mean difference in FEV_1 scores among $beta_2$ agonist-treated patients was 14% higher than among placebo-treated patients. Patients receiving placebo were more likely to discontinue treatment as a result of adverse events than were those who received a $beta_2$ agonist (relative risk [RR] = 0.49, 95% confidence interval = 0.33 to 0.73; a RR value of zero indicates no risk).

According to the drug monograph, side effects of treatment with $beta_2$ agonists that occur in more than 1% of treated adult patients include nervousness (20%), headache (7%), tachycardia (5%), heart palpitations (5%), muscle cramps (3%), and nausea (2%). Contraindications for the use of beta$_2$ agonists include current or recently terminated treatment with monoamine oxidase inhibitors (MAOIs) or tricyclic antidepressants (TCAs) because cardiovascular side effects may be amplified. Both oral and inhaled beta$_2$ agonists can provoke cardiac arrhythmias and tachycardia by stimulating beta$_2$ receptors in the heart; produce systemic vasodilation and hypotension by stimulating beta$_2$ receptors in blood vessels throughout the body; cause tremor and anxiety; and trigger life-threatening paradoxical bronchospasm. Side effects are more likely with oral formulations because these agents are taken in larger doses and have systemic rather than local activity. Although serious complications are rare at the usual inhaled dosages, the chance of cardiac side effects necessitates careful dosing in patients with probable or established heart disease.

Long-Acting Beta$_2$ Agonists

Overview. Long-acting beta$_2$ agonists provide 10–12 hours of bronchodilation, thus permitting twice-daily dosing. Their convenience improves compliance compared with the four-times-daily schedule required with albuterol and other short-acting agents. Although they are not appropriate for acute symptomatic relief, long-acting drugs may reduce the need for rescue therapy with short-acting beta$_2$ agonists. In addition to salmeterol (GlaxoSmithKline's Serevent/Aeromax) and formoterol (Yamanouchi [Tokyo, Japan]/Novartis's Foradil, AstraZeneca's Oxis Turbuhaler, Yamanouchi/Aventis Pharmaceuticals Inc.'s [Bridgewater, New Jersey] Atock), bambuterol (AstraZeneca's Bambec) is used to treat COPD though much less frequently. Because of its infrequent use in this indication, bambuterol is not discussed in detail here.

Mechanism of Action. The mechanism of action of long-acting beta$_2$ agonists is similar to that of short-acting beta$_2$ agonists. Briefly, beta$_2$ agonists bind to active beta$_2$ receptors (i.e., receptors associated with active G proteins). These G proteins initiate an intracellular signal transduction cascade (involving activation of adenylyl cyclase and the subsequent generation of cAMP that results in reduced free intracellular calcium, which induces smooth-muscle relaxation and improves breathing in COPD patients (Johnson M, 1998). However, long-acting beta$_2$ agonists are typically more lipophilic (i.e., fat-soluble) than short-acting beta$_2$ agonists (Johnson M, 1998). This difference in biochemical properties results in the deposition of long-acting beta$_2$ agonists in cellular membranes, which provides sustained delivery of the drug to the beta$_2$ adrenergic receptor. This lipophilicity also is believed to prolong the interaction of these agents with the beta$_2$ adrenergic receptor (Lewell XQ, 1992). Together, these actions result in prolonged bronchodilation relative to short-acting beta$_2$ agonists.

Formulation. Similar to short-acting beta$_2$ agonists, long-acting beta$_2$ agonists are available as inhalers, tablets, capsules, syrups, patches, and respirator (nebulizer) solutions. The MDI and DPI formulations are most commonly prescribed for the management of COPD and other respiratory disorders.

Salmeterol. Salmeterol xinafoate (GlaxoSmithKline's Serevent/Aeromax) is indicated for the treatment of asthma, exercise-induced bronchospasm, and COPD in all the major markets. Its mechanism of action is consistent with that of other $beta_2$ agonists, although it is approximately 50 times more selective for $beta_2$ adrenoreceptors than the short-acting $beta_2$ agonist albuterol/salbuterol/salbutamol. Researchers hypothesize that salmeterol interacts with the $beta_2$ adrenergic receptor at two sites (Johnson M, 1998). One receptor-binding site is located within the cellular membrane (hydrophobic) and the other binding site is located on the extracellular surface (hydrophilic). The hydrophilic site is identical to the binding site for albuterol, and consequently, the hydrophobic site is likely responsible for salmeterol's longer action.

Clinical trial results submitted during the U.S. approval process for COPD showed that salmeterol improved FEV_1 similar to the anticholinergic ipratropium but offered a more convenient twice-daily dosing schedule. Significant gains in FEV_1 occurred within 30 minutes of inhalation and peaked at 4 hours, with the therapeutic effect sustained over the next 12 hours (Mahler DA, 1999).

The regular use of salmeterol (50 µg bid) has been shown to significantly enhance peak expiratory flow rates, reduce the need for rescue bronchodilators, and improve symptom scores in patients with moderate-to-severe COPD (Ulrick CS, 1995). Salmeterol has also been found to reduce exacerbations and improve QOL, with no evidence that regular use leads to the tachyphylaxis (progressive decline in response) that can be seen with short-acting agents.

A 12-week, placebo-controlled trial compared the efficacy of salmeterol (42 µg bid), ipratropium (36 µg qid), and placebo (bid or qid) in 405 COPD patients (Rennard SI, 2001). Approximately 130 patients were randomized to each of the three treatment arms and patient characteristics were comparable across groups. Both agents improved baseline FEV_1 values by approximately 20%, whereas placebo did not affect this measure ($p = 0.001$). Patient QOL was measured using the Chronic Respiratory Disease Questionnaire (CRDQ). Baseline scores in all groups were similar, and a change of ten points or greater was considered clinically significant. A proportion of patients in all treatment arms achieved a ten-point increase in CRDQ scores (placebo, 38%; salmeterol, 46%; and ipratropium, 41%). Although these differences in CRDQ scores were not statistically significant, the difference between the salmeterol-treated group relative to the placebo-treated group approached significance ($p = 0.078$).

A separate trial involving 411 COPD patients was conducted under conditions similar to those in the aforementioned Rennard trial (Mahler DA, 1999) and yielded comparable results. Salmeterol and ipratropium improved FEV_1 values relative to placebo over the course of the trial, but in this trial, salmeterol was significantly superior to placebo ($p < 0.001$) at weeks 0, 4, 8, and 12; salmeterol was also superior to ipratropium ($p < 0.005$) at weeks 4 and 8. In this study, 46% of salmeterol-treated patients ($p = 0.002$) and 39% of ipratropium-treated patients ($p = 0.041$) achieved a ten-point increase in CRDQ scores. Both achievements are significant when compared with the 27% of placebo-treated patients who achieved the same level of improvement.

In a double-blind, placebo-controlled trial involving 144 subjects with stable COPD, salmeterol and ipratropium have been shown to have an additive benefit, eliciting improvements in FEV_1 and the rate of acute exacerbations during treatment (van Noord JA, 2000[a]). Subjects were randomized after a run-in period of 2 weeks to receive either salmeterol 50 µg twice daily, salmeterol 5 µg twice daily plus ipratropium 40 µg four times daily, or placebo for a period of 12 weeks. Salmeterol significantly increased FEV_1 (peak of 7% predicted), and the combination of salmeterol plus ipratropium elicited a greater bronchodilator response than salmeterol alone during the first six hours post-inhalation. During treatment, there were significant improvements in daytime symptom scores and morning peak expiratory flow in both the salmeterol and the salmeterol/ipratropium groups ($p < 0.001$), with an associated reduction in the use of rescue albuterol. The study's authors report that although there was added benefit from the combination therapy in improvement in airway obstruction, there was no improvement in symptom control or need for rescue medication with a short-acting $beta_2$ agonist.

A recent investigation of the functional impact of adding salmeterol and tiotropium in COPD patients found that although the combination is more efficacious than the single agents alone, salmeterol's broncholytic activity precludes its once-daily administration (Cazzola M, 2004[a]). This 20-patient pilot study tested the effects of single doses of tiotropium (18 µg), salmeterol (50 µg), and their combination on FEV_1. At 24 hours post-inhalation, the mean FEV_1 value was higher than the mean predosing value for tiotropium alone and the tiotropium/salmeterol combination but not for salmeterol alone, leaving the authors to conclude that a once-daily combination of salmeterol plus tiotropium is "inadvisable."

According to the drug monograph, side effects of salmeterol include tremor, nervousness, and heart palpitations in 1–3% of treated patients; these three side effects exhibited some dose-dependent correlation. Other side effects that occurred in 1–3% of treated patients include rhinitis, nausea, rash, urticaria, and musculoskeletal pain.

Salmeterol has been plagued by recent controversial news reports that FDA Associate Science Director David Graham has grouped it, with four other non-COPD drugs, as having the potential for higher rates of problematic side effects than were seen in clinical trials. GlaxoSmithKline vigorously contests this claim; the company asserts that the drug is safe and effective when used appropriately and in accordance with labeling and treatment guidelines (GlaxoSmithKline, press release, November 18, 2004). The company adds that mortality considerations prompted the placement of a black box warning on salmeterol's U.S. labeling but did not preclude the drug from approval and launch in the United States.

Formoterol. Formoterol (Yamanouchi/Novartis's Foradil, AstraZeneca's Oxis Turbuhaler, Yamanouchi/Aventis's Atock) (Figure 4) is available for the treatment of COPD in the United States and Europe, but not in Japan. It is also available for asthma and exercise-induced bronchospasm in patients older than six years of age.

Although formoterol induces bronchodilation via activation of the same signal transduction pathway that is activated by other $beta_2$ agonists, this agent activates

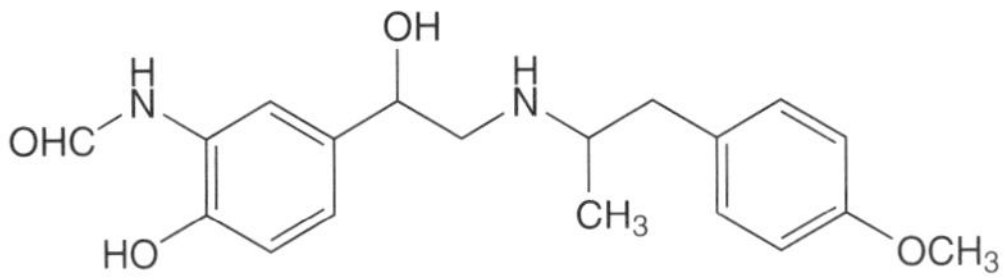

FIGURE 4. *Structure of formoterol.*

the receptor by a slightly different mechanism than that of salmeterol. Formoterol is less lipophilic than salmeterol. Because of this difference, formoterol initially accumulates in the cellular membrane and then diffuses into the extracellular space and interacts with the $beta_2$ adrenergic receptor only at the extracellular active site, activating this receptor (Johnson M, 1998). Formoterol displays an onset of action similar to that of albuterol, but its effects are longer lasting, given its deposition in the cellular membrane.

Numerous studies confirm the utility of formoterol in the management of COPD. Use of this product is associated with improved spirometry measurements (FEV_1 values); reduced cough, sputum production, and dyspnea; and improvement in QOL scores using the St. George's Respiratory Questionnaire (SGRQ) (reviewed in Friedman M, 2002). The drug has proven helpful even in some patients with a poor initial response to it (i.e., patients whose airway obstruction appears partially or poorly reversible upon initial testing), challenging the validity of bronchodilator-reversibility testing for COPD (Muir JF, 2004). (Bronchodilator-reversibility testing is a controversial means of gauging whether a patient is likely to respond to a standard dose of a bronchodilator.)

In placebo-controlled trials that pit formoterol against other active agents, this long-acting $beta_2$ agonist has been found to offer at least comparable efficacy to the anticholinergic agent ipratropium bromide and superior efficacy to the methylxanthine theophylline (Dahl R, 2001; Wadbo M, 2002[b]; Rossi A, 2002). (Ipratropium and theophylline are described in subsequent sections.)

In a study regarding the effects of 12 weeks of treatment with formoterol, ipratropium, or placebo on walking distance, lung function, symptoms, and QOL in 183 patients with moderate-to-severe nonreversible COPD, improvements in the shuttle walking test (SWT) were seen in 41%, 38%, and 20% of patients receiving formoterol (18 µg twice daily), ipratropium (80 µg three times daily), and placebo, respectively (Wadbo M, 2002[b]). (The SWT has been proposed as a more valid alternative to the conventional six-minute walking test [6MWT] as an assessment of exercise tolerance in COPD.) Both formoterol and ipratropium improved FEV_1, forced vital capacity (FVC), peak expiratory flow, and daytime dyspnea but not QOL, compared with placebo.

The aforementioned Dahl study was a 12-week, multicenter, double-blind, parallel group investigation of the comparative efficacy of inhaled formoterol (12 or 24 µg twice daily) or inhaled ipratropium bromide (40 µg four times daily) versus placebo in 780 COPD subjects. Subjects taking formoterol enjoyed improvements in FEV_1 values, symptoms, and QOL scores (Dahl R, 2001). Inhaled albuterol (100 µg/puff) was provided as rescue therapy. Subjects began the trial following a 10- to 21-day acclimation period. Subjects were excluded from the trial if they were taking corticosteroids, long-acting beta$_2$ agonists, theophylline, or anticholinergic agents; if they had recently changed treatment regimens; if they experienced lung infections within one month of trial initiation; or if they suffered from asthma. The primary end point was FEV$_1$ values; secondary end points included symptom improvement and QOL scores. Doses of 12 and 24 µg of formoterol improved FEV$_1$ values by 22.3% and 19.4%, respectively; both values were significantly better than placebo ($p = 0.001$). Formoterol treatment resulted in FEV$_1$ values that were 8.6% and 5.7% (at the 12 and 24 µg doses, respectively) greater than that observed with ipratropium ($p < 0.025$). Formoterol also significantly improved symptoms ($p \leq 0.007$) and QOL scores ($p < 0.01$) relative to placebo. Ipratropium use was not associated with improvements in symptoms or QOL scores relative to placebo.

A total of 82 patients discontinued the trial; 40 discontinuations were due to adverse events (Dahl R, 2001). Side effects occurred at similar rates in all treatment groups and most frequently included headache, tremor, and COPD exacerbation. The discontinuation rate was lowest among patients who received the 12 µg bid dose of formoterol.

Another trial examined the safety, efficacy, and tolerability of inhaled formoterol (12 or 24 µg twice daily) relative to placebo and to theophylline over 12 months (Rossi A, 2002). A total of 854 COPD patients were randomized to receive one of these four treatment regimens (approximately 200 patients per treatment group). Patients randomized to the theophylline treatment arm were treated in an open-label fashion because careful dose titration is required. Similar to the trial conducted by Dahl and colleagues, this trial demonstrated overall superior efficacy of both doses of formoterol relative to placebo at 3 and 12 months as measured by standardized area under the curve (AUC)-FEV$_1$ scores. Formoterol doses of 12 and 24 µg resulted in FEV$_1$ scores that were approximately 20% higher than those in the placebo-treated group ($p < 0.001$). Using AUC-FEV$_1$ scores as an indicator, both doses of formoterol also demonstrated efficacy superior to that of theophylline (although theophylline was also superior to placebo). However, the greatest efficacy (as measured by AUC-FEV$_1$) was observed with the lower dose of formoterol at 3 months (8.5% superior, $p = 0.005$) and 12 months (7.7% superior, $p \leq 0.026$).

Approximately two thirds of patients in each treatment arm experienced side effects, nearly half of which were considered mild (Rossi A, 2002). Adverse events occurred at similar frequencies, with the exception of nausea and vomiting, which were more common among theophylline-treated patients. Discontinuation rates were highest among theophylline-treated patients. Overall, formoterol provided safety and efficacy superior to that of placebo and theophylline.

Anticholinergics

Overview. The American Thoracic Society (ATS) views anticholinergics as first-line drugs for COPD patients needing continuous bronchodilation; guidelines established by the Global Initiative for Chronic Obstructive Lung Disease (GOLD) support this positioning (GOLD, 2005). This section provides detailed discussion of ipratropium bromide (Boehringer Ingelheim/Teijin's Atrovent, generics) and tiotropium (Boehringer Ingelheim/Pfizer's [New York, New York] Spiriva), a newcomer to the marketplace. Tiotropium launched in several European markets in 2002 and in the United States as the HandiHaler DPI formulation in 2004. Its safety, efficacy, and convenience position it to become the leading anticholinergic and, hence, the leading product indicated for COPD in the major markets. Oxitropium bromide (Boehringer Ingelheim's Oxivent/Ventilat/Tersigan, 3 M's [St. Paul, Minnesota] Tersigat, UCB, Inc. [Smyrna, Georgia] Pulsigan) has traditionally been used much less commonly than other anticholinergics because of the strong position of ipratropium and, more recently, the rapid physician uptake of tiotropium. Boehringer discontinued the product in May 2004 to avoid reformulating it to comply with CFC-banning requirements (Monthly News Review, October 13, 2003).

Mechanism of Action. Anticholinergic drugs block the effects of acetylcholine, a parasympathetic nervous system neurotransmitter that promotes bronchoconstriction. Acetylcholine, released from branches of the vagus nerve that run along the airways, binds to the M_1 and M_3 muscarinic receptors located in the smooth muscle and submucosal glands in the airways. Acetylcholine binding activates the receptors, stimulating both the contraction of smooth muscle via activation of the M_1 receptor (leading to bronchoconstriction) and the secretion of mucus from the submucosal glands via activation of the M_3 receptor. By binding to the M_1 and M_3 muscarinic receptors, anticholinergic drugs block the access of acetylcholine, thus reducing the number of activated receptors. As a result, smooth-muscle tone in the airways declines, thereby reducing bronchoconstriction and mucus secretion. However, nonselective anticholinergic agents (i.e., ipratropium and oxitropium) also inhibit the M_2 receptor, which functions as a negative regulator of acetylcholine release; this inhibition results in increased release of acetylcholine.

Anticholinergics offer the following advantages over short-acting $beta_2$ agonists:

- Anticholinergic efficacy does not appear to wane; this lack of tachyphylaxis is important because upon diagnosis, most COPD patients require chronic bronchodilator therapy.
- Inhaled anticholinergics remain primarily in the airways; because they do not cross the blood–brain barrier, dosages can be safely doubled or tripled to improve bronchodilation without concern for side effects. In COPD trials, anticholinergics have generally been well tolerated, with the most common adverse reaction being dry mouth.

Ipratropium Bromide. Ipratropium bromide (Boehringer Ingelheim/Teijin's Atrovent, generics) (Figure 5) is indicated and widely used in COPD management

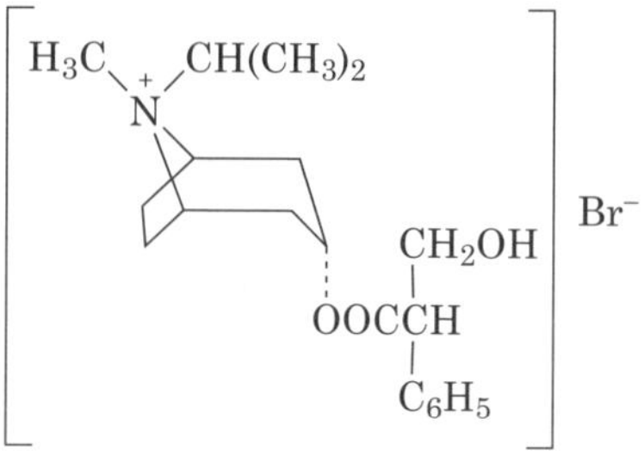

FIGURE 5. *Structure of ipratropium bromide.*

in all the major markets. Its most recent approval—in an environmentally friendly, non-chlorofluorocarbon (CFC) propellant called hydrofluoroalkane (HFA)—was approved in the United States in November 2004 for use in the maintenance treatment of bronchospasm associated with COPD. Several currently available agents are offered in MDIs that contain CFCs. The development of inhalers that contain no CFCs or hydrochlorofluorocarbons (HCFCs) is mandated through the United Nations Environment Program (UNEP) Montreal Protocol on Substances That Deplete the Ozone Layer. Phase-out of the chemicals controlled under the protocol is gradual, with HCFCs being reduced by 35% by 2004, 65% by 2010, 90% by 2015, and 99.5% by 2020, with 0.5% permitted for maintenance purposes only until 2030 (UNEP, 2000).

Ipratropium elicits bronchodilation; however, it is not selective for the M_1 and M_3 muscarinic receptors responsible for bronchoconstriction. The agent also binds to M_2 receptors, blocking the favorable bronchodilating effects of this receptor subtype.

In a 1989 study of patients with moderate-to-severe COPD, ipratropium bromide was superior to the beta$_2$ agonist, albuterol, with regard to FEV_1 and FVC at 30 minutes and at three, four, and five hours post-inhalation (Braun SR, 1989). The combination of ipratropium and albuterol provides greater bronchodilation than either drug alone (Combivent Inhalation Aerosol Study Group, 1994; Wadbo M, 2002[b]). Yet long-term studies suggest that, although effective in relieving COPD symptoms, ipratropium bromide does not modify the disease course. The multicenter, longitudinal Lung Health Study (LHS) followed nearly 6,000 smokers for five years and found that patients with moderate COPD exhibited improvements in baseline lung function after one year of ipratropium therapy, but over the subsequent four years, their FEV_1 values declined at a rate comparable to that of the placebo control group.

Side effects of ipratropium bromide include headache, dry mouth, and worsening of COPD symptoms; COPD symptoms worsen when the total daily dose of ipratropium equals or exceeds 2,000 µg. Other side effects observed with ipratropium bromide administration in more than 3% of treated patients are pain, flu-like symptoms, and pharyngitis (ipratropium drug monograph; Wadbo M, 2002[a]).

Tiotropium. Under the European Mutual Recognition Procedure, tiotropium (Boehringer Ingelheim/Pfizer's Spiriva) was approved and launched for COPD in several major European markets starting in 2002. In September 2002, although an FDA advisory panel recommended U.S. approval of tiotropium for maintenance treatment of airway constriction associated with COPD, the FDA rejected the companies' request to approve tiotropium for the relief of shortness of breath (dyspnea). In January 2004, the Spiriva HandiHaler (DPI formulation) received U.S. marketing rights for the maintenance treatment of COPD-associated bronchospasm. In October 2004, tiotropium was granted Japanese marketing approval for the treatment of COPD. The companies position the drug as the first once-daily COPD medication to provide significant and sustained improvements in lung function.

Tiotropium is roughly ten times more potent than ipratropium and has a longer duration of action. In the human lung, tiotropium binds to M_1 and M_3 receptors for extended periods but quickly disengages from M_2 receptors, thus resulting in prolonged inhibition of acetylcholine-induced airway muscle contraction. Therefore, tiotropium is considered selective for M_1 and M_3 receptors.

Single-dose and long-term studies suggest that tiotropium is fast-acting, safe, and effective for the management of COPD (Casaburi R, 2002; Littner MR, 2000; Maesen FPV, 1995). Tiotropium has been shown to offer long-term symptomatic improvement in COPD patients with and without short-term bronchodilator responses (i.e., FEV_1 improvement) (Tashkin D, 2003). This benefit has significance given that short-term bronchodilator response has been used by some physicians as a criterion for guiding the decision to prescribe long-term maintenance treatment with inhaled bronchodilators. Data from a randomized, double-blind, placebo-controlled trial also suggest that 21 days of tiotropium therapy (18 µg/day) may marginally enhance mucociliary clearance, a finding that has yet to be replicated in a large, controlled trial (Hasani A, 2004).

The long-term efficacy of tiotropium was evaluated in a one-year, randomized, placebo-controlled study involving 921 patients with COPD (Casaburi R, 2002). In addition to showing increased bronchodilation (20–25% improvement in FEV_1 values compared with 11% in placebo-treated patients), patients receiving 18 µg tiotropium once daily demonstrated reduced dyspnea, fewer exacerbations, and improved health outcomes (determined using the SGRQ and Short Form-36 [SF-36], a multi-item scale that assesses health and well-being) relative to patients receiving placebo. Patients taking tiotropium also reported using fewer "as-needed" doses of albuterol.

Multiple studies have confirmed the comparative efficacy of tiotropium over ipratropium (van Noord JA, 2000[b]; Pauwels R, 2001; Vincken W, 2002; Oostenbrink JB, 2004). The use of tiotropium or ipratropium was evaluated in two one-year, randomized, double-blind clinical trials enrolling 535 patients with COPD who were randomized into the treatment groups (Oostenbrink JB, 2004). The mean number of exacerbations per patient was reduced by 27% in the tiotropium patients compared with those treated with ipratropium. Additionally, the number of hospitalizations was reduced by 45% in the tiotropium group compared with the ipratropium-treated group. Pulmonary function measures of FEV_1 favored tiotropium: 47.6% of tiotropium-treated patients compared with 25% of ipratropium patients showed FEV_1 improvements of at least 12% over one year.

Patients were also assessed for QOL improvements using the SGRQ and the transitional dyspnea index (TDI) questionnaires. Approximately 16.6% more patients treated with tiotropium reported experiencing at least four units improvement on the SGRQ after one year compared with patients treated with ipratropium. A greater percentage of the tiotropium-treated patients experienced at least one unit of improvement on the TDI focal score over one year compared with ipratropium-treated patients—30.5% versus 16.2%, respectively.

In a one-year trial performed on behalf of the Dutch/Belgian Tiotropium Study Group, 535 patients with COPD were randomized to receive either 18 μg tiotropium once daily or 40 μg ipratropium four times daily (Vincken W, 2002). Patients receiving tiotropium had a greater increase in FEV_1 than those treated with ipratropium, an increase that was sustained over the course of the year. At the end of one year, the FEV_1 of patients in the tiotropium group (measured at 24 hours after treatment) was 120 mL above the baseline (day 1, before treatment). In contrast, patients in the ipratropium group displayed a 30 mL decline in FEV_1 (measured before the morning ipratropium dose) relative to baseline. In addition, patients receiving tiotropium experienced fewer exacerbations (35%) than those receiving ipratropium (46%). Patients in the tiotropium group reported greater improvements in dyspnea, measured by Transition Dyspnea Index (TDI), and health-related QOL, assessed by SF-36 and SGRQ.

Data from the W. Vincken study presented at the 2001 European Respiratory Society Congress in Berlin, Germany, showed that tiotropium produces greater benefits than ipratropium regardless of disease severity or the frequency of exacerbations (Pauwels R, 2001). At the end point of the 12-month study, the mean differences between tiotropium and ipratropium in changes in FEV_1 values from baseline were + 174, +128, +116, and + 59 mL for patients grouped by exacerbation frequency (0, 1, 2, >2 per year), respectively. In addition, tiotropium improved spirometry, dyspnea, and health-related QOL even in patients who did not show a predetermined, short-term response to a bronchodilator.

In addition to having better efficacy than other anticholinergics, tiotropium produces superior gains in lung function and health status compared with the long-acting beta$_2$ agonist salmeterol (Donohue JF, 2002; Brusasco V, 2003). In a six-month, randomized, multicenter, multinational trial, 623 COPD patients received 18 μg tiotropium once daily, 50 μg salmeterol twice daily, or placebo (Donohue JF, 2002). Compared with placebo treatment, the mean predose morning FEV_1 following six months of therapy increased significantly more for the tiotropium group (0.14 L) than for the salmeterol group (0.09 L; $p < 0.01$). The average 0- to 12-hour FEV_1 for tiotropium was statistically superior to that of salmeterol (difference, 0.08 L; $p < 0.001$). The increase in FEV_1 during 12 hours after the first dose of tiotropium and salmeterol was similar. By day 15 of treatment, improvements in trough FEV_1 with the drugs were seen with spirometry; at 24 weeks, trough FEV_1 had improved significantly above placebo by 137 mL in the tiotropium group and by 85 mL in the salmeterol group. The difference between tiotropium and salmeterol was also significant (52 mL, $p < 0.01$). At the end of the study, trough FVC had improved significantly over placebo—by 247 mL—in the tiotropium group ($p < 0.0001$) and by 134 mL in the salmeterol group ($p < 0.001$). Patients receiving tiotropium also demonstrated greater improvements in dyspnea and QOL (as assessed by SGRQ). Dry mouth was the most significant side effect seen with tiotropium; however, it did not affect participation in the study.

In a study of more than 1200 patients, exacerbations of COPD and health resource utilization were positively affected after six months of treatment with once-daily tiotropium but generally not with twice-daily salmeterol (the drug did have an effect on the number of hospital days associated with all causes) (Brusasco V, 2003). Tiotropium also improved health-related QOL, dyspnea, and lung function in COPD patients. These trials provide data supporting the use of tiotropium as a first-line therapy for the treatment of COPD.

Because anticholinergics and beta$_2$ agonists act on different parts of the airways, combining drugs from both classes may produce greater total bronchodilation than either agent alone. Preliminary results from a short-duration trial comparing the efficacy of tiotropium and formoterol with tiotropium alone in 95 patients (with moderate-to-severe COPD) demonstrated improved lung function with the combination (van Noord, 2003). In this open-label, randomized, crossover study, the addition of formoterol once daily to tiotropium maintenance therapy resulted in increased average FEV$_1$ and FVC spirometric measures. A double-blind, randomized pilot study explored the effects of single inhaled doses of formoterol, tiotropium, and the combination of both in 20 patients with stable COPD (Cazzola M, 2004[b]). Agents were administered on three nonconsecutive days; formoterol alone or in combination with tiotropium demonstrated a faster onset of action compared with tiotropium alone as measured by FEV$_1$. At 24 hours postdosing, FEV$_1$ measurements were significantly higher in the tiotropium and formoterol/tiotropium groups compared with formoterol alone. The findings demonstrated the different pharmacodynamic effects of formoterol (fast onset of action) and tiotropium (longer duration of action) and indicated that the two drugs can be complementary. This study was not powered for statistical significance, but initial results should lead to full-scale clinical studies.

In a retrospective analysis of one-year trials of tiotropium, the drug was associated with a reduced rate of loss of FEV$_1$ (mean decline in trough FEV$_1$ between days 8 and 344 was 58 mL/year and 12 mL/year in the placebo and tiotropium groups, respectively [$p = 0.005$]) (Anzueto A, 2005). Further long-term, prospective studies are required to confirm this observation. Boehringer Ingelheim and Pfizer initiated the Understanding Potential Long-Term Impacts on Function with Tiotropium (UPLIFT) trial—a large-scale, multiyear study of the effects of long-term treatment with tiotropium on lung function in COPD—in 2002. This study will assess the rate of lung function decline, QOL, exacerbations, hospitalizations, and mortality in up to 6000 COPD patients. The first results from UPLIFT are expected by the end of 2007.

Beta$_2$ Agonist/Anticholinergic Combination Agents

Overview. Products that use a combination of agents, such as ipratropium/albuterol (Boehringer Ingelheim's Combivent, Merck KGaA [Darmstadt, Germany]/Dey's [Napa, California] Duoneb, Valeas's [Milan, Italy] Breva) and ipratropium/fenoterol (Boehringer Ingelheim's Duovent/Berodual/Bronchodual), have become popular COPD therapies in several of the major pharmaceutical markets. Such combinations reduce the cost of therapy and allow more convenient dosing, thus improving patient compliance. They also allow for the treatment of patients with lower doses of each therapeutic agent, a characteristic that is anticipated to correlate with a reduced risk of side effects.

Mechanism of Action. Anticholinergics promote bronchodilation, primarily in the large airways, where cholinergic nerves and muscarinic receptors predominate. Beta$_2$ agonists primarily dilate the bronchioles, where the beta-adrenergic receptors abound. Because these two drug classes act on different airways, their combination should logically produce greater bronchodilation than either agent alone.

Ipratropium/Albuterol. The FDA approved the combination therapy ipratropium/albuterol (Boehringer Ingelheim's Combivent, Merck KGaA/Dey's Duoneb, Valeas's Breva) for the treatment of COPD, including chronic bronchitis and emphysema. Ipratropium/albuterol is also approved in the major European markets, except for Germany. It is specifically indicated for the treatment of bronchospasm in patients who are treated with more than one bronchodilator. This combination therapy is supplied in inhalation aerosol form.

In the Combivent Inhalation Aerosol Study Group, 1994 (CIAS), the combination of ipratropium and albuterol delivered from the same MDI produced significantly greater and longer bronchodilation in patients with stable COPD than did either agent when used individually; onset of action was as rapid as that of albuterol alone. In this 12-week, double-blind trial, 534 patients were randomized to receive the combination therapy, ipratropium alone, or albuterol alone; all agents were administered by inhalation three times daily. Patients were examined on days 1, 29, 57, and 85. Increases in FEV$_1$ values were greatest among patients who received the combination therapy (31–33%); ipratropium and albuterol alone were not as effective (24–25% and 24–27%, respectively). The combination therapy was superior to monotherapy with either agent at all examination dates (Combivent Inhalation Aerosol Study Group, 1994).

Similar results were observed in a 12-week, double-blind, randomized, controlled trial involving 833 COPD patients (Gross N, 1998). Patients in this trial received ipratropium (0.5 mg), albuterol (2.5 mg), or ipratropium/albuterol combination therapy (0.5 mg and 2.5 mg, respectively) four times daily for two weeks per regimen. Each patient continued on the final treatment regimen for the remaining six weeks of the trial. COPD patients were included in the trial if they exhibited FEV$_1$ values between 25% and 65% of expected values, were older than 40, smoked for more than ten years, required the use of a bronchodilator for three or more months prior to the initiation of the trial, and were able to walk for six minutes. Combination treatment significantly improved FEV_1 values measured within eight hours of administration relative to ipratropium (37% higher with combination, $p < 0.001$) or albuterol (24% higher with combination, $p < 0.001$) alone. Nearly half of all treated patients experienced some side effects, including pain, nausea, leg cramps, and pharyngitis, although the majority of the side effects were mild (Gross N, 1998). The rate of side effects was comparable in all treatment arms.

Ipratropium/Fenoterol. Ipratropium/fenoterol (Boehringer Ingelheim's Duovent/Berodual/Bronchodual) combines the anticholinergic agent ipratropium with the short-acting $beta_2$ agonist fenoterol. This combination therapy is indicated for the treatment of chronic bronchitis with or without asthma and for reversible bronchospasm associated with bronchial asthma.

Clinical trial data examining this combination therapy are scarce. However, because albuterol and fenoterol are $beta_2$ agonists that are somewhat similar in efficacy, the effects on lung function of ipratropium/fenoterol should rival those of ipratropium/albuterol.

Inhaled Corticosteroids

Overview. Corticosteroids (also termed *glucocorticosteroids* and *glucocorticoids*) are potent anti-inflammatory agents, typically delivered via MDI or DPI for treating respiratory disorders. In contrast to their well-established role in the treatment of asthma, inhaled corticosteroids are not approved for COPD. The GOLD guidelines recommend inhaled corticosteroids only for moderate-to-severe COPD patients with an FEV_1 less than 50% or with frequent exacerbations. Nonetheless, inhaled steroids are often used to alleviate COPD symptoms not sufficiently controlled by bronchodilators.

More than 100 studies have investigated oral and inhaled steroids in COPD. Traditionally, studies have used FEV_1 as the main outcome measure, but more recently, researchers have added exacerbation frequency and QOL as study end points. Although studies have shown a reduction in exacerbation frequency with inhaled steroid use, these agents generally fail to demonstrate significant improvements in lung function (GSK's flutcasone [Flovent/Flixotide/Atemur/Flutide], discussed next, has shown some positive effect on FEV_1, FVC, and peak expiratory flow). Approximately ten randomized, placebo-controlled, short-term studies have shown that inhaled steroids administered over a period of 3–12 weeks generally do not reduce airflow obstruction. It should be noted, however, that in several trials certain patients experienced substantial improvements in lung function, but researchers have not been able to determine which characteristics predict a responsive individual. A short challenge (i.e., up to 14 days) with oral steroids, for example, was not found to be predictive. Inhaled corticosteroids available in the major markets include fluticasone propionate

(GSK's Flovent/Flixotide/Atemur/Flutide), budesonide (AstraZeneca's Pulmicort/Pulmaxan, Novartis's Miflonide, Chiesi Pharmaceuticals's [Rockville, Maryland] Budiair), triamcinolone acetonide (Aventis's Azmacort, Wyeth's [Madison, New Jersey] Delphicort, Bristol-Myers Squibb's [North Billerica, Massachusetts] Volon), beclomethasone dipropionate (various manufacturers, generics), and flunisolide (Forest's Aerobid, Boehringer Ingelheim's Inhacort). Among these corticosteroids, fluticasone propionate, budesonide, and triamcinolone are commonly prescribed off-label for COPD.

Mechanism of Action. Corticosteroids exert their therapeutic effect by binding to glucocorticoid receptors, which are found in all cells and are abundant in the epithelium of bronchi. In this way, corticosteroids alter intracellular activities and reduce the transcription of genes that encode proteins involved in the inflammatory response (e.g., IL-1β, IL-8). By reducing the levels of these inflammation mediators, corticosteroid therapy leads to reduced levels of lymphocytes, eosinophils, macrophages, and mast cells in mucosal fluids, which are more common in asthma than in COPD. In addition, corticosteroids increase the transcription of those genes responsible for producing beta$_2$ adrenoreceptors and lipocortin 1, a protein that inhibits phospholipase A$_2$ (a proinflammatory enzyme). Corticosteroids also inhibit T-cell activation (and subsequent cytokine release), promote apoptosis of eosinophils, inhibit NO synthase, and reduce mucus secretion by submucosal gland cells; they may help restore damaged epithelium and increase the number of ciliated cells in the lungs.

Although their mechanism of action in COPD is unknown, corticosteroids likely reduce the number, activity, and chemotaxis (movement by a cell in reaction to a chemical stimulus) of inflammatory cells in the lungs and reduce airway hyperreactivity. However, neutrophils play a central role in the pathophysiology of COPD and are largely unaffected by corticosteroids.

Formulation. Corticosteroids are available in a variety of formulations: topical creams and ointments; oral tablets, capsules, and syrups; suppositories and enemas; inhalers (both MDIs and DPIs); foams; and intravenous solutions. The inhaled formulations are most commonly used for the long-term management of COPD.

Fluticasone Propionate. Fluticasone propionate (GlaxoSmithKline's Flovent/Flixotide/Atemur/Flutide) is indicated for the treatment of asthma, allergic rhinitis, dermatitis, and pruritus; its use in COPD is off-label. This corticosteroid acts via the same general mechanism of action as other corticosteroids, including alteration of intracellular activities and reducing the transcription of genes that encode proteins involved in the inflammatory response.

A multicenter study examined the effects of fluticasone propionate (500 µg twice daily) versus placebo in 281 COPD patients for six months (Paggiaro PL, 1998). By the end of the study period, patients receiving fluticasone propionate exhibited significant improvement in several lung parameters, including FEV$_1$, FVC, and peak expiratory flow. In addition, moderate or severe exacerbations, median daily cough, and sputum volume were significantly lower, and exercise capacity significantly improved in the fluticasone propionate group.

Results from the Inhaled Steroids in Obstructive Lung Disease in Europe (ISOLDE) study suggested that fluticasone propionate (500 µg bid) for three years reduced the yearly rate of disease exacerbations by 26% relative to placebo (Burge PS, 2000). More than 750 subjects were enrolled in the trial, with 376 receiving fluticasone propionate and 375 receiving placebo.

A post hoc analysis of the ISOLDE study was conducted to determine whether COPD patients with mild disease or moderate-to-severe disease are more likely to benefit from fluticasone propionate (Jones PW, 2003). Approximately half of the patients in each treatment arm suffered from mild disease (FEV_1 values $\geq$ 50% of predicted values) and the remainder suffered from moderate-to-severe disease (FEV_1 values $<$ 50% of predicted values). In this study, COPD patients with moderate-to-severe disease experienced more than 1.5 exacerbations per patient per year; patients with mild disease experienced less than 1 exacerbation per patient per year. Although fluticasone propionate reduced the incidence of exacerbations in both groups of patients, the effect was significant ($p = 0.022$) in patients with moderate-to-severe disease. These results suggest that patients with more severe disease may benefit from fluticasone propionate treatment more than patients with mild disease. However, this difference may be attributable to the higher incidence of exacerbations in more severe disease.

Fluticasone was recently investigated for its potential ability to prevent irreversible obstruction in COPD (van Grunsven, 2003). In the Detection, Intervention, and Monitoring Program of COPD and Asthma (DIMCA) study, 48 patients were randomized to receive fluticasone (250 µg twice daily) or placebo, with the therapies assessed for their effects on pre- and postbronchodilator FEV_1, PC20 histamine challenge, functional status, and occurrence of acute exacerbations. After three months, the pre- and postbronchodilator FEV_1 values had increased 174 mL and 125 mL, respectively, in the fluticasone group relative to placebo. However, the main outcome measure—postbronchodilator decline in FEV_1—was not positively affected by fluticasone use.

Budesonide. Budesonide (AstraZeneca's Pulmicort/Pulmaxan, Novartis's Miflonide) (Figure 6) is indicated for the treatment of allergic rhinitis, asthma, Crohn's disease, and ulcerative colitis. It is used off-label for COPD. This corticosteroid acts via the same general mechanism of action as other corticosteroids, including alteration of intracellular activities and reducing the transcription of genes that encode proteins involved in the inflammatory response.

The positive findings from Paggiaro's international study of fluticasone seem to point toward a role for inhaled corticosteroids in the long-term treatment of COPD (Paggiaro PL, 1998). Fluticasone-treated patients exhibited significant improvement in FEV_1, FVC, and peak expiratory flow, as well as both moderate and severe exacerbations. In addition, median daily cough and sputum volume were significantly lower, and exercise capacity was significantly improved. However, results from two subsequently published three-year studies of budesonide argue otherwise. Both the European Respiratory Society Study on Chronic Obstructive

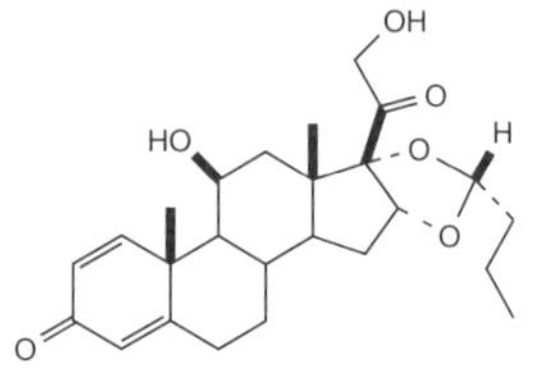

FIGURE 6. *Structure of budesonide.*

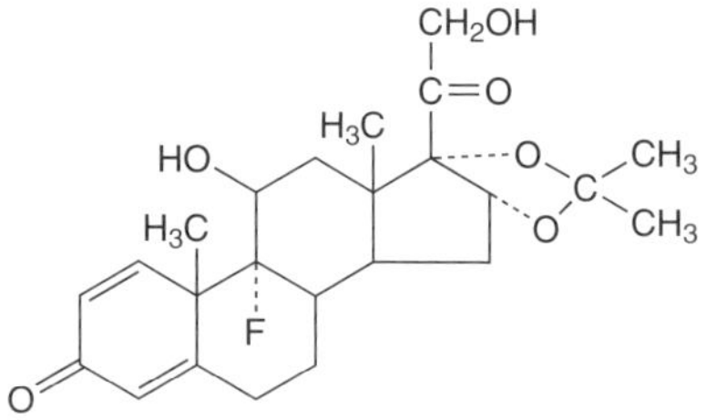

FIGURE 7. *Structure of triamcinolone acetonide.*

Pulmonary Disease (EUROSCOP) and an arm of the Copenhagen City Heart Study (CCHS) found that inhaled budesonide (800 µg daily) had no effect on the rate of FEV_1 decline in patients with mild-to-moderate COPD (Pauwels RA, 1999; Vestbo J, 1999). The findings from EUROSCOP and CCHS threatened to close the door on the use of corticosteroids in stable COPD. However, the ISOLDE results, while showing only modest improvements in FEV_1 among patients treated with fluticasone, also reinforced the drug's ability to significantly reduce the yearly rate of disease exacerbations. This latter benefit has reignited debate on the potential role of corticosteroids in COPD.

Triamcinolone Acetonide. Triamcinolone acetonide (Aventis's Azmacort, Wyeth's Delphicort, Bristol-Myers Squibb's Volon) (Figure 7) is indicated for the treatment of more than 20 indications, including immune and inflammatory diseases and disorders, musculoskeletal diseases, viral infections, and ocular diseases. It is used off-label for COPD. This corticosteroid acts via the same general mechanism of action as other corticosteroids, including alteration of intracellular activities and reducing the transcription of genes that encode proteins involved in the inflammatory response.

In December 2000, results from the Lung Health Study II (LHS II) were released (Lung Health Study Research Group, 2000). In this randomized trial, which sought to study the effects of inhaled corticosteroids on disease progression in patients with mild-to-moderate COPD, 1116 patients received either triamcinolone acetonide or placebo for a mean duration of 40 months. The researchers found that the drug did not significantly reduce the decline in FEV_1 or FVC. However, the treatment group experienced less dyspnea and fewer hospitalizations for respiratory symptoms than did patients in the placebo group. The treatment was associated with greater bone demineralization and more skin bruising compared with placebo.

Corticosteroid/Beta$_2$ Agonist Combination Products

Overview. Two corticosteroid/long-acting beta$_2$ agonist combination agents are available for COPD in most of the major markets: fluticasone/salmeterol (GlaxoSmithKline's Seretide/Advair/Advair Diskus/Atmadisc/Viani) and budesonide/formoterol (AstraZeneca's Symbicort). See the "Emerging Therapies" section for discussion of corticosteroid/beta$_2$ agonist combination agents in development for COPD. GlaxoSmithKline's Advair Diskus 250/50—the Seretide Accuhaler—was approved in the United States in November 2003 for the treatment of COPD associated with chronic bronchitis; trial data on the drug in patients with emphysema-predominant COPD are lacking, however. A 2004 meta-analysis of combined, single-inhaler treatment with a corticosteroid plus long-acting beta$_2$ agonist in more than 4000 patients found that compared with placebo, combinations offer clinically meaningful differences in health-related QOL, symptoms, and exacerbations (Nannini L, 2004). Individual trials of two commonly used corticosteroid/beta$_2$ combinations (single or multiple inhalers) are discussed in subsequent sections.

Mechanism of Action. Corticosteroids exert their therapeutic effect by binding to glucocorticoid receptors, which are found in all cells and are abundant in the epithelium of bronchi. In this way, corticosteroids alter intracellular activities and reduce the transcription of genes that encode proteins involved in the inflammatory response, including the cytokines interleukin-1β and interleukin-3, -4, -5, -6, and -8; TNF-α; granulocyte-monocyte colony-stimulating factor (GM-CSF); and regulated on activation normal T-cell expressed and secreted (RANTES). By lowering the levels of these inflammation mediators, corticosteroid therapy reduces levels of lymphocytes, eosinophils, macrophages, and mast cells in mucosal fluids, which are more common in asthma than in COPD. In addition, corticosteroids increase the transcription of those genes responsible for producing beta$_2$ adrenoreceptors and lipocortin 1, a protein that inhibits phospholipase A$_2$ (a proinflammatory enzyme). Corticosteroids also inhibit T-cell activation (and subsequent cytokine release), promote apoptosis of eosinophils, inhibit NO synthase, and reduce mucus secretion by submucosal gland cells, and they help restore damaged epithelium and increase the number of ciliated cells in the lungs.

Although their mechanism of action in COPD is unknown, corticosteroids likely reduce the number, activity, and chemotaxis of inflammatory cells in the lungs and ease airway hyperreactivity. However, although neutrophils play a central role in the pathophysiology of COPD, they are largely unaffected by corticosteroids.

The mechanism of action of long-acting $beta_2$ agonists is similar to that of short-acting $beta_2$ agonists. $Beta_2$ agonists bind to active $beta_2$ receptors—that is, receptors associated with active G proteins. These G proteins initiate an intracellular signal transduction cascade (involving activation of adenylyl cyclase and the subsequent generation of cAMP) that results in reduced free intracellular calcium, which induces smooth-muscle relaxation and improves breathing in COPD patients (Johnson M, 1998). However, long-acting $beta_2$ agonists are typically more lipophilic (fat-soluble) than short-acting $beta_2$ agonists (Johnson M, 1998). This difference in biochemical properties results in the deposition of long-acting $beta_2$ agonists in cellular membranes, thereby providing sustained delivery of the drug to the $beta_2$ adrenergic receptor. This lipophilicity also is believed to prolong the interaction of these agents with the $beta_2$ adrenergic receptor (Lewell XQ, 1992). Together, these actions prolong bronchodilation relative to short-acting $beta_2$ agonists.

Fluticasone/Salmeterol. GlaxoSmithKline launched its combination fluticasone/salmeterol inhaler for asthma in Europe as Seretide in 2000 and in the United States as Advair in 2001 (the Advair Inhaler and Advair Diskus products both contain salmeterol and fluticasone at varying strengths, but their different delivery mechanisms warrant different dosing—two puffs twice daily for the Advair Inhaler versus one inhalation twice daily for Advair Diskus). In November 2003, the FDA approved GlaxoSmithKline's fluticasone/salmeterol propionate combination therapy in a dose of 250 µg fluticasone/50 µg salmeterol (Advair Diskus 250/50) for COPD associated with chronic bronchitis.

A large (691-patient), placebo-controlled trial examined combined fluticasone (500 µg) and salmeterol (50 µg) delivered via the Diskus device (Mahler DA, 2002). After 24 weeks of treatment, a significantly greater increase in predose FEV_1 with the combination of agents versus salmeterol alone or placebo (156 mL, 107 mL, and -4 mL, respectively) and a significantly greater increase in two-hour postdose FEV_1 with the combination compared with fluticasone alone or placebo (261 mL, 138 mL, and 28 mL, respectively) was observed. Additionally, the combination of agents was associated with greater improvement in a measure of dyspnea (the Transition Dyspnea Index) compared with fluticasone or placebo, prompting the study's authors to conclude that the combination improves lung function and reduces the severity of dyspnea compared with individual components or placebo.

Results from a multicenter, randomized, double-blind, placebo-controlled 24-week trial involving 723 COPD patients suggest that combination therapy with salmeterol and fluticasone is superior to placebo and to either agent used alone (Hanania NA, 2003). At the trial's end point (the last on-treatment, post-baseline assessment), combination therapy significantly ($p \leq 0.012$) increased the morning predose FEV_1 (165 mL) compared with salmeterol (91 mL) and placebo (1 mL) and significantly ($p \leq 0.001$) increased the two-hour postdose FEV_1 (281 mL) compared with fluticasone (147 mL) and placebo (58 mL). Compared with placebo, fluticasone plus salmeterol combination therapy significantly improved dyspnea, QOL, and symptoms of chronic bronchitis. Adverse events were comparable across treatment groups, with the exception of oral candidiasis, which occurred most frequently in fluticasone-treated patients (either as a monotherapy or in combination with salmeterol).

In the Trial of Inhaled Steroids and Long-Acting $Beta_2$ Agonists (TRISTAN), a randomized, year-long trial of salmeterol and fluticasone in 1465 COPD patients, the combination of these two agents was found to offer better control of symptoms and lung function, without an increased risk for side effects, than with either agent alone (Calverley P, 2003). Although all active treatments improved lung function, symptoms, and health status, the combination of salmeterol (50 μg twice daily) and fluticasone (500 μg twice daily) significantly improved pretreatment FEV_1—the study's primary efficacy measure—over placebo (treatment difference 133 mL; $p < 0.0001$) and salmeterol (treatment difference 73 mL; $p < 0.0001$) or fluticasone (treatment difference 95 mL; $p < 0.0001$) separately. Investigators found a similar frequency in side effects (which were generally well tolerated) among all treatments.

A single-blind crossover randomized study of the bronchodilator effect of an inhaled combination of fluticasone/salmeterol (250 μg/50 μg) and budesonide/formoterol (400 μg/12 μg) in 16 patients with moderate-to-severe COPD found both combinations to be effective in reducing airflow obstruction (Cazzola M, 2003). The budesonide/formoterol combination returned maximum improvement in FEV_1 above baseline more quickly than did the fluticasone/salmeterol combination (120 minutes versus 300 minutes, respectively). This difference was attenuated at 720 minutes, however, when increases in FEV_1 over baseline values were equivalent.

The combination of fluticasone and salmeterol resulted in greater lung function control and symptom management compared with ipratropium/albuterol (Donohue JF, 2004), but to bolster support for the use of fluticasone/salmeterol use as maintenance therapy in COPD, GlaxoSmithKline released data from the COPD and Seretide: A Multicentre Intervention and Characterization (COSMIC) study at the 100th annual meeting of the American Thoracic Society in Orlando in May 2004 (Wouters EFM, 2004). Data from this three-month, 373-patient study showed that upon discontinuation of fluticasone/salmeterol therapy (and switch to 12 months of maintenance on salmeterol alone), COPD patients experienced an immediate and dramatic change in health status, as measured by shortness of breath within two days (scale 0–4; mean difference 0.17, $p < 0.001$), sustained reductions in FEV_1, increases in disturbed sleep nights (mean difference 6%, $p < 0.001$), and mild exacerbations (1.3 for salmeterol versus 0.6 for fluticasone/salmeterol, $p = 0.020$).

GlaxoSmithKline is conducting more studies of this combination therapy in the reduction of dyspnea, exacerbations, and hyperinflation. Inhaled corticosteroids and long-acting bronchodilators have been shown to reduce symptoms and exacerbations in COPD patients, but the Toward a Revolution in COPD Health (TORCH) study, a randomized, placebo-controlled, 6200-subject trial, is the first to assess three years of treatment with salmeterol and fluticasone, alone or in combination, on mortality in such patients. Secondary end points of the trial will assess the rate of exacerbations and health status, need for long-term oxygen therapy, and change in lung function among study subjects. Results of the study are expected in 2006.

Budesonide/Formoterol. AstraZeneca launched its combination budesonide/formoterol inhaler (Symbicort Turbuhaler) in Europe for the treatment of asthma in 2001. In February 2003, it completed the European Union Mutual Recognition Procedure for approval of the drug in patients with severe COPD (i.e., FEV_1 <50% predicted) and a history of repeated exacerbations that cannot be controlled by long-acting $beta_2$ agonists alone. The company will not file for U.S. approval of the Turbuhaler formulation. Instead, a powdered MDI is in development for asthma and COPD.

In two 12-month studies of budesonide/formoterol in patients with an FEV_1 of 50% or lower than predicted normal and a history of exacerbations, the combination significantly reduced exacerbation risk, improved lung function, and provided rapid and sustained symptom relief (Calverley PMA, 2003; Szafranski W, 2003). Compared with formoterol treatment alone, the budesonide/formoterol combination prolonged the time to first exacerbations and reduced exacerbation risk and the need for intervention with oral steroids by 30%.

In the Calverley study of 1022 COPD patients, treatment was intensified initially with the oral steroid prednisolone (30 mg/day) and inhaled formoterol Turbuhaler (9 µg twice daily) for two weeks to optimize patient health status (Calverley PMA, 2003). Then, patients were randomized to receive the combination product Symbicort (320/9 µg twice daily), budesonide alone (400 µg twice daily), formoterol alone (9 µg twice daily), or placebo. Symbicort consistently showed FEV_1 improvement throughout the duration of the trial, while FEV_1 declined with all other treatments. The combination significantly reduced exacerbation risk compared with monotherapy or placebo, prolonging the time to first exacerbation requiring medical intervention by 158, 100, and 76 days more than placebo, formoterol alone, and budesonide alone, respectively. The combination also reduced the rate of oral steroid use during exacerbations by 28%, 30%, and 45% versus budesonide, formoterol, and placebo, respectively. Improvements in health-related QOL were also superior with the combination treatment.

In a randomized, double-blind, placebo-controlled study, 812 patients were randomized to receive Symbicort (160 µg /4.5 µg twice daily), budesonide alone (200 µg twice daily), formoterol alone (4.5 µg twice daily), or placebo, after a two-week run-in period devoid of all maintenance medications save terbutaline (Szafranski W, 2003). Combined treatment was associated with a 23% and 24% reduction in the number of severe exacerbations compared with formoterol monotherapy and placebo, respectively. The combination also significantly improved FEV_1 — by 9% and 15% compared with budesonide and placebo, respectively — and symptom scores (breathlessness, cough, chest tightness, and nighttime awakenings) within the first week versus all other treatment arms (an effect maintained over 12 months versus budesonide and placebo).

Methylxanthines

Overview. Xanthine derivatives, including methylxanthine, have been used for decades as bronchodilators. Theophylline (various manufacturers and generics) is the most widely used methylxanthine, but aminophylline (GlaxoSmithKline's Phyllocontin, generics) is also used to treat COPD. The use of methylxanthines for the treatment of COPD has declined with the introduction of safer, more effective agents (e.g., $beta_2$ agonists, anticholinergics).

Mechanism of Action. Methylxanthines in general, and theophylline in particular, likely have several mechanisms of action, but which ones are responsible for the bronchodilating effect is unclear. Some researchers believe that this effect is mediated by the inhibition of phosphodiesterase (PDE) isoenzymes, particularly PDE3 and PDE4, which degrade cAMP and cyclic nucleotide metabolism (cGMP). Inhibition of these enzymes maintains intracellular levels of cAMP and cGMP. The subsequent generation of cAMP results in reduced free intracellular calcium, which in turn induces smooth-muscle relaxation and improves breathing.

Theophylline. Used to treat asthma for more than 50 years, theophylline (Figure 8) is the most frequently prescribed oral bronchodilator for chronic COPD management. It is indicated for the treatment of symptoms of airflow obstruction associated with chronic asthma and other chronic lung diseases (e.g., emphysema, chronic bronchitis). Theophylline monotherapy can be particularly useful in people who are unable to use MDIs properly. However, because of its propensity for side effects, theophylline is considered a third-line drug, added to improve airflow in patients who remain symptomatic while taking optimal doses of inhaled anticholinergics and $beta_2$ agonists.

In addition to inhibiting PDEs, theophylline displays anti-inflammatory and immunomodulating activities. It is a nonselective antagonist of adenosine receptors found on the surface of some cells, including mast cells. Theophylline prevents mast cells from releasing mediators that trigger allergic inflammatory reactions. Adenosine-receptor antagonism by theophylline increases ventilation during hypoxia and reduces respiratory muscle fatigue. Theophylline may also block the effects of inflammatory mediators such as leukotriene B4 (LTB_4), IL-8, and TNF-α and it may increase the production of the anti-inflammatory cytokine IL-10. Interestingly, theophylline apparently exerts most of its anti-inflammatory

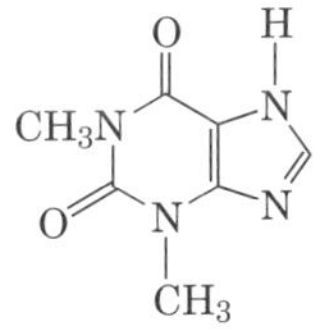

FIGURE 8. *Structure of theophylline.*

and immunomodulating effects (as opposed to its bronchodilating effects) at relatively low plasma concentrations. Yet the drug may cause notable side effects, described further in this section.

Theophylline improves FEV and exercise performance, reduces dyspnea, and, in some COPD patients, elicits a subjective feeling of improved well-being. Although most data suggest that the drug produces only minimal changes in pulmonary function, some researchers maintain that improvement correlates directly with the length of treatment. Unlike inhaled bronchodilator therapy, which achieves its full effect within a few minutes to hours of dosing, the bronchodilator action of theophylline is generally achieved after prolonged (i.e., two to six weeks) treatment. Theophylline therapy may be especially helpful in preventing nocturnal bronchospasm in COPD patients. Plus, because of its ability to reduce pulmonary vascular resistance and increase cardiac output, theophylline may improve QOL in COPD patients with concurrent cardiac disease or cor pulmonale (enlargement and strain or failure of the right side of the heart due to increased blood flow resistance through damaged lungs).

Theophylline is associated with numerous side effects: nausea, vomiting, increased ventilatory drive, and ventricular arrhythmias (all of which are presumably consequences of nonspecific PDE isoenzyme inhibition); as well as tremor, sinus tachycardia, increased gastric acid secretion, diuresis, insomnia, and anxiety (all of which are likely the result of adenosine-receptor antagonism). Theophylline also has the potential for adverse interactions with commonly used drugs such as antibiotics. Because of its narrow therapeutic index, theophylline requires careful titration via routine blood monitoring to avoid the occurrence of adverse effects. Side effects are largely avoidable if serum theophylline levels are maintained in the 10–15 µg/mL range.

Mucolytic Agents

Overview. In the early stages of COPD in smokers, airway secretions have relatively low viscosity and are easily cleared by mucociliary action. Over many years, continued airway irritation by noxious particles impairs mucociliary clearance, resulting in mucus retention and the subsequent accumulation in the airways of inflammatory cells and cellular debris that thickens mucus and further impedes clearance. Viscous mucus traps bacteria and other microbes, thus intensifying inflammation and contributing to airflow obstruction and tissue damage.

Various agents have been used for mucolysis. These agents include aerosolized mixtures of ascorbic acid, copper sulfate, and sodium percarbonate, as well as lung surfactants and several proteolytic agents (e.g., Genentech Inc. [South San Francisco, California] dornase alpha [Pulmozyme], a recombinant form of deoxyribonuclease [DNase]). These agents are often expensive and sometimes have limited availability.

Mechanism of Action. Mucolytic agents clear mucus by liquefying sputum. Although clearing secretions can be a significant problem for COPD patients, little evidence shows that thinning mucus (mucolysis) by liquefying sputum improves lung function. Furthermore, current methods of sputum volume measurement cannot distinguish the source of the collected secretion. Thus, it is impossible to determine if mucolytic agents are clearing mucus from the lower respiratory tract as intended or from the upper respiratory tract and mouth; the latter would be less effective in relieving COPD symptoms.

N-Acetylcysteine. One of the longest-used mucolytics is N-acetylcysteine, which has been on the market for more than three decades. Although this agent thins secretions in patients with chronic bronchitis, it neither affects sputum volume nor improves airflow, and it can induce bronchoconstriction. A systematic review of the effects of oral mucolytic drug use in COPD found that regular oral mucolytic therapy as prophylaxis for a duration of at least two months reduces acute exacerbations and days of illness in patients with stable chronic bronchitis and COPD (Poole PJ, 2001). The majority of the studies included in this review involved N-acetylcysteine. The review provided the impetus for investigating whether mucolytics reduce not only the frequency (prophylaxis) but also the severity and duration (treatment) of acute exacerbation. Yet in a randomized, double-blind, placebo-controlled trial, N-acetylcysteine (with corticosteroids and bronchodilators) failed to modify the outcome in acute exacerbations of COPD (Black PN, 2004).

Alpha₁-Antitrypsin Augmentation

Overview. Alpha$_1$-antitrypsin (AAT) is a serum glycoprotein encoded on chromosome 14, produced by the liver, and found in the lungs. A deficiency in AAT, a naturally occurring (hereditary) disorder that needs treatment and can lead to emphysema, is the only known genetic abnormality linked to the development of COPD. When present in sufficient quantities, AAT inhibits the activity of enzymes implicated in emphysema. Supplementation with AAT, a preparation of purified human alpha$_1$-proteinase inhibitor (alpha$_1$-PI), is occasionally used in patients with emphysema. Because AAT is extracted from human plasma, recipients of this therapy face a small risk of contracting bloodborne infections such as hepatitis B, Creutzfeld-Jacob disease (a rare neurodegenerative disorder), and HIV. The safety record of Bayer Pharmaceutical's (West Haven, Connecticut) Prolastin has been excellent, but the manufacturer has withdrawn batches of AAT when it became known that some donors may have been exposed to Creutzfeld-Jacob disease.

Mechanism of Action. AAT is secreted by infiltrating neutrophils into the lungs of emphysema patients and is largely responsible for the destruction of elastase in the lungs, resulting in reduced lung elasticity (Khan H, 2002). Administration of AAT minimizes the elastin-degrading activity of neutrophil elastase, thereby slowing the rate of decline in lung function. (Naturally present in the lungs, AAT, when administered to diseased lungs, may help slow further deterioration.)

Partially Purified Human Alpha₁-Antitrypsin. Partially purified human AAT (Bayer's Prolastin) is indicated for the treatment of emphysema patients with AAT deficiency. It has been available in the United States and some European markets for more than 60 years. AAT augmentation therapy is appropriate in nonsmoking, younger patients with severe AAT deficiency and associated emphysema. No other AAT agent has reached the market, although several companies are developing other AAT formulations.

Prolastin has been shown to increase AAT concentration in the airways, but whether treatment prevents emphysema progression is unknown. No long-term controlled trials of Prolastin have been performed because of the relatively small number of people with AAT deficiency and the slow clinical course of emphysema. However, data from the U.S. National Institutes of Health (NIH) registry of patients with severe AAT deficiency indicate that AAT therapy has some efficacy in preserving lung function. AAT augmentation, however, not only poses the risk inherent with plasma-derived products but is also extremely expensive—annual treatment for a 70 kg (155 lb) person costs an estimated $40,000.

Other Therapies

Smoking Cessation. Smoking cessation is the first and most important intervention in COPD treatment and the only strategy proven to slow long-term decline in FEV_1. According to the landmark Lung Health Study (LHS), smokers who quit regain a fraction of lost lung function and subsequently lose function at the same rate as those who had never smoked (Anthonisen NR, 1994). Follow-up data 11 years after the LHS reveal that continued abstinence from smoking slows the decline in lung function by 50% in COPD patients (Anthonisen NR, 2002).

Unfortunately, prolonged abstinence from smoking is exceedingly difficult to sustain. Each year, less than 10% of the nearly 20 million people in the United States who quit smoking "cold turkey" are able to remain smoke-free, according to an epidemiological study of U.S. tobacco use (Fiore MC, 1992). More than 50% of recidivism occurs within the first week, when nicotine withdrawal symptoms are most intense.

Nicotine replacement via skin patch, chewing gum, nasal spray, lozenge, or inhaler improves smoking cessation rates; for example, 12-week transdermal nicotine treatment results in 20–30% success. Non-nicotine pharmacotherapies (e.g., GlaxoSmithKline's bupropion [Zyban]) have also been extensively investigated for their effectiveness in eliciting smoking cessation. A review of the effects of behavioral interventions (e.g., counseling), pharmacotherapy (nicotine replacement therapy and non-nicotine therapy), and combinations of both found that a 12-week course of bupropion sustained-release (SR) combined with individual counseling failed to offer significant improvements in prolonged (12-month) smoking abstinence rates compared with no intervention (Wagena EJ, 2004). However, a meta-analysis of the effectiveness of various antidepressant agents for smoking cessation revealed that although some drugs (bupropion and nortriptyline [Novartis's Pamelor, generics]) were useful in promoting smoking cessation, other antidepressants (e.g., selective serotonin reuptake inhibitors [SSRIs]) were not (Hughes JR, 2004). Compared with placebo, bupropion or nortriptyline, when used as the only pharmacotherapy, both approximately doubled the odds of continued smoking abstinence at 12 months (19.3% bupropion versus 10.2% placebo; 18.5% nortriptyline versus 7.6% placebo) (Hughes JR, 2004).

The most effective strategies for long-term smoking abstinence appear to include some form of nicotine replacement therapy. In one assessment, adjunctive nicotine replacement therapy plus bupropion improved smoking cessation rates at 12 months compared with either therapy alone (Hughes JR, 2000). For instance, in four randomized, placebo-controlled studies, 300 mg/day of bupropion for 7–12 weeks elicited higher 12-month abstinent rates than placebo (20% versus 8%, respectively). Nicotine replacement therapy combined with intensive behavioral therapy results in significantly higher efficacy over a five-year period compared with no intervention (Wagena EJ, 2004). Nicotine patches in combination with cognitive-behavioral techniques for smoking cessation show benefits five years after treatment; one trial at a private, specialized smoking cessation clinic found a 33.1% rate of abstinence (continuous abstinence for the previous 12 months) (Garcia-Vera MP, 2004).

Oxygen Therapy. Oxygen therapy is the only intervention proven to increase life expectancy in COPD. This survival benefit, however, extends only to patients with severe disease characterized by hypoxemia (low blood oxygen levels) as determined by arterial blood gas measurement. According to the findings of two large trials, long-term oxygen supplementation in such individuals can reverse hypoxemia-induced polycythemia (abnormal elevation of red blood cells), increase body weight, reduce cor pulmonale, improve mental function, and enhance the ability to perform most activities of daily living (Tarpy SP, 1995). On the other hand, oxygen therapy in patients with mild-to-moderate COPD without hypoxemia has no effect on symptoms, function, or survival, making patient selection particularly important with this therapy.

Pulmonary Rehabilitation. Pulmonary rehabilitation refers to education and exercise training techniques designed to improve patients' QOL and reduce the burden of COPD on the health care system. Comprehensive programs provide respiratory, physical, and occupational therapy; nutritional assistance; and psychosocial and vocational rehabilitation.

Evidence indicates that pulmonary rehabilitation is an important component of COPD management. Two meta-analyses of clinical trials of pulmonary rehabilitation for COPD found that, although such programs did not affect lung function, health-related QOL and exercise capacity improved and dyspnea declined, resulting in fewer hospital admissions (Cambach W, 1999; Lacasse Y, 1996). In addition, patients reported an improved sense of well-being and less anxiety after completing these programs. Nonetheless, assessing the cost-effectiveness of pulmonary rehabilitation poses problems because the benefits are modest on average and the therapeutic effort may be large. Although exercise training is likely responsible for the improvement, it is not entirely clear which components of a particular program are responsible.

Pulmonary rehabilitation is increasingly provided in an outpatient setting. Programs vary considerably in frequency, duration, and activities, but the "best" ones last several weeks, use a multidisciplinary approach, involve both patients and their families, and have a long-term maintenance component.

Surgery. Despite advances in medical therapy, a significant number of patients with advanced COPD face a miserable existence and are at high risk of death. This subgroup includes patients with an FEV_1 less than 45% of predicted value who remain symptomatic despite the following measures:

- Smoking cessation.
- Optimal use of inhaled bronchodilators, antibiotics for acute bacterial infections, and inhaled or oral corticosteroids.
- Use of supplemental oxygen.
- Pulmonary rehabilitation.

These individuals may be appropriate candidates for surgical treatment—either lung volume reduction surgery (LVRS) or lung transplantation.

Lung Volume Reduction Surgery. Surgery for bullous emphysema was performed as early as the 1940s, but new techniques of LVRS (also known as reduction pneumoplasty, lung shaving, or lung contouring) have expanded the application of this therapy to patients with more diffuse forms of the disease. Modern LVRS involves bilateral removal (via scalpel or laser) of up to approximately one third of the worst areas of emphysematous lung by peripheral resection. The proposed benefits of LVRS are the following:

- Restoration of elastic recoil in the small airways, leading to a reduction in airway resistance.
- Improved ventilation-perfusion in the remaining lung tissue.
- Return of the diaphragm to a more favorable length to optimize pressure generation.

Randomized controlled trials—albeit small—showed that LVRS was efficacious in improving spirometric values, exercise capacity, and health status (Criner GJ, 1999; Geddes D, 2000; Goldstein RS, 2003). In most studies, bilateral LVRS resulted in 20–40% increases in FVC and FEV_1 and 10–20% reductions in total lung capacity and residual volume. Unilateral LVRS resulted in the same qualitative physiological changes, but they were of less magnitude. Operative mortality is extremely variable; most investigators reported rates of 5–9%. Some researchers suggest that in patients with severe emphysema, LVRS may ease symptoms and improve physiological parameters of respiratory mechanics at rest and during exercise (Geddes D, 2000).

Data from the five-year, multicenter, U.S. National Emphysema Treatment Trial (NETT), a study jointly sponsored by the National Heart, Lung and Blood Institute (NHLBI), Centers for Medicare & Medicaid Services (CMS), and Agency for Healthcare Research and Quality (AHRQ) study, have legitimized bilateral LVRS as a potential treatment for a subgroup of emphysema patients—specifically, those with diseased tissue localized to the upper lobes of the lungs and low baseline exercise capacity. Patients meeting these criteria are typically those for whom insurers and government agencies cover LVRS costs. Overall, NETT data have helped elucidate the impact of LVRS on survival (i.e., LVRS offers no survival advantage over medical therapy alone) and physiological improvements more than two years post-treatment (i.e., exercise capacity after 24 months had improved by more than ten watts [a measure of workload performed] in 16% of patients in the surgery group, as compared with 3% of patients in the medical-therapy group) (Fishman A, 2003).

Enrollment for this Phase III trial began in late 1997; follow-up on the last recruited patients was conducted in December 2002. Emphysema patients with substantially reduced ability to function were enrolled in the study if they were nonsmokers devoid of certain conditions (e.g., recent unstable angina) and had not undergone thoracic or cardiac surgeries that could influence survival or interfere with trial participation. In total, 3777 patients were evaluated for possible inclusion in, and 1218 were selected for, the trial. After a six- to ten-week rehabilitation program (including optimized medications, oxygen as needed, exercise, and guidance in effective breathing methods), patients were randomized to continue rehabilitation ($n = 610$) or to have LVRS in addition to continued medical treatment ($n = 608$). Five hundred and eighty patients eventually received surgery and 562 received routine medical care (Fishman A, 2003).

Patients were evaluated for response to treatment at six months, one year, and every year thereafter until the conclusion of NETT. Researchers measured lung function, QOL scores, dyspnea, exercise capacity, and survival, illness, and hospitalization rates. Approximately 95% of patients in each group received treatment as directed. Among study participants, 749 (371 in the surgery group and 378 in the medical group) were followed for at least 24 months (Fishman A, 2003; NETT Research group, 2003). Overall, patients in the surgical group showed improvements over the medical group in exercise capacity (15% versus 3%, respectively, with improvements of at least ten watts) and QOL at 24 months (33% versus 9%); a subgroup of surgical patients with upper-lobe emphysema with low exercise capacity at baseline fared best compared with medically treated patients of similar profile (30% versus 0%, and 48% versus 10%, respectively, showed improvement in exercise capacity and QOL measures). Both non-high-risk surgical survivors—who initially saw improvements in lung function, exercise capacity on a bicycle, distance walked in six minutes, dyspnea, and QOL—and medically treated patients saw their various scores decline by the two-year mark to pre-LVRS levels in the surgical group and to below baseline levels for the medically treated patients.

Overall mortality was the same for surgically and medically treated groups over the long-term follow-up. However, 90-day mortality among surgically treated patients as a whole (7.9%) was significantly higher than the 1.3% rate seen in the medically treated patients. The lowest 90-day mortality rate among surgically treated patients was found in a subgroup of patients with upper-lobe emphysema with or without low exercise capacity (2.9%). Complete data from NETT supported a previously published interim analysis that revealed that patients with a low FEV_1 (less than 20% predicted) with either homogenous emphysema on CT scan or very low carbon monoxide diffusing capacity are at high risk of death after surgery (NETT Research Group, 2001; NETT Research Group 2003); in this group, 90-day mortality was 28%, sufficiently high for researchers to recommend use of this "high risk" classification as exclusion criteria for future LVRS procedures. Additionally, more surgically treated patients than medically treated patients required hospitalization or nursing home placement for the first eight months after treatment assignment.

A prospective economic analysis conducted by NETT researchers over three years of follow-up found that although one-year post-treatment costs are higher for LVRS patients than the costs of medical treatment alone, total medical care costs between surgically and medically treated groups were equivalent in year 3 (NETT Research Group, 2003. Investigators concluded that LVRS's benefits would have to be maintained in the long-term if the procedure is to be considered comparably good value as other surgical interventions (e.g., coronary artery bypass graft [CABG], which costs an estimated $60,000-$70,000 per procedure).

Lung Transplantation. Generally, patients younger than 55–60 who have end-stage COPD may be candidates for single- or double-lung transplantation. At specialized U.S. centers, the three-year survival rate is approximately 60%; morbidity and mortality are caused primarily by chronic rejection of donor lungs. The availability of lung transplantation varies among the major markets, but overall, the procedure is performed infrequently given the scarcity of donor organs and the high cost of surgery (approximately $150,000–$200,000). In several markets, lung transplantation is reserved for AAT-deficient patients with diffuse emphysema because these patients tend to be younger and, owing to both age and disease etiology, have a greater chance for survival.

EMERGING THERAPIES

Of the current research and development (R&D) initiatives for chronic obstructive pulmonary disease (COPD), agents from two classes of drugs hold the greatest commercial promise: Once-daily long-acting $beta_2$ agonists offer a theoretical improvement over currently marketed long-acting $beta_2$ agonists, and phosphodiesterase 4 (PDE4) inhibitors represent a novel approach to treatment. Several companies are also developing combination long-acting beta$_2$ agonist/inhaled corticosteroid products. Other emerging drugs discussed in this section (e.g., protease inhibitors, mucolytics) lack data demonstrating that they provide notable improvements over existing therapies or are able to slow COPD progression. Early investigations are also being conducted on a host of anti-inflammatory classes: purinoreceptor (P2X) receptor antagonists/ion channel blockers, chemokine antagonists, selective nitric oxide (NO) synthesis inhibitors, interleukin-8 (IL-8) inhibitors, and early-stage "nitro-steroids."

Table 3 presents the most notable therapies in development for the management of COPD. As a result of the United Nations Environment Program (UNEP) Montreal Protocol, which mandates the phasing out of chlorofluorocarbon (CFC)-containing propellants in inhalers, several non-CFC-containing reformulations of existing agents (e.g., formoterol [Novartis's Foradil]) have entered or will soon enter respiratory markets; these reformulations are discussed in the "Current Therapies" section. This section also does not discuss short-acting beta$_2$ agonists or other agents that would be used as rescue medication.

Long-Acting Beta$_2$ Agonists

Overview. Researchers are investigating once-daily long-acting beta$_2$ agonists for their greater convenience and, in theory, better side-effect profiles than marketed agents such as salmeterol (GlaxoSmithKline's Serevent/Aeromax) and formoterol (Yamanouchi/Novartis's Foradil, AstraZeneca's Oxis Turbuhaler, Yamanouchi/Sanofi-Aventis's Atock). The most advanced of these agents is Sepracor's arformoterol, for which two pivotal Phase III trials in COPD have been completed. Several agents are in earlier stages of development—some progressing as far as Phase II trials for COPD in at least one of the major markets. However, published clinical trial results to date are lacking, thus precluding a detailed discussion of the agents' potential in COPD. For instance, among Chiesi's ongoing respiratory R&D initiatives are European Phase II investigations of an inhaled formulation of the dual beta$_2$ and beta$_3$ agonist CHF-4226 (formerly TA-2005), which was in-licensed from Tanabe Seiyaku (Osaka, Japan), and an inhaled formoterol/corticosteroid combination for asthma and COPD. As part of a joint agreement to develop long-acting beta$_2$ agonists, GlaxoSmithKline and Theravance are conducting Phase II COPD and asthma trials of several potential candidates, including GSK-159797, GSK-597901, and 678007. Although both GSK-159797 and GSK-597901 have demonstrated expected increases in FEV$_1$ in asthma patients, data on any of the compounds in COPD patients are sparse (Theravance, press release, December 4, 2003).

The COPD drug market is increasingly competitive owing to the emergence of tiotropium (Boehringer Ingelheim/Pfizer's Spiriva), the uptake of already approved long-acting beta$_2$ agonists, and the availability of combination agents in the major markets. Once-daily administration of a beta$_2$ agonist that has an efficacy and side-effect profile comparable to that of currently marketed long-acting beta$_2$ agonists (which are prescribed twice daily) would be an attractive option

TABLE 3. Emerging Therapies in Development for Chronic Obstructive Pulmonary Disease

Compound	Development Phase	Marketing Company
***Long-acting beta*$_{2\ agonists}$**		
Arformoterol		
United States	III	Sepracor
Europe	—	—
Japan	—	—
QAB-149		
United States	II	Novartis
Europe	II	Novartis
Japan	—	—
***Long-acting beta*$_{2\ agonist/corticosteroidcombinations}$**		
GSK-159797/GSK-685698		
United States	II	GlaxoSmithKline
Europe	II	GlaxoSmithKline
Japan	—	—
Anticholinergicss		
AD-237		
United States	II	Vectura/Arakis
Europe	II	Vectura/Arakis
Japan	—	—
Phosphodiesterase 4 inhibitors		
Roflumilast		
United States	III	Altana
Europe	PR	Altana
Japan	II/III	Altana/Tanabe
Cilomilast		
United States	PR(3)	GlaxoSmithKline
Europe	III	GlaxoSmithKline
Japan	—	—
Arofylline		
United States	II/III	Almirall Prodesfarma
Europe	II/III	Almirall Prodesfarma
Japan	—	—
AWD-12–281		
United States	—	—
Europe	II	GlaxoSmithKline
Japan	—	—
Leukotriene antagonists		
Amelubant (BIIL-284)		
United States	—	—
Europe	II	Boehringer Ingelheim
Japan	—	—
Protease inhibitors		
Midesteine		
United States	—	—
Europe	III	Medea Research
Japan	—	—

TABLE 3. (*continued*)

Compound	Development Phase	Marketing Company
Mucolytic agents		
ML-03		
United States	II	Milkhaus Laboratory
Europe	—	—
Japan	—	—
Promoters of elastin synthesis		
R-667		
United States	—	—
Europe	II	Roche
Japan	—	—

GlaxoSmithKline was granted an approvable letter for cilomilast from the FDA in October 2003; approval is pending submission of suitable data from an additional Phase III trial in COPD.

PR = Preregistered.

in the bronchodilator market. Indeed, development of a once-daily long-acting beta$_2$ agonist that could be combined in a single inhaler with tiotropium would be a marketing coup for its producer.

Mechanism of Action. The mechanism of action of long-acting beta$_2$ agonists is similar to that of short-acting beta$_2$ agonists. Briefly, beta$_2$ agonists bind to active beta$_2$ receptors—that is, receptors associated with active G proteins. These G proteins initiate an intracellular signal transduction cascade involving activation of adenylyl cyclase and the subsequent generation of cyclic adenine monophosphate (cAMP), resulting in reduced free intracellular calcium, which induces smooth-muscle relaxation and improves breathing in COPD patients (Johnson M, 1998). However, long-acting beta$_2$ agonists are typically more lipophilic (fat-soluble) than short-acting beta$_2$ agonists (Johnson M, 1998). This difference in biochemical properties results in the deposition of long-acting beta$_2$ agonists in cellular membranes, which provides sustained delivery of the drug to the beta$_2$ adrenergic receptor. This lipophilicity is believed to prolong the interaction of these agents with the beta$_2$ adrenergic receptor (Lewell XQ, 1992). Together, these actions result in prolonged bronchodilation relative to short-acting beta$_2$ agonists.

Arformoterol. Sepracor's arformoterol (R,R-formoterol), a single-isomer version of formoterol (Novartis's Foradil, AstraZeneca's Oxis) in an inhaled solution, is in Phase III development in the United States for the treatment of bronchospasm in COPD patients. It has remained in Phase III development for COPD since 2001. In a first-quarter earnings conference call on April 27, 2004, Sepracor reported that it is investigating both once- and twice-daily administration of arformoterol in trials. In 2003, Sepracor announced the results of one of two pivotal, 12-week, Phase III trials of arformoterol in COPD; the company reported the completion of the second such trial in October 2004 (Sepracor, press release, October

26, 2004). Further published quantitative data on these studies involving a total of 1325 patients are limited, although Sepracor has indicated that arformoterol significantly improved FEV_1 immediately postdose and for up to 24 hours and improved symptoms such as dyspnea compared with placebo.

Sepracor's assessment of arformoterol in its Phase II program for obstructive airway disease included patients with asthma and COPD. However, the degree of bronchodilation seen in asthmatic patients is typically higher than in COPD patients, so it is likely that the change in FEV_1 seen in COPD patients would be less than the 24–27% change from baseline seen in arformoterol's Phase II 340-patient asthma trial (Arformoterol, 2004).

Formoterol has two asymmetric carbon atoms in the molecule, making four stereoisomers possible. (Stereoisomers are differing forms of amino acids that have the same molecular formula but different configurations; pairs of stereoisomers are called enantiomers.) The commercially available form of formoterol is a mixture of R,R- and S,S-formoterol. In vitro evidence indicates that the R,R-enantiomer is 1000 times more potent than the S,S-enantiomer—a noteworthy finding given the belief that the S-enantiomer of short-acting $beta_2$ agonists may contribute to some of their adverse effects (e.g., increased airway reactivity to spasmogens) (Trofast J, 1991; Chapman ID, 1992). Pharmacological studies reveal that the bronchodilator activity of formoterol resides in the R,R-enantiomer. In theory, arformoterol may provide greater potency and offer reduced adverse effects compared with the racemic mixture.

QAB-149. Novartis $beta_2$ agonist QAB-149 is in Phase IIb development for COPD and asthma, in both oral and inhaled formulations. Phase III trials of QAB-149 are due to commence in 2006.

A randomized, double-blind, Phase II trial of the inhaled formulation of QAB-149, which uses SkyePharma's SkyeHaler DPI technology, was initiated in July 2004. In January 2005, Novartis reported that the drug showed "strong efficacy" and safety in both COPD and asthma. The Phase IIb trial is investigating the efficacy and safety of four doses of QAB-149 (50 μg, 100 μg, 200 μg, and 400 μg) delivered via a multiple-dose inhaler, and one dose of the drug (400 μg) delivered via a single-dose inhaler, in patients with COPD. Prior Phase II trials of QAB-149 in asthma and COPD patients demonstrated that the agent is efficacious, safe, and well tolerated (Novartis, press release, November 19, 2003).

Long-Acting Beta₂ Agonist/Corticosteroid Combinations

Overview. As reported in the "Current Therapies" section, a 2004 meta-analysis of combined treatment with a corticosteroid plus a long-acting $beta_2$ agonist in more than 4000 patients found that, compared with placebo, combinations offer clinically meaningful differences in health-related quality of life (QOL), symptoms, and exacerbations (Nannini L, 2004). Such combination agents represent attractive therapeutic options—particularly in light of inhaled corticosteroids' ability to reduce exacerbation rates—for patients with moderate-to-severe COPD who need more continuous bronchodilation.

Several long-acting beta$_2$ agonist/corticosteroid combinations are under investigation. Novartis and Schering-Plough are jointly developing a single-inhaler product that combines two currently available agents, formoterol and mometasone furoate (Schering-Plough's Asmanex). There are also a number of combinations clustered in Phase II or earlier investigation, including several GlaxoSmithKline (GSK) agents. The discussion here focuses on GSK-159797/GSK-685698, for which more data have been made available.

Mechanism of Action. The combination of a long-acting beta$_2$ agonist and inhaled corticosteroid offers a more convenient means for opening the airways and reducing inflammation. Beta$_2$ agonists bind to active beta$_2$ receptors—G proteins—which initiate an intracellular signal transduction cascade involving activation of adenylyl cyclase and the subsequent generation of cyclic adenine monophosphate (cAMP). This process results in reduced free intracellular calcium, which induces smooth-muscle relaxation and improves breathing in COPD patients (Johnson M, 1998).

Corticosteroids exert their therapeutic effect by binding to glucocorticoid receptors in the epithelium of bronchi, thus altering intracellular activities and reducing the transcription of genes that encode proteins involved in the inflammatory response (e.g., cytokines such as interleukin-8 [IL-8], tumor necrosis factor alpha [TNF-α]). By lowering the levels of these inflammation mediators, corticosteroid therapy reduces the levels of lymphocytes, eosinophils, macrophages, and mast cells in mucosal fluids, all of which are more common in asthma. In addition, corticosteroids increase the transcription of those genes responsible for producing beta$_2$ adrenoreceptors and lipocortin 1, a protein that inhibits phospholipase A$_2$ (a proinflammatory enzyme). Corticosteroids also inhibit T-cell activation (and subsequent cytokine release), promote apoptosis of eosinophils, inhibit nitric oxide (NO) synthase, and reduce mucus secretion, and they help restore damaged epithelium and increase the number of ciliated cells in the lungs.

Corticosteroids are likely to reduce the number, activity, and chemotaxis (movement by a cell in reaction to a chemical stimulus) of inflammatory cells in the lungs and ease airway hyperreactivity. However, neutrophils play a central role in the pathophysiology of COPD and are largely unaffected by corticosteroids; thus, many COPD patients have a suboptimal response to treatment with corticosteroids.

GSK-159797/GSK-685698. With several long-acting beta$_2$ agonist/corticosteroid initiatives under way, GSK is conducting Phase II trials of several possible such combinations. Of these, GSK has provided information (albeit limited) on the GSK-159797/GSK-685698 combination, which teams a once-daily corticosteroid that GSK refers to as more potent than other inhaled steroids (GlaxoSmithKline, press release, December 3, 2003) with its investigatory long-acting beta$_2$ agonist (GSK-159797). The company is billing the combination as the successor to Advair (fluticasone/salmeterol), based on data that showed GSK-159797's greater effect than that of salmeterol on FEV_1 24 hours postdose and GSK-685698's ability to remain in the lungs for twice as long as fluticasone (GlaxoSmithKline, press release, December 3, 2003).

Anticholinergics

Overview. Tiotropium's initial commercial success, together with factors such as the increasing prevalence of COPD and the convergence of national and international guidelines on the benefits of anticholinergics as first-line drugs for COPD patients needing continuous bronchodilation, has contributed to the search for other effective agents in this class. Vectura (Chippenham, United Kingdom)/Arakis's (Babraham, United Kingdom) AD-237, GSK's GSK-202405, and Almirall Prodesfarma's (Barcelona, Spain) LAS-34273 and LAS-35201 are all anticholinergics in development for COPD. All are in Phase II development except for LAS-35201, which is in Phase I.

Mechanism of Action. Anticholinergic agents block the effects of acetylcholine, a parasympathetic nervous system neurotransmitter that promotes bronchoconstriction. Acetylcholine, released from branches of the vagus nerve that run along the airways, binds to the M_1 and M_3 muscarinic receptors located in the smooth muscle and submucosal glands in the airways. Acetylcholine binding activates the receptors, stimulating both the contraction of smooth muscle via activation of the M_1 receptor (leading to bronchoconstriction) and the secretion of mucus from the submucosal glands via activation of the M_3 receptor. By binding to the M_1 and M_3 muscarinic receptors, anticholinergic drugs block the access of acetylcholine, thus reducing the number of activated receptors. As a result, smooth-muscle tone in the airways declines, thereby reducing bronchoconstriction and mucus secretion. Inhibition of M_2 receptors, as seen with the nonselective anticholinergics ipratropium bromide (Boehringer Ingelheim/Teijin's Atrovent, generics) and oxitropium (Boehringer Ingelheim's Oxivent/Ventilat/Tersigan, 3M's Tersigat, UCB's Pulsigan), results in increased acetylcholine release (the M_2 receptor functions as a negative regulator of acetylcholine release).

AD-237. Vectura and Arakis are using the proprietary PowderHale technology for the codevelopment of a dry-powder inhaler (DPI) formulation of AD-237, a long-acting anticholinergic that the companies report is already marketed for another, unspecified indication in the United States and Europe. Phase IIa trials in COPD were completed in May 2004 in the two regions; Phase IIb trials are to be conducted in the second half of 2005, with results expected in the first half of 2006.

A 45-subject, double-blind, placebo-controlled Phase IIa study investigated the safety and efficacy of 20 µg, 125 µg, 250 µg, and 400 µg doses of AD-237. The drug offered statistically significant improvements in FEV_1 over a 32-hour period compared with placebo, as well as few side effects (Vectura, press release, May

18, 2004). However, it is not yet clear that Vectura's PowderHale technology, which the companies claim optimizes the drug via targeted deep lung penetration, will provide any added benefit in terms of improved efficacy or fewer systemic side effects.

Phosphodiesterase 4 Inhibitors

Overview. Because COPD is characterized by inflammation of the airways, several pharmaceutical companies are seeking to develop safe and effective anti-inflammatory treatments. Theophylline, a methylxanthine, is a nonspecific inhibitor of phosphodiesterase (PDE) and is often relegated to second- or third-line status owing to its relatively poor efficacy and safety and tolerability profile. However, PDE inhibition research has been focused on targeting individual PDE enzymes (each with distinct activities and tissue distributions) in hopes of improving on these attributes.

Research has focused on developing specific PDE4 inhibitors that effectively suppress airway inflammation and have improved side-effect profiles compared with that of theophylline. Initial data from clinical trials with selective PDE4 inhibitors were somewhat disappointing; agents demonstrated limited efficacy and substantial emetic and/or cardiovascular side effects. Improved understanding of the molecular biology of PDEs, however, has led to the synthesis of second-generation agents with an improved risk/benefit ratio, making cardiovascular and central nervous system side effects less of an issue. Yet gastrointestinal (GI) side effects, including nausea, vomiting, and dyspepsia, remain possible dose-limiting problems with many PDE4 drugs. Differences in individual PDE4 inhibitors are thought to be determined, at least in part, by a therapeutic ratio of selectivity for receptor subtypes; of the four isoenzymes encoded by the PDE4 gene (PDE4A, PDE4B, PDE4C, and PDE4D), the PDE4B and PDE4D isoenzymes are responsible for anti-inflammatory effects and emesis, respectively (Lipworth BJ, 2005).

Several PDE4 inhibitors are in clinical trials for COPD and asthma. In February 2003, Celgene announced at the BIO CEO and Investor Conference 2003 in New York that CC-1088, a thalidomide analogue and PDE4 inhibitor, would be compared with two of Celgene's other PDE4 inhibitors (CC-5048 and CC-1004) for either Crohn's disease or COPD; trial results for COPD remain to be reported. Ono Pharmaceuticals is developing the oral PDE4 inhibitor ONO-6126. According to Ono's 2004 annual report, ONO-6126 has entered Phase II trials for bronchial asthma in Europe and Japan and Phase II trials for COPD in the United States. In March 2005, Icos reported that a Phase II trial of its PDE4 agent, IC-485, did not meet the primary end point of improving lung function (Icos, press release, March 23, 2005).

The short length of trials typically conducted for COPD agents—and particularly for anti-inflammatories—presents a hurdle to showing long-term benefit of PDE4 inhibitors for this indication. Indeed, GSK's cilomilast (Ariflo), discussed later in this section, is undergoing an additional Phase III study in the United

States to provide long-term efficacy data (six months to one year) as an FDA condition of approval. Drugs may not always be able to elicit a short-term increase in FEV$_1$ but may gradually show other positive effects (e.g., disease-modifying benefits of long-term anti-inflammatory activity).

Late-phase PDE4 inhibitors have been shown to reduce disease exacerbations. Clinical trials for COPD frequently involve patients with severe disease who have marked, irreversible lung damage. Because anti-inflammatory treatments may demonstrate better efficacy in patients with mild-to-moderate disease, these agents may work best in a segment of the COPD population that is often not diagnosed or drug-treated.

Mechanism of Action. A novel approach to COPD, PDE4 inhibitors provide both bronchodilation and anti-inflammatory effects by blocking the activity of inflammatory mediators (e.g., leukotrienes). Specifically, cyclic adenosine monophosphate (cAMP) and cyclic guanosine monophosphate (cGMP) are generated within cells following the activation of certain cellular receptors, such as beta adrenergic receptors. These cyclic nucleotides then activate smooth-muscle relaxation and bronchodilation in the pulmonary arteries and airways. Beta$_2$ adrenergic receptor activation by natural ligands or beta$_2$ agonists leads to the generation of cAMP and results in bronchodilation. Eventually, cAMP and cGMP are degraded, returning the cell to an inactive state. PDE isoenzymes, particularly PDE3 and PDE4, normally degrade cAMP and cGMP, and inhibition of PDE action will maintain intracellular levels of cAMP and cGMP, thereby prolonging the duration of bronchodilation. The main PDE expressed by neutrophils, macrophages, and CD8 + T cells is PDE4. Aside from promoting relaxation of smooth muscle, PDE4 inhibition suppresses activation of inflammatory cells and modulates the activity of pulmonary nerves (Friedman M, 2003).

Roflumilast. Roflumilast (ALTANA, Inc. [Melville, New York]/Tanabe's Daxas), an oral PDE4 inhibitor, is preregistered for COPD in Europe. The European filing was submitted in February 2004, supported by six-month data from the pivotal RECORD study (Altana, press release, February 13, 2004). Roflumilast is in Phase III investigation for COPD in the United States, where plans for an early 2005 NDA submission were scuttled due to slower-than-anticipated enrollment in an additional trial required to support the U.S. submission dossier (Altana, press release, October 28, 2004). The 12-month, long-term efficacy study in COPD—the 1100-patient OPUS trial—will examine roflumilast's effect on acute disease exacerbations, as well as its effects on pulmonary function and QOL. The trial's projected completion date is July 2005 (National Institutes of Health Clinical Trials Database [OPUS Study], http://clinicaltrials.gov/ct/show/NCT00076089?order=1, accessed March 7, 2005).

In Japan, where an Altana/Tanabe codevelopment and commercialization agreement covers the drug, roflumilast is in Phase II/III trials for COPD, and Tanabe plans to file an NDA for the drug in 2006 (Pharma Marketletter, October 18, 2004).

Results from the double-blind, placebo-controlled Phase III RECORD trial involving 1400 COPD patients were reported at several respiratory association meetings, including the Annual Meeting of the American Thoracic Society in Orlando, Florida, in May 2004; the German Congress for Pneumology, in Frankfurt, Germany, in March 2004; and at the 13th Annual Congress of the European Respiratory Society in Vienna, Austria, in September 2003. The efficacy of roflumilast was greatest at four weeks; the gains in FEV_1 then began to decline at a rate similar to that seen in placebo-treated patients, suggesting that the drug may not slow disease progression (DiMarco F, 2003). In addition, results show that the bronchodilation achieved by this agent is lower than that of beta$_2$ agonists or anticholinergics. Data from the RECORD cohort presented at both the first and second Strategic Resources Institute (SRI) Phosphodiesterases in Drug Discovery and Development conference in November 2003 and November 2004, respectively, showed that, despite improvements in FEV_1, the QOL of COPD patients taking roflumilast remained unchanged during the trial. However, roflumilast treatment significantly reduced the exacerbation rate, from a "rate-per-patient" of 1.13 with placebo to 1.03 and 0.75 with roflumilast doses of 250 µg and 500 µg, respectively. Side effects seen with roflumilast treatment (250 µg and 500 µg) were generally mild or moderate in severity and included diarrhea (2.3% and 6.1%), nausea (1.0% and 3.2%), headache (0.7% and 1.8%), and abdominal pain (0.2% and 1.6%) (Bundschuh DS, 2003).

According to results reported at the March 2004 SMi Group's Chronic Obstructive Pulmonary Disease meeting in London (PDE presentation), roflumilast treatment (250 µg and 500 µg) offers significant improvements from baseline over placebo in the measures on the St. George's Respiratory Questionnaire (SGRQ), a standardized self-completed questionnaire for measuring impaired health and perceived well-being (i.e., QOL) in airways disease (Bredenbröker D, 2004). The incidence of diarrhea (6%), nausea (3%), abdominal pain (3%), headache (2%), and weight loss (2%) reached significance as compared with placebo.

Preclinical data reveal that roflumilast has high bioavailability and a half-life of 15 hours (longer than cilomilast's 7-hour half-life, described in the subsequent section), which may give the drug an edge as a once-daily PDE4 therapy. Compared with cilomilast, roflumilast has an improved therapeutic ratio, with greater selectivity for PDE4B than PDE4D isoenzymes (Lipworth BJ, 2005). Because the maximum dose of cilomilast is limited by dose-related toxicity, trials of cilomilast have investigated the benefits of giving the drug twice daily, whereas roflumilast is being developed as a once-daily agent. However, side effects (such as nausea and diarrhea [Bredenbröker D, 2002]) also are a concern with roflumilast.

The presentation at the 2004 SMi conference in London also reported that gains in FEV_1 scores were greater in roflumilast-treated patients compared with placebo than in cilomilast-treated patients compared with placebo. Although these results suggest that roflumilast may have greater efficacy than cilomilast, head-to-head trials are required to truly compare the efficacy of these agents.

Cilomilast. In October 2003, GSK received an approvable letter from the FDA for cilomilast (Ariflo), an orally available, second-generation PDE4 inhibitor. The letter follows a nonfavorable assessment by an FDA advisory committee, which questioned the below-target improvement in FEV_1 (30–40 mL below the goal of 120 mL) set for three pivotal placebo-controlled trials of cilomilast. Formal approval is pending completion of an additional study demonstrating long-term efficacy of cilomilast in COPD; the requirement pushes back approval to 2006 at earliest. Cilomilast is in Phase III trials in Europe for COPD and asthma and Phase II trials in Japan for asthma.

Cilomilast has had mixed clinical trial results. By 2003, four pivotal, placebo-controlled, Phase III trials had been performed involving a total of 2263 COPD patients; two of these trials demonstrated efficacy. GSK presented Phase III data from one of these trials at the meeting of the ATS in May 2001. In this U.S. Phase III trial of twice-daily cilomilast (15 mg orally) versus placebo in 2058 stable COPD patients, cilomilast was associated with improvements in lung function (approximately 10 mL increases in FEV_1 compared with a 30 mL decline in FEV_1 in placebo-treated patients) and fewer exacerbations (Edelson JD, 2001). In late 2000, initial Phase III results of cilomilast in COPD patients indicated that the drug was associated with clinical benefit (SmithKline Beecham, press release, October 31, 2000); however, its failure to significantly improve FEV_1 in a European Phase III trial prompted the need for additional confirmation (GSK Ariflo long-term … , 2003). Therefore, the FDA requested a repeat of the U.S. arm of cilomilast's Phase III trial.

Previous Phase II trials in COPD patients had also shown lung function improvements (e.g., 11% and 7% increases in FEV_1 and FVC, respectively) over baseline and improvements in QOL measures (Giembycz MA, 2001). However, some side effects (e.g., nausea, diarrhea, abdominal pain) also appeared. No drug interactions were reported.

In a Phase II study involving 424 COPD patients who responded poorly to bronchodilator therapy (i.e., nonreversible airway disease), 15 mg cilomilast twice daily produced statistically significant improvements in FEV_1 relative to placebo over a six-week period: 130 mL for cilomilast compared with -30 mL for placebo (Compton CH, 2001). No significant improvements in QOL were observed in the short time frame of this trial. However, results from another Phase II trial conducted in 264 patients with COPD suggested that COPD patients with nonreversible airway disease did not respond to treatment with cilomilast at 12 weeks (Reisner C, 2003). In this multicenter, randomized, double-blind trial, 156 COPD patients with nonreversible airway disease and 108 patients who were responsive to bronchodilator therapy were randomized to receive either cilomilast or placebo for 12 weeks. Patients with reversible COPD who received cilomilast ($n = 69$) experienced a 12% mean increase in FEV_1 compared with placebo-treated patients ($n = 39$); whereas patients with nonreversible airway disease ($n = 105$) did not experience a net increase in FEV_1 compared with placebo-treated patients ($n = 51$). Together, these data suggest that reversible COPD patients are potentially more likely to benefit from treatment with cilomilast. However, longer-term trials may demonstrate efficacy in both subsets of COPD patients.

One factor inhibiting the therapeutic potential of cilomilast is that the high doses required with this agent cause dose-limiting toxicities.

Arofylline. Although it has been in Phase III development for bronchitis since 2003 (Phase III development for asthma began in 1997, with no current development for the indication), Almirall Prodesfarma has not released any significant new information to reflect a change in development status for its selective PDE4 inhibitor, arofylline. The drug is reportedly still in Phase II/III trials in the United States and Europe for COPD.

Phase II results for arofylline show improvement in lung function for patients with moderate-to-severe COPD (*Scrip*, May 18, 2001:2644). In this study, 141 patients received either 90 mg of arofylline once daily or placebo. After three months, patients in the arofylline group had a 9% increase in FEV_1 over baseline. Patients receiving arofylline also experienced fewer exacerbations than did those receiving placebo (15.3% and 35.4%, respectively). Phase II studies for COPD were expected to be complete by the end of 2002, but no development information has been reported since 2001.

AWD-12–281. Elbion AG (Radebeul, Germany) and GSK are developing AWD-12–281 (GSK-842470), an inhaled 5-hydroxyindole PDE4 inhibitor that, if approved, will be marketed and distributed by GSK. AWD-12–281 is in Phase II trials for COPD, as confirmed by Elbion at the BIO-Europe 2004 meeting in Cologne, Germany, in November 2004 (*R&D Focus Drug News*, November 29, 2004).

Phase I data for AWD-12–281 in COPD were presented in November 2004 at the Second SRI Phosphodiesterases in Drug Discovery and Development conference, held in Philadelphia. Doses of up to 40 mg/kg/day were reportedly safe and well tolerated, with an adverse event rate similar to that of placebo.

Preclinical data have been reported in various animal models of asthma and COPD. One study compared the anti-inflammatory and bronchodilatory properties of AWD-12–281 with those of corticosteroids (Kuss H, 2003). In rats, intratracheal (i.t.) administration of AWD-12–281 inhibited late-phase infiltration of eosinophils into the lung (as measured by examining the bronchioalveolar lavage fluid [BALF]) to a degree that was comparable to that of the corticosteroid beclomethasone. In the lipopolysaccharide-induced lung neutrophilia model (a model for COPD), AWD-12–281 demonstrated anti-inflammatory effects in several animals. In pigs, AWD-12–281 demonstrated efficacy comparable to that of beclomethasone, and AWD-12–281 demonstrated a lower emetic potential than roflumilast. Further study of this agent for the treatment of COPD is warranted.

Leukotriene Antagonists

Overview. Leukotriene antagonists are nonsteroidal anti-inflammatory agents indicated for the treatment of asthma. Although they inhibit leukotriene D4, which has not been shown to be involved in the inflammation associated with

COPD, the continued demand for better anti-inflammatory approaches in COPD has fueled a limited number of development initiatives.

Pranlukast (Ono Pharmaceutical Company [Osaka, Japan] Onon) is in Phase II development for COPD in Japan, but no data have been reported on its safety or efficacy for the indication. Boehringer Ingelheim's amelubant (formerly BIIL-284), for which Phase I data are available, appears to have stalled in this phase of development. Several studies have been conducted on zafirlukast (AstraZeneca's Accolate) in COPD patients, resulting in moderately beneficial but typically short-lived increases in FEV_1 compared with $beta_2$ agonist therapy (Cazzola M, 2000; Cazzola M, 2001; Nannini LJ Jr., 2003). The company does not report the drug being formally in development for COPD.

Mechanism of Action. The primary leukotriene involved in the pathogenesis of COPD is leukotriene B4, a potent neutrophil chemoattractant produced by alveolar macrophages and present in the sputum of COPD patients. As previously mentioned, many leukotriene antagonists block the action of leukotriene D4, which has not been shown to be involved in the development of pulmonary inflammation seen in COPD. But small studies—such as those examining the efficacy of the leukotriene B4 agonist zafirlukast; salmeterol; and a combination of both agents—found that subgroups of patients had a better response to the combination than to salmeterol alone (Cazzola M, 2000; Cazzola M, 2001). Such findings have spurred continued (albeit limited) research into the potential of leukotriene antagonists in COPD.

Amelubant. Boehringer Ingelheim's amelubant (BIIL-284) (Figure 9) is the most advanced leukotriene B4 antagonist in clinical development. Amelubant is a pro-drug; metabolites of this compound (BIIL-260 and BIIL-315) antagonize the leukotriene B4 receptor. In June 2002, Boehringer Ingelheim received orphan drug status for this agent in the treatment of cystic fibrosis.

Phase I trials conducted in Germany were completed in 1998, and results from this trial were reported at the COPD: New Developments and Therapeutic Opportunities meeting at the National Heart and Lung Institute, London, in June 1999. Study subjects received various doses of the agent, ranging from 2.0 µg to 750 mg, all of which were well tolerated. The dose-dependent inhibition of neutrophil Mac-1, an adhesion molecule involved in the inflammatory response, was also observed. Higher doses of amelubant (2.5–75 mg) blocked the action of leukotriene B4 for up to 40 hours and correlated with the plasma levels of the active metabolites of amelubant. Further development of this agent for COPD has not been reported despite these promising results.

Protease Inhibitors

Overview. Early-phase development initiatives for protease inhibitors in COPD are ongoing. For example, AstraZeneca has multiple protease inhibitors in pre-clinical development.

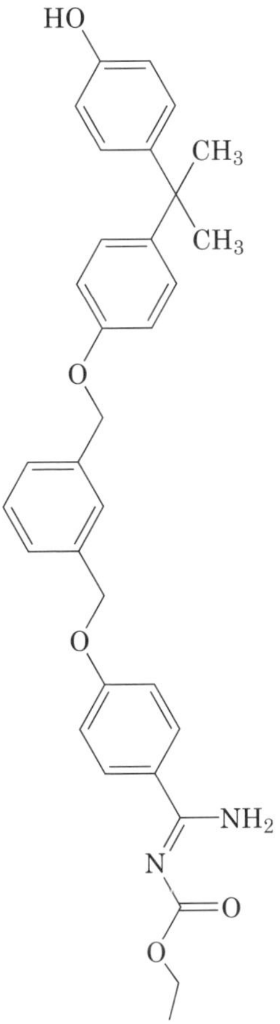

FIGURE 9. Structure of BIIL-284.

Partially purified, plasma-derived human alpha$_1$-antitrypsin (AAT) (Bayer's Prolastin), the first elastase inhibitor therapy developed for COPD, is approved for use in patients with emphysema caused by congenital AAT deficiency and is under investigation for other COPD patients. AAT supplementation has only a marginal effect on the rate of decline in lung function, according to many small clinical trials, and there is no evidence that AAT supplementation can block the progression of COPD in patients with normal AAT plasma concentrations. AAT is also expensive, requires weekly injection, and has inherent safety issues related to the large number of donors required to generate this plasma-derived product.

Alpha Therapeutics's (Los Angeles, California) AAT product (A$_1$ PI [Aralast]) is marketed in the United States for the treatment of emphysema in patients with congenital AAT deficiency. The drug, which is a plasma-derived alpha$_1$-proteinase inhibitor, was approved by the FDA in January 2003 as an augmentation therapy in AAT-deficient patients with evidence of emphysema. Baxter was announced as the worldwide distributor of the AAT therapy (Alpha Therapeutics, press release, January 9, 2003). In October 2003, Alpha Therapeutics was acquired by Baxter Healthcare Corporation (Deerfield, Illinois), including all assets related to the AAT therapy (Baxter Healthcare, press release, October 21, 2003). This agent may find off-label use in non-AAT-deficient emphysema patients. However, issues voiced about Bayer's Prolastin are relevant here; high cost, safety concerns, and limited efficacy will likely limit the market uptake of this agent.

Recombinant AAT formulations delivered directly to the lungs—such as PPL Therapeutics (Midlothian, United Kingdom)/Bayer's recombinant AAT (recAAT) and Aventis Behring/Nektar Therapeutics's (Huntsville, Alabama) alpha$_1$-proteinase inhibitor (API)—would provide a more convenient route of administration and may be less expensive to manufacture than Prolastin. However, these agents have not lived up to their initial promise. PPL Therapeutics and Bayer were developing an aerosol formulation of recombinant AAT therapy, recAAT. Phase II trials of the agent in patients with emphysema and congenital AAT deficiency have been conducted in the United States and Europe. In June 1999, the FDA awarded recAAT orphan drug status for congenital emphysema; a positive opinion for EU orphan drug designation was issued in May 2001. Phase III trials were to be initiated in 2003, but the program was suspended in June 2003, a decision largely based on the anticipated cost of continued development and the decision not to build a purification plant to extract recombinant AAT (Bayer Biological Products, press release, June 18, 2003).

ZLB Behring (King of Prussia, Pennsylvania) (formerly Aventis Behring and Centeon) and Nektar Therapeutics (formerly Inhale Therapeutic Systems) were collaborating to develop a DPI formulation of ZLB Behring's API product (the intravenous formulation, Zemaira, was launched in 2004 in the United States). Phase Ib U.S. trials in patients with AAT-deficient emphysema were completed in 2001 (Aventis Behring, press release, April 10, 2001). API was well tolerated at all doses tested. Inhaled API received orphan drug designation from the FDA in 2000 and orphan medicinal product designation from the European Commission in 2001. In November 2003, however, Nektar announced that its collaboration with Aventis Behring would be terminated (Nektar Therapeutics, press release, November 5, 2003).

Other protease inhibitors that have attracted attention include agents that inhibit matrix-metalloproteinases (MMPs), which are proteases capable of degrading all the components of the extracellular matrix of lung parenchyma, including elastin, collagen, and fibronectin. These agents could potentially halt impairment of lung function and slow disease progression. Other investigators are studying inhibitors of cathepsin, an enzyme with elastolytic activity; serum protease inhibitors (serpins) such as elafin, an elastase-specific inhibitor; and secretory leukoprotease inhibitors, which appear to be major inhibitors of elastase activity in the airways.

Mechanism of Action. Compelling evidence suggests that the lung damage associated with COPD results from an imbalance between proteases, including neutrophil elastase and MMPs that digest elastin and other structural proteins, and protective antiproteases such as AAT. Theoretically, therapies capable of either inhibiting these proteolytic enzymes or increasing the quantity of antiproteases should restore this balance, thus halting lung tissue destruction and progressive airflow obstruction.

Midesteine. Medea Research's (Port Jefferson Station, New York) elastase inhibitor, midesteine, is listed as being in Phase III trials in Italy for the treatment of emphysema; however, little information has been made available on this agent. Results from a double-blind, placebo-controlled trial in former smokers with COPD suggested that midesteine (500 mg bid) for at least four weeks was not associated with significant side effects. These patients also exhibited significant reductions in urinary desmosine, a marker for the degradation of mature elastin, suggesting that the drug was able to reduce elastin breakdown in the lungs of these patients (Luisetti, M, 1996).

Mucolytic Agents

Overview. Continued airway irritation by tobacco over many years impairs mucociliary clearance, resulting in the retention of mucus and the subsequent accumulation of inflammatory cells and cellular debris in the airways that thickens mucus and further impedes clearance. In addition, viscous mucus traps bacteria and other microbes, thus intensifying inflammation and contributing to airflow obstruction and tissue damage. Mucolytic agents help reduce the viscosity of mucus, clearing mucus from the lung. Most agents in this class are in development for cystic fibrosis—a genetic disorder associated with highly viscous mucus production, including in the lungs and gastrointestinal tract. Few agents are in late-stage development for COPD.

Mechanism of Action. Mucolytic agents clear mucus by liquefying sputum. Although clearing secretions can be a significant problem for COPD patients, little evidence exists to show that thinning mucus (mucolysis) by liquefying sputum improves lung function. Furthermore, current methods of sputum volume measurement cannot distinguish the source of the collected secretion. Therefore, it is impossible to determine whether mucolytic agents are clearing mucus from the lower respiratory tract, as intended, or from the upper respiratory tract and mouth; the latter would be less effective in relieving COPD symptoms. Mucolytics are widely used in Europe, but few such agents have received approval in the United States.

ML-03. Milkhaus Laboratory, Inc.'s (Boxford, Massachusetts) ML-03 (HP-3) appears stalled in Phase II development for COPD in the United States. Results of two Phase II trials—one in patients with chronic bronchitis and one in patients with COPD—showed ML-03 increased expectoration and produced significant improvements in objective tests of pulmonary function and physical performance capacity compared with placebo (Milkhaus Laboratory, press release, February 25, 1999). However, no further trial data have been reported. The most recent update of drugs in development from the Pharmaceutical Research and Manufacturers of America (PhRMA) indicates only that Phase II trials of the drug have been completed. Whether ML-03 can truly improve pulmonary function and physical performance capacity or prevent mucus formation, which is difficult to objectively measure, remains unclear.

Promoters of Elastin Synthesis

Overview. Elastin is an integral component of lung tissue that is partially responsible for the elasticity of this organ. Elastin degradation correlates with a loss in lung function due to compromised elasticity. Therapeutic agents that promote elastin synthesis in the lungs may slow or stop the progressive functional decline in COPD patients and may potentially reverse some of the underlying tissue destruction associated with advanced disease.

The National Heart, Lung and Blood Institute (NHLBI) has completed the Feasibility of Retinoic Acid Treatment in Emphysema (FORTE) study, for which the objectives were to identify optimal patient populations, appropriate retinoids, doses, dosing schedules, routes of administration, and outcome measures. Preliminary results of FORTE were presented at the May 2004 American Thoracic Society meeting in Orlando, Florida. Participants in the FORTE study were randomized to receive all-trans-retinoic acid (ATRA) in high-dose (1 mg/kg bid), ATRA in low dose (0.5 mg/kg bid), 13-cis retinoic acid (13cRA; dose of 1 mg/kg/day), or placebo. In the study, retinoic acid treatment as given showed no evidence of rapidly or substantially reversing or improving emphysema. Furthermore, researchers believe that the ATRA formulations may have caused a reduction in the ability of the lungs to transport oxygen to the blood during treatment with the agent. Researchers indicate that the results do not preclude future successes with other forms of retinoic acid.

Roche (Basel, Switzerland) has not disclosed whether its all-trans-retinoic acid, Vesanoid, has progressed beyond Phase II development for emphysema. This agent was launched in January 2001 for leukemia in several countries, including the United States, France, Germany, the United Kingdom, and Japan. Preclinical studies offer conflicting conclusions whether all-trans-retinoic-acid is able to reverse emphysema in mice and rats (Maden M, 2004; Fujita M, 2004). A pilot study involving 30 patients with emphysema was performed to assess the safety and feasibility of 25 mg/m^2 all-trans-retinoic acid treatment administered twice daily for three months (Mao JT, 2002). Although the agent was well tolerated, no benefits over placebo were found in the short trial, as assessed by measurements of pulmonary lung function, CT, and responses to the SGRQ. Further studies would have to be conducted to determine if higher doses of all-trans-retinoic acid or longer treatment regimens would induce positive changes in lung function or repair tissue damage.

Mechanism of Action. The mechanism by which retinoic acid encourages alveolar development is unclear, but researchers suspect that by forming new alveoli, this drug may cause gene expression to revert to that of an earlier period of lung development during which alveoli normally form.

Preclinical research on all-trans-retinoic acid suggests a mode of therapy that may actually reverse lung damage. In rat and hamster models of elastase-induced emphysema, treatment with retinoic acid reduced the amount of damaged lung tissue that was caused by the loss of lung elastic recoil and completely reversed other anatomic characteristics of the disease by forming new, smaller alveoli (Massaro GD, 1997).

R-667. Roche is developing R-667 (Ro-330074), an orally available retinoic acid receptor gamma (RARγ) agonist that displays 100-fold selectivity for this receptor compared with the two other RAR receptors, RARα and RARβ. Roche's development pipeline listed R-667 in continued Phase II trials in late 2004. The company reports that proof-of-concept data from a Phase II trial of the drug's efficacy, safety, and tolerability in emphysema patients will be available in the second half of 2006.

Results from a Phase I trial in patients with emphysema were presented in July 2003 at the New Drugs for Respiratory Diseases, Fifth International Conference in San Diego. The agent was well tolerated over a range of doses; skin irritation was the most frequently reported side effect. In preclinical studies, the agent purportedly demonstrated an ability to regenerate lung tissue and restore lung function. If results from Phase II trials in patients with lung disease mirror the preclinical results obtained in rodent models of lung disease, then this agent may address the underlying mechanisms of disease rather than merely address COPD symptoms.

REFERENCES

American Thoracic Society (ATS). Definitions, epidemiology, pathophysiology, diagnosis, and staging. *American Journal of Respiratory and Critical Care Medicine*. 1995; **152**:S78–S121.

American Thoracic Society. Standards for the diagnosis and care of patients with chronic obstructive pulmonary disease. *American Journal of Respiratory and Critical Care Medicine*. 1995;**152**:S78–S121.

American Lung Association (ALA). *Trends in Chronic Bronchitis and Emphysema: Morbidity and Mortality*. Epidemiology and Statistics Unit. February 2000.

American Lung Association (ALA). *Trends in Chronic Bronchitis and Emphysema: Morbidity and Mortality*. Epidemiology and Statistics Unit. March 2001. www.lungusa.org/data/copd/copd1.pdf. Accessed November 15, 2001.

Anthonisen NR, et al. Effects of smoking intervention and the use of an inhaled anticholinergic bronchodilator on the rate of decline of FEV$_1$. The Lung Health Study. *Journal of the American Medical Association*. 1994;**272**:1497–1505.

Anthonisen NR, et al. Smoking and lung function of Lung Health Study participants after 11 years. *American Journal of Respiratory and Critical Care Medicine*. 2002; **166**:675–679.

Anzueto A, Menjoge SS, Kesten S. Changes in FEV_1 over time in one-year clinical trials of tiotropium in COPD. *American Journal of Respiratory and Critical Care Medicine*. 2001;**16e**:A280.

Anzueto A. One-year analysis of longitudinal changes in spirometry in patients with COPD receiving tiotropium. *Pulm Pharmacol Ther*. 2005;**18**(2):75–81.

Arformoterol: (R,R)-Eformoterol, (R,R)-Formoterol, Arformoterol Tartrate, Eformoterol-Sepracor, Formoterol-Sepracor, R,R-Eformoterol, R,R-Formoterol. *Drugs in R&D*. 2004;**5**(1):25–27(3).

Arofylline looks good in COPD. *Scrip*. PJB Publications, Ltd.; May 18, 2001;**2644**: 25.

Bakke S, et al. Prevalence of obstructive lung disease in a general population: relation to occupational title and exposure to some airborne agents. *Thorax*. 1991;**46**:863–870.

Barbera JA, et al. Mechanisms of worsening gas exchange during acute exacerbations of chronic obstructive pulmonary disease. *European Respiratory Journal*. 1997;**10**:1285–1291.

Barnes PJ. Chronic obstructive pulmonary disease: new opportunities for drug development *Trends in Pharmacological Sciences*. 1998;**19**:415–423.

Barnes PJ. Chronic obstructive pulmonary disease. *New England Journal of Medicine*. 2000;**343**:269–280.

Barnes PJ. Tiotropium bromide. *Expert Opinion on Investigative Drugs*. 2001;**10**:733–740.

Barnes PJ. Small airways in COPD. *New England Journal of Medicine*. 2004;**350**(26):2635–2637.

Bartolome R, et al. Standards for the Diagnosis and Care of Patients with Chronic Pulmonary Disease. American Thoracic Society guidance. *Am J Respir Crit Care Med*. 1995;**152**(5 Pt 2):77–121S.

Benhamou D, et al. Rapid onset of bronchodilation in COPD: a placebo-controlled study comparing formoterol (Foradil Aerolizer) with salbutamol (Ventodisk). *Respiratory Medicine*. 2001;**95**:817–821.

Bredenbroker D, et al. Safety of once-daily roflumilast, a new, orally active, selective phosphodiesterase 4 inhibitor, in patients with COPD. The American Thoracic Society International Conference; May 19–22, 2002; Abstract C92.

Brahman SS. Asthma in the elderly. *American Review of Respiratory Disease*. 1991; **143**:336–340.

Brantly, M., T. Nukiwa, and R. G. Crystal. 1988. Molecular basis of alpha,-antitrypsin deficiency. *Am. J. Med*. **84**:13–31.

Braun SR, et al. A comparison of the effect of ipratropium and albuterol in the treatment of chronic obstructive airway disease. *Archives of Internal Medicine*. 1989;**149**:544–547.

Bredenbroker D, et al. Safety of once-daily roflumilast, a new, orally active, selective phosphodiesterase 4 inhibitor, in patients with COPD. The American Thoracic Society International Conference; May 19–22, 2002; Abstract C92.

Bresnitz EA. Epidemiology of advanced lung disease in the United States. *Clinics in Chest Medicine*. 1997;**18**:421–433.

Bridgewood A, et al. *Living in Britain: Results from the 1998 General Household Survey*. Office for National Statistics. Social Service Division. The Stationary Office: London. 2000.

Brotons B, et al. Prevalence of chronic obstructive lung disease and asthma. A cross-sectional study. *Archivos de Bronconeumologia*. 1994;**30**:149–152.

Brusasco V, et al. Health outcomes following treatment for six months with once daily tiotropium compared with twice daily salmeterol in patients with COPD. *Thorax*. 2003;**58**:399–404.

Buist AS, Vollmer WM. Smoking and other risk factors. In: Murray JF, Nadel JA, eds. *Textbook of respiratory medicine*; Philadelphia: WB Saunders: 1994:1259–1287.

Buist AS. The US Lung Health Study. *Respirology*. 1997;**2**:303–307.

Bundschuh DS. Strategic Research Institute conference, Phosphodieasterases in Disease, November 13–14, 2003.

Burge PS, et al. Randomised, double blind, placebo controlled study of fluticasone propionate in patients with moderate to severe chronic obstructive pulmonary disease: the ISOLDE trial. *British Medical Journal*. 2000;**320**:1297–1303.

Burrows B, et al. The course and prognosis of different forms of chronic airways obstruction in a sample from the general population. *New England Journal of Medicine*. 1987;**317**:1309–1314.

Calverly P, et al. Combined salmeterol and fluticasone in the treatment of chronic obstructive pulmonary disease: a randomised controlled trial. *Lancet*. 2003;**361**(9356):449–456.

Calverley PMA. Effect of budesonide/formoterol on severe exacerbations and lung function in moderate to severe COPD. *European Respiratory Journal*. 2003;**22**:912–919.

Cambach W, et al. The long-term effects of pulmonary rehabilitation in patients with asthma and chronic obstructive pulmonary disease: a research synthesis. *Archives of Physical Medicine and Rehabilitation*. 1999;**80**:103–111.

Casaburi R, et al. A long-term evaluation of once-daily inhaled tiotropium in chronic obstructive pulmonary disease. *European Respiratory Journal*. 2002;**19**:217–224.

Cazzola M, et al. Lung function improvement in smokers suffering from COPD with zafirlukast, a CysLT(1)-receptor antagonist. *Pulm Pharmacol Ther*. 2000;**13**(6):301–305.

Cazzola M, et al. Comparison of the bronchodilating effect of salmeterol and zafirlukast in combination with that of their use as single treatments in asthma and chronic obstructive pulmonary disease. *Respiration*. 2001;**68**(5):452–459.

Cazzola M, et al. Bronchodilator effect of an inhaled combination therapy with salmeterol + fluticasone and formoterol + budesonide in patients with COPD. *Respir Med*. 2003; **97**(5):453–457.

Cazzola M, et al. The functional impact of adding salmeterol and tiotropium in patients with stable COPD. *Respir Med*. 2004;**98**(12):1214–1221. [a]

Cazzola M, et al. The pharmacodynamic effects of single inhaled doses of formoterol, tiotropium and their combination in patients with COPD. *Pulm Pharmacol Ther*. 2004;**17**(1):35–39. [b]

Celli BR, et al. Population impact of different definitions of airway obstruction. *European Respiratory Journal*. 2003;**22**:268–273.

Centre de Recherche D'Etude de Documentation en Economie de la Sante (CREDES). Sante, soins et protection sociale en 2000. Paris, France, 2001.

Chapman ID, et al. Active enantiomers may cause adverse effects in asthma. *Trends in Pharmacological Sciences*. 1992;**13**(6):231–232.

Chen Y. Genetics and pulmonary medicine. 10:Genetic epidemiology of pulmonary function. *Thorax*. 1999;**54**:818–824.

Chen JC, et al. Worldwide epidemiology of chronic obstructive pulmonary disease. *Current Opinion in Pulmonary Medicine*. 1999;**5**:93–99.

Combivent Inhalation Aerosol Study Group. In chronic obstructive pulmonary disease, a combination of ipratropium and albuterol is more effective than either agent alone: an 85-day multicenter trial. *Chest*. 1994;**105**:1411–1419.

Compton CH, et al. Cilomilast, a selective phophodiesterase-4 inhibitor for treatment of patients with chronic obstructive pulmonary disease: a randomised, dose-ranging study. *Lancet*. 2001;**358**:265–270.

Coultas DB, et al. The health impact of undiagnosed airflow obstruction in a national sample of United States adults. *American Journal of Respiratory and Critical Care Medicine*. 2001;**164**:372–377.

Criner GJ, et al. Prospective randomized trial comparing bilateral lung volume reduction surgery to pulmonary rehabilitation in severe chronic obstructive pulmonary disease. *Am J Respir Crit Care Medicine*. 1999;**160**:2018–2027.

Critics diagnose systemic maladies of FDA. *OMB Watch*. November 30, 2004. www.ombwatch.org/article/archive/219.

Croxton TL, et al. Future research directions in chronic obstructive pulmonary disease. *American Journal of Respiratory and Critical Care Medicine*. 2002;**165**:838–844.

Dahl R, et al. Inhaled formoterol dry powder versus ipratropium bromide in chronic obstructive pulmonary disease. *American Journal of Respiratory and Critical Care Medicine*. 2001;**164**:778–784.

Dayal HH, et al. Passive smoking in obstructive respiratory disease in an industrialized urban population. *Environ Res*. 1994;**65**:161–171.

Dennis SM, et al. Regular inhaled salbutamol and asthma control: the TRUST randomised trial. *Lancet*. 2000;**355**:1675–1679.

de Serres FJ. Worldwide racial and ethnic distribution of alpha1-antitrypsin deficiency: summary of an analysis of published genetic epidemiological surveys. *Chest*. 2002;**122**(5):1818–1829.

Dhala A, et al. Respiratory health consequences of environmental tobacco smoke. *Med Clin North Am*. 2004;**88**(6):1535–1552.

Dickinson JA, et al. Screening older patients for obstructive airways disease in a semi-rural practice. *Thorax*. 1999;**54**:501–505.

DiMarco F, et al. Onset of action of tiotropium (TIO) + formoterol (FOR) in patients with stable COPD. 13th Annual Congress of the European Respiratory Society; Sept. 27–Oct. 1, 2003.

Donohue JF, et al. A 6-month, placebo-controlled study comparing lung function and health status changes in COPD patients treated with tiotropium or salmeterol. *Chest*. 2002;**122**:47–55.

Donohue JF, et al. A short-term comparison of fluticasone propionate/salmeterol with ipratropium bromide/albuterol for the treatment of COPD. Treatments in Respiratory Medicine. 2004;**3**(3):173–181.

Dow L. Asthma versus chronic obstructive pulmonary disease—exploring why "reversibility versus irreversibility" is no longer an appropriate approach. *Clinical and Experimental Allergy*. 1999;**29**:739–743.

Edelman NH, et al. Chronic obstructive pulmonary disease; task force on research and education for the prevention and control of respiratory diseases. *Chest*. 1992;**102**:243S–256S.

Edelson JD, et al. Cilomilast, a selective phosphodiesterase-4 inhibitor for treatment of patients with chronic obstructive pulmonary disease: a randomized, dose-ranging study. *Lancet*. 2001;**358**:265–270.

Faulkner MA, et al. Pharmacologic Treatment of Chronic Obstructive Pulmonary Disease: Past, Present, and Future. *Pharmacotherapy*, 2003;**23**(10):1300–1315.

Feenstra TL, et al. The impact of aging and smoking on the future burden of chronic obstructive pulmonary disease: a model analysis in the Netherlands. *American Journal of Respiratory and Critical Care Medicine*. 2001;**164**:590–596.

Ferguson GT. Management of COPD. Early identification and active intervention are crucial. *Postgraduate Medicine*. 1998;**103**:129–141.

Fiore MC. Trends in cigarette smoking in the United States. The epidemiology of tobacco use. *Medical Clinics of North America*. 1992;**76**:289–303.

Fishman A, et al. National Emphysema Treatment Trial Research Group. A randomized trial comparing lung-volume-reduction surgery with medical therapy for severe emphysema. *New England Journal of Medicine*. 2003;**348**:2059–2073.

Fletcher CM, et al. *The Natural History of Chronic Bronchitis and Emphysema: An 8-Year Study of Working Men in London*; Oxford, United Kingdom: Oxford University Press: 1976.

Friedman M, et al. Formoterol therapy for chronic obstructive pulmonary disease: a review of the literature. *Pharmacotherapy*. 2002;**22**:1129–1139.

Friedman M. Future treatment strategies for COPD. *Clin Cornerstone*. 2003;**5**(1):45–51.

Friedman M, et al. Healthcare costs with tiotropium plus usual care versus usual care alone following 1 year of treatment in patients with chronic obstructive pulmonary disorder (COPD). *Pharmacoeconomics*, 2004;**22**(11):741–749.

Fujita M, et al. Retinoic acid fails to reverse emphysema in adult mouse models. *Thorax*. 2004;**59**(3):224–230.

Fukuchi Y, et al. Prevalence of chronic obstructive pulmonary disease in Japan: results from the Nippon COPD epidemiology (NICE) study. *European Respiratory Journal*. 2001;**18**(suppl):275S.

Fukuchi Y. The epidemiology of COPD. *COPD Frontier*. 2003;**2**(1):8–12.

Gallus S, et al. Smoking in Italy 2003, with a focus on the young. *Tumori*. 2004; **90**(2):171–174.

Garcia-Vera MP. Clinical utility of the combination of cognitive-behavioral techniques with nicotine patches as a smoking-cessation treatment: five-year results of the "Ex-Moker" program. *J Subst Abuse Treat*. 2004;**27**(4):325–333.

Geddes D, et al. Effect of lung-volume-reduction surgery in patients with severe emphysema. *New England Journal of Medicine*. 2000;**343**:239–245.

German Federal Statistical Office. Federal Health Monitoring System (GFSO). www.gbe-bund.de. Accessed November 11, 2004.

Giembycz MA. Cilomilast: a second generation phosphodiesterase 4 inhibitor for asthma and chronic obstructive pulmonary disease. *Expert Opinions on Investigatory Drugs*. 2001;**10**:1361–1379.

Global Initiative for Chronic Obstructive Lung Disease (GOLD). GOLD Workshop Report. National Institutes of Health. National Heart, Lung, and Blood Institute (NHLBI): Bethesda, MD. 2001. Available at www.goldcopd.com. Accessed October 1, 2003.

Goldstein RS, et al. Influence of lung volume reduction surgery (LVRS) on health related quality of life in patients with chronic obstructive pulmonary disease. *Thorax* 2003; **58**:405–410.

Gross N, et al. Inhalation by nebulization of albuterol-ipratropium combination (Dey Combination) is superior to either agent used alone in the treatment of chronic obstructive pulmonary disease. *Respiration*. 1998;**65**:354–362.

GSK Ariflo long-term efficacy trials needed for COPD approval—FDA Cmte. *Pink Sheet*. 2003;**65**:36(24).

GSK Flovent/Advair Diskus needs more COPD data; Serevent cleared for COPD. *Pink Sheet*. FDC Reports; April 1, 2002;**64**: 13.

Gurkan F, et al. The effect of passive smoking on the development of respiratory syncytial virus bronchiolitis. *Eur J Epidemiol*. 2000;**16**:465–468.

Halbert RJ, et al. Interpreting COPD prevalence estimates: what is the true burden of disease? *Chest*. 2003;**123**(5):1684–1692.

Hanania NA, et al. The efficacy and safety of fluticasone propionate (250 microg)/salmeterol (50 microg) combined in the Diskus inhaler for the treatment of COPD. *Chest*. 2003;**124**:834–843.

Hankinson JL, et al. Spirometric reference values from a sample of the general US population. *American Journal of Respiratory and Critical Care Medicine*. 1999;**159**:179–187.

Hasani A, et al. The effect of inhaled tiotropium bromide on lung mucociliary clearance in patients with COPD. *Chest*. 2004;**125**(5):1726–1734.

Hasselgren M, et al. Estimated prevalences of respiratory symptoms, asthma and chronic obstructive pulmonary disease related to detection rate in primary health care. *Scandinavian Journal of Primary Health Care*. 2001;**19**:54–57.

Hogg JC, et al. The nature of small-airway obstruction in chronic obstructive pulmonary disease. *New England Journal of Medicine*. 2004;**350**(26):2645–2653.

Hubbard RC, Crystal RG. Antiproteases. In: Crystal RB, West JB, Barnes PJ, Cherniak NS, Weibel ER, eds. *The Lung: Scientific Foundations*; New York: Raven Press: 1991:1755–1787.

Hughes JR, et al. Antidepressants for smoking cessation. *The Cochrane Database of Systematic Reviews* 2004, Issue 4, Art. No.:CD000031. DOI:10:1002/14651858.

Hughes JR, et al. Anxiolytics and antidepressants for smoking cessation. *Cochrane Library*. 2000; Issue 2.

Hughes JR, et al. Antidepressants for smoking cessation. *The Cochrane Database of Systematic Reviews* 2004, Issue 4, Art. No.: CD000031. DOI:10:1002/14651858.

Hurd S. The impact of COPD on lung health worldwide: epidemiology and incidence. *Chest*. 2000;**117**;(2):1S–4S.

Instituto Nacional de Estatistica (INEbase). http://www.ine.es/inebase/indexi.html. Accessed November 14, 2004.

Izumi T. Chronic obstructive pulmonary disease in Japan. *Current Opinions in Pulmonary Medicine*. 2002;**8**:102–105.

Jaen A, et al. Prevalence of chronic bronchitis, asthma and airflow limitation in a general population sample of Catalonia (Spain). *European Respiratory Journal*. 1995;**8**(suppl 19):107.

Jaen A, et al. Prevalence of chronic bronchitis, asthma and airflow limitation in an urban-industrial area of Catalonia. *Archivos de Bronconeumologia*. 1999;**35**:122–128.

Johnson M. β_2-adrenoreceptor agonists: optimal pharmacological profile. *The Role of β_2-Agonists in Asthma Management*. The Medicine Group, Oxford; 1983: 6–8.

Johnson M. The β-adrenoreceptor. *American Journal of Respiratory and Critical Care Medicine*. 1998;**158**:S146–S153.

Jones PW, et al. Disease severity and the effect of fluticasone propionate on chronic obstructive pulmonary disease exacerbations. *European Respiratory Journal*. 2003; **21**:68–73.

Jordan LM, et al. Chronic obstructive pulmonary disease in the general population: an epidemiological study in Guipuzcoa (Spain). *Archivos de Bronconeumologia*. 1998; **34**:23–27.

Khan H, et al. Alpha-1 antitrypsin deficiency in emphysema. *The Journal of the Association of Physicians of India*. 2002;**50**:579–582.

Kozak LJ, et al. National Hospital Discharge Survey: 2000 Annual Summary with detailed diagnosis and procedure data. National Center for Health Statistics. *Vital and Health Statistics*. 2002;**13**(153).

Kuss H, et al. In vivo efficacy in airway disease models of N-(3,5-dichloropyrid-4-yl)-[1-(4-fluorobenzyl)-5-hydroxy-indole-3-yl]-glyoxylic acid amide (AWD 12–281), a selective phosphodiesterase 4 inhibitor for inhaled administration. *Journal of Pharmacology and Experimental Therapeutics*. 2003;**307**:373–385.

Lacasse Y, et al. Meta-analysis of respiratory rehabilitation in chronic obstructive pulmonary disease. *Lancet*. 1996;**348**:1115–1119.

Lacasse Y, et al. Trends in the epidemiology of COPD in Canada, 1980 to 1995. COPD and Rehabilitation Committee of the Canadian Thoracic Society. *Chest*. 1999;**116**:306–313.

Lange P, et al. Chronic obstructive lung disease in Copenhagen: cross-sectional epidemiological aspects. *Journal of Internal Medicine*. 1989;**226**:25–32.

Laurell CB, Eriksson S. The electrophoretic alpha-1 globulin pattern of serum in alpha-1 antitrypsin deficiency. *Scand J Clin Lab Invest*. 1963;**15**:123–140.

Leichtl S, et al. Dose-related efficacy of once-daily roflumilast, a new, orally active, selective phosphodiesterase 4 inhibitor, in chronic obstructive pulmonary disease. The American Thoracic Society International Conference; May 19–22, 2002; Abstract 326.

Leuenberger P, et al. Passive smoking exposure in adults and chronic respiratory symptoms (SAPALDIA Study). Swiss Study on Air Pollution and Lung Diseases in Adults. SAPALDIA Team. *Am J Respir Crit Care Med*. 1994;**150**:1222–1228.

Lewell XQ. A model of the adrenergic beta$_2$ receptor and binding sites for agonist and antagonist. *Drug Design and Discovery*. 1992;**9**:29–48.

Lipworth BJ. Phosphodiesterase-4 inhibitors for asthma and chronic obstructive pulmonary disease. *Lancet*. 2005;**365**(9454):167–175.

Littlejohns P, et al. Prevalence and diagnosis of chronic respiratory symptoms in adults. *British Medical Journal*. 1989;**298**(6687):1556–1560.

Littner MR, et al. Long-acting bronchodilation with once-daily dosing of tiotropium (Spiriva) in stable chronic obstructive pulmonary disease. *Am J Respir Crit Care Med*. 2000;**161**:1136–1142.

Luisetti M, et al. MR 889, a neutrophil elastase inhibitor, in patients with chronic obstructive pulmonary disease: a double-blind, randomized, placebo-controlled clinical trial. *European Respiratory Journal*. July 1996;**9**:1482–1486.

Lundback B, et al. Obstructive lung disease in northern Sweden: respiratory symptoms assessed in a postal survey. *European Respiratory Journal*. 1991;**4**:257–266.

Lung Health Study Research Group. Effect of inhaled triamcinolone on the decline in pulmonary function in chronic obstructive pulmonary disease. *New England Journal of Medicine*. 2000;**343**:1902–1909.

Maden M, Hind M. Retinoic acid in alveolar development, maintenance and regeneration. *Philos Trans R Soc Lond B Biol Sci*. 2004;**359**(1445):799–808. Review.

Maesen FPV, et al. Tiotropium bromide, a new long-acting antimuscarinic bronchodilator: a pharmacodynamic study in patients with chronic obstructive pulmonary disease (COPD). Dutch Study Group. *European Respiratory Journal*. 1995;**8**:1506–1513.

Mahler DA, et al. Efficacy of salmeterol xinafoate in the treatment of COPD. *Chest*. 1999;**115**:957–965.

Mahler DA, et al. Effectiveness of fluticasone propionate and salmeterol combination delivered via the Diskus device in the treatment of chronic obstructive pulmonary disease. *Am J Respir Crit Car Med*. 2002;**166**(6):1084–1091.

Mannino DM, et al. Obstructive lung disease and low lung function in adults in the United States. *Archives of Internal Medicine*. 2000;**160**:1683–1689.

Mannino DM, et al. Chronic obstructive pulmonary disease—United States, 1971–2000. *Mortality and Morbidity Weekly Report Surveillance Summary*. 2002;**51**(6):1–16. [a]

Mannino DM. COPD. Epidemiology, prevalence, morbidity and mortality, and disease heterogeneity. *Chest*. 2002;**121**(5)(suppl):121–126. [b]

Mao JT, et al. A pilot study of all-trans-retinoic acid for the treatment of human emphysema. *American Journal of Respiratory and Critical Care Medicine*. 2002;**165**:718–723.

Massaro GD, Massaro D. Retinoic acid treatment abrogates elastase-induced pulmonary emphysema in rats. *Nature Medicine*. 1997;**3**:675–677.

McConnochie KM, Roghmann KJ. Parental smoking, presence of older siblings, and family history of asthma increase risk of bronchiolitis. *Am J Dis Child*. 1986;**140**:806–812.

McElvaney NG, Crystal RG. Inherited susceptibility of the lung to proteolytic injury. In: Crystal RG, West JB, Weibel ER, Barnes PJ, eds. *The lung: scientific foundations*. Philadelphia: Lippincott-Raven; 1997:2537–2553.

Ministry of Health, Labor, and Welfare (MHLW). The MHLW National Nutrition Survey (with smoking rates from the Japan Tobacco Survey). 2001. www.health-net.or.jp/kenkonet/tobacco/product/pd090000.html. (In Japanese.) Accessed November 14, 2001.

Ministry of Health, Labor, and Welfare (MHLW). MHLW report on smoking prevalence and smoking health related issues—1999. Available at wwwdbtk.mhlw.go.jp/toukei/kouhyo/indexkk_ 3_ 2.html. (In Japanese). Accessed 11/14/04.

Molarius A, et al. Trends in cigarette smoking in 36 populations from the early 1980s to the mid-1990s: findings from the WHO MONICA Project. *American Journal of Public Health*. 2001;**91**:206–212.

Montnemery P, et al. Prevalence of obstructive lung diseases and respiratory symptoms in southern Sweden. *Respiratory Medicine*. 1998;**92**:1337–1345.

Morkjaroenpong V, et al. Environmental tobacco smoke exposure and nocturnal symptoms among inner-city children with asthma. *J Allergy Clin Immunol* (2002) **110**:147–153.

Muir JF, et al. FEV$_1$ reversibility does not adequately predict effect of formoterol via Aerolizer in chronic obstructive pulmonary disease. *International Journal of Clinical Practice*. 2004;**58**(5):457.

Nannini LJ Jr, Flores DM. Bronchodilator effect of zafirlukast in subjects with chronic obstructive pulmonary disease. *Pulm Pharmacol Ther*. 2003;**16**(5):307–311.

Nannini L, et al. Combined corticosteroid and longacting beta-agonist in one inhaler for chronic obstructive pulmonary disease (Cochrane Review). *The Cochrane Library*. 2004; Issue 4.

National Center for Health Statistics [NCHS]. Vital and Health Statistics. Summary Health Statistics for U.S. Adults: National Health interview Survey, 2002. U.S. Department of Health and Human Services, Centers for Disease Control and Prevention, Division of Health Interview Statistics, National Center for Health Statistics, Hyattsville, Maryland, 2004. Available at www.cdc.gov/nchs/products/pubs/pubd/series/sr10/ser10.htm. Accessed 11/14/04.

National Center for Health Statistics (NCHS). The Third National Health and Nutrition Examination Survey, NHANES III, 1988–94 on CD-ROM. National Center for Health Statistics, Centers for Disease Control and Prevention, Hyattsville, Maryland, 1997; CD-ROM Series 11, No. 1.

National Center for Health Statistics (NCHS). Data file documentation. National Health Interview Survey, 1994 (machine readable data file and documentation). National Center for Health Statistics, Centers for Disease Control and Prevention, Hyattsville, Maryland, 1999. www.cdc.gov/tobacco. Accessed November 14, 2001.

National Center for Health Statistics (NCHS). Data file documentation, National Health Interview Survey, 1996 (machine readable data file and documentation). National Center for Health Statistics, Centers for Disease Control and Prevention, Hyattsville, Maryland, 1999. www.cdc.gov/nchs/data. Accessed November 14, 2001.

National Center for Health Statistics (NCHS). *NHIS Survey Description*. U.S. Division of Health Interview Statistics, National Center for Health Statistics, Centers for Disease Control and Prevention, Hyattsville, Maryland, 2001. www.cdc.gov/nchs/nhis. Accessed November 14, 2001.

National Emphysema Treatment Trial Research Group. Cost effectiveness of lung-volume-reduction surgery for patients with severe emphysema. *New England Journal of Medicine*. 2003;**348**:2092–2102.

NETT Research Group. Patients at high risk of death after lung-volume reduction surgery. *New England Journal of Medicine*. 2001;**345**:1075–1083.

Oostenbrink JB, et al. One-year cost-effectiveness of tiotropium versus ipratropium to treat chronic obstructive pulmonary disease. *European Respiratory Journal*. 2004; **23**(2):241–249.

OPUS Study: Effect of roflumilast on exacerbation rate in patients with chronic obstructive pulmonary disease. http://clinicaltrials.gov/ct/show/NCT00076089?order=1, accessed March 7, 2005.

Orie NGM, et al. The host factor in bronchitis. In: Orie NGM, Sluiter JH, eds. *Bronchitis: an International Symposium*. Assen, Netherlands: Royal van Gorcum, 1961;43–59.

Paggiaro PL, et al. Multicentre randomised placebo-controlled trial of inhaled fluticasone propionate in patients with chronic obstructive pulmonary disease. International COPD Study Group. *Lancet*. 1998;**351**:773–780.

Patient Survey 1996, Statistics and Information Dept., Minister's Secretariat, Ministry of Health, Labor and Welfare. wwwdbtk.mhlw.go.jp/toukei/data/150/1996/gaikyou/0002480/g16.html.

Pauwels RA, et al. Long-term treatment with inhaled budesonide in persons with mild chronic obstructive pulmonary disease who continue smoking. *New England Journal of Medicine*. 1999;**340**:1948–1953.

Pauwels R, et al. Tiotropium: COPD exacerbations and decline in FEV1. The Annual Congress of the European Respiratory Society; September 22–26, 2001; Abstract 3252.

Petty TL. Definition, epidemiology, course, and prognosis of COPD. *Clin Cornerstone*. 2003;**5**(1):1–10.

Population Division of the Department of Economic and Social Affairs of the United Nations Secretariat. *World Population Prospects: The 2000 Revision*. Disk 2: Extensive Set (United Nations publication, Sales No. E.01.XIII.13), 2001.

Population Division of the Department of Economic and Social Affairs of the United Nations Secretariat. *World Population Prospects: The 2002 Revision*, vol. II, The Sex and Age Distribution of Populations (United Nations publication, Sales No. E.03.XIII.7), 2003.

Ram FS, Sestini P. Regular inhaled short acting beta$_2$ agonists for the management of stable chronic obstructive pulmonary disease: Cochrane systematic review and meta-analysis. *Thorax*. 2003;**58**:580–584.

Reisner C, et al. Cilomilast is efficacious in chronic obstructive pulmonary disease (COPD). European Respiratory Society, September 28, 2003. Abstract P530.

Rennard S, et al. Impact of COPD in North America and Europe in 2000: subjects' perspective of Confronting COPD International Survey. *European Respiratory Journal*. 2002;**20**(4):799–805.

Rennard SI, et al. Use of a long-acting inhaled B2-adrenergic agonist, salmeterol xinafoate, in patients with chronic obstructive pulmonary disease. *American Journal of Respiratory and Critical Care Medicine*. 2001;**163**:1087–1092.

Rennard SI. Pathogenesis of COPD. *Clin Cornerstone*. 2003;**5**(1):11–16.

Renwick DS, et al. Prevalence and treatment of chronic airways obstruction in adults over the age of 45 years. *Thorax*. 1996;**51**:164–168.

Roche N. Guidelines versus clinical practice in the treatment of chronic obstructive pulmonary disease. *European Respiratory Journal*. 2001;**18**:903–908.

Rossi A, et al. Comparison of the efficacy, tolerability, and safety of formoterol dry powder and oral, slow-release theophylline in the treatment of COPD. *Chest*. 2002;**121**:1058–1069.

Ryu JH, et al. Obstructive lung diseases: COPD, asthma, and many imitators. *Mayo Clinic Proceedings*. 2001;**76**:1144–1153.

Sethi JM, Rochester CL. Smoking and chronic obstructive pulmonary disease. *Clinics in Chest Medicine*. 2000;**21**:67–86.

Shapiro SD. The pathogenesis of emphysema: the elastase:antielastase hypothesis 30 years later. *Proc Assoc Am Physicians*. 1995;**107**:346–352.

Siafakas NM, et al. ERS Consensus Statement. Optimal assessment and management of chronic obstructive pulmonary disease (COPD). *European Respiratory Journal*. 1995;**8**:1398–1420.

Silverman EK, Speizer FE. Risk factors for the development of chronic obstructive pulmonary disease. *Med Clin North Am*. 1996;**80**:501–522.

Silverman EK. Genetic epidemiology of COPD. *Chest*. 2002;**121**(3 suppl):1S–6S.

SMi Conference presentation, PDE 4 Inhibitors, Second Chronic Obstructive Pulmonary Disease meeting, March 10, 2004, London, UK. www.smi-online.co.uk.

Sobradillo V, et al. Geographic variations in prevalence and underdiagnosis of COPD. *Chest*. 2000;**118**:981–989.

Stang P, et al. The prevalence of COPD: using smoking rates to estimate disease frequency in the general population. *Chest*. 2000;**117**:354S–359S.

Szafranski W, et al. Efficacy and safety of budesonide/formoterol in the management of chronic obstructive pulmonary disease. *European Respiratory Journal*. 2003;**21**(1):74–81.

Tarpy SP, Celli BR. Long-term oxygen therapy. *New England Journal of Medicine*. 1995;**333**:710–714.

Tashkin D, Kesten S. Long-term treatment benefits with tiotropium in COPD patients with an without short-term bronchodilator responses. *Chest*. 2003;**123**(5):1441–1449.

Tata LJ, et al. Does influenza vaccination increase consultations, corticosteroid prescriptions, or exacerbations in subjects with asthma or chronic obstructive pulmonary disease? *Thorax*. 2003;**58**:835–839.

Trofast J, et al. Steric aspects of agonism and antagonism at beta-adrenoreceptors: synthesis of and pharmacological experiments with the enantiomers of formoterol and their diastereomers. *Chirality*. 1991;**3**(6):443–450.

Ulrick CS. Efficacy of inhaled salmeterol in the management of smokers with chronic obstructive pulmonary disease: a single centre randomized, double blind, placebo controlled, crossover study. *Thorax*. 1995;**50**:750–754.

United Kingdom Department of Health (UKDOH). Statistics on Smoking: England, 2003. www.publications.doh.gov.uk/public/sb0321.htm. Accessed November 14, 2004.

U.S. Surgeon General. *The Health Consequences of Smoking—Chronic Obstructive Pulmonary Disease: A Report of the U.S. Surgeon General*. Washington, D.C.: U.S. Department of Health and Human Services; Publication No. 84-50205, 1984.

Van Grunsven P, et al. Short- and long-term efficacy of fluticasone proprionate in subjects with early signs and symptoms of chronic obstructive pulmonary disease. Results of the DIMCA study. *Respir Med*. 2003;**97**(12):1303–1312.

van Noord JA, et al. Long-term treatment of chronic obstructive pulmonary disease with salmeterol and the additive effect of ipratropium. *European Respiratory Journal*. 2000;**15**:878–885. [a]

van Noord JA, et al. A randomized controlled comparison of tiotropium and ipratropium in the treatment of chronic obstructive pulmonary disease. The Dutch tiotropium study group. *Thorax*. 2000;**55**:289–294. [b]

van Noord JA, et al. Comparison of once daily tiotropium, twice daily formoterol and the free combination, once daily, in patients with COPD [abstract]. *Am J Respir Crit Care Med*. 2003;**167**:A320.

van Noord JA, et al. Tiotropium maintenance therapy in patients with COPD and the 24-h spirometric benefit of adding once or twice daily formoterol during 2-week treatment periods. *American Thoracic Society Abstracts* [ATS Abstracts 2 View] May 2003; Abstract D82.

van Noord JA, et al. Tiotropium maintenance therapy in patients with COPD and the 24-h spirometric benefit of adding once or twice daily formoterol during 2-week treatment periods [abstract]. *Am J Respir Crit Care Med*. 2004;**167**:A95.

Vathenen AS, et al. High-dose inhaled albuterol in severe chronic airflow limitation. *The American Review of Respiratory Disease*. 1988;**138**:850–855.

Vestbo J, et al. Long-term effect of inhaled budesonide in mild and moderate chronic obstructive pulmonary disease: a randomised controlled trial. *Lancet*. 1999;**353**(9167): 1819–1823.

Viegi G, et al. Prevalence rates of respiratory symptoms in Italian general population samples exposed to different levels of air pollution. *Environmental Health Perspectives*. 1991;**94**:95–99.

Viegi G, et al. Prevalence rates of respiratory symptoms and diseases in general population samples of North and Central Italy. *International Journal of Tuberculosis and Lung Diseases*. 1999;**3**:1034–1042.

Viegi G, et al. Prevalence of airways obstruction in a general population: European Respiratory Society vs. American Thoracic Society definition. *Chest*. 2000;**117**:339S–345S.

Viegi G, et al. Epidemiology of chronic obstructive pulmonary disease (COPD). *Respiration*. 2001;**68**:4–19.

Vincken W, et al. Improved health outcomes in patients with COPD during one year's treatment with tiotropium. *European Respiratory Journal*. 2002;**19**:209–216.

von Hertzen L, et al. Airway obstruction in relation to symptoms in chronic respiratory disease—a nationally representative population study. *Respiratory Medicine*. 2000;**94**:356–363.

Wadbo M, et al. Effects of formoterol and ipratropium bromide in COPD: a 3-month placebo-controlled study. *European Respiratory Journal*. 2002;**20**(5):1138–1146.

Wagena EJ, et al. The efficacy of smoking cessation strategies in people with chronic obstructive pulmonary disease: results from a systematic review. *Respir Med*. 2004; **98**(9):805–815.

Wouters EFM. Economic analysis of the Confronting COPD survey: an overview of results. *Respiratory Medicine*. 2003;**97**:S3–S14.

Wouters EFM et al. One year withdrawal of fluticasone after three months treatment with combined salmeterol/fluticasone in COPD: results of the COSMIC study. American Thoracic Society Annual Conference, May 25. 2004; poster 515.

Yano E, et al. Health effects of volcanic ash: a repeat study. *Archives of Environmental Health*. 1990;**45**:367.

GASTROINTESTINAL

Irritable Bowel Syndrome

ETIOLOGY AND PATHOPHYSIOLOGY

Introduction

Irritable bowel syndrome (IBS) is a functional gastrointestinal (GI) disorder of the intestines that is associated with abdominal pain, disturbed defecation (constipation/diarrhea), and/or bloatedness. The condition is the most common disorder that gastroenterologists diagnose and one regularly encountered in general practice (Camilleri M, 2001). However, despite the high prevalence of IBS, the condition's etiology and pathophysiology remain poorly characterized, making development of agents to relieve patients' symptoms a daunting task for the pharmaceutical industry. Few notable breakthroughs have been made in therapy for IBS patients in the last decade, with the exception of the 5-HT receptor modulator class. To fully comprehend the scientific knowledge regarding altered GI motility and increased visceral sensitivity in IBS, it is essential to outline the basic structures of the GI tract and the innervation of these structures, as discussed in the next section.

Wiley Handbook of Current and Emerging Drug Therapies, Volumes 5–8
Copyright © 2007 Decision Resources, Inc. Published by John Wiley & Sons, Inc.

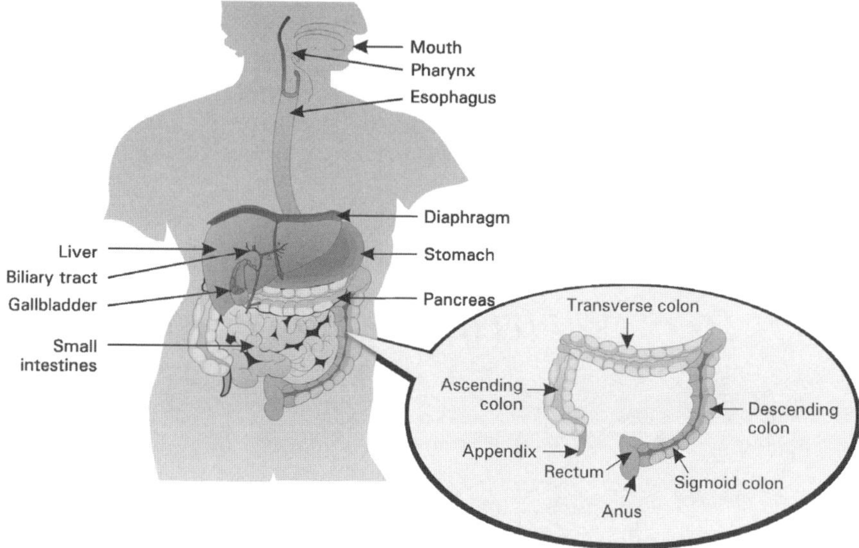

FIGURE 1. *The gastrointestinal system.*

Anatomy

Structures of the Gastrointestinal Tract. The GI tract consists of the alimentary canal (from the mouth to the anus) and glandular organs that secrete digestive substances into the canal. Figure 1 illustrates the major constituent organs of the GI tract. The organs of interest in the study of IBS are the small and large intestines. After food has been mechanically ground and mixed with gastric fluids, the resulting chyme is pushed into the small intestine. The small intestine consists of three segments—the duodenum, the jejunum, and the ileum—and its main role is to break down food and absorb nutrients. Biliary and pancreatic secretions mix with food in the duodenum, further digesting the material already mixed with gastric fluids. Food then passes into the jejunum, where the majority of digestion and absorption occurs. Through the extensive multilayered and folded surface of the jejunal mucosa, nutrients, water, ions, and enzymes are absorbed from the digested material into the bloodstream. The ileum then retrieves certain water-soluble vitamins and secretes hormones that influence further GI activity.

Unused material then enters the large intestine (also called the colon) through the ileocecal valve, which allows only one-way transit of material, blocking colonic bacteria from entering the small intestine. The large intestine consists of four segments: the ascending, transverse, descending, and sigmoid colons. The colonic phase of digestion is responsible for further reabsorption of water and ions, and the process usually reduces 2 L of content down to 200 mL each day. Waste material resulting from this process moves through the colon into the rectum, where the increased intralumenal pressure stimulates the urge to defecate.

The small and large intestines both accomplish the task of digestion through two types of smooth-muscle contractions: (1) segmenting contractions, which mix lumenal contents, and (2) propagating contractions, which move material through the intestine. These contractions are created by the multilayered musculature of both organs. In both intestines, layers of smooth muscle are arranged to constrict the intestinal circumference and shorten intestinal length upon contraction. Figure 2 shows a cross section of the intestinal walls, including musculature and innervation.

Innervation of the Gastrointestinal Tract. The autonomic nervous system, which controls all involuntary body systems, regulates the contractility of smooth muscle in the GI tract. Three components of the autonomic nervous system—the sympathetic, parasympathetic, and enteric nervous systems—are the primary instigators of intestinal contractions.

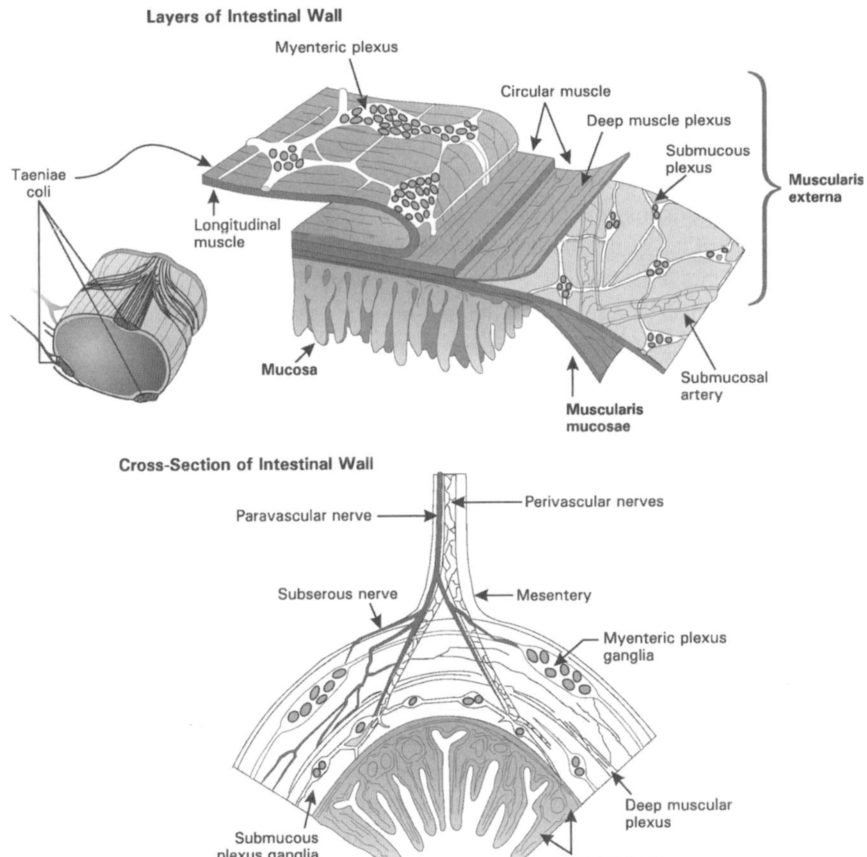

FIGURE 2. *Musculature and innervation of intestinal walls.*

The sympathetic nervous system is generally responsible for accelerating or intensifying bodily functions, as in the "fight or flight" response to stress, but it works to slow GI function during stress. Sympathetic system nerves release adrenergic neurotransmitters, mainly epinephrine and norepinephrine. The parasympathetic nervous system works in opposition to the sympathetic system. Through release of the neurotransmitter acetylcholine, the parasympathetic system slows most bodily activities while increasing GI activity.

The third component of the GI-related autonomic system is the enteric nervous system (ENS), or "brain in the gut." This network of neurons permeates the organs of the GI tract and resembles the brain in many ways. It is protected by a blood-myenteric barrier akin to the blood–brain barrier, and the ENS neurons are the same types (sensory neurons, interneurons, and motor neurons) found in the brain. Also, chemical regulation of the ENS is accomplished with the same neurotransmitters and neuropeptides found in the central nervous system (CNS). The ENS controls smooth-muscle contraction, blood flow, transport of water and nutrients, and fluid secretion from the GI tract.

The neural cells of the ENS are found in ganglia within the walls of the digestive tract, organized into ganglionated plexuses. Two plexuses are predominant in the ENS: (1) the myenteric (Auerbach's) plexus, which is found between the longitudinal and circular muscle layers of GI organs, and (2) the submucosal plexus, which is found mainly in the small and large intestines and is sandwiched between the circular musculature and the mucosa.

The neural transmission lines between the ENS and the CNS constitute the brain-gut axis. The sympathetic, parasympathetic, and enteric nervous systems communicate via bidirectional traffic; that is, signals from the brain cause GI activity, and sensory input from the gut is sent back to the brain. Via these neural pathways, external and cognitive stimuli can affect GI motility, sensation, and secretion. Conversely, visceral activity can affect mood, behavior, and the perception of pain. Figure 3 depicts a heuristic model of the brain-gut axis.

The ENS communicates with higher brain centers (e.g., the hypothalamus, cerebral cortex) responsible for regulating GI function. Although the brain is responsible for initiating numerous GI functions, the ENS has a stand-alone capability that allows it to control GI function independently. The integrated ENS circuitry has a library of "programs" that it can employ for basic GI function. ENS-controlled functions in the intestines include power propulsion (large movements of material) toward the anus, postprandial mixing, and oral-directed movement (vomiting) of food in response to intestinal distress.

Much of the brain-gut communication that controls GI function is managed through endogenous chemicals. The nerves of the ENS react primarily to acetylcholine, as well as to other excitatory transmitters such as tachykinins, substance P (neurokinin A), serotonin (5-HT), neuropeptide K, and neuropeptide gamma. Inhibitory transmitters (those that slow GI function and neurons' receptivity) include nitric oxide, adenosine triphosphate (ATP), and vasoactive intestinal protein (VIP).

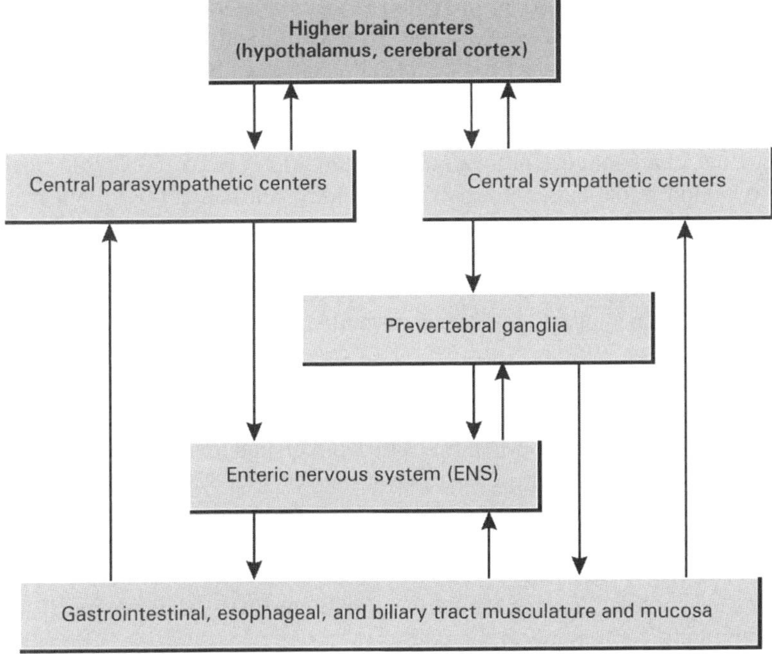

FIGURE 3. *Heuristic model of the brain-gut axis.*

Pathophysiology

IBS patients clearly exhibit disordered motor patterns throughout the GI tract, particularly in the small and large intestines. Although past and current research points to an association between IBS symptoms and abnormal contractility, a causal link has not yet been definitively established. Because abnormal contractility has not yet been clearly linked with symptoms, and because IBS patients often experience pain during normal motor activity, researchers also have looked at a hyperalgesic (heightened sensitivity to pain) model to explain abdominal pain in IBS. These two models are discussed in the following sections.

Altered Gastrointestinal Motility. In the large intestine (or colon), three types of myoelectric activity regulate the contraction of smooth muscle. First, slow waves regulate the frequencies of phasic contractions. Second, spike potentials elevate the membrane potential above the threshold needed for contraction. Spike potentials can be either of two types: short spike bursts (SSBs), which last 5–15 seconds in phase with slow waves, or long spike bursts (LSBs), which last up to a minute and are unrelated to slow waves. Both types of spike bursts trigger segmenting contractions, and LSBs also produce some propagating contractions in both the oral and anal directions. The third myoelectric pattern is high-amplitude contraction, called the giant migrating contraction, which occurs once or twice daily and facilitates mass movements of feces and defecation.

Research reveals that, when the colon is unstimulated (i.e., in a fasting state), no clear difference exists between the myoelectric activity in IBS patients and that in people without IBS. The stimulated colon normally exhibits spike potential and contractile activity 10 minutes after ingestion of a meal, and such activity usually ceases within 50–60 minutes. In IBS patients, however, rectosigmoid contractions can continue for up to three hours after a meal. This prolongation is more common in patients with diarrhea-predominant IBS (D-IBS), but it is also seen in patients with constipation-predominant IBS (C-IBS). IBS patients also exhibit myoelectric activity in the colon after a sham feeding (when patients are made to believe they will receive a meal but are denied food at the last moment). This phenomenon suggests that the abnormal contractions may have their origin in the CNS control centers.

The role of abnormal myoelectric and motor activity in the small intestine in the pathogenesis of IBS symptoms is less clear than that of abnormal colonic activity. The small intestine exhibits three motor patterns: (1) migrating motor complexes (MMCs), which occur cyclically every 90–120 minutes in both the stomach and small intestine, and which clear the gut of undigested debris; (2) discrete clustered contractions (DCCs), which are bursts of phasic contractions every minute; and (3) prolonged propagating contractions (PPCs), which are intense ileal contractions that empty the small intestine's contents, much like the giant migrating contraction in the colon.

Some IBS patients exhibit postprandial (following a meal) MMC abnormalities. In this subset of patients, MMCs occur more frequently in D-IBS patients and are of weaker intensity in C-IBS patients. Some motility studies have shown that abnormal small intestine contractions correlate with abdominal pain (Evans PR, 1996), but such results have not been satisfactorily duplicated.

Visceral Sensitivity. The distension and contraction of the GI tract that accompany digestion occur below the threshold of perception. Normally, pain in the gut registers only when it reaches a point that reflects significant risk of damage to tissue or organs. IBS patients, however, have heightened visceral sensitivity, and they experience abdominal pain in response to normal gut stimuli.

IBS patients also complain of visceral pain when the GI tract is unstimulated. The MMCs of the small intestine occur cyclically, even during the fasting state, and people without IBS are rarely aware of their occurrence. Research has shown that nearly half of IBS patients experience discomfort during postprandial and fasting-state MMCs. In the large intestine, fasting-state SSB activity is associated with abdominal pain in C-IBS patients (Kellow JE, 1999).

Researchers have proposed several mechanisms to explain abnormal visceral sensitivity in IBS patients. Altered receptor sensitivity in the gut is one likely cause. Neurogastroenterologic studies suggest that such altered sensitivity may occur when the ENS "recruits" silent nociceptors. These receptors register pain in the GI tract when it reaches the thresholds that indicate trauma, such as severe distension or perforation, as opposed to normal function. In IBS patients, silent nociceptors may function constantly and react to stimuli that are below the normal threshold.

Increased excitability of the GI neural system is another possible explanation for enhanced pain perception in IBS patients. Studies have found that repeated balloon distension of the colon produces hypersensitivity during subsequent inflations. The locus of hypersensitivity is the dorsal horn neurons in the spine and brain stem, suggesting that the afferent pathways are to blame for the phenomenon. More recent experimental results also implicate the afferent pathways in the pelvis. Two types of afferent fibers populate this region: 75–80% of fibers respond to all distending pressures and do not inform the CNS of painful stimuli; the remaining 20–25% respond to high-intensity distending pressures, which are usually encoded as pain. Repeated colonic distension causes both low- and high-intensity receptor fibers to be activated at low distension pressures, resulting in symptoms of pain. Researchers still do not understand why the high-intensity fibers become hyperactivated during repeated distension.

Altered CNS modulation is the third major hypothesis used to explain hyperalgesia in IBS. The CNS and ENS communicate bidirectionally; the gut acts on CNS commands and then relays information back to the CNS, influencing subsequent input from the brain. The disappearance of IBS symptoms during sleep and the increase of propagating contraction velocity shortly after awakening support the role of abnormal CNS modulation. Evaluation of cerebral activity using positron-emission tomography (PET) scans has also differentiated IBS patients from normal subjects. Rectal balloon inflation normally produces activity in the anterior cingulate cortex, but in IBS patients, the prefrontal cortex becomes activated. Abnormal CNS activity may be explained by psychopathology; the areas of the prefrontal cortex activated in IBS patients are also responsible for hypervigilance (excessive attention paid to normal bodily functions) and anxiety.

Etiology

Given researchers' incomplete understanding of any physiological abnormalities underlying IBS, it should come as no surprise that the causes of the disorder are not well established. However, some theories have come to the fore as possible etiological mechanisms, including those that are outlined in the following sections.

Psychopathology. Historically, IBS has been treated as an affliction of hypochondriacs; little attention was given to comorbid psychiatric conditions. As the interplay between the CNS and ENS became better known, however, the psychopathology of IBS emerged as an area of interest. Some research has shown a correlation between IBS and comorbid psychiatric disorders. One study found that a lifetime history of major psychiatric illness was present in 94% of IBS patients, and more than 80% were psychiatrically ill at the time of the study, most with anxiety and mood disorders (Lydiard NB, 1993). However, the data on causal links are contradictory. Part of the difficulty in establishing the psychopathology of IBS is the "chicken or egg" phenomenon. Studies have not been able thus far to conclude whether psychiatric illnesses predate or emerge simultaneously with the development of IBS, or if IBS predisposes patients to subsequent development of psychiatric illness.

Most theoretical models describing the psychopathology of IBS can be reduced to a "vicious circle." In IBS patients, stress to the GI tract causes activation of areas of the brain not activated in normal individuals. These areas, such as the prefrontal cortex and locus ceruleus, are highly associated with anxiety and mood disorders. The preexistence of psychiatric disorders potentially causes hyperreactivity of these areas, and they then may overstimulate the gut in response.

In addition to defined psychiatric disorders, chronic and/or severe stress affects symptom intensity in IBS. Research has found that IBS patients report more stressful events, more changes in stool pattern relating to stress, and higher reactivity to stress than do controls. One study also showed that 60–66% of IBS patients had experienced stressful life events prior to onset of the condition, compared with 25% of controls (Creed FH, 1988). Stress also seems to prolong the duration of IBS episodes, according to a 16-month longitudinal study in Australia. A majority (76%) of clinical outcomes were dependent on stress during the 16-month follow-up period, exposure to one or more stressors produced no clinical improvement in symptoms, and exposure to no stressors correlated with improved symptoms (Bennett EJ, 1998).

The high incidence of posttraumatic stress disorder (PTSD) in IBS patients has led to study of a possible link between IBS and abuse. The association between prior physical and/or sexual abuse and IBS was first demonstrated in a 1990 study (Drossman DA, 1993). Among IBS patients in a referral gastroenterology practice, the incidence of physical/sexual abuse was 50%. However, other researchers argued that the link between IBS and a history of abuse was largely explained by psychological factors (Talley NJ, 1998). When the researchers controlled for neuroticism and psychiatric disorders, they found no correlation between prior and/or current abuse and IBS.

Postinfectious Irritable Bowel Syndrome. One area of research that has garnered renewed attention is the role of infectious enteritis in the development of IBS. Although a recent history of acute infectious diarrhea preceding the onset of IBS symptoms is not common to all patients, an association has been found in approximately one-third of patients across studies. In prospective studies of patients with infectious diarrhea, researchers have found increased risk of developing IBS symptoms (relative risk 6.6–10.1) in the year postinfection (Ilnyckyj A, 1999; Parry SD, 2002). A small study of 38 patients involved in two outbreaks of salmonella food poisoning found similar results: 12 patients (32%) had persisting bowel symptoms 12 months after the acute infection (McKendrick MW, 1994).

Several hypotheses have been put forth to explain the link between acute GI infections and the development of IBS. Because some studies have found an increased risk of IBS associated with increased severity of GI infection, some researchers believe higher degrees of mucosal permeation may be at fault. The more invasive the organism, the more likely that damage to mucosal nerves will occur. Another possible explanation is a residual inflammatory response, such as was found in one study of patients following acute campylobacter infection (Spiller RC, 2000). The treatment of GI infections may also be to blame—some researchers contend that antibiotics alter the gut flora and predispose patients to bowel dysfunction.

Inflammatory Mediators. Inflammation of the intestines has been shown to cause changes in GI motility and the excitability of ENS neurons. When intestinal inflammation occurs, levels of substance P increase and levels of acetylcholine and noradrenaline decrease, reducing muscle contractility. Early research into possible the inflammatory pathogenesis of IBS included one study that found IBS-like symptoms expressed in inflammatory bowel disease (IBD) patients in remission (Isgar B, 1983). More recent work has found evidence of increased mast cells in IBS patients' colons (O'Sullivan M, 2000), and full-thickness biopsies of the jejunum of IBS patients uncovered low-grade infiltration of lymphocytes in the myenteric plexus in nine of ten patients (Törnblom H, 2002).

Two general theories attempt to explain inflammation's role in IBS. First, inflammatory processes themselves may be at fault, as in the proposed role of mast cells in the small and large intestine. Mast cells identify and "remember" toxic substances, and they play a key role in allergic GI reactions. If such cells are either too numerous or too active in the GI tract of IBS patients, they may stimulate allergic responses to otherwise normal stimuli.

The second theory is that residual damage to the gut prompts the development of IBS in the postinflammatory period. In the jejunal biopsy study mentioned earlier, for example, IBS patients all showed evidence of neuronal degeneration that could have a perpetuating effect on ENS signaling and thereby influence IBS symptoms. This hypothesis has also been put forth to explain the data showing a 25–30% overlap between IBS and celiac disease patients. The latter suffer from gluten intolerance that, through an inflammatory process in the small intestine, causes GI symptoms similar to D-IBS. A study screened D-IBS patients for serum and duodenal markers of celiac disease and found 30–35% expressed antibodies that are markers for latent/potential celiac disease (Wahnschaffe U, 2001). Because patients with latent disease generally do not have active celiac disease symptoms but do show evidence of inflammatory damage in the GI tract, these results may point to a subset of IBS patients who have developed postinflammation abnormalities resulting from celiac disease.

CURRENT THERAPIES

No cure is available for irritable bowel syndrome (IBS), but symptoms can often be effectively managed by educating the patient about the condition and suggesting dietary modifications, with or without introducing pharmacological therapy. Available pharmacotherapy for IBS is intended primarily to restore normal bowel function and reduce abdominal pain. Some patients clearly have one predominant motility symptom (diarrhea [D-IBS] or constipation [C-IBS]); others have mixed motility symptoms (M-IBS) that can make the design of a treatment regimen difficult. Some commonly used agents for the treatment of IBS, such as antidiarrheals and laxatives, are available over-the-counter (OTC) as well as in prescription formulations. Prior to consulting a physician, many patients attempt to manage their condition through self-medication with OTC therapies.

This section outlines the principal drug classes used in the treatment of IBS (5-HT receptor modulators, laxatives, antidiarrheals, antispasmodics, and antidepressants). Table 1 summarizes the most commonly used agents within these classes. Nonpharmacological approaches to the treatment of IBS are also available in the seven major pharmaceutical markets (United States, France, Germany, Italy, Spain, United Kingdom, and Japan). In some patients, the psychological nature of IBS (some research has shown a correlation between IBS and comorbid psychiatric disorders) requires the use of psychological therapies, including cognitive-behavioral therapy and hypnosis. Generally, these treatment approaches are used in a minority of patients with severe refractory disease; therefore, they are not discussed further here.

5-HT Receptor Modulators

Overview. The majority of the body's serotonin (5-hydroxytryptamine, 5-HT) is found in the gastrointestinal (GI) tract. When the large intestine is distended by digested material, release of serotonin stimulates the peristaltic reflex. At least five subtypes of serotonin receptors are present throughout the GI organs. Because serotonin binds differently to each subtype, the same chemical can produce multiple effects in the gut. The receptor subtypes of most interest in IBS research are 5-HT_3 and 5-HT_4 receptors. 5-HT_3 receptors are located on the enteric nervous system (ENS) neurons throughout the GI tract and on the ends of afferent neurons that transmit signals from the gut to the central nervous system (CNS). Serotonin acting on these receptors is excitatory, so it enhances motility and visceral sensation.

Agents targeting the 5-HT_3 receptor include alosetron (GlaxoSmithKline's [Brentford, Middlesex, United Kingdom] Lotronex), ondansetron (GlaxoSmithKline's Zofran), and granisetron (Roche's [Basel, Switzerland] Kytrill). However, despite the use of ondansetron and granisetron as antiemetics in the United States for several years, only alosetron has FDA approval for IBS because of the more comprehensive clinical trial data for this agent (Michoki RJ, 2000). 5-HT_4 receptors are also excited when bound to serotonin, but they are mostly located in neurons in smooth muscle. They are found throughout the GI tract's musculature as well as in cardiac smooth muscle. Tegaserod (Novartis's [Basel, Switzerland] Zelmac/Zelnorm) is currently the only marketed 5-HT_4 modulator for IBS.

Mechanism of Action. Agents in the 5-HT receptor modulator class stimulate or inhibit the activity of 5-HT receptors in the gut, reducing visceral pain sensations and altering intestinal transit in IBS patients.

TABLE 1. Current Therapies Used for Irritable Bowel Syndrome

Agent	Company/Brand	Daily Dose	Availability
5-HT receptor modulators			
Alosetron	GlaxoSmithKline's Lotronex	2 mg	US
Tegaserod	Novartis's Zelmac/Zelnorm	12 mg	US
Laxatives			
Fiber			
Psyllium	Procter & Gamble's Metamucil/Regulan, generics	2–15 g	US, F, G, I, S, UK
Methylcellulose	GlaxoSmithKline's Citrucel, Edigen's Muciplasma, generics	15–30 g	US, S, UK, J
Calcium	Wyeth's FiberCon, Numark	1–5 g	US, F, G, I, S, UK, J
polycarbophil	Laboratories' Equalactin, generics		
Osmotics			
Lactulose	Solvay's Duphalac/Bifiteral, generics	10–40 g	US, F, G, I, S, UK, J
Polyethylene glycol	Braintree's Miralax, Norgine's	17 g	US, F, G, I, S, UK
(PEG)	Klean-prep		
Motor stimulants			
Senna	Purdue Fredrick's Senokot, Woelm's Depuran, generics	20–60 mg	US, F, G, I, S, UK, J
Bisacodyl	Novartis/Boehringer Ingelheim's Dulcolax, generics	5–15 mg	US, F, G, I, S, UK, J
Sodium picosulfate	Boehringer Ingelheim's Laxoberal, Omegin's Darmel Pico	6–10 mg	G, I, J
Antidiarrheals			
Loperamide	McNeil's Imodium, Janssen-Cilag's Linguial, generics	8–16 mg	US, F, G, I, S, UK, J
Diphenoxylate	Pfizer's Lomotil, Sanofi-Synthélabo's Diarsed, generics	15–20 mg	US, F, S, UK
Antispasmodics			
Anticholinergics			
Hyoscyamine sulfate	Schwarz Pharma's Levsin, Boehringer Ingelheim's Buscopan, generics	1.10–2.25 mg	US, G, I, S, UK, J
Dicyclomine	Aventis's Bentyl, Florizel's Merbentyl, generics	30–120 mg	US, UK, J
Cimetropium bromide	Yamanouchi's Alginor	100–150 mg	I
Calcium-channel blockers			
Pinaverium bromide	Solvay's Dicetel/Edicet	450 mg	F, I, S
Other antispasmodics			

(continued overleaf)

TABLE 1. (continued)

Agent	Company/Brand	Daily Dose	Availability
Mebeverine	Solvay's Duspatalin/Colofac, generics	400–800 mg	F, G, I, S, UK
Trimebutine	Pfizer/Sigma Tau's Debridat, generics	600 mg	F, I, S, J
Antidepressants			
Tricyclic antidepressants			
Imipramine	Novartis/Mallinckrodt's Tofranil, generics	100 mg maximum	US, F, G, I, S, UK, J
Amitriptyline	AstraZeneca's Elavil, Roche's Laroxyl, generics	75 mg maximum	US, F, G, I, S, UK, J
Desipramine	Novartis's Pertofan, Aventis's Nopramin, generics	100 mg maximum	US, F, G, I
Selective serotonin reuptake inhibitors			
Fluoxetine	Eli Lilly's Prozac, generics	10 mg	US, F, G, I, S, UK
Paroxetine	GlaxoSmithKline's Paxil	10 mg	US, F, G, I, S, UK, J
Sertraline	Pfizer's Zoloft	50 mg	US, F, G, I, S, UK

US = United States; F = France; G = Germany; I = Italy; S = Spain; UK = United Kingdom; J = Japan.

FIGURE 4. Structure of alosetron (X = N).

Alosetron. Alosetron (GlaxoSmithKline's Lotronex) (Figure 4), an orally active 5-HT receptor modulator, was approved for the treatment of IBS in March 2000 in the United States for use only in women with diarrhea-predominant IBS (D-IBS). However, in November 2000, it was withdrawn from the market following well-publicized reports of ischemic colitis and five related deaths. In late 2002, alosetron was reintroduced in the United States under an extensive risk management program that requires the participation of physicians, patients, and pharmacists and calls for several additional safety and efficacy studies. The agent is available for specific use in female patients with severe D-IBS. Further development of the drug has been discontinued in all of the other major markets, although alosetron could potentially become available outside the United States, following an initial period of monitoring (Lembo A, 2003).

Alosetron selectively antagonizes 5-HT$_3$ receptors, leading to a slowing of gastric motility and providing relief for patients with D-IBS. The agent also reduces the transmission of afferent signals from the gut to the brain. Selective 5-HT$_3$ antagonists are the most efficacious of the 5-HT receptor modulators against visceral pain.

Early clinical investigations revealed a heightened efficacy of alosetron in women; hence, large-scale clinical investigations have enrolled women only. One preliminary investigation involving 622 male patients did show a significant improvement in IBS symptoms based on treatment with 1 mg alosetron, given twice daily, compared with placebo; however, efficacy has not been investigated further in the male population (Lembo A, 2003).

Trials have focused on females because of the availability of positive data to support further investigations and because this group has a high prevalence of IBS (Lembo A, 2003). In May 1999, during Digestive Disease Week, data were presented from two large-scale, multicenter, randomized, double-blind, placebo-controlled trials conducted in the United States. Women with D-IBS were given 1 mg alosetron twice daily for 12 weeks. The results of one of these trials were published in early 2000. The agent demonstrated moderate efficacy against diarrhea in IBS patients, although a significant placebo effect was observed: 41% of patients receiving alosetron reported adequate relief of abdominal pain and discomfort at 12 weeks, compared with 29% of the placebo group (Camilleri M, 2000). Alosetron also increased stool firmness and significantly reduced urgency and stool frequency in treated patients.

A trial involving 801 women with D-IBS who had unsatisfactory control over bowel urgency found that alosetron improved control (Lembo T, 2001). The patients were randomized to receive either 1 mg of alosetron or placebo twice daily for 12 weeks. On completion of the trial, the patients treated with alosetron had a significantly greater number of days with satisfactory control of bowel urgency compared with those on placebo. In addition, a significantly higher percentage of patients treated with alosetron (76%) showed overall improvement in IBS symptoms compared with those on placebo (44%).

A European trial compared alosetron with the commonly used smooth-muscle relaxant mebeverine (Solvay's [Brussels, Belgium] generics) in the relief of IBS symptoms (Jones RH, 1999). The study enrolled 623 women with D-IBS who received either alosetron (1 mg, twice daily) or mebeverine (135 mg, three times daily) for 12 weeks. In the third month, 58% of the patients taking alosetron reported pain-free days compared with 48% on mebeverine. Alosetron recipients also had fewer days with urgency and reduced mean stool frequency, and they had increased firmness of stool. This study has been criticized for using only half the normal daily dose of mebeverine.

Constipation is the most commonly reported adverse side effect with alosetron treatment, occurring in 20–30% of patients receiving therapy. However, it is the development of more sinister side effects such as ischemic colitis that have led to the agent's limited availability and use. The incidence of ischemic colitis was 1:750 in clinical investigations; in each case, patients recovered without significant complications (Lembo A, 2003). However, in November 2000, at the time of the drug's withdrawal from the market, 84 cases of ischemic colitis had been reported, and 2 deaths occurred; 54 of these patients required hospitalization and 11 required surgery. Three deaths from small bowel ischemia were also attributed to the drug. Most importantly, this agent causes fatalities without much of a warning signal (Moynihan R, 2002).

Following reapproval, as part of the risk management plan for alosetron, physicians who intend to prescribe the agent must participate in a program that requires them to self-test their ability to diagnose and treat IBS and recognize and manage complications of constipation and ischemic colitis. Pharmacists can distribute bottles of only 30 tablets at one time, during which time the physician must assess the patient's response. If the patient fails to respond to therapy within four weeks, no further medication is provided. These restrictions make alosetron a highly inconvenient therapy for both patient and physician. The risk management program for alosetron also requires GlaxoSmithKline to conduct Phase IV postmarketing studies to further test the drug's safety and efficacy. The randomized, double-blind, placebo-controlled studies will evaluate the effect of lower doses of alosetron and assess its use specifically during episodes of diarrhea on an as-needed basis.

Tegaserod. Tegaserod (Novartis's Zelmac/Zelnorm), another orally active 5-HT receptor partial agonist, has been developed in the United States and Europe for the treatment of C-IBS. The agent is also being developed for the potential treatment of other functional GI disorders, such as gastroesophageal reflux disease (GERD), chronic constipation, and functional dyspepsia. In February 2000, Novartis submitted an approval request for tegaserod to the FDA and the European Agency for the Evaluation of Medicinal Products (EMEA). In June 2000, the FDA's Gastrointestinal Drugs Advisory Committee recommended tegaserod for treating female IBS patients. However, one year later, the FDA issued a nonapprovable letter, citing concerns about the rate of abdominal surgeries in tegaserod-treated patients. Novartis appealed the FDA's decision and successfully argued that the small increase was not related to the drug. In July 2002, the FDA approved tegaserod for the short-term (12-week) treatment of women with IBS.

Tegaserod's development in Europe also faltered when Novartis voluntarily withdrew its marketing submission to the EMEA in May 2001. Reportedly, the EMEA's Committee for Proprietary Medicinal Products (CPMP) was not convinced of the drug's efficacy and expressed concern about the methodology used in some preclinical trials. Clinical investigations are under way to support European approval of this agent. Novartis began recruitment of 2,500 C-IBS female patients in late 2002 for a multinational clinical study that will compare tegaserod treatment with placebo during two four-week treatment periods separated by a treatment-free period of 2–12 weeks.

Tegaserod is a 5-HT$_4$ receptor partial agonist that binds with high affinity to human 5-HT$_4$ receptors. By acting as an agonist at neuronal 5-HT$_4$ receptors, the compound triggers the release of further neurotransmitters, such as calcitonin gene-related peptide, from sensory neurons in the GI tract, stimulating the peristaltic reflex and intestinal secretion as well as inhibiting visceral sensitivity.

Several large-scale clinical studies have assessed tegaserod's efficacy. One randomized, double-blind, multicenter study investigated the safety and efficacy of tegaserod in 1,519 women with C-IBS (Novick J, 2002). Patients were randomized to receive either 6 mg tegaserod twice daily ($n = 767$) or placebo ($n = 752$) daily for 12 weeks. Efficacy was evaluated by the Subject's Global Assessment of Relief (SGA), which measures patients' overall well-being and their symptoms of abdominal pain, discomfort, and constipation. The tegaserod-treated group experienced relief of IBS symptoms, as measured by significant improvements in SGA, compared with those on placebo. Mild, transient diarrhea was the only adverse event reported (6.4% tegaserod, 2.9% placebo).

A 12-week randomized, double-blind, multicenter study involving 801 patients with C-IBS investigated doses of 2 mg and 6 mg tegaserod twice daily versus placebo (Müller-Lissner SA, 2001[b]). Patients treated with tegaserod showed statistically significant relief of overall IBS symptoms (12.7% in the 2 mg group and 11.8% in the 6 mg group). Individual IBS symptoms assessed daily also showed significant improvement. Investigators noted that the tegaserod-treated patients experienced a reduction in abdominal pain/discomfort, an increase in the number of bowel movements, an improvement in stool consistency, and a reduction in the number of days with significant bloating. The incidence of adverse events in this study was similar in both groups, although patients treated with tegaserod experienced transient diarrhea more frequently than did those receiving placebo.

Studies of tegaserod have been carried out primarily in Western populations. One large-scale study investigated the agent in 520 patients with C-IBS in the Asia/Pacific region (Kellow J, 2003). Patients were randomized to receive 6 mg of tegaserod ($n = 259$) or placebo ($n = 261$) twice daily for 12 weeks. The study's primary end point was relief of IBS symptoms. The mean proportion of patients with overall satisfactory relief of symptoms was significantly greater in the tegaserod group (62%) than in the placebo group (44%). Clinically relevant effects of the drug were seen as early as one week into the study. Headache was the common side effect associated with tegaserod treatment. Also, significantly more patients in the tegaserod group experienced diarrhea than did those in the placebo group.

A 12-month study assessed tegaserod's long-term tolerability (Tougas G, 2002). The multicenter, open-label study was conducted with flexible dose titration of tegaserod in outpatients with C-IBS. Of 579 C-IBS patients treated with tegaserod, 304 completed the trial. The most common adverse events, attributable to tegaserod at any dose, were mild and transient diarrhea (10.1%), headache (8.3%), abdominal pain (7.4%), and flatulence (5.5%). Twenty-five patients (4.4%) reported serious adverse events, which led to discontinuation by six patients, and one patient suffered from acute abdominal pain that was attributed to tegaserod. No other tegaserod-related side effects were detected.

One of the FDA's primary reasons for initially rejecting tegaserod's approval was concern about the increased rate of abdominal surgeries in tegaserod- versus placebo-treated patients. In the clinical trial data submitted by Novartis to the

FDA, 0.3% of tegaserod-treated patients underwent abdominal surgery, compared with 0.2% of the placebo group. The most common procedure was gallbladder surgery (cholecystectomy), performed on 0.2% and 0.1% of patients receiving tegaserod and placebo, respectively. As one of the conditions of approval, the FDA has asked Novartis to conduct further studies regarding both the intermittent and long-term use of tegaserod.

The FDA has evaluated data from postmarketing surveillance of tegaserod and, in response, has updated the labeling of the product. Warnings about the potential for severe diarrhea, which state that a small number of patients (0.04%) experience clinically significant diarrhea while taking the product, are now included. The label's precautions section also has a note on ischemic colitis and other forms of intestinal ischemia; however, the label states that no causal link between such conditions and tegaserod has been found. Novartis highlights that the number of probable ischemic colitis cases (16) reported in postmarketing surveillance for tegaserod is in line with the expected incidence of ischemic colitis in the general population, reported as 4.5–44 per 100 000 people (Higgens PD, 2004).

Laxatives

Overview. Laxatives are commonly used to relieve constipation in patients with IBS. Because of its safety, efficacy, and low cost, fiber is often used as a first-line laxative therapy. Patients can increase their dietary fiber intake or take fiber supplements. Sources of dietary fiber include fruits, vegetables, and whole grains. Some high-fiber foods (particularly those containing bran fiber) can cause gas and bloating, so patients may opt for less flatulogenic fiber-rich foods, such as potatoes. Several fiber supplements are readily available OTC for treating IBS. The most commonly used supplements are soluble fibers (bran, psyllium, pectin) and insoluble fibers (methylcellulose, calcium polycarbophil). Given the small sample sizes and a large placebo effect (60–70% of patients in control groups have responded favorably to placebo), controlled studies involving fiber have generally failed to clarify its therapeutic effect in the overall IBS population (Camilleri M, 2002). Regardless, physicians recommend increased fiber intake for the majority of IBS patients. No one form of fiber has proved more efficacious than another in treating IBS in clinical studies, so the choice of agent is usually left to patient preference based on palatability and side effects.

Stronger laxative agents such as the osmotic laxatives and the motor stimulants are also available if required. This section discusses the most commonly used agents.

Mechanism of Action. Laxatives increase the transit of food through the human intestine via several mechanisms. These mechanisms include increasing the amount of nonabsorbable solid residue (bulk) in the feces, increasing the water content of the feces, altering feces consistency to make them softer, and stimulating gastric motility and secretion.

Formulation. Several formulations of laxatives are available, including powder, syrup, and tablet formulations for oral use and suppository formulations.

Psyllium. Psyllium (Procter & Gamble's [Cinicinnati, Ohio] Metamucil/Regulan, generics), also called isphagula, is soluble fiber derived from the seed husks of plants of the plantago genus. All fibers, both soluble and insoluble, release short-chain fatty acids (SCFAs), which increase the rate at which water is secreted by the intestinal mucosa. High levels of SCFAs also reduce rectosigmoid pressure, lower transit time, and increase stool mass. Bacterial mass increases with fiber level, promoting quicker bacterial fermentation of stool. Fiber tends to "normalize" stool frequency, not only by speeding colonic transit when it has been abnormally long (constipation) but also by slowing transit when it has been abnormally short (diarrhea). When taken with water, psyllium, which consists mainly of indigestible polysaccharides in a powder form, increases fecal mass, softens stool, and stimulates peristalsis, helping relieve constipation.

Clinical data regarding the use of psyllium in IBS patients are limited. A small placebo-controlled, double-blind, crossover study involving 20 patients with IBS investigated the effect of psyllium on whole gut transit time (Jalihal A, 1990). Patients treated with the agent showed significant ($p < 0.001$) improvement over those taking placebo in global symptoms of IBS and satisfying bowel movements. Researchers observed a correlation between improvement in well-being and the number of days of satisfying bowel movements, but they saw no correlation with regard to indices of pain, stool frequency, and changes in transit time. This study demonstrates that easing bowel dissatisfaction is a key reason behind psyllium's therapeutic success.

In another double-blind, placebo-controlled study, 80 patients with IBS were given psyllium (Prior A, 1987). Based on patients' SGAs, 82% of psyllium-treated patients compared with 53% of placebo-treated patients judged treatment satisfactory. Bowel habit was unchanged in the placebo group, while constipation in the treated group improved significantly. Transit time also significantly increased in those treated with psyllium compared with those on placebo. No treatment effect was observed with respect to abdominal pain and bloating.

Common problems associated with the use of psyllium observed in clinical investigations include flatulence, bloating, and temporary cramping. In some cases, these effects led to a patient's withdrawal from therapy.

Methylcellulose. Methylcellulose (GlaxoSmithKline's Citrucel, Edigen's [Madrid, Spain] Muciplasma, generics) is another plant polysaccharide. This drug can be obtained both OTC and by prescription in either powder or tablet form in the United States, Europe, and Japan. This agent is an insoluble fiber that has similar actions to psyllium; it increases fecal mass, softens the stool, and stimulates peristalsis.

Although clinical data are lacking to support the use of methylcellulose to treat IBS, the agent is used in this patient population. Some patients experience flatulence with methylcellulose, although this side effect is less common than with psyllium.

Calcium Polycarbophil. Calcium polycarbophil (Wyeth's [Madison, New Jersey] FiberCon, Numark Laboratories's Equalactin, generics) is available in tablet form. Although it has been available OTC in Europe and the United States for years, calcium polycarbophil was not launched in Japan until October 2000 and is available only as a prescription product. Calcium polycarbophil is an insoluble fiber that increases fecal mass, softens the stool, and stimulates peristalsis.

Clinical data highlighting the actions of calcium polycarbophil in patients with IBS are limited. One randomized, double-blind, crossover study investigated a 6 g daily dose of calcium polycarbophil versus placebo in 23 patients with IBS (Toskes PP, 1993). Seventy-one percent of the patients indicated that calcium polycarbophil was better than placebo for symptom relief. Statistically significant improvements in ease of stool passage were observed in the calcium polycarbophil group. Patients given polycarbophil reported less nausea, pain, and bloating compared with those given placebo.

Calcium polycarbophil is commonly associated with flatulence, but, as with methylcellulose, the side effect is less common than it is with psyllium.

Lactulose. Lactulose (Solvay's Duphalac/Bifiteral, generics) is an osmotic laxative; the agent is a synthetic disaccharide made up of fructose and galactose and is available in both syrup and powder formulations. Colonic bacteria metabolize lactulose, primarily into lactic acid, which is an SCFA similar to that produced by fiber. Lactic acid acidifies the intestinal crypt, producing the osmotic effect of drawing water into the colon.

As with the previously described methylcellulose, no clinical data support the use of lactulose in IBS patients. Nevertheless, the agent is commonly prescribed for this indication. Physicians recommend that patients start with a low dose of lactulose and increase to the minimum necessary for therapeutic effect. Lactulose's effects include flatulence, cramps, diarrhea, and electrolyte disturbances. The agent is not intended for long-term use. Because it accelerates colonic transit, it can interfere with the absorption of other drugs—a troublesome problem, particularly in elderly patients who may be taking a host of medications for other conditions.

Polyethylene Glycol. Polyethylene glycol (PEG) (Braintree Laboratories's [Braintree, Massachusetts] Miralax, Norgine's [Amsterdam, the Netherlands] Klean-prep) is available in both powder and tablet form; it is odorless and flavorless, making it more palatable for patients than other laxatives. PEG, another osmotic laxative, is a high-molecular-weight compound that is metabolically inert and is not susceptible to fermentation. PEG can significantly increase the number of bowel movements in constipated patients and greatly improve stool consistency and ease of passage.

PEG solutions may be better tolerated in IBS patients than other osmotic laxatives because they are associated with less bloating, although no randomized, controlled studies of PEG in patients with IBS have been carried out to date to support this hypothesis (Talley NJ, 2003).

Senna. Senna (Purdue Frederick's [Stamford, Connecticut] Senokot, Woelm's [Freitag, Germany] Depuran, generics) is derived from the seeds and leaves of plants in the cassia genus. Senna is a member of the motor stimulant laxative group, which increases peristalsis in the gut via stimulation of the gut mucosa, through activation of local reflexes. Senna has laxative activity because it contains derivatives of anthracene (e.g., emodin); these derivatives normally combine with glycosides. As the agent passes into the human colon unchanged, bacteria hydrolyze the glycoside component, releasing the active derivative, which is then absorbed and directly stimulates nerve endings in the myenteric plexus, increasing smooth-muscle activity and defecation. The laxative action of a single oral dose usually takes about eight hours.

Clinical data describing the actions of senna in the IBS population are not available. However, motor stimulant agents are known to induce abdominal pain and, in extreme cases, damage the myenteric plexus (Talley NJ, 2003).

Bisacodyl. The motor stimulant laxative bisacodyl (Boehringer Ingelheim's [Ingelheim, Germany] Dulcolax, generics) is a diphenylmethane similar to the phenolphthalein laxatives that were withdrawn from the market in 1997. Research showed that phenolphthalein was carcinogenic in animal models, but no evidence to date suggests that all diphenylmethanes promote tumor growth. This agent can be administered orally or as a suppository.

Bisacodyl's mechanism of action mirrors that of senna. It increases peristalsis in the gut via stimulation of the gut mucosa, through activation of local reflexes. Laxative effects occur within 6–12 hours postdosing.

Clinical data on the use of this agent in the IBS population are not available; as with senna, the adverse effects associated with motor stimulants should be considered.

Sodium Picosulfate. Sodium picosulfate (Boehringer Ingelheim's Laxoberal, Omegin's [Gottmadingen, Germany] Darmel Pico) is also a member of the motor stimulant laxative group. The agent is available in tablet form. It has limited availability in the major pharmaceutical markets.

This agent's mechanism of action is similar to that of both senna and bisacodyl. It increases peristalsis in the gut via stimulation of the gut mucosa, through activation of local reflexes.

Clinical data examining this agent's efficacy in the IBS population are not available. Like all motor stimulants, sodium picosulfate should be used with caution given the potential for adverse side effects.

Antidiarrheals

Overview. Diarrhea is one of the most socially restrictive symptoms associated with IBS. Also, chronic diarrhea carries the possibility of dehydration, which, in severe cases, may lead to a patient being hospitalized for intravenous fluid and electrolyte replenishment. In general, patients suffering from D-IBS use antidiarrheal agents on an as-needed basis; only in cases of severe D-IBS are antidiarrheals used on a consistent dosage schedule.

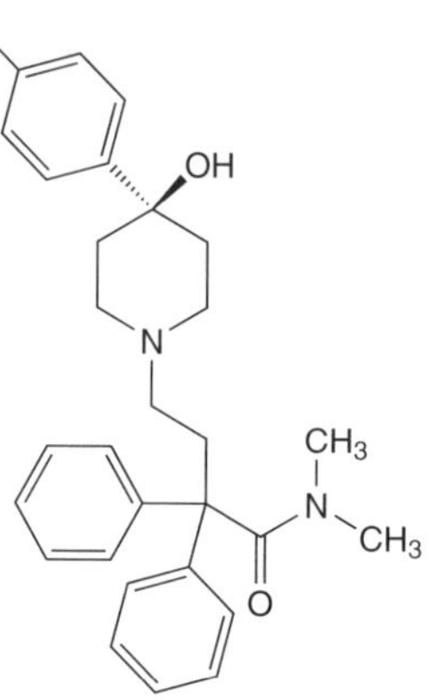

FIGURE 5. *Structure of loperamide.*

Mechanism of Action. Antidiarrheals reduce colonic transit, typically through direct action on the smooth muscle of the GI tract. This action increases the bulk, density, and viscosity of the feces and prevents excessive loss of electrolytes and fluids. Most antidiarrheals prescribed for IBS patients are active at opiate receptors in the GI tract, which control smooth-muscle contractility.

Formulation. Antidiarrheal agents are given orally, in either a tablet or syrup formulation.

Loperamide. Loperamide (Ortho-McNeil's [Raritan, New Jersey] Imodium, Janssen-Cilag [Issy-Les-Moulineaux, France] Linguial, generics) (Figure 5) is an orally active antidiarrheal available both OTC and by prescription. This agent is an antiperistaltic (it reduces contractility) that exerts an opioid-like effect by activating opioid receptors on circular and longitudinal muscles of the intestines. This action reduces smooth-muscle contractions and increases transit time. Loperamide's secondary mechanisms of action enhance intestinal water and ion absorption, probably as a result of slower transit time, and strengthen rectal sphincter tone. The agent does not produce opiate dependency because it cannot cross the blood–brain barrier (Camilleri M, 2001).

A randomized, double-blind study compared loperamide with placebo in the treatment of IBS (Efskind PS, 1996). Ninety patients received standard dosing of loperamide or placebo for five weeks. During the course of the study, the loperamide group experienced an improved stool consistency (32%), reduced defecation (36%), and reduced overall intensity of pain, although some patients in the loperamide group reported an increase in abdominal pain during the night. A meta-analysis of four clinical trials of IBS patients found that loperamide reduces diarrhea symptoms, including a statistically significant improvement in stool frequency and consistency (Jailwala J, 2000). Clinical studies of loperamide have failed to demonstrate its efficacy in improving fecal urgency or abdominal distension.

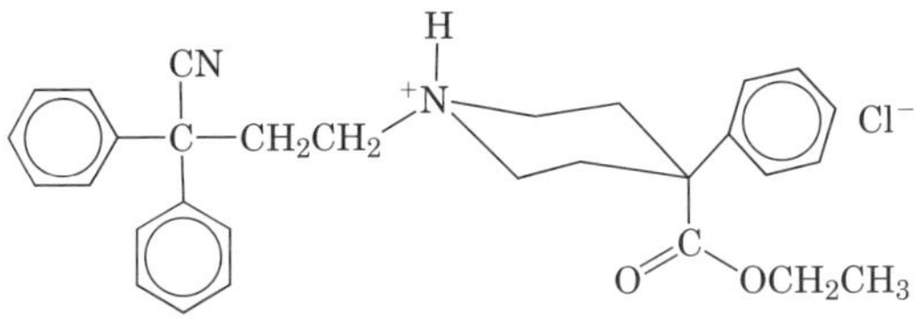

FIGURE 6. Structure of diphenoxylate.

Loperamide's side effects are infrequent and mild; however, treatment may exacerbate symptoms of constipation in patients who have M-IBS. Use of a liquid formulation of loperamide may reduce the potential for developing constipation (Camilleri M, 2001).

Diphenoxylate. The antidiarrheal diphenoxylate (Pfizer's [New York, New York] Lomotil, Sanofi-Synthelabo's [New York, New York] Diarsed, generics) (Figure 6) is available in tablet form by prescription in combination with atropine (generic) in the United States and Europe. Diphenoxylate reduces intestinal motility by activating the mu-opioid receptor in colonic smooth muscle. Its inhibitory effect on intestinal smooth muscle reduces propulsion and peristaltic action and increases transit time. Because diphenoxylate can cross the blood–brain barrier, it has significant opioid activity, and higher doses can cause dependence. Atropine is added to diphenoxylate in the prescription formulation to discourage opiate abuse and relax stomach spasms.

Clinical data regarding the efficacy of diphenoxylate-atropine in patients with IBS are not available. However, diphenoxylate must be used with extreme caution in patients with liver disease; in such cases, it can cause hepatic coma. Atropine's side effects, which are similar to those of cholinergic agents, include dizziness, insomnia, headache, glaucoma, and tachycardia; the latter two side effects limit use of this combination in elderly patients (Camilleri M, 2001).

Antispasmodics

Overview. Antispasmodic agents are used primarily for the treatment of pain symptoms in patients with IBS. The primary agents in the antispasmodic group are anticholinergics (e.g., hyoscyamine sulfate [Schwarz Pharma's (Milwaukee, Wisconsin) Levsin, Boehringer Ingelheim's Buscopan, generics], dicyclomine [Aventis Pharmaceuticals, Inc.'s (Bridgewater, New Jersey) Bentyl, Florizel's (United Kingdom) Merbentyl, generics], cimetropium bromide [Yamanouchi Pharmaceutical (Tokyo, Japan) Alginor]), and the calcium-channel blockers (CCBs), such as pinaverium bromide (Solvay's Dicetel/Edicet). The anticholinergics are the most commonly prescribed antispasmodics in the United States. In Europe and Japan, other antispasmodics that act more specifically in the gut are used to treat IBS. These alternative agents are mostly papaverine derivatives (mebeverine [Solvay's Duspatalin/Colofac, generics]) and enkephalin-like agents (trimebutine [Pfizer/Sigma Tau's (Rome, Italy) Debridat, generics]).

A meta-analysis of five antispasmodics (anticholinergics and others) showed a 64% reduction in abdominal pain with these agents, compared with a 45% reduction for placebo (Jailwala J, 2000). Data regarding the effect of antispasmodics on colonic transit times are contradictory, but some agents have been shown to modestly improve diarrhea symptoms in IBS.

Mechanism of Action. Antispasmodic agents reduce the spontaneous activity of the intestinal smooth muscle. Relaxation of the smooth muscle, in turn, reduces pain symptoms experienced by IBS patients (Brandt LJ, 2002).

Formulation. Agents in the antispasmodic class are available in oral, sublingual, and injectable formulations, although the injectable formulations are not used in IBS therapy.

Hyoscyamine Sulfate. Hyoscyamine sulfate (Schwarz Pharma's Levsin, Boehringer Ingelheim's Buscopan, generics) is a commonly prescribed antispasmodic and a member of the anticholinergic group. The agent is available in an oral and sublingual formulation.

Anticholinergic agents exert their effects by inhibiting the actions of acetylcholine on postganglionic parasympathetic acetylcholine receptors. Hyoscyamine exhibits anticholinergic effects in smooth muscle, cardiac muscle, and the exocrine glands. Because hyoscyamine (Figure 7) works on systemic cholinergic receptors, it is indicated for a variety of conditions: it reduces tremor and muscle stiffness in Parkinson's disease patients, it relaxes smooth muscles in the bladder to treat incontinence, and it inhibits gastric contractions when used for peptic ulcer treatment. In IBS, hyoscyamine inhibits GI propulsive motility and controls excessive secretion in the upper GI tract (esophagus and stomach).

Detailed clinical investigations into the efficacy of hyoscyamine in IBS patients are lacking. However, like all anticholinergics, hyoscyamine sulfate is able to cross the blood–brain barrier and reach the central nervous system (CNS), often triggering side effects such as dry mouth, blurred vision, and urinary retention. Because of the potential for adverse side effects, hyoscyamine is prescribed to patients on an as-needed basis only.

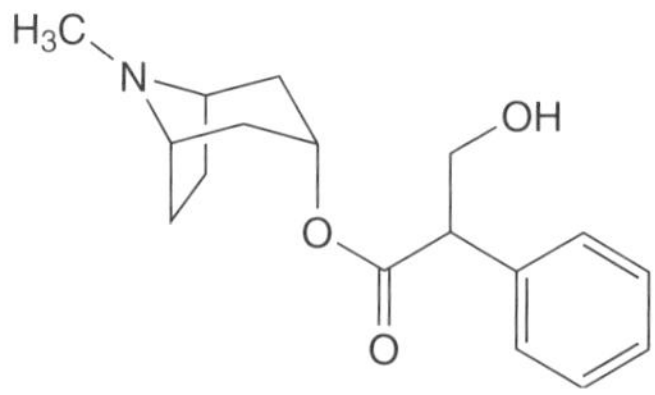

FIGURE 7. *Structure of hyoscyamine.*

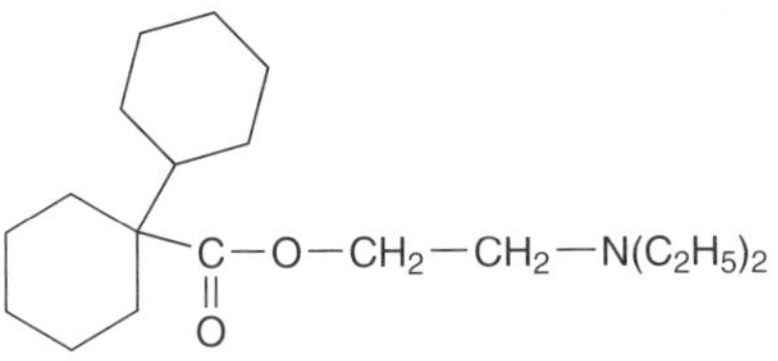

$C-O-CH_2-CH_2-N(C_2H_5)_2$

FIGURE 8. Structure of dicyclomine.

Dicyclomine. Dicyclomine (Aventis's Bentyl, Florizel's Merbentyl, generics) (Figure 8) is another oral anticholinergic agent. Dicyclomine is more selective than hyoscyamine; it inhibits smooth-muscle spasms only in the GI tract. Like hyoscyamine, dicyclomine reduces tone and motility of GI smooth muscle by blocking acetylcholine receptors. Animal models suggest it also inhibits bradykinin- and histamine-induced spasms in the ileum of the small intestine.

In a study of 100 patients conducted more than 20 years ago, 82% of IBS patients demonstrated improvement in pain symptoms, compared with 55% of placebo patients (Page JG, 1981). No recent trials have examined the use of this agent in IBS patients.

Although dicyclomine is more specific than other anticholinergics, it produces the same side effects. Approximately 60% of patients experience negative anticholinergic side effects, primarily dry mouth and dizziness.

Cimetropium Bromide. Cimetropium bromide (Yamanouchi's Alginor) is an oral anticholinergic, antispasmodic agent. This agent inhibits smooth-muscle contraction in the gut and relieves pain by inhibiting the action of acetylcholine on its receptors.

Several studies demonstrate the agent is efficacious at reducing symptoms in IBS patients. A randomized, double-blind, placebo-controlled trial involving 48 patients with IBS investigated the effects of 50 mg cimetropium bromide given twice daily for six months (Centonze V, 1988). Pain scores fell by an average of 16% in the placebo group compared with 87% in the cimetropium bromide group. Twenty patients (87%) in the cimetropium bromide group reported a global improvement in their condition versus 5 patients (24%) in the placebo group. Forty-eight percent of the treated population reported side effects (dry mouth and lethargy), but none of these patients withdrew from the investigation.

Another placebo-controlled study evaluated 70 C-IBS and D-IBS patients with bowel alterations and episodes of abdominal pain lasting for at least two months (Dobrilla G, 1990). At three months, the frequency of abdominal pain dropped 86% in the cimetropium group, compared with 50% in the placebo group. The improvements over placebo seen in the cimetropium group were statistically significant for both pain frequency and severity.

Despite cimetropium bromide's efficacy with respect to pain relief in IBS, the agent has very limited availability in the major markets.

Pinaverium Bromide. Pinaverium bromide (Solvay's Dicetel/Edicet) is an antispasmodic with CCB activity. Intestinal contractions depend, in part, on the activity of calcium ion channels. CCBs inhibit postprandial colonic motility and relax the smooth muscle of the biliary and GI tracts.

A randomized, double-bind, placebo-controlled trial of pinaverium was conducted in Argentina (Awad R, 1995). The study enrolled 40 female patients who received either 50 mg of pinaverium twice daily or placebo with food. Results showed that pinaverium relieved constipation, diarrhea, and pain symptoms and was moderately effective against distension.

An open-label trial conducted in India found pinaverium to be efficacious in 61 patients with IBS (Jayanthi V, 1998). Treatment with the agent resulted in a 49% decline in abdominal pain, a 74% improvement in stool consistency, a 71% decline in urgency, and a 64% decline in the presence of mucus in the stool. However, the results of this study must be considered with caution because of the open nature of the trial design.

A study involving 91 patients with D-IBS compared pinaverium with the antispasmodic agent mebeverine (discussed in the next section) (Lu CL, 2000). Patients were randomized to receive 50 mg pinaverium or 100 mg mebeverine twice daily for two weeks. Daily defecation was markedly reduced following treatment with both agents, and stool consistency improved. Both drugs similarly improved patients' global well-being (73.4% improvement for pinaverium and 71.8% improvement for mebeverine). Only pinaverium significantly prolonged colonic transit time, a fact that may explain the agent's relative success in patients suffering from D-IBS.

Pinaverium's side effects, which are similar to those of other CCBs, include dizziness, nausea, and hypotension. The agent is contraindicated in patients with kidney or liver dysfunction.

Mebeverine. Mebeverine (Solvay's Duspatalin/Colofac, generics) (Figure 9) is one of the most popular IBS therapies in European markets. The agent is even available OTC (as Solvay's Colofac IBS) in tablet form in the United Kingdom.

Mebeverine is a papaverine derivative that acts on opiate receptors to relax smooth muscle. It slows colonic motility, reduces intraluminal pressure in the bowel, and has a modest effect on abdominal pain and distension. Mebeverine has

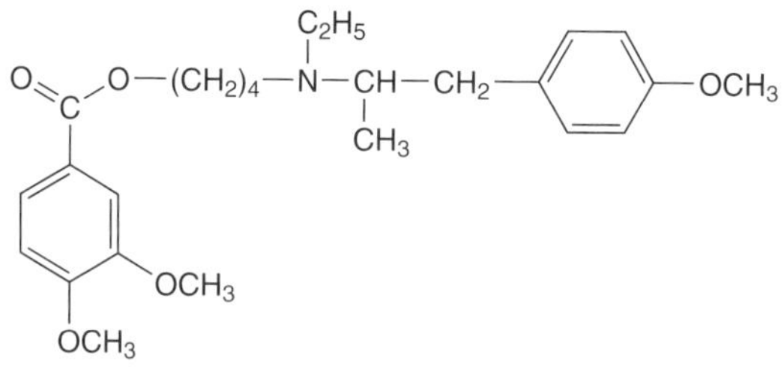

FIGURE 9. *Structure of mebeverine.*

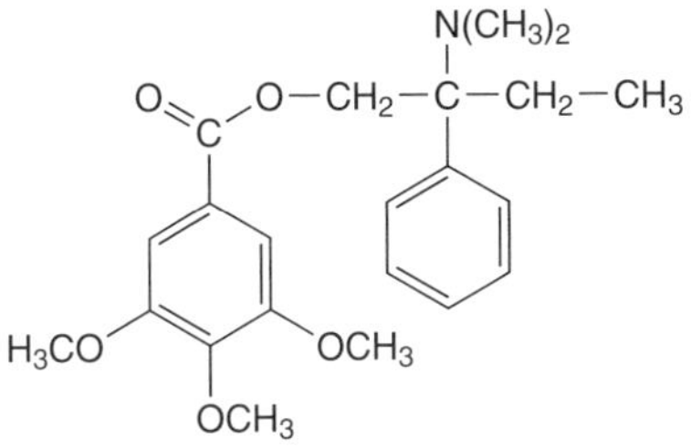

FIGURE 10. *Structure of trimebutine.*

alternating prokinetic and antispasmodic effects in the small intestine, increasing motor activity while simultaneously reducing the proportion of migrating motor complexes (MMCs).

Mebeverine produced favorable results in a Belgian study involving 60 C-IBS and D-IBS patients (Van Outryve M, 1995). Patients received either 270 mg of mebeverine three times per day or 400 mg of the sustained-release formulation twice per day. After six weeks of treatment, 80% of patients from both groups reported significant improvement, and 40% of patients were symptom-free.

Mebeverine's side effects—which include dizziness, tachycardia, and anorexia—are rare.

Trimebutine. Trimebutine (Pfizer/Sigma Tau's Debridat, generics) (Figure 10), available in tablet form, is an alternative antispasmodic agent and a peripherally acting enkephalin. This agent has affinity for the mu, kappa, and delta opiate receptors in the GI tract, and it regulates the release of motilin, vasoactive intestinal peptide, and gastrin. Trimebutine is active throughout the GI tract, where it accelerates gastric emptying and stimulates motility in the small intestine. Its effects in the colon include reduction (by 45–75%) of long spike burst action (LSB) and helping synchronize electrophysiological spikes and contractions. In constipated patients, trimebutine nearly doubles colonic transit rates.

Trimebutine's utility is generally limited to C-IBS patients because its primary therapeutic benefit is a decline in colonic transit time. However, clinical investigations have demonstrated that trimebutine is effective in patients with IBS and GERD (Kountouras J, 2002). Certain studies with trimebutine have also shown some alleviation of pain, but in a meta-analysis of muscle-relaxant trials in IBS, trimebutine ranked six among seven agents (Poynard T, 1994). Because trimebutine acts as a peripheral opioid antagonist, it poses no risk of dependence.

Antidepressants

Overview. Initially, the use of antidepressants was proposed for the large proportion of IBS patients who also suffered from clinical depression, but it was subsequently discovered that antidepressants, independent of their mood-modulating effects, have neuromodulatory and analgesic properties that make them useful in treating IBS itself. These effects are usually seen at dosages that are subtherapeutic for the treatment of psychiatric disorders, and they occur more quickly than mood elevation.

Most of the antidepressants used in IBS treatment are from one of two drug classes: tricyclic antidepressants (TCAs) and selective serotonin reuptake inhibitors (SSRIs). Although SSRIs are more popular in the treatment of depression, TCAs represent the majority of antidepressant use for IBS symptoms, mainly because their use is better documented in clinical trials of IBS, while very few randomized, blinded trials have tested SSRI use in IBS. However, statistical and patient-selection methods from favorable studies of TCAs in IBS have been called into question, so the utility of TCAs has not yet been adequately proved.

The three most commonly prescribed TCAs for IBS are the tertiary amines amitriptyline (AstraZeneca's [Wilmington, Delaware] Elavil, Roche's Laroxyl, generics) and imipramine (Novartis/Mallinkrodt's [Hazelwood, Missouri] Tofranil, generics) and the secondary amine desipramine (Novartis's Pertofan, Aventis's Nopramin, generics). Other TCAs such as trimipramine (Aventis's Surmontil) have also been shown to be effective at reducing abdominal pain in IBS patients (Camilleri M, 2000). Generally, the TCAs are interchangeable in the treatment of IBS; the choice of agent depends mostly on physician preference. The most commonly prescribed SSRIs for IBS are fluoxetine (Eli Lilly and Company's [Indianapolis, Indiana] Prozac, generics), paroxetine (GlaxoSmithKline's Paxil), and sertraline (Pfizer's Zoloft). Because no single SSRI has demonstrated better efficacy than others, the choice of agent is often determined by the physician's familiarity with a particular agent.

Mechanism of Action. The exact mechanism by which antidepressants alleviate IBS symptoms is unclear. These agents may regulate the afferent pathways from the gut to the brain, thereby rectifying the abnormal sensation of pain. Another hypothesis is that antidepressants directly modulate the effect of serotonin (an important chemical regulator of GI function, as discussed earlier in the "5-HT Receptor Modulators" section) in the gut. In D-IBS patients, the anticholinergic side effects of some antidepressants cause constipation, an effect that helps combat the predominant diarrhea symptoms.

Imipramine. Imipramine (Novartis/Mallinckrodt's Tofranil, generics) (Figure 11) is a frequently prescribed TCA used in the treatment of IBS. TCAs block the synaptic reuptake of serotonin and norepinephrine, and they are potent blockers of cholinergic and histaminergic receptors. Imipramine's mechanism of action is not entirely understood, but, like all TCAs, it definitely blocks the reuptake of serotonin and norepinephrine. Secondary actions, such as anticholinergic and antiadrenergic effects, have led to its use in IBS and childhood enuresis.

A study of imipramine showed that it modulates small intestine function both in D-IBS patients and in controls (Gorard DA, 1995). Fourteen patients (eight controls, six with D-IBS) took imipramine for five days, and, while the periodicity of migrating motor complexes (MMCs) was not affected, phase 3 MMC speed was slowed in all participants. Another study compared imipramine with the

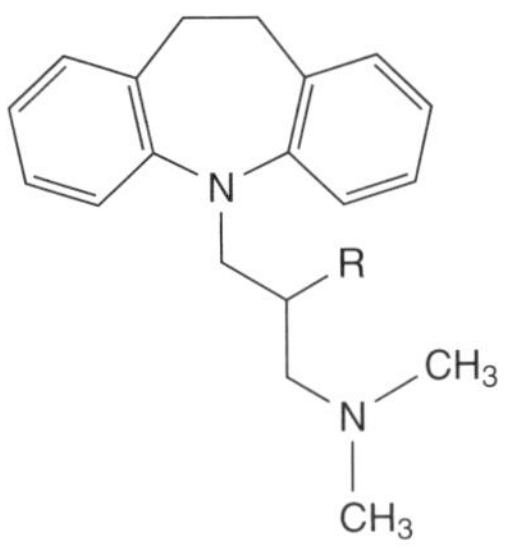

FIGURE 11. *Structure of imipramine (R = H).*

SSRI paroxetine (GlaxoSmithKline's Paxil) and found that, although both agents slowed orocecal transit (from mouth to end of small intestine), only imipramine prolonged whole-gut transit times to relieve diarrhea (Gorard DA, 1994).

Like all TCAs, imipramine is associated with numerous adverse side effects that often cause compliance problems; up to 40% of patients treated with TCAs discontinue therapy or switch to another agent (Talley NJ, 2003). TCAs' adverse effects are related to their action on multiple receptor sites throughout the CNS. Because TCAs block the histaminergic receptors, they often cause weight gain and sedation. These agents also block cholinergic receptors; thus, to avoid additional anticholinergic effects (dry mouth, blurred vision, constipation), physicians should be cautious in prescribing TCAs with other anticholinergic agents such as dicyclomine and hyoscyamine. To circumvent these side effects, physicians often start with very low doses and scale up to the minimum dose that proves therapeutic for IBS symptoms. TCAs cannot be used concurrently with monoamine oxidase inhibitors (MAOIs) because of the risk of hypertensive crisis.

Amitriptyline. Like all TCAs, amitriptyline (AstraZeneca's Elavil, Roche's Laroxyl, generics) (Figure 12) inhibits the reuptake of serotonin and norepinephrine, but it might have lower activity in the CNS than other agents in this class, making it more gut-specific. Like its active metabolite nortriptyline (Novartis's Pamelor, generics), which has also been shown to reduce abdominal pain in IBS patients when given in combination with fluphenazine (Bristol-Myers [North Billerica, Massachusetts] Squibb's Prolixin, generics), amitriptyline exhibits stronger anticholinergic effects than other TCAs, but it does not inhibit norepinephrine reuptake as strongly (Camilleri M, 2001).

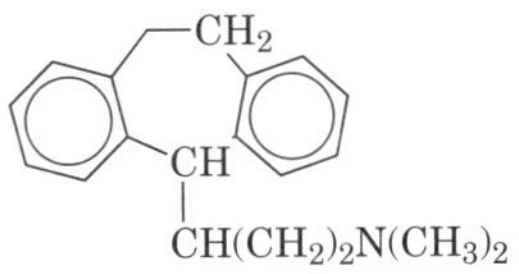

FIGURE 12. *Structure of amitriptyline.*

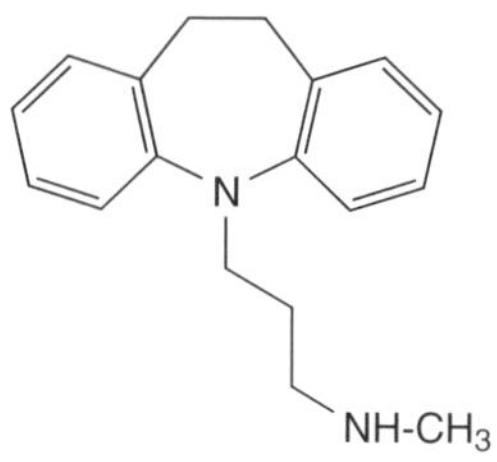

FIGURE 13. *Structure of desipramine.*

Clinical data on the use of amitriptyline in IBS patients are scarce. However, in one controlled study, investigators reported an improvement in global well-being, abdominal pain, and bowel pattern following treatment with amitriptyline (Hasler WL, 2003). They also identified young age and extroversion as predictors of drug response.

As is the case for all TCAs, a high incidence of side effects as a direct result of amitriptyline drug therapy often results in patients discontinuing treatment (Montgomery SA, 1989).

Desipramine. Desipramine (Novartis's Pertofan, Aventis's Nopramin, generics) Figure 13) is the active metabolite of imipramine. Compared with other TCAs, desipramine is the strongest and most selective inhibitor of norepinephrine reuptake. The compound works on both the CNS and ENS, where it blocks serotonergic, cholinergic, and adrenergic receptors. In the dorsal nerve fibers, desipramine alleviates pain symptoms of IBS by reducing the response of mechanosensitive afferent nerves. Desipramine is useful primarily in treating D-IBS; its slowing of transit times would exacerbate constipation in C-IBS.

A comparative study of desipramine, atropine, and placebo showed the greatest benefit with desipramine (Greenbaum DS, 1987). A four-week observation period followed three six-week test periods in this investigation. Among 28 IBS patients (19 with D-IBS, 9 with C-IBS), desipramine reduced stool frequency, diarrhea, and abdominal pain and slowed contractions in the D-IBS patients significantly more than did atropine or placebo.

In an earlier study, which pooled C-IBS and D-IBS patients into a single group, desipramine showed a benefit in pain reduction but not in alleviating bowel irregularity. Thus, although the benefit of desipramine in regulating motility is in question, the agent is clearly efficacious against IBS pain symptoms.

Fluoxetine. Fluoxetine (Eli Lilly's Prozac, generics) (Figure 14) was the first SSRI introduced to the market (in 1987). The agent is widely used for depression in the United States and Europe but is not yet approved in Japan.

Like all SSRIs, fluoxetine acts by inhibiting the reuptake of serotonin at the neuronal synapses. Unlike TCAs, SSRIs have little or no effect on norepinephrine reuptake, nor do they have an effect on the cholinergic, histaminergic, and adrenergic receptors. Because SSRIs are highly selective for serotonergic receptors,

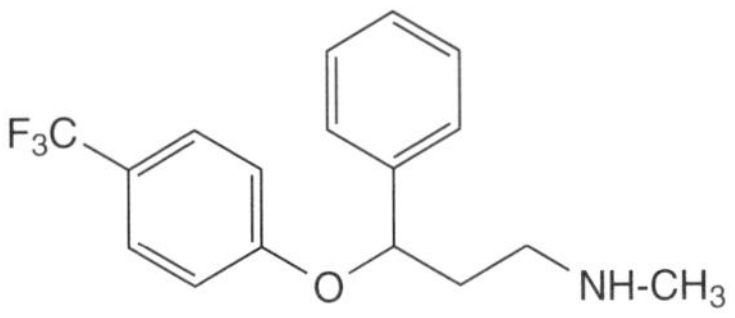

FIGURE 14. *Structure of fluoxetine.*

they have almost no anticholinergic or sedating side effects. This factor makes SSRIs more tolerable for patients with C-IBS (the anticholinergic side effects of TCAs can cause or worsen constipation). In IBS management, SSRIs are used primarily to relieve pain and to improve motility, but the mechanism by which SSRIs achieve these effects in IBS is unknown.

No controlled studies have analyzed fluoxetine's efficacy in IBS, but some physicians use it off-label for IBS patients. One study showed treatment with fluoxetine caused a slight but significant reduction in IBS symptoms (Kuiken SD, 2002).

Among the SSRIs, fluoxetine has the longest half-life, a factor that offers an advantage in the case of missed doses. All of the SSRIs discussed in this section, including fluoxetine, have similar side effects, of which the most troubling is sexual dysfunction in both women and men. However, SSRIs typically cause sexual dysfunction at the higher doses used in treating depression, so this side effect is not as likely to affect IBS patients taking psychiatrically subtherapeutic doses.

Paroxetine. Paroxetine (GlaxoSmithKline's Paxil) (Figure 15) is a commonly used SSRI in the treatment of anxiety disorders and social phobia, in addition to depression. Its mechanism of action is similar to that of fluoxetine, inhibiting the reuptake of serotonin at the neuronal synapses.

A study of paroxetine's effect on the small intestine found that it caused more frequent MMCs and increased the propagation velocity of phase 3 contractions (Gorard DA, 1994). However, this same study (cited earlier in the discussion of imipramine) found that, although paroxetine increases orocecal transit, it has no

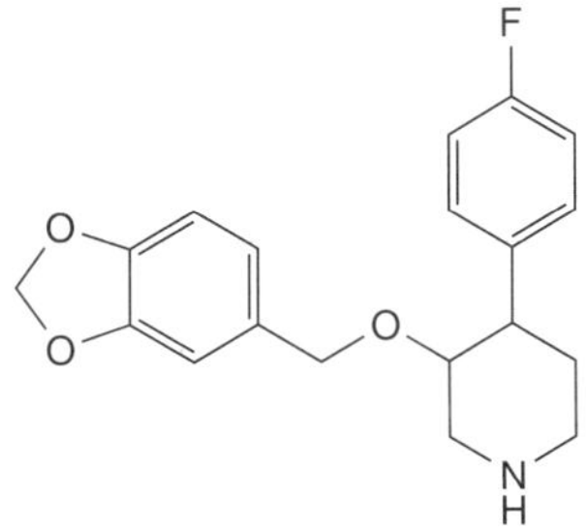

FIGURE 15. *Structure of paroxetine.*

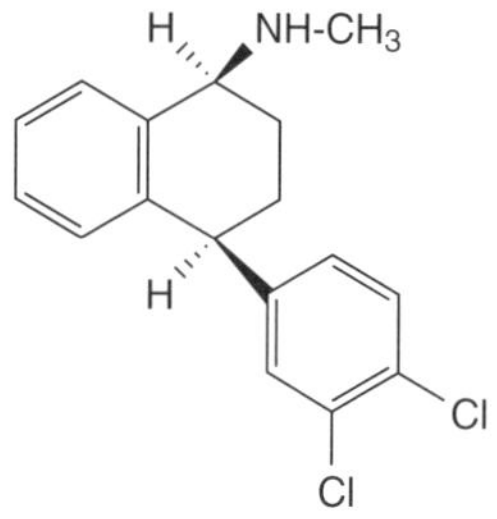

FIGURE 16. *Structure of sertraline.*

effect on whole-gut transit time. The demonstrated action of paroxetine on the small intestine suggests that it could be useful for IBS patients suffering from constipation, but the clinical results are not entirely conclusive.

Sertraline. Sertraline (Pfizer's Zoloft) (Figure 16) is effective as an antidepressant, but, among the three SSRIs discussed here, it has the least scientific data concerning use in IBS. Some reports indicate that sertraline can reduce IBS symptoms, including pain, and that it is associated with fewer side effects. Like all SSRIs, this agent acts by inhibiting the reuptake of serotonin at the neuronal synapses.

EMERGING THERAPIES

The investigation of novel compounds for the treatment of irritable bowel syndrome (IBS) remains a challenging area of R&D for both the biotechnology and pharmaceutical industries. The problem stems from the lack of understanding of the etiology and pathophysiology of this common functional gastrointestinal (GI) disorder. Because the majority of current therapies for IBS address abnormal motility more effectively than they do pain, most IBS drug development in recent years has focused on therapies for visceral hypersensitivity. This approach has proved very difficult because the exact pathways involved in visceral sensitivity in IBS have not been fully characterized.

The agents at the most advanced stages of development for IBS are in the following drug classes: 5-HT receptor modulators, tachykinin receptor antagonists, cholecystokinin (CCK) A receptor antagonists, opioid receptor modulators, corticotropin-releasing factor (CRF) receptor antagonists, and chloride-channel activators. In preclinical development are agents that target somatostatin receptors, antagonize the actions of motilin, modulate ion-channel activity, and inhibit the activity of the transcription factor NFκB. These novel approaches have the potential to combat both abdominal pain and motility abnormalities in IBS. However, further discussion of these early-stage compounds is not within the scope of this section, which focuses on compounds in clinical development. Table 2 lists the drug therapies in later-stage development for IBS.

TABLE 2. Emerging Therapies in Development for Irritable Bowel Syndrome

Compound	Development Phase	Marketing Company
5-HT receptor modulators		
Cilansetron		
United States	D	Solvay
Europe	III	Solvay
Japan	—	—
Renzapride		
United States	II	Alizyme
Europe	II	Alizyme
Japan	—	—
E-3620		
United States	—	—
Europe	—	—
Japan	II	Eisai
Tachykinin receptor antagonists		
Nepadutant		
United States	—	—
Europe	II	Menarini
Japan	—	—
Saredutant		
United States	—	—
Europe	II	Sanofi-Synthélabo
Japan	—	—
Talnetant		
United States	—	—
Europe	II	GlaxoSmithKline
Japan	—	—
Cholecystokinin A receptor antagonists		
Dexloxiglumide		
United States	D	Forest Laboratories/RottaPharm
Europe	III	RottaPharm
Japan	—	—
Opioid receptor modulators		
PTI-901		
United States	D	Pain Therapeutics
Europe	—	—
Japan	—	—
Asimadoline		
United States	—	—
Europe	II	Merck KGaA
Japan	—	—
Corticotrophin-releasing factor receptor antagonists		
NBI-34041		
United States	—	—
Europe	I	Neurocrine Biosciences
Japan	—	—
Chloride-channel activators		
SPI-0211 (RU-0211)		
United States	II	Sucampo Pharmaceuticals
Europe	—	—
Japan	—	—

D = Discontinued.

5-HT Receptor Modulators

Overview. Clinical research has shown that modulation of 5-HT_3 and 5-HT_4 receptors affects visceral pain sensation and intestinal transit. The serotonin (5-HT) receptor modulator drug class has received the majority of IBS researchers' attention for nearly a decade. However, early agents in this class—alosetron (GlaxoSmithKline's Lotronex) and tegaserod (Novartis's Zelnorm/Zelmac)—have encountered considerable opposition during the approval process as a result of safety concerns revealed during clinical trials and postmarketing studies. These agents have been approved in the United States, but their prescription (particularly prescription of alosetron) is tightly regulated. In addition, because 5-HT receptor modulators have specificity for a single motility symptom (either diarrhea or constipation), more than 50% of the IBS population is necessarily excluded from treatment with any given 5-HT modulator.

The challenge for emerging agents within this class is to demonstrate significant improvements in both efficacy and safety over existing agents to gain wider approval. Several companies are pursuing 5-HT receptor modulators for the treatment of IBS. GlaxoSmithKline (GSK), Mitsubishi-Tokyo Pharmaceuticals (Tokyo, Japan), Pharmagene (Royston, Hertfordshire, United Kingdom), and Meiji Seika Kaisha (Tokyo, Japan) have discovery-phase programs, while Solvay, Alizyme PLC (Cambridge, United Kingdom), and Eisai Inc. (Teaneck, New Jersey) have agents in later-stage development.

Mechanism of Action. Agents in the 5-HT receptor modulator class stimulate or inhibit the activity of 5-HT receptors in the gut, reducing visceral pain sensations and altering intestinal transit in IBS patients.

Cilansetron. Cilansetron is a 5-HT receptor modulator being developed by Solvay in the United States and Europe for the treatment of diarrhea-predominant IBS (D-IBS) in both men and women. Like the currently marketed alosetron, the agent antagonizes 5-HT_3 receptors, thereby slowing gastric motility and providing relief for patients with D-IBS. The agent also reduces the transmission of afferent signals from the gut to the brain. Cilansetron is preregistered in Europe, where in June 2005, the Medicines and Healthcare Products Regulatory Agency (MHRA) of the United Kingdom (the reference member state under the European Union [EU] mutual recognition procedure) requested data from further clinical trials of the drug in IBS. In the United States, clinical data supporting a new drug application (NDA) for cilansetron were based on efficacy and safety studies in approximately 4000 D-IBS patients, and Solvay reports that its NDA submission included an appropriate-use program—not unlike that of alosetron in the United States—that is based on collaboration with physicians, pharmacists, patients, and risk-minimization experts. However, the FDA issued a non-approvable letter for cilansetron in April 2005, requesting, as did European regulators, that further clinical trials be conducted as a prerequisite to IBS approval. Solvay reported in November 2005 that it was discontinuing registration activity for cilansetron in the United States rather than undergo additional trials of the drug.

In May 2002, at the Digestive Disease Week meeting in San Francisco, the results of two clinical studies evaluating the efficacy of cilansetron were reported (Caras S, 2002). The two 12-week, double-blind, placebo-controlled studies were conducted in the United States ($n = 471$; doses: 1, 2, 8, 16 mg three times daily [t.i.d.]) and in Canada and Europe ($n = 435$; doses: 1, 2, 4, 16 mg t.i.d.) with male and female patients. D-IBS patients were selected according to the Rome I criteria, and efficacy was measured via response to a weekly questionnaire addressing the adequate relief of IBS symptoms (abdominal pain/discomfort, abnormal bowel habits). At the start of the trial, subjects were categorized by the severity of their IBS symptoms: approximately 76% of responders had active IBS symptoms during the two weeks prior to the start of the study, 13% of patients experienced some symptoms, and approximately 8% experienced no symptoms. Among the patients who had active symptoms, the efficacy benefit (measured as adequate global symptom relief) of cilansetron was significantly greater (25–41%) than that with placebo. Among the patients who experienced some symptoms, cilansetron (2 mg) demonstrated a 29% efficacy benefit compared with placebo. Cilansetron's efficacy in the patients who experienced no symptoms prior to the study was more difficult to discern. The active symptom group, at the start of the study, may represent a more severely ill population that responds well to cilansetron treatment. This study demonstrates that cilansetron is efficacious in relieving symptoms associated with D-IBS. Furthermore, it is effective in both male and female patients, a factor that will position cilansetron as a significant competitor to alosetron, which is not approved for use in the male population (Camilleri M, 2000).

Solvay's Phase III clinical trials program in collaboration with Quintiles Inc. (South San Francisco, California) has recruited more than 4000 D-IBS patients from more than 700 study centers around the world. In October 2003, the company announced that "headline" results from the first two efficacy studies in this program show convincing evidence that patients benefit from treatment with cilansetron. The medical community eagerly awaits publication of further data.

Any 5-HT$_3$ receptor antagonist must demonstrate significant benefits over alosetron with respect to efficacy and safety to make an impact on the IBS market. The key issue for cilansetron will be its adverse-events profile. With the exception of constipation, no significant adverse events such as ischemic colitis (associated with alosetron use) were reported in the studies presented at the 2002 Digestive Disease Week meeting. Data from long-term studies are needed to assess whether cilansetron is safer than alosetron; without this evidence, the agent may experience difficulties during the approval process in the United States and Europe. In particular, cilansetron's ability to differentiate itself from other agents in this class has raised questions, given that all 5-HT$_3$ receptor antagonists are pharmacologically similar (Stacher G, 2001).

Renzapride. Renzapride is a 5-HT receptor modulator in development by Alizyme in Europe and the United States. The agent was initially being developed by SmithKline Beecham, but Alizyme gained full ownership of the compound following SmithKline Beecham's merger with Glaxo Wellcome. Patient recruitment for Phase III trials began in late 2005.

Renzapride differs from currently marketed 5-HT receptor modulators because it has a distinctive pharmacology. The compound displays both 5-HT_3 receptor antagonist and 5-HT_4 receptor agonist effects; normally, these two actions oppose each other. Inhibition of 5-HT_3 receptors slows gastric motility and reduces transmission of afferent signals between the gut and the brain; stimulation of 5-HT_4 receptors triggers peristalsis in the gut. This multireceptor action potentially normalizes motility in IBS patients. Studies suggest that, overall, renzapride may be a more potent 5-HT_4 receptor agonist than 5-HT_3 receptor antagonist; its net effect is to accelerate motility. However, in a Japanese study comparing renzapride with a more selective 5-HT_4 receptor agonist in early clinical development (YM-53389), renzapride was less effective in facilitating lower GI propulsion (Nagakura Y, 1999). The authors suggest this relative weakness stems from renzapride's conflicting 5-HT_3 receptor antagonism. Because it acts at both receptor subtypes, renzapride has the potential to treat more than one subtype of IBS; studies are being carried out in patients with both constipation predominant IBS (C-IBS) and mixed-symptom IBS (M-IBS).

In October 2000, Alizyme announced preliminary results of a Phase IIa trial. The single-blind, placebo-controlled trial involved 20 patients (12 female, 8 male) with C-IBS. Statistical data from the trial have not been released, but the company claims that renzapride improved colonic motility and GI transit time better than placebo (Alizyme, press release, October 16, 2000). Animal models have shown that renzapride is also a potent stimulator of gastric emptying, but it is unknown if this action directly affects whole-gut transit time in IBS patients.

In April 2003, Alizyme announced the preliminary results of a Phase IIb clinical study. The randomized, double-blind, placebo-controlled, parallel-group, dose-ranging study involved 510 C-IBS patients recruited from general practices in the United Kingdom. The researchers compared the efficacy and safety of three once-daily doses of renzapride (1, 2, and 4 mg/day) and placebo over a 12-week period, following a two-week run-in period. The primary end point was the patients' weekly assessment of abdominal pain and discomfort during weeks 5–12 of the treatment protocol. Patients were classified as responders if they recorded adequate relief in 75% of the weeks of treatment. Treatment with renzapride increased the responder rate for adequate relief of abdominal pain and discomfort by 9% over treatment with placebo, and it increased bowel movements (statistically significant at 2 and 4 mg/day) and improved stool consistency (statistically significant at 4 mg/day). The study demonstrated that renzapride was well tolerated and had no clinically relevant side effects. The most common adverse events were diarrhea (25.2%) and headache (17.8%), compared with 9.6% and 13.6%, respectively, in the placebo arm (Alizyme, press release, April 24, 2003).

In September 2003, Alizyme announced preliminary data from a Phase II trial involving 168 M-IBS patients. This randomized, double-blind, placebo-controlled, dose-ranging study—the first of its kind in an M-IBS population—was carried out in hospitals in the United Kingdom. As with the C-IBS study, the investigators compared the efficacy and safety of three doses of renzapride (1, 2, and 4 mg/day) with placebo. The study lasted eight weeks and had a two-week run-in period. The primary end point was satisfactory relief of IBS on more than 50% of days during treatment. At the optimum dose (2 mg/day), up to 14% more patients receiving renzapride, at any one time (average 6% more over the treatment period), were classified as responders compared with those receiving placebo. The proportion of responders increased to 18% (average 8% more over the treatment period) when data from female patients alone were analyzed. The daily responder rate in the two-week run-up period was approximately 30% for all groups. It increased to 57% in the 2 mg/day renzapride group compared with 43% in the placebo group (Alizyme, press release, September 24, 2003).

Renzapride will launch into a highly competitive marketplace for 5-HT receptor modulators. The agent will be in direct competition with the selective 5-HT$_4$ receptor agonist tegaserod for the treatment of C-IBS patients, but it may hold some advantage over tegaserod in that its 5-HT$_3$ receptor antagonist action could help mediate visceral pain. Selective 5-HT$_4$ receptor agonists like tegaserod are not as effective against the pain symptoms of IBS. Renzapride's efficacy in the M-IBS population could be the key to its success; if the agent gains approval for both C-IBS and M-IBS, it will have a larger target population than either of the currently marketed 5-HT modulators (tegaserod and alosetron). Further large-scale trials are needed to assess the agent's efficacy in this population, and long-term-use investigations are needed to evaluate the compound's safety, an important issue for agents in this drug class in view of previous regulatory issues.

Alizyme recently filed a new patent application as a result of developments in various features of the commercial manufacturing process for renzapride. If the company is granted the patent, renzapride's patent life could be extended to 2023. A patent extension would be extremely useful in this case because of Alizyme's need to find a licensing partner, a task that may delay the compound's entry to the marketplace.

E-3620. Eisai is developing E-3620, an agent in Phase II clinical trials in Japan for IBS, gastric motility disorders, and gastritis. Like renzapride, E-3620 is a dual 5-HT$_3$ antagonist/5-HT$_4$ agonist. In 1999, the company reported that treatment with E-3620 is associated with an improvement in the symptoms of diarrhea and the sense of fullness and anorexia associated with chronic gastritis and IBS.

Tachykinin Receptor Antagonists

Overview. The role of the neurokinins (tachykinins)—substance P, neurokinin A, and neurokinin B—in the pathogenesis of IBS has been the subject of considerable investigation and debate within the scientific community. Many companies have taken an interest in this research area over the last decade, but no tachykinin receptor antagonists have yet reached the market. Pfizer has an NK$_1$ receptor antagonist (CP-122721) and both Menarini Group (Florence, Italy) and Solvay have NK$_2$ receptor antagonists in preclinical development. Sanofi-Synthélabo is developing a dual NK_2/NK_3 antagonist for IBS. The following sections discuss tachykinin receptor antagonists in clinical trials.

Mechanism of Action. All of the tachykinins act as full agonists at the tachykinin receptors NK_1, NK_2, and NK_3. Activation of these receptors in the GI tract is associated with altered GI motility, inflammation, secretion, and visceral hypersensitivity—all features of IBS. Agents antagonizing the actions of tachykinins at tachykinin receptors in the GI tract relax the GI smooth muscle, thereby inhibiting contractions and, theoretically, controlling pain related to muscle spasms.

Nepadutant. Menarini is developing the NK_2 receptor antagonist nepadutant for the treatment of visceral hypersensitivity in IBS and asthma. The compound is in Phase IIa trials for IBS in Belgium and Sweden.

Results from in vitro studies show nepadutant to be a potent, competitive, and reversible antagonist at human NK_2 receptors (Patacchini R, 2001). Animal studies also suggest that nepadutant can reduce rectal hyperalgesia but has little effect on normal sensation. These results indicate that tachykinin NK_2 receptor antagonists might not produce visceral analgesia in all patients, like opiates do, but rather they can correct visceral hyperalgesia in patients with abnormal GI sensitivity (Toulouse M, 2000).

Saredutant. Sanofi-Synthélabo is developing the tachykinin antagonist saredutant as a potential oral treatment for visceral hypersensitivity in IBS; the compound is also in development for depression. In May 2003, the company announced that saredutant had entered Phase IIb clinical trials for IBS in France. This agent has a mechanism of action similar to that of nepadutant—both target NK_2 receptors.

Preclinical studies of the drug were presented at the 2002 Digestive Disease Week meeting (Gaultier E, 2002). One mg/kg of saredutant given intraperitonealy reduced trimitrobenzene-sulfonate-induced rectal pain by 54%. Drug treatment did not affect colonic retention time, suggesting that saredutant could be used to treat visceral pain without causing constipation. Few data are available concerning saredutant's tolerability; one author reported that a potential adverse event in IBS patients treated with the agent may be mild frontal headache (Van Schoor J, 1998).

Talnetant. Talnetant is a selective NK_3 antagonist under development by GSK in Europe. The agent is in Phase II clinical trials for IBS, schizophrenia, and urinary incontinence.

Preclinical data for talnetant were presented at the 2002 Digestive Disease Week. Researchers carried out electrophysiological recordings of intrinsic primary afferent neuron activity in guinea pig ileum (Furness JB, 2002). At a concentration of 100 nM, talnetant had no effect on neuronal excitability, but it significantly reduced the amplitude of slow excitatory postsynaptic potential (EPSP) from 10.5 mV to 2.5 mV. It also reduced the ascending and descending reflexes induced by distension.

Cholecystokinin A Receptor Antagonists

Overview. Cholecystokinin (CCK), a neurohormonal peptide found in both the central and enteric nervous systems, is involved in the regulation of GI motility and secretion. Development activity with regard to antagonists at CCK receptors is limited. The only compound in the later stages of development is Rotta Pharmaceuticals (Wall, New Jersey) dexloxiglumide, which recently encountered problems with respect to efficacy in clinical trials.

Mechanism of Action. Although its physiological role is not well defined, CCK is believed to act on neuronal and smooth-muscle receptors. CCK is often found in conjunction with—and appears to act much like—substance P, which stimulates GI smooth-muscle contraction. The peptide is also thought to act as a neurotransmitter of pain signals through actions on NK receptors. Researchers have noted elevated plasma levels of CCK in patients with chronic pancreatitis and abdominal pain (Miyasaka K, 2003); these effects are believed to be mediated predominantly through CCK_1 receptors. Agents antagonizing the actions of CCK at CCK_1 receptors in the gut potentially reduce abdominal pain symptoms in IBS patients.

Dexloxiglumide. In August 2000, Forest Laboratories, Inc. (New York, New York) entered into an agreement with the Italian company RottaPharm (specifically, Rotta Research Lab, a branch of RottaPharm) to develop and market the CCK_1 receptor antagonist dexloxiglumide for the treatment of motility abnormalities and pain in patients with C-IBS in the United States. Forest conducted two Phase III trials involving more than 1,400 IBS female patients in the United States. These trials were completed in mid 2003, and a U.S. launch was expected for 2004. However, in October 2003, Forest discontinued development of dexloxiglumide in the United States for C-IBS because the trial failed to show significant efficacy over placebo. Despite this setback, RottaPharm is continuing Phase III trials for C-IBS, pancreatitis, and GI motility disease in Italy.

In a Phase II, placebo-controlled, double-blind study in Europe involving 469 IBS patients, C-IBS and D-IBS subjects were randomized to receive either dexloxiglumide (200 mg three times daily) or placebo for 12 weeks. Dexloxiglumide was more effective than placebo in relieving IBS symptoms, and both treatments were well tolerated. The proportion of responders was higher with dexloxiglumide than with placebo, reaching statistical significance in all patients regardless of their IBS subgroup (59% versus 45% for placebo) and in C-IBS patients specifically (60% versus 43% for placebo). In the C-IBS subjects, dexloxiglumide was also significantly more effective than placebo in terms of the number of pain- and bloating-free days, reductions in straining and incomplete evacuation, and improved global well-being (D'Amato M, 1999).

The primary end point in both Phase III studies conducted in the United States was the Subject's Global Assessment of Relief (SGA), which measures abdominal discomfort, pain, and altered bowel habits as perceived by the patient. Preliminary results reported by Forest suggest that development was discontinued because of dexloxiglumide's lack of significant efficacy over placebo; however, a trend toward efficacy was observed in both trials. Importantly, dexloxiglumide was well tolerated and was not associated with an increased incidence of gallstones, a hypothesized side effect of CCK antagonists.

Opioid Receptor Modulators

Overview. Opioids are a family of receptors and ligands that profoundly affect the neural circuits that modulate pain and motility in the gut. Both agonists and antagonists at the various opioid receptors represented in the periphery (kappa, mu, delta, and sigma) are under investigation for the treatment of IBS. Pfizer has an agent in preclinical development (JO-2871, a sigma opioid receptor modulator and novel antidiarrheal), while both GSK (UK-321130, a delta opioid antagonist) and Eli Lilly (alvimopan, a mu receptor antagonist) have compounds in Phase I development for IBS. Compounds targeting opioid receptors in the later stages of development are targeting pain symptoms.

Mechanism of Action. Modulation of opioid receptors in the gut is associated with improvements in IBS symptoms, including reduced visceral hypersensitivity and modulated GI motility.

PTI-901. Pain Therapeutics (South San Francisco, California) had been developing a low-dose formulation of the opioid antagonist naltrexone hydrochloride for the potential treatment of IBS, the drug had advanced to Phase III clinical trials in the United States. The company had hoped to capitalize on PTI-901's unique mechanism of restoring the balance of opioid activity in the gut through antagonism of opioid receptors. (Some researchers believe that an imbalance of opioid activity in the gut—triggered by the release of intrinsic opioids from neurons in the gut, metabolic disorders, or emotional stress—contributes to IBS symptoms [Pain Therapeutics, press release, November 25, 2003]). However, Pain Therapeutics discontinued development of PTI-901 in December 2005 after data from a randomized, double-blinded, multicenter U.S. study in 600 women showed that the drug provided no meaningful benefit after three months of treatment compared with placebo (Pain Therapeutics, press release, December 9, 2005).

Clinical information on the actions of PTI-901 in IBS patients is limited. A pilot study assessing the agent's safety and efficacy was carried out in Israel. In this open-label study, 50 patients diagnosed with IBS were treated with 0.5 mg of PTI-901 daily for four weeks. According to the study results released in May 2003, the response to treatment rate was 76.5% ($n = 17$) in males and 75.0% ($n = 25$) in females. Patients given PTI-901 reported a 193% ($n = 37$) increase in the number of pain-free days at week 4 compared with baseline. They also reported improvements in bowel urgency, stool consistency, and number of stool-free days. The study found PTI-901 to be safe and well tolerated (Pain Therapeutics, press release, October 15, 2003).

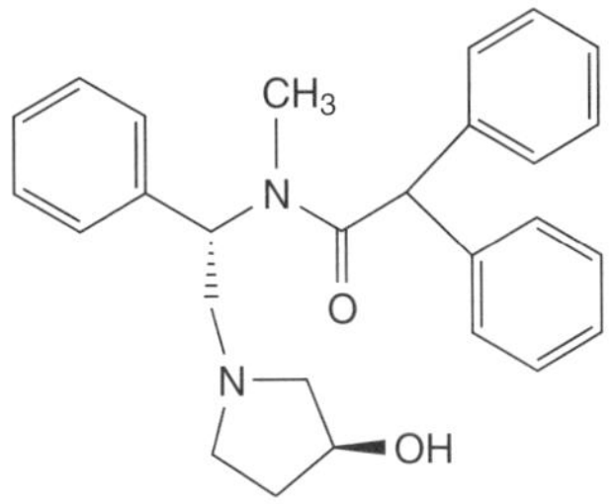

FIGURE 17. Structure of asimadoline.

Asimadoline. In June 2005, Tioga Pharmaceuticals (San Diego, California), under license from Merck KGaA, was seeking funding to conduct its own Phase IIb efficacy trials of asimadoline (Figure 17), a kappa opioid agonist being developed as an IBS treatment (Merck [Whitehouse Station, New Jersey] KGaA had conducted a Phase IIa study of the drug in 2002). In June 2005, the companies reported that Tioga Pharmaceuticals would be funded by Forward Ventures, a San Diego-based venture capital firm, while additional funds to conduct Phase IIb trials would be raised (*Business Wire*, press release, June 15, 2005).

According to Tioga Pharmaceuticals, asimadoline is a peripherally active analgesic that amplifies the body's own pain protection mechanisms and inhibits the release of substance P. Opioid kappa receptors are located on sensory afferent pathways and thought to be involved in visceral nociception. Agents that target these receptors can, theoretically, reduce pain without affecting gut motility (Michocki RJ, 2000).

A randomized, double-blind, placebo-controlled study involving 20 females with IBS and a pain threshold below 32 mmHg (millimeters of mercury) compared 0.5 mg of oral asimadoline with placebo (Delvaux M, 2003). Following treatment, the patients were subject to a series of left colonic distensions (5–40 mmHg pressure). Results showed that asimadoline significantly reduced the intensity of abdominal pain. The effects observed were more pronounced at intermediate pressure distension steps, and the mean pain score was significantly lower at 20, 25, and 30 mmHg distension with respect to placebo. Asimadoline was well tolerated, and no serious adverse events were reported.

Corticotropin-Releasing Factor Receptor Antagonists

Overview. Corticotropin-releasing factor (CRF) is a peptide that functions as a neurotransmitter in the brain. It plays a critical role in coordinating the body's overall response to stress, and it interacts with two known receptor subtypes, CRF_1 and CRF_2. Two companies that are investigating CRF receptor antagonists for IBS are Research Corporation Technologies (Tucson, Arizona), which has a compound in preclinical development, and Neurocrine Biosciences, Inc. (San Diego, California) which has an agent in Phase I clinical trials. The latter agent is discussed in detail here.

Mechanism of Action. Preclinical models have demonstrated that selective CRF_1 receptor antagonists can block stress responses. Consequently, this mechanism may be a good target for drugs to improve the symptoms of such conditions as anxiety, depression, and functional GI disease.

NBI-34041. Neurocrine Biosciences is developing NBI-34041 for the potential treatment of IBS, anxiety, and depression. The compound is in Phase I clinical trials for all three indications. NBI-34041 is the lead in a series of compounds targeting the CRF_1 receptor. Preclinical models have demonstrated that selective CRF_1 receptor antagonists can block stress responses. Neurocrine was originally developing the agent in collaboration with GSK, but the compound is no longer included in the latter's pipeline.

According to preliminary results from a Phase I dose-escalation study, the agent demonstrates rapid absorption and good dose proportionality, and its plasma half-life supports a once-daily dosing schedule (Neurocrine, press release, March 8, 2001).

Chloride-Channel Activators

Overview. Investigation into novel approaches to combat altered GI motility in IBS is relatively limited; the majority of R&D programs are heavily focused on relieving IBS-associated pain. The following paragraphs discuss one compound, a chloride-channel activator, under investigation for the potential relief of constipation.

Mechanism of Action. Activation of chloride channels in GI epithelial cells increases intestinal water secretion, potentially boosting gut motility and relieving constipation (Talley NJ, 2002).

SPI-0211. Sucampo Pharmaceuticals (Bethesda, Maryland) is developing SPI-0211, a chloride-channel activator, for the potential treatment of constipation and IBS in the United States. In April 2003, Sucampo announced that it had launched a Phase II clinical trial in the United States to evaluate SPI-0211's safety and efficacy in 200 C-IBS patients.

SPI-0211 is a bicyclic fatty acid that activates CIC-2 chloride channels located on the gut epithelium, increasing intestinal water. The results of a multicenter, randomized, placebo-controlled study involving 242 patients with constipation were presented at the 2003 Digestive Disease Week meeting. The researchers administered 24 µg of SPI-0211 twice daily for four weeks. Patients who received SPI-0211 experienced a significant increase in the frequency of spontaneous bowel movements; within 24 hours of treatment, 57% of these patients experienced spontaneous bowel movements compared with 37% of the placebo group. The SPI-0211-treated patients also experienced improvements in stool consistency and straining. Adverse events, including headache, nausea, and diarrhea, were more commonly reported in the drug-treated group, but, overall, SPI-0211 was safe and well tolerated (Sucampo, press release, May 19, 2003).

In January 2004, Sucampo announced the completion of a second Phase III clinical study of SPI-0211. The study involved 237 constipated patients in 20 centers across the United States. According to the company, the results duplicated the significant results of the first efficacy study (Sucampo, press release, January 12, 2004).

REFERENCES

Agreus L, et al. Identifying dyspepsia and irritable bowel syndrome: the value of pain or discomfort and bowel habit descriptors. *Scandinavian Journal of Gastroenterology*. 2000;**35**:142–151.

Awad R, et al. The irritable bowel syndrome treatment using pinaverium bromide as a calcium-channel blocker. *Acta Gastro-Enterologica Lationamerica*. 1995;**25**:137–144.

Balboa A, Mearin F. Epidemiological characteristics and socioeconomic importance of irritable bowel syndrome. *Revista Espanola de Enfermedades Digestivas*. 2000;**92**(12):806–819.

Bennett EJ, et al. Level of chronic life stress predicts clinical outcome in irritable bowel syndrome. *Gut*. 1998;**43**:256–261.

Bennett G, Talley NJ. Irritable bowel syndrome in the elderly. *Best Practice and Research Clinical Gastroenterology*. 2002;**16**(1):63–76.

Bommelaer G. Epidemiologie des troubles fonctionnels intestinaux dans une population apparemment saine. *Gastroenterology and Clinical Biology*. 1986;**10**(7):7–12.

Bommelaer G, et al. Epidemiologie du syndrome de l'intestin irritable. *Gastroenterology and Clinical Biology*. 1990;**14**:9–12.

Bommelaer G, et al. Prevalence of irritable bowel syndrome in the French population according to the Rome I criteria. *Gastroenterological Clinical Biology*. 2002;**26**:1118–1123.

Borum ML. Physician perception of IBS management in women and men. *Digestive Diseases and Sciences*. 2002;**47**(1):236–237.

Boyce PM, et al. Irritable bowel syndrome according to varying diagnostic criteria: are the new Rome II criteria unnecessarily restrictive for research and practice? *American Journal of Gastroenterology*. 2000;**95**(11):3176–3183.

Brandt LJ, et al. Systematic review on the management of irritable bowel syndrome in North America. *American Journal of Gastroenterology*. 2002;**97**(suppl 11):S7–S26.

Camilleri M, et al. Efficacy and safety of alosetron in women with irritable bowel syndrome: a randomised, placebo-controlled trial. *Lancet*. 2000;**355**:1035–1040.

Camilleri M. Management of the irritable bowel syndrome. *Gastroenterology*. 2001;**120**:652–668.

Camilleri M, et al. Clinical perspectives, mechanisms, diagnosis, and management of irritable bowel syndrome. *Alimentary Pharmacology and Therapeutics*. 2002;**8**:1407–1430.

Caras S, et al. Cilansetron shows an increase in adequate relief rate in nonconstipated IBS subjects who respond as having no adequate relief at baseline. *Gastroenterology*. 2002;**122**(suppl 1):A550.

Cash BD, et al. The utility of diagnostic tests in irritable bowel syndrome patients: a systematic review. *American Journal of Gastroenterology*. 2002;**97**(11):2812–2819. Review.

Centonze V, et al. Oral cimetropium bromide, a new antimuscarinic drug, for long-term treatment of irritable bowel syndrome. *American Journal of Gastroenterology*. 1988:**83**:1262–1266.

Chey WD, et al. Utility of the Rome I and Rome II criteria for irritable bowel syndrome in U.S. women. *American Journal of Gastroenterology*. 2002;**97**(11):2803–2811.

Creed FH, et al. Functional abdominal pain, psychiatric illness, and life events. *Gut*. 1988;**29**:235–242.

D'Amato M, et al. The CCKA receptor antagonist dexloxiglumide in the treatment of IBS. Digestive Disease Week; May 16–19, 1999; Orlando, FL. Abstract 1249.

Delvaux M, et al. Functional bowel disorders and irritable bowel syndrome in Europe. *Alimentary Pharmacology*. 2003;**18**(suppl 3):75–79.

Dobrilla G, et al. Long-term treatment of irritable bowel syndrome with cimetropium bromide: a double-blind placebo-controlled clinical trial. *Gut*. 1990;**31**:355–358.

Drossman DA. U.S. Householder Survey of Functional Gastrointestinal Disorders: prevalence, sociodemography, and health impact. *Digestive Diseases and Sciences*. 1993;**38**(9):1569–1580.

Drossman DA, ed. The Functional Gastrointestinal Disorders, 2nd Edition. McLean, VA: Degnon Associates; 2000.

Efskind PS, et al. A double-blind placebo-controlled trial with loperamide in irritable bowel syndrome. *Scandinavian Journal of Gastroenterology*. 1996;**31**:463–468.

Evans PR, et al. Jejunal sensorimotor dysfunction in irritable bowel syndrome: clinical and psychological features. *Gastroenterology*. 1996;**110**:393–404.

Fennerty MB. IBS: challenges in diagnosis. *Medscape Gastroenterology*. 2003;**5**(2). Posted September 22, 2003. Accessed October 1, 2003.

Furness JB, et al. NK_3 receptor antagonism by talnetant (SB-223412) suggests a role for NK_3 receptors in enteric reflexes evoked by relatively intense stimuli. *Gastroenterology*. 2002;**122**(suppl 1):A256.

Gorard DA, et al. Influence of antidepressants on whole gut and orocecal transit times in health and irritable bowel syndrome. *Alimentary Pharmacology and Therapeutics*. 1994;**8**(2):159–166.

Gorard DA, et al. Effect of a tricyclic antidepressant on small intestinal motility in health and diarrhea-predominant irritable bowel syndrome. *Digestive Diseases and Sciences*. 1995;**40**(1):86–95.

Greenbaum DS, et al. Effects of desipramine on irritable bowel syndrome compared with atropine and placebo. *Digestive Diseases and Sciences*. 1987;**32**(3):257–266.

Hahn BA, et al. Impact of irritable bowel syndrome on quality of life and resource use in the United States and United Kingdom. *Digestion*. 1999;**60**:77–81.

Hamm LR, et al. Additional investigations fail to alter the diagnosis of irritable bowel syndrome in subjects fulfilling the Rome criteria. *American Journal of Gastroenterology*. 1999;**94**(5):1279–1282.

Hasler WL. Pharmacotherapy for intestinal motor and sensory disorders. *Gastroenterology Clinics*. 2003;**32**:1–19.

Heaton KW. How bad are the symptoms and bowel dysfunction of patients with the irritable bowel syndrome? A prospective, controlled study with emphasis on stool form. *Gut*. 1991;**32**:73–79.

Heaton KW. Symptoms of irritable bowel syndrome in a British urban community: consulters and nonconsulters. *Gastroenterology*. 1992;**102**:1962–1967.

Higgens PD, et al. Systematic review: the epidemiology of ischemic colitis. *Alimentary Pharmacology and Therapeutics*. 2004;**19**(7):729–738.

Holton KB. Irritable bowel syndrome: minimize testing, let symptoms guide treatment. *Journal of Family Practice*. 2003;**52**:942–950.

Hungin APS, et al. Irritable bowel syndrome (IBS): prevalence and impact in the U.S.A.-- the Truth in IBS (T-IBS) Survey. *American Journal of Gastroenterology*. 2002;**97**(2):S280–S281.

Hungin APS, et al. The prevalence, patterns, and impact of irritable bowel syndrome: an international survey of 40,000 subjects. *Alimentary Pharmacology Therapeutics*. 2003;**17**:643–650.

Ilnyckyj A, et al. Association of travel-related diarrhea (TD) with irritable bowel syndrome (IBS): is postinfectious IBS a true entity? *Gastroenterology*. 1999;**116**(4 part 2):A1011.

Isgar B, et al. Symptoms of irritable bowel syndrome in ulcerative colitis in remission. *Gut*. 1983;**24**:190–192.

Jackson JL, et al. Treatment of functional gastrointestinal disorders with tricyclic antidepressant medications: a meta-analysis. *American Journal of Medicine*. 2000;**108**:65–72.

Jailwala J, et al. Pharmacologic treatments of irritable bowel syndrome: a systematic review of randomized clinical trials. *Annals of Internal Medicine*. 2000;**133**:136–147.

Jalihal A, Kurian G. Ispaghula therapy in irritable bowel syndrome: improvement in overall well-being is related to reduction in bowel dissatisfaction. *Journal of Gastroenterology and Hepatology*. 1990;**5**:507–513.

Jayanthi V, et al. Role of pinaverium bromide in South Indian patients with irritable bowel syndrome. *Journal of the Association of Indian Physicians*. 1998;**46**:369–371.

Jones RH, Lydeard S. Irritable bowel syndrome in the general population. *British Medical Journal*. 1992;**304**:87–90.

Jones RH, et al. Alosetron relieves pain and improves bowel function compared with mebeverine in female nonconstipated irritable bowel syndrome patients. *Alimentary Pharmacology and Therapeutics*. 1999;**11**:1419–1427.

Kawamura A, et al. Prevalence of irritable bowel syndrome and its relationship with *Helicobacter pylori* infection in a Japanese population. *American Journal of Gastroenterology*. 2001;**96**(6):1946. Letter.

Kawamura A. Data acquisition. Personal communication on January 9, 2003.

Kellow JE, et al. Principles of applied neurogastroenterology: physiology/motility-sensation. *Gut*. 1999;**45**(suppl II):II17–II24.

Kellow J, et al. An Asia-Pacific, double-blind, placebo-controlled, randomized study to evaluate the efficacy, safety, and tolerability of tegaserod in patients with irritable bowel syndrome. *Gut*. 2003;**52**:671–676.

Kountouras J, et al. Efficacy of trimebutine therapy in patients with gastroesophageal reflux disease and irritable bowel syndrome. *Hepato-Gastroenterology*. 2002;**49**:193–197.

Kuiken SD. Fluoxetine (Prozac) for the treatment of irritable bowel syndrome: a randomized, controlled clinical trial. *Gastroenterology*. 2002;**122**:W1024. Abstract.

Lembo A, et al. Alosetron in irritable bowel syndrome. *Drugs*. 2003;**63**:1895–1905.

Lembo T, et al. Symptoms and visceral perception in patients with pain-predominant irritable bowel syndrome. *American Journal of Gastroenterology*. 1999;**94**:1320–1326.

Lembo T, et al. Alosetron controls bowel urgency and provides global symptom improvement in women with diarrhea-predominant irritable bowel syndrome. *American Journal of Gastroenterology*. 2001;**96**:2662–2670.

Lu CL, et al. Effect of a calcium-channel blocker and antispasmodic in diarrhea-predominant irritable bowel syndrome. *Journal of Gastroenterology and Hepatology*. 2000;**15**:925–930.

Lydiard NB, et al. Prevalence of psychiatric disorders in irritable bowel syndrome. *Psychosomatics*. 1993;**34**:229–234.

Lynn RB. Irritable bowel syndrome: managing the patient with abdominal pain and altered bowel habits. *Medical Clinics of North America*. 1995;**79**(2):375–390.

Matteo N, et al. Prevalence of irritable bowel syndrome in Italy: a population-based study. *Gastroenterology*. 2001;**120**(5):(suppl 1) A230. Abstract.

Mayer EA, et al. Review article: gender-related differences in functional gastrointestinal disorders. *Alimentary Pharmacology and Therapeutics*. 1999;**12**(suppl 2):65–69.

McKendrick MW, Read NW. Irritable bowel syndrome: postsalmonella infection. *Journal of Infection*. 1994;**29**:1–3.

Mearin F, et al. Irritable bowel syndrome prevalence varies enormously depending on the employed diagnostic criteria: comparison of Rome II versus previous criteria in a general population. *Scandinavian Journal of Gastroenterology*. 2001;**36**(11):1155–1161.

Mertz HR. Irritable bowel syndrome. *New England Journal of Medicine* 2003;**349**:2136–2146.

Michocki RJ, et al. Treatment innovations for irritable bowel syndrome. *Special Report for the American Pharmaceutical Association*. 2000.

Miyasaka K, Funakoshi A. Cholecystokinin and cholecystokinin receptors. *Journal of Gastroenterology*. 2003;**38**:1–13.

Montgomery SA, et al. Why do amitryptiline and dothiepin appear to be so dangerous in overdose? *Acta Psychiatry Scandinavian Supplement*. 1989;**354**:47–53.

Moynihan R. FDA advisers warn of more deaths if drug is relaunched. *British Medical Journal*. 2002;**325**:561.

Müller-Lissner SA, et al. Epidemiological aspects of irritable bowel syndrome in Europe and North America. *Digestion*. 2001;**64**(3):200–204 [a].

Müller-Lissner SA, et al. Tegaserod, a 5-HT$_4$ receptor partial agonist, relieves symptoms in irritable bowel syndrome patients with abdominal pain, bloating, and constipation. *Alimentary Pharmacology Therapeutics*. 2001;**15**:1655–1666 [b].

Nagakura Y, et al. Pharmacological properties of a novel gastroprokinetic benzamide selective for human 5-HT$_4$ receptor versus human 5-HT$_3$ receptor. *Pharmacology Research*. 1999;**39**(5):375–382.

Novick J, et al. A randomized, double-blind, placebo-controlled trial of tegaserod in female patients suffering from irritable bowel syndrome with constipation. *Alimentary Pharmacology Therapeutics*. 2002;**16**:1877–1888.

Olden KW. Diagnosis of irritable bowel syndrome. *Gastroenterology*. 2002;**122**(6):1701–1714.

O' Sullivan M, et al. Increased mast cells in the irritable bowel syndrome. *Neurogastroenterology and Motility*. 2000;**12**:449–457.

Page JG, Dirnberger GM. Treatment of the irritable bowel syndrome with Bentyl (dicyclomine hydrochloride). *Journal of Clinical Gastroenterology*. 1981;**3**(2):153–156.

Parry SD, et al. Does infectious diarrhea (ID) predispose people to functional gastrointestinal disorders (FGIDs): a prospective community case-control study. *Gut*. 2002;**50**(suppl II):A1(001).

Patacchini R, et al. Peripheral tachykinin receptors as targets for new drugs. *European Journal of Pharmacology*. 2001;**429**:13–21.

Piai G, et al. Long-term treatment of irritable bowel syndrome with cimetropium bromide, a new antimuscarinic compound. *Current Therapeutic Research*. 1987;**41**:967–977.

Population Division of the Department of Economic and Social Affairs of the United Nations Secretariat. *World Population Prospects: The 2002 Revision*, vol. I, *Comprehensive Tables* (United Nations publication, Sales No. E.03.XIII.6); and *World Population Prospects: The 2002 Revision*, vol. II, *The Sex and Age Distribution of Populations* (United Nations publication, Sales No. E.03.XIII.7), 2003.

Poynard T, et al. Meta-analysis of smooth-muscle relaxants in the treatment of irritable bowel syndrome. *Alimentary Pharmacological Therapy*. 1994;**8**:499–510.

Poynard T, et al. Meta-analysis of smooth-muscle relaxants in the treatment of irritable bowel syndrome. *Alimentary Pharmacological Therapy*. 2001;**15**:355–361.

Prior A, Whorwell PJ. Double-blind study of ispaghula in irritable bowel syndrome. *Gut*. 1987;**28**:1510–1513.

Saito YA, et al. A comparison of the Rome and Manning criteria for case identification in epidemiological investigations of irritable bowel syndrome. *American Journal of Gastroenterology*. 2000;**95**(10):2816–2824.

Saito YA, et al. The epidemiology of irritable bowel syndrome in North America: a systematic review. *American Journal of Gastroenterology*. 2002;**97**(8):1910–1915.

Schlemper RJ, et al. Peptic ulcer, non-ulcer dyspepsia, and irritable bowel syndrome in the Netherlands and Japan. *Scandinavian Journal of Gastroenterology*. 1993;**2000**:33–41.

Schmulson M, et al. Symptom differences in moderate to severe IBS patients based on predominant bowel habit. *American Journal of Gastroenterology*. 1999;**94**(10):2929–2935.

Spiller RC, et al. Increased rectal mucosal enteroendocrine cells, T lymphocytes, and increased gut permeability following acute campylobacter enteritis and in postdysenteric irritable bowel syndrome. *Gut*. 2000;**47**:804–811.

Stacher G. Cilansetron Solvay. *Current Opinion in Investigational Drugs*. 2001;**2**(10):1432–1436.

Talley NJ. Irritable bowel syndrome in a community: symptom subgroups, risk factors, and health care utilization. *American Journal of Epidemiology*. 1995;**142**:76–83.

Talley NJ, et al. Predictors of health care seeking for irritable bowel syndrome: a population-based study. *Gut*. 1997;**41**:394–398.

Talley NJ, et al. Is the association between irritable bowel syndrome and abuse explained by neuroticism? A population-based study. *Gut*. 1998;**42**:47–53.

Talley NJ. Gastrointestinal symptoms and subjects cluster into distinct upper and lower groupings in the community: a four-nations study. *American Journal of Gastroenterology*. 2000;**95**(6):1439–1447.

Talley NJ, Spiller R. Irritable bowel syndrome: a little understood organic bowel disease? *Lancet*. 2002;**360**:555–564.

Talley NJ. Evaluation of drug treatment in irritable bowel syndrome. *British Journal of Clinical Pharmacology*. 2003;**56**:362–369.

Talley NJ. New therapeutic insights into irritable bowel syndrome. Digestive Disease Week 2001. (www.medscape.com/viewprogram/551_ pnt, Accessed January 2004).

Tanum L, Malt UF. A new pharmacologic treatment of functional gastrointestinal disorder. A double-blind placebo-controlled study with mianserin. *Scandinavian Journal of Gastroenterology*. 1996;**31**(4):318–325.

Thompson WG. Gender differences in irritable bowel symptoms. *European Journal of Gastroenterology and Hepatology*. 1997;**9**(3):299–302 [a].

Thompson WG, et al. Irritable bowel syndrome: the view from general practice. *European Journal of Gastroenterology and Hepatology*. 1997;**9**(7):689–692 [b].

Thompson WG. The road to Rome. *Gut*. 1999;**45**(suppl 2):1180.

Thompson WG. Irritable bowel syndrome in general practice: prevalence, characteristics, and referral. *Gut*. 2000;**46**(1):78–82.

Törnblom H, et al. Full-thickness biopsy of the jejunum reveals inflammation and enteric neuropathy in irritable bowel syndrome. *Gastroenterology*. 2002;**123**:1972–1979.

Toskes PP, et al. Calcium polycarbophil compared with placebo in irritable bowel syndrome. *Alimentary Pharmacology and Therapeutics*. 1993;**7**:87–92.

Tougas G, et al. Long-term safety of tegaserod in patients with constipation-predominant irritable bowel syndrome. *Alimentary Pharmacology and Therapeutics*. 2002;**10**:1701–1708.

Toulouse M, et al. Role of tachykinin NK_2 receptors in normal and altered rectal sensitivity in rats. *British Journal of Pharmacology*. 2000;**129**:193–199.

Van Outryve M, et al. A double-blind crossover comparison study of the safety and efficacy of mebeverine sustained release in the treatment of irritable bowel syndrome. *Journal of Clinical Pharmacy and Therapeutics*. 1995;**20**(5):277–282.

Van Schoor J, et al. The effect of the NK_2 tachykinin receptor antagonist SR-48968 (saredutant) on neurokinin A-induced bronchoconstriction in asthmatics. *European Respiratory Journal: Official Journal of the European Society for Clinical Respiratory Physiology*. 1998;**12**:17–23.

Viera AJ. Management of irritable bowel syndrome. *American Family Physician*. 2002;**66**:1867–1874.

Wahnschaffe U, et al. Celiac disease-like abnormalities in a subgroup of patients with irritable bowel syndrome. *Gastroenterology*. 2001;**121**:1329–1338.

Whitehead WE, et al. Impact of irritable bowel syndrome on quality of life. *Digestive Diseases and Sciences*. 1996;**41**:2248–2253.

Cumulative Index of Drug and Molecule Names, Volumes 1–8

Boldface roman numerals indicate the volume in which the entry appears.

17-Allylaminogeldanamycin (17AAG), **I:**415, 420, **II:**619, 138

3-AP, **II:**138

5-alpha-reductase inhibitors (5-ARIs), **VII:**267, 279–283, 290, 293–294

5-Azacytidine, **I:**425

A-6, **II:**138, **VIII:**54, 56

A-74187, **V:**225

A-443654, **VIII:**49

A-674563, **VIII:**49

A-790742, **V:**145

A-I Milano (ApoA-IM), **VI:**470

AA-10025, **VII:**326

AAB-001, **V:**367

AAE-581, **III:**251

Aβ inhibitors, **V:**349

Abacavir, **IV:**90, 283, 301, **V:**113, 114, 122–125, 135–136, 140–141

Abacavir/lamivudine regimen, **V:**114, 123, 125, 140

Abacavir/lamivudine/zidovudine regimen, **V:**113, 114, 122, 125, 135–136

Abarelix, **II:**240

Abatacept, **II:**682, 688, 689, **VIII:**175–176

Abbokinase, **V:**203, **VII:**202, 222–223

Abciximab, **I:**65, **V:**193, 221, 222, **VI:**423, 437–438

Abetimus sodium, **VIII:**176–177

ABI-007, **II:**138, 143, **IV:**109

Abilify, **V:**269, 343, 399, 416, 421–422, **VI:**314, 316, 328–330

Abraxane, **II:**138, 143, **IV:**109

ABT-089, **V:**294, **VI:** 336, 348

ABT-510, **II:**65

ABT-627, **VIII:**54, 56

ABT-737, **VIII:**47, 49

ABT-751, **I:**486, 500

ABT-773, **III:**479

ABT-874 (formerly J-695), **II:**539, 547

ABT-306552, **VI:**596

ABthrax, **IV:**277, 284, 285

ABX-EGF, **VIII:**37, 38

AC-2993, **IV:**28

AC-3933, **V:**351

AC-2993 LAR, **III:**389

ACA-125, **II:**140

ACAM1000, **IV:**72

ACAM2000, **IV:**72

Acarbose, **III:**144, 342, 350, 367–369

ACC-001, **V:**353, 367–368, **VI:**106, 117

Accolate, **II:**403, 460

Accupril, **III:**14, **V:** 16

Accuprin, **VII:**28–29

Accupro, **III:**14, **V:**16, **VII:**28–29

Accutane, **IV:**107, **VIII:**166

Acebutolol, 656

EXEL-9820, **IV:**281

Exemestane, **I:**278

Exemestane, single agent, **I:**230, 255

Exenatide, **III:**343, 374–376, 379, 388, 391, 392

Exenatide LAR, **III:**389, 390

Exenatidec, **IV:**28

Exisulind, **II:**74–76

Expectorants, **IV:**182

Extended release formulation of metformin, **III:**355

Extended release nicotinic acid, **III:**54, 78

Extended spectrum β-lactam, **III:**583–585

Extended spectrum β-lactam antibiotic, **III:**583–585, 587, 588

Extended spectrum penicillins, **III:**445, 449, 450, 452, 453, 517, 518, 521

Exubera, **III:**298, 301, 303, 304, 394–396, 398, 399

EYE-001, **III:**26, 27

Ezeterol, **III:**54, 67–69, 75–77, 83, 155

Ezetimibe, **III:**53, 54, 67–69, 75–77, 83, 139, 155, 173

5-Fluorouracil (5-FU), **I:**224, 225, 231, 232, 234, 307, 310–313, 328, 329, 376, 447, 452–455, 457–460, 462, 463, 465, 466, 469–473, 476–481, 488, 494, 497, **II:**155, 184–191, 197, 199–201, 203, 348

Fabrazyme, **IV:**203, 313

Factive, **III:**473, 475, 477

Factor VIIa, **IV:**286

Famotidine, **I:**61

Famoxin, **IV:**293

Farmarubicin, **I:**226, **II:**313, 316, 317, 320, 321, 326, 349

Farmitrexat, **I:**225

Farmorubicin, **I:**162, 174, **II:**310, 313, 316, 317, 320, 321, 349

Farmorubicina, **II:**313, 316, 317, 320, 321, 326, 349

Farnesyl protein transferase inhibitors, **I:**485

Farnesyl transferase inhibitors, **I:**189, 423, 424, 491, 492, **II:**617, 626, 627, 8, 60, 206, 207, 277

Faslodex, **I:**230, 256

Fastic, **III:**342, 365

Fastin, **III:**191, 192, 197, 198, 204

Femara, **I:**230, 253

Femora, **I:**230, 253

Fenfluramine, **III:**190, 198, 204

Fenofibrate, **III:**53, 72, 73, 93, 94, 139, 157

Fenretinide, **II:**141, 333, 353

Fenticonazole, **IV:**185

Feron, **III:**648, 665

Fexofenadine, **I:**11, **II:**380, 381, 384–390, 392

Fialuridine, **I:**38

Fibrates (fibric acid derivatives), **III:**53, 54, 71–75, 93, 94, 139, 141, 157

Fildesin, **I:**83, 534, 541, 544

Filgrastim, **IV:**105, 106

Finasteride, **II:**254, 278

Fiorinal, **IV:**110

First-generation antihistamines, **II:**383, 389

Fivasa, **II:**520, 521, 533

Fixed-dose combinations, **III:**342

FK-228, **II:**139

Flagyl, **II:**510, 531, 532, **III:**576, 601, 602

Flagyl IV, **III:**576, 601, 602

Flavopiridol, **I:**376

Flixonase, **II:**380, 382, 396, 397, 399, 400, 402, 406, 411, 413, 414

Flixotide, **II:**443, 448–452, 458, 459, 462, 473

Flonase, **II:**380, 382, 396, 397, 399, 400, 402, 406, 411, 413, 414

Florone, **II:**592

Flovent, **II:**443, 448–452, 458, 459, 462, 473

Floxapen, **III:**575, 581

Floxin, **III:**464, 465

Floxuridine, **I:**452

Flucloxacillin, **III:**575, 581, 711

Fludar, **I:**350

Fludara, **I:**349, 350, 354–359, 361, 362, 364–367, 372, 373, 376, 379, 381